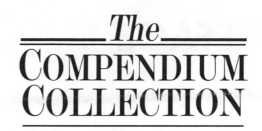

D0927263

GASTROENTEROLOGY

IN PRACTICE

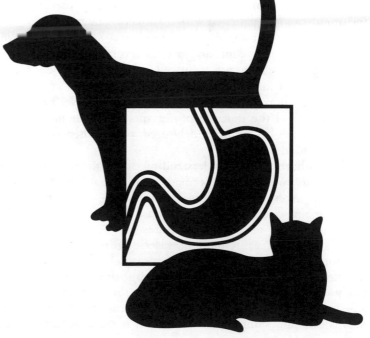

Published by Veterinary Learning Systems
Trenton, New Jersey

ISBN 1-884254-10-1

PREFACE

During the last decade, more progress has probably been made in our understanding of the causes, pathogenesis, diagnosis, and treatment of gastrointestinal disease in small animals than in any other period in history. Many of these advances are documented in this collection.

Esophageal disease, particularly megaesophagus, remains one of the greatest challenges to the clinician. With the development of the acetylcholine receptor antibody test, Dr. Diane Shelton and her colleagues have demonstrated that up to 20% of patients with what is currently diagnosed as idiopathic megaesophagus actually have focal myasthenia gravis.[1] What, however, of those patients whose disease is still idiopathic? What is the cause of esophageal dilatation and how can we better diagnose and treat the condition? Treatment with pyridostigmine and immunosuppressants has little influence on the progress of focal myasthenia gravis, and for most patients with megaesophagus, we have a limited number of medical options. Sadly, the best of these still appears to be feeding the patient in an elevated position. Calcium channel blockers show some therapeutic promise but much work remains to be done with these drugs.[2]

Important advances have also been made in our understanding of canine and feline gastric disease. This situation has been helped by the advent of endoscopy to the extent that gastroscopy and mucosal biopsy are now routine in many practices. In the past decade, there has also been a much better understanding of the physical and chemical parameters that protect the gastric mucosa (the so-called "gastric mucosal barrier"). Nonetheless, ulcer disease (which is reviewed in this book by Dr. Karen Moreland) is still widespread. Endoscopy is the key to diagnosis of ulcer disease and once diagnosed, treatment can be facilitated with a variety of new drugs that rapidly protect the gastric mucosa and reverse the disease process. The clinician now has several H_2-receptor antagonists to choose from, including cimetidine, ranitidine, and famotidine; the new proton pump antagonist omeprazole, which has added a new level of protection; and the mucosal protectants sucralfate and misoprostil are becoming widely used as their benefits are understood.

We also have a better understanding of gastric motility disorders, which are described in this book by Dr. Jean Hall. Accurate diagnosis of these diseases regrettably remains one of exclusion, because there is no reliable and simple test that quantitates gastric motility. Scintigraphic measurement of gastric emptying and electrogastrography (the cutaneous measurement of gastric electrical activity) are possibilities, but these tests are likely to be confined to research centers for the foreseeable future. Whereas specific diagnosis of motility disorders is difficult, symptomatic treatment is facilitated by metoclopramide and will be further enhanced when cisapride is approved by the FDA. Seemingly available everywhere but in the United States, this potent promotility drug (which stimulates and coordinates canine and feline gastric, small intestinal, and colonic motility) is revolutionizing the treatment of a variety of motility diseases.

Although most motility disorders are better understood, gastric dilatation-volvulus (GDV) remains as frustrating and enigmatic as ever. There are more dogs surviving GDV now than there were 10 years ago, but this is largely the result of improvements in surgical technique and postoperative care as described in this book by Drs. Mike Leib and Robert Martin. We are still, however, far from understanding the cause of GDV. Indeed, it is probable that no single cause exists but, rather like heart disease in humans, a number of genetic, environmental, and dietary risk factors combine to initiate the cycle of aerophagia and impaired gastric emptying and eructation that eventually lead to gastric dilatation. Defining these risk factors remains one of our biggest challenges.

We have also learned a great deal about small intestinal disease. The two big "diseases" of the past decade are plasmacytic lymphocytic enteritis and small intestinal bacterial overgrowth. Although these two conditions are regarded as diseases from the point of view of treatment, both are probably a manifestation of disrupted enteric defense mechanisms. Dr. Todd Tams gives an elegant description of the state of the art with regard to diagnosis and treatment of plasmacytic lymphocytic enteritis and Dr. Al Jergens takes the process a step further with a detailed description of the disorder in cats. Both authors also share their frustrations about defining the cause of what is now the most common chronic enteropathy seen in small animal practice. Recent advances in our knowledge of intestinal immunity and mucosal defense mechanisms have, however, allowed a better understanding of the potential mechanisms of plasmacytic enteritis and, perhaps, a glimpse into tomorrow's therapy.

Our knowledge of small intestinal bacterial overgrowth (SIBO) follows a parallel course. Although SIBO is a treatable component of a variety of chronic enteric diseases, we are only now beginning to realize how widespread the disorder is.[3] Although the mechanisms that control the growth of enteric flora are well understood, we have no idea of how they are disrupted to allow overgrowth in dogs and cats. When these processes are understood, we will perhaps be able to provide more rational therapy.

Colonic disease has also come into better focus during the past decade. We now realize, for example, that most of what was once called "idiopathic" or "chronic active" colitis is, in fact, an extension or an alternative manifestation of plasmacytic lymphocytic enteritis. We also appreciate that, in many animals, the disease appears to be caused by a sensitivity to dietary protein and can be ameliorated, although seldom cured, by a change to a novel dietary protein.[4]

Some colonic diseases have been more resistant to elucidation. For example, idiopathic megacolon with secondary obstipation in cats remains as much of an enigma as ever. The disease appears to be a disorder of smooth muscle function rather than one of defective innervation but the exact pathophysiologic mechanisms continue to be elusive.[5] Treatment of megacolon has been revolutionized by using lactulose as an osmotic laxative with the option of subtotal colectomy.[6] If anecdotal reports from Canada and Europe are to be believed, however, cisapride (which appears to stimulate colonic motility in afflicted cats) will dramatically reduce the number of animals undergoing surgery for megacolon.

The causes of pancreatic disease remain as elusive as ever. In this book, Drs. Mike Schaer and Kenny Simpson accurately portray the current state of the art with regard to diagnosis and treatment. The problem is that although more dogs with acute pancreatitis are surviving now than at any time in history, we still have no reliable means of diagnosis or prophylaxis. Pancreatic biopsy remains the gold standard for diagnosing pancreatitis but few of us wish to resort to this as a routine diagnostic technique. Serum lipase and amylase measurements are woefully inadequate as a diagnostic test; dogs can die from acute pancreatitis with absolutely normal amylase and lipase levels. With the recent discovery that the canine stomach contains large quantities of lipase,[7] we have learned that both plasmacytic lymphocytic and eosinophilic gastritis can mimic pancreatitis, right down to dramatically elevated serum amylase and lipase activity. We can only hope that the analysis of trypsin-activation peptide, currently undergoing clinical evaluation, will prove to be a more sensitive test.

Recent advances in veterinary medicine have contributed to a more complete understanding of exocrine pancreatic insufficiency (EPI). Indeed, if I had to name the most significant accomplishment in gastroenterology in the past decade, it would have to be the development, testing, and clinical application of the trypsinogen-like immunoreactivity test (the TLI test) by Drs. David Williams and Roger Batt for the diagnosis of exocrine pancreatic insufficiency. The basis of this and other gut function tests are reviewed by these authors in this book. Thanks to these two investigators, an accurate diagnosis of EPI now requires only a single blood sample taken after an overnight fast. Clients need no longer bear the expense of inappropriately prescribed enzyme replacement therapy. We can only hope that the next decade will bring a better understanding of the cause of pancreatic acinar atrophy, the major cause of the clinical syndrome of EPI.

We have also seen progress in our understanding of liver disease during the past decade. The histopathologic spectrum of both canine and feline liver disease is now well defined, and thanks to the work of Drs. Sharon Center and Denny Meyer (whose work is chronicled here), we have a very good idea of the meaning of the various liver tests and how to interpret them for a variety of hepatic diseases. Recently developed test kits have made the measurement of fasting and postprandial serum bile acid concentrations and the assessment of blood ammonia routine in veterinary practice. Biopsy of the liver is usually indicated if liver function tests are abnormal. Veterinary pathologists are becoming more adroit at interpreting minuscule biopsy samples and are also beginning to place their diagnoses into relatively well-accepted histologic categories, which helps the clinician choose appropriate treatment.

Clinicians are also becoming much better at suspecting and diagnosing portocaval shunts and realizing that the disease is almost as common in cats as in dogs. Successful surgical therapy or medical management with diet and lactulose for this disorder is now routine.

Clinicians have also become much better at recognizing the early stages of liver disease and are instituting much more aggressive therapy. The recent understanding of the benefits of treatment with ursodeoxycholic acid appears to have had a significant impact on morbidity in a variety of chronic liver diseases.

Despite these advances, I am pessimistic about progress made in liver disease. With the exception of congenitally acquired portosystemic shunts, we cannot accurately state the cause of any other chronic canine or feline liver disease. We know that copper accumulates in the liver of Bedlington terriers as well as in the liver of a variety of other breeds, but the relationships between copper accumulation and hepatic pathology have not been defined. And what about cholangiohepatitis, hepatic fibrosis, cirrhosis, "chronic active hepatitis," lipidosis, and so on? What are the causes of these diseases? The elucidation of the causes of liver disease remains our greatest challenge in small animal gastroenterology.

Although the past decade has been an exciting one in small animal gastroenterology, I believe the best is yet to come.

Colin F. Burrows, BVetMed, PhD,
MRCVS, Diplomate ACVIM

REFERENCES

1. Shelton GD, Willard MD, Cardinet GH, Lindstrom J: Acquired myasthenia gravis: Selective involvement of esophageal, pharyngeal, and facial muscles. J Vet Int Med 4:281–284, 1990.
2. Chandra NC, McLeod CG, Hess JL: Nitedipine: Attempting therapeutic option for the treatment of megaesophagus in adult dogs. JAAHA 25:175–179, 1989.
3. Rutgers HC, Lamport A, et al: Bacterial overgrowth in dogs with chronic intestinal disease. J Vet Int Med 7:133, 1993.
4. Nelson RW, et al: Nutritional management of idiopathic chronic colitis in the dog. J Vet Int Med 2:133–137, 1988.
5. Washabau R: Feline colonic motility: Function and dysfunction. Proc ACVIM 637–639, 1991.
6. Bright RM, Burrows CF, Goring R, et al: Subtotal colectomy for treatment of acquired megacolon in the dog and cat. JAVMA 188:1412–1416, 1986.
7. Carriere F, et al: Dog gastric lipase: Stimulation of its secretion in vivo and cytolocalization in mucous pit cells. Gastroenterology 102:1535–1545, 1992.

CONTENTS

INTESTINAL DISEASES

PANCREATIC DISEASES

LIVER DISEASES

SURGERY

TRAUMA/EMERGENCIES

UPPER GASTROINTESTINAL DISEASES

INFECTIONS

MISCELLANEOUS DISORDERS

New Approaches to Malabsorption in Dogs

Roger M. Batt, BVSc, MSc, PhD, MRCVS
Department of Veterinary Pathology
University of Liverpool
Liverpool, England

Many abnormalities affecting the pancreas or the small intestine can result in chronic malabsorption by interfering with the degradative or absorptive phases in the handling of one or more nutrients. Clinical signs depend on the duration and the severity of the disease and can include chronic diarrhea, poor weight gain, or weight loss. Because these signs are relatively nonspecific and because in some cases there might be no signs (such as diarrhea) to draw attention to the gastrointestinal tract, accurate diagnostic tests are essential in distinguishing between the various conditions that can result in malabsorption.

Preliminary diagnostic steps must include routine examination of feces, blood, and urine to rule out intestinal parasites, pathogenic bacteria, and systemic disorders. Subsequent investigations of dogs with possible malabsorption typically include digestion and absorption tests and biopsy of the small intestine; the results can be misleading, however. Erroneous diagnosis of exocrine pancreatic insufficiency (EPI) is one problem, which is compounded by the limitations of routine functional and morphologic studies in detecting small intestinal disease.

New procedures have been introduced to help overcome these difficulties. Assay of serum trypsin like immunoreactivity (TLI) has been established for the accurate diagnosis of EPI, and assays of serum folate and vitamin B_{12} have been validated for the identification of chronic small intestinal disease. In addition to these diagnostic procedures, which can be used routinely, biochemical analysis of peroral jejunal biopsies has been used as a research tool to assist characterization and to promote a better understanding of the pathogenesis of canine enteropathies.

In this article, potential abnormalities that can result in malabsorption are considered and diagnostic problems are discussed. These new approaches are illustrated by the description of three distinct enteropathies, which have been characterized by the application of predominantly biochemical criteria to the analysis of peroral jejunal biopsies.

Defects Resulting in Malabsorption
Nature of the Mucosal Barrier

The small intestine is a tube, the luminal surface area of which is enhanced by villi lined by a sheet of absorptive epithelial cells—the enterocytes (Figure 1). These cells contain organelles common to other cells, such as mitochondria and lysosomes; in addition, the brush border is a specialized region of the plasma membrane that plays an important role in the absorption and the digestion of specific dietary constituents. To gain access to the enterocytes, and from there to the intercellular spaces and then to the blood, ingested nutrients must pass through this brush-border barrier. Knowledge of the structure of the brush-border membrane therefore is fundamental to understanding the various abnormalities that can result in malabsorption.[1]

The brush-border membrane consists of a phospholipid barrier containing specific enzyme and carrier proteins (Figure 2). The enzyme proteins involved in the terminal stages of the degradation of some nutrients are positioned at the surface. The carrier proteins are buried deeper in the membrane. Water-soluble molecules, including the products of carbohydrate and protein digestion, cannot dissolve in the phospholipid barrier and thus must use specific transport or carrier proteins to cross the membrane. Because there are specific carriers for monosaccharides, larger carbohydrates must be degraded. This is achieved by enzymes secreted into the gastrointestinal tract and by enzymes located at the luminal surface of the brush-border membrane (Figure 3).

Starch usually is the major carbohydrate in the diet and consists of straight (amylose) and branched (amylopectin) chains of glucose. These are split by α-amylase (predominantly from the pancreas) into maltose, maltotriose, and α-limit dextrin. These products are subsequently hydrolyzed by brush-border maltase (glucoamylase) and α-dextrinase (isomaltase) to release glucose, which then is transported across the membrane by glucose carriers. Dietary sucrose is hydrolyzed at the brush border into fructose and glucose, which then cross the membrane on their respective carriers. Lactose is split by brush-border lactase into glucose

and galactose, which cross the membrane independently on glucose carriers.

Protein digestion and absorption follow an overall pattern similar to that for large carbohydrates (such as starch); but there are differences between the two, particularly the ability of dipeptides (but not disaccharides) to cross the brush-border membrane. The first steps of protein degradation (Figure 4) occur in the lumen by the action of proteolytic enzymes from the stomach (pepsin) and the pancreas (trypsin, chymotrypsin, carboxypeptidase, and elastase) to form short-chain oligopeptides, dipeptides, and amino acids. The oligopeptides subsequently

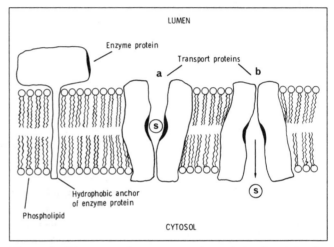

Figure 2—Diagrammatic representation of the brush-border membrane, illustrating the relationships between the phospholipid bilayer, an enzyme protein, and a carrier protein; the possible functioning of the latter in the transport of a water-soluble molecule (*S*) across the membrane (*a* and *b*) also is illustrated.

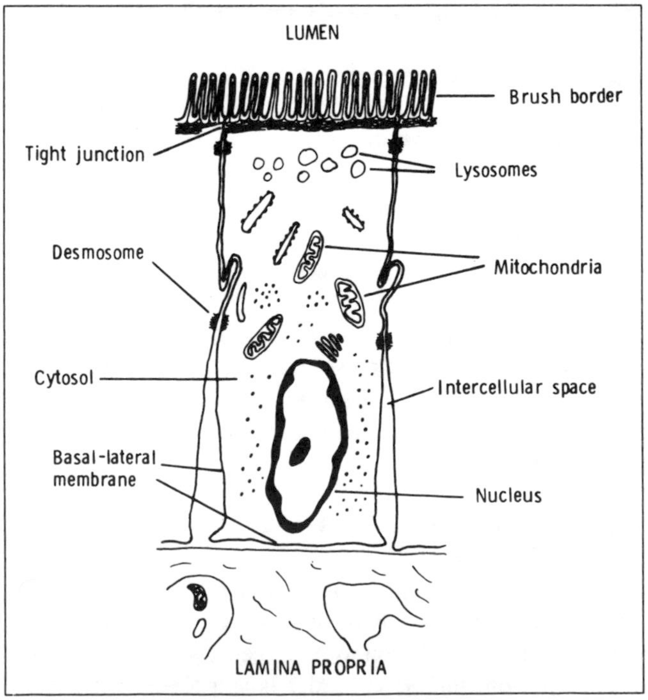

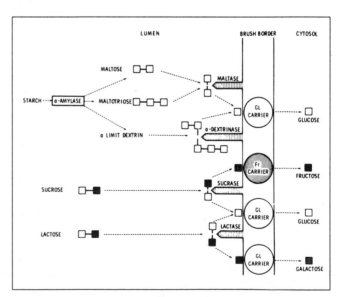

Figure 3—Diagrammatic representation of carbohydrate digestion and absorption. Carbohydrates are split by pancreatic amylase and/or intestinal brush-border enzymes to release monosaccharides, which then can cross the membrane on glucose (*GL*) or fructose (*Fr*) carriers.

Figure 1—Schematic representation of an enterocyte.

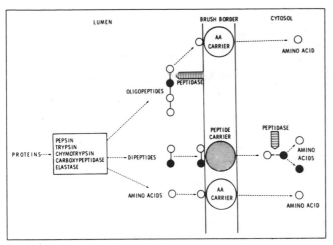

Figure 4—Diagrammatic representation of protein digestion and absorption. Protein is degraded by proteolytic enzymes from the stomach and the pancreas and by brush-border peptidases to release dipeptides and amino acids, which then can cross the membrane on peptide or amino acid (*AA*) carriers, respectively.

are hydrolyzed at the brush-border surface by peptidases, and the dipeptides and amino acids cross the membrane on specific carrier proteins. Dipeptides within the enterocytes then are split by cytosolic dipeptidase activity to release free amino acids. The brush-border plays an additional role in this degradative sequence because enteropeptidase (enterokinase) activity is localized there and is responsible for the conversion of trysinogen (the inactive proenzyme secreted by the pancreas) to trypsin, which subsequently activates chymotrypsin, carboxypeptidase, and elastase.

Fat-soluble molecules do not need a specific mechanism to cross the brush-border barrier; they pass through the phospholipid bilayer by passive diffusion. Prior degradation of relatively large lipids is essential, however. Fats are emulsified and squirted by the stomach into the duodenum to be mixed with bile and pancreatic juice. Triglycerides usually are the main dietary lipid, and these are degraded by pancreatic lipase at the surface of the emulsified lipid droplets to release monoglycerides and free fatty acids primarily (Figure 5). For efficient absorption, these products must be presented to the brush-border membrane in mixed micelles formed by interaction with conjugated bile salts. The monoglycerides and fatty acids then cross the brush border by passive diffusion, but the conjugated bile salts remain in the lumen to form further mixed micelles and eventually are absorbed by specific carriers present only in the ileum.

Malabsorption

Malabsorption can be a consequence of interference with any of the mechanisms responsible for the degradation or the subsequent absorption of one or more nutrients. The potential abnormalities can be determined from a knowledge of the normal mechanisms described (Figures 3 to 5). The main conditions are summarized in Table I.

EPI can have particularly serious consequences because

the pancreas plays a crucial role in the initial stages of digestion of the main dietary constituents. The pancreas has a considerable functional reserve, but when this is depleted (for example, because of acinar atrophy in dogs[2,3]) the intraluminal concentrations of α-amylase, pancreatic proteases, and lipase fall below critical levels. The result is relatively severe malabsorption of starches, proteins, and triglycerides.

Small intestinal disease also can result in malabsorption of many nutrients by interference with the number or the function of individual enterocytes. A secondary deficiency of brush-border enzymes and of carrier proteins and a reduction in surface area might be a consequence of villous atrophy and/or damage to microvilli. An important distinction from the primary brush-border deficiencies is that this secondary damage usually is much less specific and can result in malabsorption of various dietary constituents (Table I). A loss of carrier proteins is particularly important because for many molecules the rate-limiting step at the brush border is transport not digestion. Nevertheless, a loss of brush-border enzymes can result in malabsorption if their activities are reduced sufficiently. The clinical consequences of small intestinal disease depend on the severity and the extent of damage along the small intestine; in general, intestinal disease in dogs results in less-marked malabsorption than that typical of EPI.

In contrast with secondary damage to the mucosa, specific biochemical abnormalities of the brush-border membrane can occur in the absence of morphologic damage and will result in malabsorption of specific molecules (Table I). These conditions are well described in humans,[1] but only milk intolerance associated with lactase deficiency has been documented in dogs.[4]

Diagnosis of Exocrine Pancreatic Insufficiency

In the past, limitations of routine diagnostic procedures probably have been responsible for a gross exaggeration of

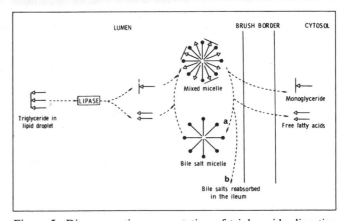

Figure 5—Diagrammatic representation of triglyceride digestion and absorption. Triglycerides are split by pancreatic lipase to release monoglycerides and free fatty acids, which interact with conjugated bile salts and present at the brush border as mixed micelles. The monoglycerides and the free fatty acids then cross the membrane by passive diffusion, while bile salts (*a*) form further mixed micelles or (*b*) are reabsorbed in the ileum.

TABLE I
Principal Enzyme and Carrier-Protein Deficiencies

Condition	Deficiency	Malabsorption
Exocrine pancreatic insufficiency	α-amylase	Starch
	Proteolytic enzymes	Protein
	Lipase	Triglycerides
Small intestinal disease (secondary deficiencies)	Disaccharidase	Disaccharides
	Sugar carriers	Monosaccharides
	Brush-border peptidase	Oligopeptides
	Peptide and amino acid carriers	Peptides and amino acids
	Reduced surface area	Lipid
Brush-border membrane disease (primary deficiencies)	Lactase	Lactose
	Sucrase-α-dextrinase	Sucrose, α-limit dextrins
	Glucose-galactose carrier	Glucose, galactose
	Enterokinase	Protein
	Amino acid carrier	None

the prevalence of EPI, and this has contributed to a failure to recognize small intestinal disease. Typically, EPI in dogs results from acinar atrophy that causes a severe depletion of functional exocrine tissue.[2,3] Diagnosis depends on the demonstration of a deficiency of pancreatic enzymes. As an indirect approach, the demonstration of starch and lipid malabsorption can suggest pancreatic amylase and lipase deficiencies, respectively; but because the absorption of these nutrients also depends on extrapancreatic factors (Figures 3 and 5), these findings alone do not support a definitive diagnosis of EPI.

A more direct approach is to assay the pancreatic enzymes. A common test is based on the estimation of fecal trypsin activity—for example, by gelatin digestion or by enzyme assay—but the results can be extremely misleading.[4,5] One problem is that the degradation of pancreatic enzymes begins at the time of secretion; residual fecal activity depends on many factors, particularly the speed of transit through the gut. Consequently, a normal dog might have low fecal trypsin activity, a fact that can result in the erroneous diagnosis of EPI in a patient with a normal pancreas.

Accurate diagnosis can be made by the assay of pancreatic enzymes in the lumen of the proximal small intestine. To avoid duodenal intubation, this can be achieved in vivo for chymotrypsin by giving the synthetic substrate N-benzoyl-L-tyrosyl-para-aminobenzoic acid (BT-PABA, bentiromide) orally and subsequent assay of PABA in blood or urine.[6-10] Although this test has simplified the diagnosis of EPI in dogs greatly, widespread application of the procedure is likely to be limited by practical constraints, including the cost of bentiromide, the need for multiple blood samplings or a metabolism cage for urine collection, and the availability of PABA assay. Misleading results can occur as a consequence of delayed gastric emptying or the malabsorption of free PABA because of severe small intestinal disease.[10]

As an alternative approach, a radioimmunoassay re-

cently has been developed for accurate detection of EPI by the analysis of a single blood sample.[11] This assay for serum TLI detects trypsinogen that normally leaks from the pancreas into the blood. In dogs with EPI resulting from acinar atrophy, functional exocrine tissue is depleted severely[2,3]; consequently serum TLI concentrations are extremely low, clearly distinguishing EPI from other causes of malabsorption (Figure 6). This assay has been established in the United Kingdom by the author and now also is available in the United States.[a,11]

Investigation of Chronic Small Intestinal Disease

Once a diagnosis of EPI has been excluded, considerable difficulties remain in achieving an accurate diagnosis of small intestinal disease; these include the limitations of routine screening procedures (particularly the xylose absorption test), the relative inaccessibility of the small intestine to biopsy and, frequently, the absence of obvious histologic changes in the mucosa. Indeed, it is now apparent that the intestinal diseases that have been described morphologically and reported previously in dogs[12-17] are extreme examples and are not representative of the most common conditions, which can escape detection easily. These diagnostic problems have been tackled by the assay of serum folate and vitamin B_{12} concentrations,[18] by the introduction of a peroral biopsy technique,[19] and by the application of predominantly biochemical criteria to the objective assessment of intestinal damage.[20]

Because the rate-limiting step at the brush border is transport and not digestion for most molecules, assessment of absorptive function is useful as a screening test for small intestinal disease. Oral xylose (which is absorbed primarily in the jejunum on a monosaccharide carrier) and the subsequent measurement of blood xylose concentrations[21] have been used extensively, can be combined with the ben-

[a]For more information on this assay, contact Dr. David A. Williams, College of Veterinary Medicine, J126, JHMHC, University of Florida, Gainesville, FL 32610.

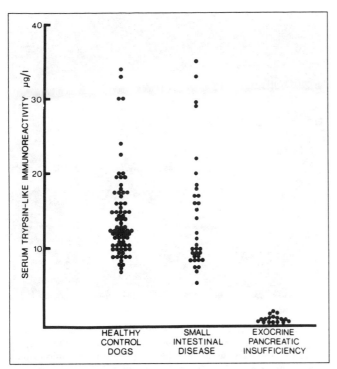

Figure 6—Serum TLI concentrations in clinically healthy dogs, dogs with small intestinal disease, and dogs with EPI.

tiromide test,[9,10] and provide a useful indirect assessment of proximal small intestinal function. Complicating factors, however—such as a slow rate of gastric emptying and bacterial metabolism of xylose—can give an erroneously low result. A more important problem is that it is not uncommon for xylose absorption to be normal in dogs with small intestinal disease; certain enteropathies thus can be overlooked easily.

In humans, abnormalities of the jejunum and the ileum can result in defective absorption of dietary folate and vitamin B_{12}, respectively, and therefore can be associated with reduced levels of these vitamins in the serum.[22,23] Similarly, in dogs, the assay of serum folate and vitamin B_{12} concentrations has provided valuable information that has contributed to the detection and the interpretation of previously unrecognized enteropathies.[18,24-26] These conditions have been characterized by the application of predominantly biochemical criteria to the analysis of peroral jejunal biopsies.[20] This new approach is illustrated in the following sections, which summarize the main findings in three of these diseases.

Enteropathy Resembling Chronic Tropical Sprue in Humans
Clinical Description

Enteropathy resembling chronic tropical sprue apparently is relatively uncommon and represents an extreme example of chronic small intestinal disease in dogs.[24] The condition has been described in a Shetland sheepdog and in three German shepherds, aged five to nine years, with histories of severe chronic diarrhea and weight loss for at least four months. Figure 7 shows that low serum folate concentrations were accompanied by an apparent reduction in xylose absorption, findings consistent with interference with the normal structure and functions of the proximal small intestinal mucosa.

Low serum vitamin B_{12} concentrations indicated that the functional mucosal damage also might have involved the distal small intestine, which is the main site of vitamin B_{12} absorption in dogs.[27] Malabsorption of vitamin B_{12} resulting from factors that include the binding of the vitamin by bacteria cannot be excluded because bacteriologic studies were not performed in these dogs. These abnormalities, particularly the vitamin deficiencies, are relatively nonspecific and merely reflect damage to the small intestinal mucosa; nevertheless, the findings are shared by tropical sprue syndrome in humans[23,28] and permit the initial identification of this disease in dogs.[24]

Mucosal Abnormalities

The morphologic appearance of jejunal biopsies from affected animals (Figure 8) indicates that this condition represents a relatively severe enteropathy in dogs. There is distinct partial villous atrophy accompanied by variable infiltration with lymphocytes and plasma cells in the lamina propria. The severity of damage is emphasized by the objective assessment of the mucosal changes via quantitative enzymology. In contrast with the other two canine enteropathies considered in this article, Figure 9 demonstrates decreased activity of many brush-border enzymes (excluding only γ-glutamyl transferase), a finding consistent with the relatively nonspecific functional and structural abnormalities discussed.

Subcellular fractionation emphasized the loss of brush-

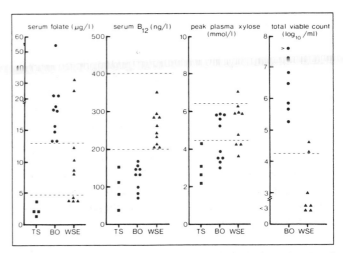

Figure 7—Serum folate and vitamin B_{12} concentrations, results of xylose absorption test, and total viable bacterial counts in the duodenal juice of dogs with small intestinal disease. *TS* = enteropathy resembling chronic tropical sprue, *BO* = bacterial overgrowth in the German shepherd, and *WSE* = wheat-sensitive enteropathy in the Irish setter. Dotted lines define control ranges or upper control values for bacterial counts. Open circle denotes patient given parenteral B_{12}. Vitamins quantitated by microbiologic assay.[18]

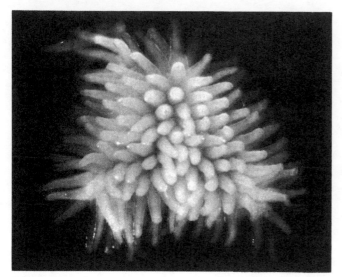

Figure 8A

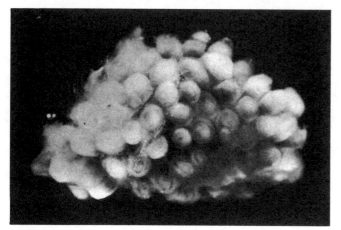

Figure 8B

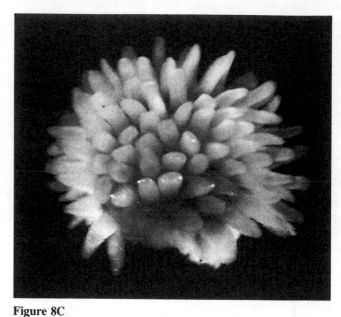

Figure 8C

Figure 8—Dissecting-microscope appearance of jejunal biopsies from (**A**) a control dog, showing normal tall, fingerlike villi; (**B**) a German shepherd with enteropathy resembling chronic tropical sprue; and (**C**) an Irish setter, demonstrating some blunting of villi. (×20)

border enzyme activities and demonstrated that biochemical abnormalities were not confined to the microvilli (Figure 10). There was a large increase in soluble N-acetyl-β-glucosaminidase activity, indicative of enhanced lysosomal fragility. In addition, a considerable increase in the activity of TRIS-resistant α-glucosidase indicated a proliferation of the endoplasmic reticulum and an enhanced rate of protein synthesis by the mucosa. In contrast with these distinct abnormalities, the activities and density distributions of marker enzymes for basolateral membranes (5' nucleotidase) and mitochondria (malate dehydrogenase) were unaffected (Figure 10).

Pathophysiologic Mechanisms

The clinical signs of severe diarrhea and weight loss in the affected dogs might have been related to malabsorption of many nutrients because a loss of brush-border enzymes and carrier proteins can result, for example, in interference with the normal handling of carbohydrates and proteins (Figures 3 and 4). Partially degraded molecules remaining in the lumen can present a relatively high osmotic load to

the distal small intestine and—together with other factors, including active secretion and diminished absorption of fluid and electrolytes—can contribute to the watery diarrhea.

The literature contains detailed discussion of the many similarities between this naturally occurring enteropathy in dogs and chronic tropical sprue in humans and of the differences between this canine condition and celiac disease (gluten-sensitive enteropathy) in humans.[24] Tropical sprue has been well documented in many parts of the world; although epidemiologic studies have implicated an infective cause,[29] no specific agent has been identified. Jejunal colonization with enteropathogenic bacteria, perhaps resulting from defective host resistance, might play a role in the pathogenesis of tropical sprue[30-32]; but colonization is not a constant feature of the disease, and no primary immunologic abnormality has been demonstrated. In dogs, however, it is conceivable that these relatively serious mucosal changes could arise as a consequence of long-standing bacterial overgrowth, a disorder recently recognized in German shepherds.[25,33]

Enteropathy and Bacterial Overgrowth in German Shepherds
Clinical Description

Enteropathy associated with bacterial overgrowth has been described in a series of 10 German shepherds, one nine years of age and the others between five months and two years.[25] All 10 had a history of intermittent diarrhea, with or without loss of weight, and had exhibited clinical signs for at least three months—in two cases, since they were one year old; in the others, since they were approxi-

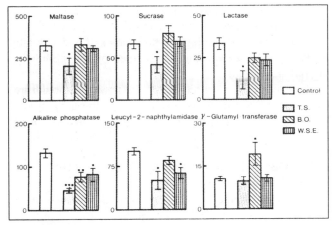

Figure 9—Activities (mU/mg protein) of brush-border enzymes in jejunal biopsies from control dogs (≥12) and patients with small intestinal disease. *TS* = enteropathy resembling chronic tropical sprue, *BO* = bacterial overgrowth in the German shepherd, and *WSE* = wheat-sensitive enteropathy in the Irish setter. Data are expressed as mean ± SEM. Statistical differences between control and affected groups are as follows: $*P<0.05$; $**P<0.01$; $***P<0.001$.

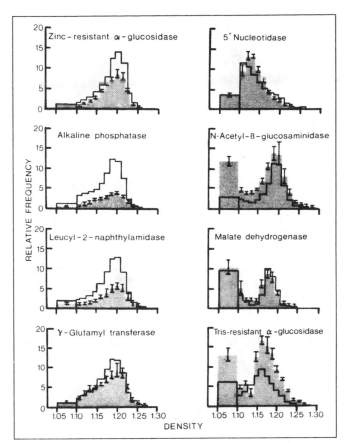

Figure 10—Subcellular fractionation of postnuclear supernatants from jejunal biopsy homogenates of dogs with enteropathy resembling chronic tropical sprue (*shaded area*) compared with controls (*solid line*). The density span—1.05 to 1.10—represents soluble enzyme activity. For each enzyme, the areas of the distributions are proportional to enzyme-specific activity (mU/mg protein). For further details, consult Reference 24.

mately two months old. Figure 7 demonstrates that serum folate concentrations were elevated and (with the exception of one patient given parenteral vitamin B_{12}) serum vitamin B_{12} concentrations were reduced, whereas only five dogs had an apparent reduction in xylose absorption.

Because many enteric bacteria have the ability to synthesize folate (which subsequently is absorbed by the jejunum) yet bind vitamin B_{12}, making it unavailable for transport, these findings suggested bacterial overgrowth in the proximal small intestine.[33] Indeed, bacterial overgrowth was confirmed by quantitative and qualitative bacteriologic examination of duodenal juice obtained from seven of the dogs, which demonstrated viable counts of greater than 10^5 organisms/ml (Figure 7). Most frequently, the overgrowth comprised bacteria of the normal flora (particularly *Escherichia coli* and enterococci), but these occasionally were accompanied by bacteria rarely present in the proximal small intestines of normal dogs (particularly *Clostridium* spp.).

Mucosal Abnormalities

Examination of peroral jejunal biopsies by dissecting and light microscopy revealed minimal changes apart from partial villous atrophy in biopsies from two dogs. There were striking biochemical changes in the mucosa, however, particularly in the brush border, where there were distinct but selective alterations in the activities of specific marker enzymes. Figure 9 demonstrates that there were no changes in the activities of the disaccharidases maltase, sucrase, and lactase or of the peptidase leucyl-2-naphthylamidase. In marked contrast, the specific activity of alkaline phosphatase was reduced significantly. Subcellular fractionation demonstrated a marked loss, particularly of the main brush-border component of enzyme activity (Figure 11), whereas γ-glutamyl transferase activity was increased.

Figure 11 also demonstrates that soluble components of N-acetyl-β-glucosaminidase and malate dehydrogenase were increased, providing indirect evidence for enhanced lysosomal fragility and mitochondrial disruption, respectively. In contrast, basolateral membrane (5' nucleotidase) and endoplasmic reticular (TRIS-resistant α-glucosidase) enzymes were relatively unaffected.

Pathophysiologic Mechanisms

In agreement with the findings in these German shepherds, histologic changes frequently are minimal in bacterial overgrowth because of the blind-loop syndrome in humans and in experimental animals[25]; however, biochemical changes apparently vary and depend on the numbers and the types of bacteria isolated. Indeed, the brush-border changes in these patients differ significantly from those described in the experimental blind-loop syndrome, in which considerably increased numbers of obligate anaerobes are present and might be directly responsible for disaccharidase deficiencies by their release from[34] or destruction in[35] the membrane.

The specific loss of alkaline phosphatase from the brush borders of these German shepherds might result from di-

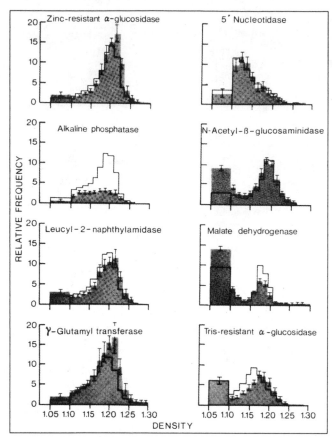

Figure 11—Subcellular fractionation of postnuclear supernatants from jejunal biopsy homogenates of dogs with bacterial overgrowth (*shaded area*) compared with controls (*solid line*). The density span—1.05 to 1.10—represents soluble enzyme activity. For each enzyme, the areas of the distributions are proportional to enzyme-specific activity (mU/mg protein). For further details, consult Reference 25.

rect damage by bacteria or their secreted products or from the bacterial metabolism of intraluminal contents into potentially toxic products (for example, deconjugated bile salts and hydroxy fatty acids).[36] These can have a direct effect on the enzyme or can act by perturbation of the associated membrane phospholipids. Other factors, such as a decrease in the rate of enzyme synthesis, can be responsible for the decreased activity of alkaline phosphatase in the microvillous membrane. The increased activity of γ-glutamyl transferase has been documented in the human blind-loop syndrome, and it has been speculated that this finding might reflect enhanced proliferative activity.[37]

The findings in these German shepherds demonstrate that bacterial colonization of the proximal small intestine can be associated with specific alterations in microvillous-membrane proteins; the findings also provide biochemical evidence for intracellular damage to the enterocytes. This mucosal injury and the intraluminal disturbances that are a direct consequence of the overgrowth can contribute to a malabsorption of dietary constituents, resulting in clinical disease. The relatively subtle nature of the mucosal abnormalities, however, suggests that intraluminal effects might be especially significant. The latter might include bacterial deconjugation of bile salts, which can interfere with effective micelle formation and can result in malabsorption of lipid (Figure 5). Deconjugated bile salts and hydroxy fatty acids might be responsible for diarrhea by the stimulation of colonic secretion.[36]

The cause of the overgrowth is unknown. Although impaired motility cannot be excluded, preliminary studies have suggested a possible underlying immunologic disorder in the breed[38] and have failed to show achlorhydria.

Wheat-Sensitive Enteropathy in Irish Setters
Clinical Description

A specific enteropathy has been described in a series of 10 Irish setters, one seven years of age and the others between seven months and two years.[26] The main clinical sign was poor weight gain or weight loss, accompanied in eight dogs by intermittent chronic diarrhea with onset typically between four and seven months of age. Figure 7 shows that serum folate concentration was low in four of the dogs, three of which also had reduced xylose absorption—findings consistent with disease of the proximal small intestine. This indirect evidence of functional disturbance was not a feature of the majority of the affected animals, consistent with the severity and apparently patchy nature of the morphologic changes. Normal serum folate might have been maintained in spite of defective folate transport by folate of bacterial origin, but this is unlikely because no marked overgrowth ($>10^5$ organisms/ml) was demonstrated in the duodenal juice obtained from seven of the dogs (Figure 7).

Bacteria might have contributed to the elevated serum folate concentrations found in two dogs[18,33]; however, duodenal juice from one of these was cultured and failed to confirm this possibility. Further evidence against long-standing overgrowth was provided by the normal serum vitamin B_{12} concentrations found in all cases (Figure 7), in marked contrast with the reduced levels in the German shepherds with bacterial overgrowth. The normal serum concentrations of vitamin B_{12} also suggested that the enteropathy was confined to the proximal small intestine, although a patchy disease of the ileum that did not interfere significantly with vitamin B_{12} absorption could not be excluded.

Mucosal Abnormalities

Morphologic changes in the mucosa were variable and apparently were patchy within individual patients. The most consistent abnormality was partial villous atrophy, less severe than that of the enteropathy resembling chronic tropical sprue and typified by the appearance of the biopsy in Figure 8C. A biopsy from one dog exhibited extremely severe subtotal villous atrophy, a typical feature of celiac disease.[26] This appearance was a rare manifestation of the disease in these dogs, however, and cannot be considered pathognomonic for celiac disease because similar changes have been observed occasionally in other disorders, including cow's milk protein intolerance[39,40] and soybean intolerance[41] in children.

Quantitative biochemical assessment of organelle pathology provided clear evidence of specific brush-border abnormalities in jejunal biopsies from the affected animals. Figure 9 demonstrates that the specific activities of alkaline phosphatase and of the peptidase leucyl-2-naphthylamidase were decreased selectively, although the activities of the disaccharidases and of γ-glutamyl transferase were unaltered. These changes contrast markedly with the generalized brush-border abnormalities associated with the more severe morphologic damage in the enteropathy resembling tropical sprue and with the selective decrease in brush-border alkaline phosphatase in bacterial overgrowth (Figure 9).

Demonstration of Wheat Sensitivity

The possibility of a dietary sensitivity in these Irish setters was supported by the considerable clinical improvement of all six dogs treated with a cereal-free diet; the possibility was pursued by breeding a litter from two affected dogs.[42,43] Jejunal biopsies from all eight progeny, on a normal diet, revealed partial villous atrophy and age-related biochemical abnormalities. In biopsies from the first four dogs at eight months of age, activities of alkaline phosphatase and leucyl-2-naphthylamidase were almost undetectable and disaccharidases (not shown) were unaltered (Figure 12). In contrast, analytic subcellular fractionation of biopsies obtained at nine months of age from the second four dogs demonstrated that specific activities reflected a major deficiency of brush-border alkaline phosphatase and apparently normal brush-border leucyl-2-naphthylamidase accompanied by elevated soluble activity.

Further investigation of the first four dogs demonstrated recovery of morphologic and biochemical parameters after five months on a cereal-free diet. Relapse on subsequent challenge with wheat flour for three months was characterized by patchy partial villous atrophy and a severe loss of brush-border alkaline phosphatase activity (Figure 12). In contrast, although the main brush-border peak of leucyl-2-naphthylamidase was spread into the lighter fractions, there were no adverse effects on the specific activities of leucyl-2-naphthylamidase or of disaccharidases (not shown).

Pathophysiologic Mechanisms

These findings document a wheat-sensitive enteropathy in Irish setters and suggest that the disorder might be an age-related abnormality affecting specific brush-border enzymes.[42,43] Although no definitive function has been ascribed to alkaline phosphatase, an abnormality of leucyl-2-naphthylamidase (aminopeptidase N)—the most abundant brush-border peptidase—might be particularly important during a critical growth phase. This might contribute to a malabsorption of proteins (Figure 4) and also might result in defective degradation of potentially toxic gliadin (wheat protein) peptides. The latter might permit the development of hypersensitivity (perhaps involving mast cells), as suggested for celiac disease,[44] so that relatively small concentrations of peptide might be adequate to trigger enterocyte damage and to cause villous atrophy despite the subsequent

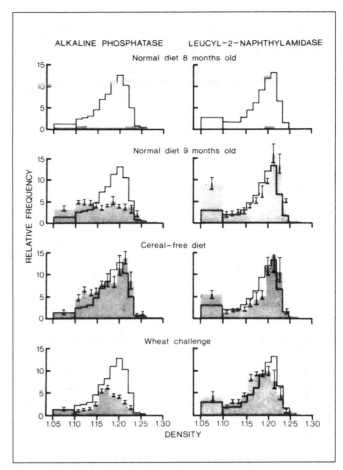

Figure 12—Subcellular fractionation of postnuclear supernatants from jejunal biopsy homogenates of Irish setters with wheat-sensitive enteropathy (*shaded area*) compared with controls (*solid line*). The density span—1.05 to 1.10—represents soluble enzyme activity. For each enzyme, the areas of the distributions are proportional to enzyme-specific activity (mU/mg protein).

appearance of peptidase activity. At present, this possibility remains speculative and the pathogenesis of this wheat-sensitive enteropathy in Irish setters is undefined.

Summary of Approach to Malabsorption
Diagnosis

When intestinal parasites, pathogenic bacteria, and systemic disorders are ruled out, the accurate assessment of exocrine pancreatic function should be the next objective in investigating dogs with possible malabsorption. This can be achieved, for example, by the assay of serum TLI in a single serum sample. Assessment should be performed to eliminate a diagnosis of EPI before the possibility of an intestinal disorder is considered. Subsequently, the estimations of serum folate and vitamin B_{12} concentrations can provide valuable information to assist the identification of small intestinal disease and to provide an initial assessment of the probable nature of the mucosal changes.

The three enteropathies described initially were differentiated primarily by the assay of serum folate and vitamin B_{12} concentrations.[18] Normal results do not exclude the possibility of small intestinal disease, however, because alterations in serum concentrations of these vitamins depend on the nature, the extent, and the duration of a mucosal abnormality. This is illustrated clearly by the disparate folate results in the Irish setters with patchy enteropathy. In addition, although bacterial overgrowth in the proximal small intestine typically can be associated with elevated serum folate and reduced vitamin B_{12} concentrations, this is not an inevitable sequela; it is influenced, for example, by the numbers and types of microorganisms present.[33]

These vitamin estimations do not eliminate the need for prior assessment of exocrine pancreatic function because EPI can interfere with the interpretation of the results, as can inadequate dietary intake or therapeutic giving of these vitamins.[18] Nevertheless, the potential value of these vitamin estimations for the detection and interpretation of small intestinal diseases in dogs cannot be overemphasized. Microbiologic assays for these vitamins were used in the studies described, however, commercial radioisotope kits—which require less technical skill—are available. Kits from different manufacturers vary in sensitivity and specificity but can be used routinely for dogs when appropriate reference ranges are established for a specific kit.

The introduction of a peroral biopsy procedure[19] and the application of predominantly biochemical criteria to the analysis of jejunal biopsies[20] have facilitated the detection and characterization of previously unrecognized canine enteropathies. Although these cannot be considered to be routine diagnostic procedures, this approach permits the validation of serum folate and vitamin B_{12} estimations for the investigation of intestinal disease and improves understanding of the pathogenesis of canine enteropathies. The peroral biopsy technique facilitates sequential studies after dietary manipulation or other treatments and consequently has proven to be particularly valuable, for example, in permitting definitive description of wheat-sensitive enteropathy in Irish setters.

Treatment

Treatment of EPI is relatively straightforward and involves lifelong replacement therapy by the addition of pancreatic enzymes (e.g., Viokase®-V—A. H. Robins) to a low-fat diet. Bacterial overgrowth can accompany EPI in some dogs; if response to replacement therapy alone is poor, this condition should be suspected and treated.

Effective treatment of small intestinal disease in dogs depends on the nature of the disorder, but frequently a practical approach to therapy is largely empirical. Initially, the possibility of dietary sensitivity should be explored because dietary modification can result in rapid improvement with no additional treatment. Although a rational explanation for the success of a particular diet might not be apparent, exclusion diets proven to be particularly helpful include lamb or cottage cheese with potato or rice. The exclusion of cereal might be the critical factor in certain cases because this should help patients with wheat-sensitive enteropathy, a problem unlikely to be confined to Irish setters. A low fat content probably will help in the management of dogs with bacterial overgrowth because bacterial metabolism of fat—for example, to hydroxy fatty acids—might contribute to clinical signs, particularly causing diarrhea by the stimulation of fluid secretion.

Oral glucocorticoids, especially prednisolone (0.5 mg/kg body weight, repeated every 12 hours for a month, followed by a reducing dose), have assisted in certain cases of small intestinal disease, including in dogs with enteropathies resembling chronic tropical sprue in humans. Beneficial effects might be a consequence of immunosuppression or might result from the direct action of glucocorticoids to increase the absorptive and digestive capacities of enterocytes by the induction of specific functional proteins.[45] Oral broad-spectrum antibiotic therapy—for example, with oxytetracycline (10 mg/kg body weight, repeated every eight hours) for periods of 7 to 28 days—has been effective in German shepherds with bacterial overgrowth. Alternative possibilities are metronidazole (10 mg/kg body weight, repeated every 12 hours) and tylosin (10 mg/kg body weight, repeated every eight hours). Repeated treatment might be necessary because the underlying reason for the colonization probably will not resolve.

Finally, supplementation with vitamins—particularly oral folate (e.g., 5 mg/day for one to six months) and parenteral vitamin B_{12} (e.g., 500 μg/month for six months)—might help in the treatment of small intestinal disease because deficiencies of these vitamins can be important in the pathogenesis of specific mucosal lesions. Folate and vitamin B_{12} are involved in DNA replication; consequently, the rapid cell turnover in the small intestine is particularly vulnerable to reduced availability of these nutrients.

As the understanding of specific enteropathies progresses, it might become possible to develop a more rational approach to the treatment and the prevention of chronic small intestinal disease in dogs.

Acknowledgments

For financial support during the course of these studies, the author thanks the Wellcome Trust, the British Small Animal Veterinary Association Clinical Studies Trust Fund, the Canine Supporters Charity, and various breed societies, including the German Shepherd Dog League and the Irish Setter Breeders Club. Figures 1–5, 7, 9, and Table I are used with permission from References 1 and 46; Figures 8A, 8B, and 10 from Reference 24; Figure 8C from Reference 26; and Figure 11 from Reference 25.

REFERENCES

1. Batt RM: The molecular basis of malabsorption. *J Small Anim Pract* 21:555–569, 1980.
2. Anderson NV, Low DG: Juvenile atrophy of the canine pancreas. *Anim Hosp* 1:101–109, 1965.
3. Hill FWG, Osborne AD, Kidder DE: Pancreatic degenerative atrophy in dogs. *J Comp Pathol* 81:321–330, 1971.
4. Hill FWG: Malabsorption syndrome in the dog: A study of thirty-eight cases. *J Small Anim Pract* 13:575–594, 1972.

5. Burrows CF, Merritt AM, Chiapella AM: Determination of fecal fat and trypsin output in the evaluation of chronic canine diarrhea. *JAVMA* 174:62–66, 1979

6. Freudiger U, Bigler B: Die Diagnose der chronischen exokrinen Pankreasinsuffizienz mit dem PABA-Test. *Kleintier-Praxis* 22:73–84, 1977.

7. Strombeck DR: New method for evaluation of chymotrypsin deficiency in dogs. *JAVMA* 173:1319–1323, 1978.

8. Batt RM, Bush BM, Peters TJ: A new test for the diagnosis of exocrine pancreatic insufficiency in the dog. *J Small Anim Pract* 20:185–192, 1979.

9. Rogers WA, Stradley RP, Sherding RG, et al: Simultaneous evaluation of pancreatic exocrine function and intestinal absorptive function in dogs with chronic diarrhea. *JAVMA* 177:1128–1131, 1980.

10. Batt RM, Mann LC: The specificity of the BT-PABA test for the diagnosis of exocrine pancreatic insufficiency in the dog. *Vet Rec* 108:303–307, 1981.

11. Williams DA, Batt RM: Diagnosis of canine exocrine pancreatic insufficiency by the assay of serum trypsin-like immunoreactivity. *J Small Anim Pract* 24:583–588, 1983.

12. Vernon DF: Idiopathic sprue in a dog. *JAVMA* 140:1062–1067, 1962.

13. Kaneko JJ, Moulton JE, Brodey RS, Perryman VD: Malabsorption syndrome resembling nontropical sprue in dogs. *JAVMA* 146:463–473, 1965.

14. Campbell RSF, Brobst D, Bisgard G: Intestinal lymphangectasia in a dog. *JAVMA* 153:1050–1054, 1968.

15. Finco DR, Duncan JR, Schall WD, et al: Chronic enteric disease and hypoproteinemia in 9 dogs. *JAVMA* 163:262–271, 1973.

16. Hill FWG, Kelly DF: Naturally occurring intestinal malabsorption in the dog. *Am J Dig Dis* 19:649–665, 1974.

17. Flesja K, Yri T: Protein-losing enteropathy in the Lundehund. *J Small Anim Pract* 18:11–23, 1977.

18. Batt RM, Morgan JO: Role of serum folate and vitamin B_{12} concentrations in the differentiation of small intestinal abnormalities in the dog. *Res Vet Sci* 32:17–22, 1982.

19. Batt RM: Techniques for single and multiple peroral jejunal biopsy in the dog. *J Small Anim Pract* 20:259–268, 1979.

20. Batt RM, Peters TJ: Subcellular fractionation studies on peroral jejunal biopsies from the dog. *Res Vet Sci* 25:94–100, 1978.

21. Hill FWG, Kidder DE, Frew J: A xylose absorption test for the dog. *Vet Rec* 87:250–255, 1970.

22. Stewart JS, Pollock DJ, Hoffbrand AV, et al: A study of proximal and distal intestinal structure and absorptive function in idiopathic steatorrhoea. *Q J Med* 36:425–444, 1967.

23. Hoffbrand AV, Necheles TF, Maldonado N, et al: Malabsorption of folate polyglutamates in tropical sprue. *Br Med J* 2:543–547, 1969.

24. Batt RM, Bush BM, Peters TJ: Subcellular biochemical studies of a naturally occurring enteropathy in the dog resembling chronic tropical sprue in human beings. *Am J Vet Res* 44:1492–1496, 1983.

25. Batt RM, Carter MW, Peters TJ: Biochemical changes in the jejunal mucosa of dogs with a naturally occurring enteropathy associated with bacterial overgrowth. *Gut* 25:816–823, 1984.

26. Batt RM, Carter MW, McLean L: Morphologic and biochemical studies of a naturally occurring enteropathy in the Irish setter dog: A comparison with coeliac disease in man. *Res Vet Sci* 37:339–346, 1984.

27. Fleming WH, King ER, Galloway RA, Roche JJ: The site of absorption of orally administered Co^{60} labelled vitamin B_{12} in dogs: The effect of dose. *Gastroenterology* 42.164–168, 1962.

28. Corcino JJ, Reisenauer AM, Halsted CH: Jejunal perfusion of simple and conjugated folates in tropical sprue. *J Clin Invest* 58:298–305, 1976.

29. Dean AG, Jones TC: Seasonal gastroenteritis and malabsorption at an American military base in the Philippines. I. Clinical and epidemiologic investigations of the acute illness. *Am J Epidemiol* 95:111–127, 1972.

30. Gorbach SL, Banwell JG, Jacobs B, et al: Tropical sprue and malnutrition in West Bengal. I. Intestinal microflora and absorption. *Am J Clin Nutr* 23:1545–1558, 1970.

31. Gorbach SL: Intestinal microflora. *Gastroenterology* 60:1110–1129, 1971.

32. Klipstein FA, Holdman LV, Corcino JJ, Moore WEC: Enterotoxigenic intestinal bacteria in tropical sprue. *Ann Intern Med* 79:632–641, 1973.

33. Batt RM, Needham JR, Carter MW: Bacterial overgrowth associated with a naturally occurring enteropathy in the German shepherd dog. *Res Vet Sci* 35:42–46, 1983.

34. Jonas A, Krishnan C, Forstner G: Pathogenesis of mucosal injury in the blood loop syndrome. Release of disaccharidases from brush-border membranes by extracts of bacteria obtained from intestinal blind loops in rats. *Gastroenterology* 75:791–795, 1978.

35. Riepe SP, Goldstein J, Alpers DH: Effect of secreted *Bacteroides* proteases on human intestinal brush-border hydrolases. *J Clin Invest* 66:314–322, 1980.

36. King CE, Toskes PP: Small intestine bacterial overgrowth. *Gastroenterology* 76:1035–1055, 1979.

37. Schjønsby H, Anderson K-J, Nordgard K, Skagen DW: Enzymatic activities in jejunal biopsy specimens from patients with the stagnant-loop syndrome. *Scand J Gastroenterol* 18:599–602, 1983.

38. Whitbread TJ, Batt RM, Garthwaite G: A relative deficiency of serum IgA in the German shepherd dog: A breed abnormality. *Res Vet Sci* 37:350–352, 1984.

39. Kruitunen P, Rapola J, Savilahti E, Visakorpi JK: Response of the jejunal mucosa to cow's milk in the malabsorption syndrome with cow's milk intolerance. A light- and electron-microscopic study. *Acta Paediatr Scand* 62:585–595, 1973.

40. Fontaine JL, Navarro J: Small intestinal biopsy in cow's milk protein allergy in infancy. *Arch Dis Child* 50:357–362, 1975.

41. Ament ME, Rubin CE: Soy protein—Another cause of the flat intestinal lesion. *Gastroenterology* 62:227–234, 1972.

42. Batt RM, McLean L, Loughran M: Specific brush-border abnormalities associated with a wheat-sensitive enteropathy (WSE) in the Irish setter dog. *Gastroenterology* 86:1021, 1984.

43. Batt RM, Carter MW, McLean L: Wheat-sensitive enteropathy in Irish setter dogs. Possible age-related brush-border abnormalities. *Res Vet Sci* 39:80–83, 1985.

44. Marsh MN: Morphologic expression of immunologically-mediated change and injury within the human small intestinal mucosa, in Batt RM, Lawrence TLJ (eds): *Function and Dysfunction of the Small Intestine*. Liverpool, Liverpool University Press, 1984, pp 167–198.

45. Batt RM, Scott J: Response of the small intestinal mucosa to oral glucocorticoids. *Scand J Gastroenterol [Suppl 74]* 17:75–88, 1982.

46. Batt RM: Small intestinal disease in the dog. *J Small Anim Pract* 26:707–718, 1984.

Management of Fecal Impaction

KEY FACTS

- Fecal impaction (or constipation) is defined as a condition in which bowel movements are infrequent or incomplete.
- A thorough diagnostic evaluation before and during treatment of fecal impaction is essential to the proper management of afflicted dogs and cats.
- Successful management of fecal impaction can be complicated by either long- and short-term effects or age-related alterations in internal organ function.
- Prevention, which is often provided by adequate dietary fiber intake and regular exercise, is advisable because treatment can often be frustrating.

Louisiana State University
Johnny D. Hoskins, DVM, PhD

ALTHOUGH fecal impaction is common, clinical presentation of the disorder varies and has many potential complications. Furthermore, the pathophysiology of fecal impaction is complex and poorly understood. Fecal impaction, which is the same as constipation, is a condition of infrequent or incomplete bowel movements. The colon is the primary target organ of fecal impaction. The excretory function of the colon is incompletely understood, partially because the techniques used to study colonic function are neither sensitive nor reproducible.[1,2] Because treatment of fecal impaction can often be frustrating, prevention is advisable.

PATHOPHYSIOLOGY OF FECAL IMPACTION

Most of the current understanding of the pathophysiology of fecal impaction has been derived from human medical literature. Limited information regarding the pathophysiologic mechanisms of fecal impaction is available for dogs or cats; therefore, most of the following discussion is based on the human medical literature.

The excretory function of the colon is influenced by both systemic and local factors that affect colonic motility. The colon of dogs, cats, and humans has three types of muscular activity: rhythmic segmentation waves, peristaltic waves, and giant migrating contractions. Rhythmic segmentation waves mix the contents of the stool, but these waves can also impede propulsion. An increase in segmentation-wave activity may therefore predispose an animal to constipation.[3] Peristaltic waves, which occur regularly throughout the day, are responsible for the aboral movement of feces in the colon.[4] Giant migrating contractions, which occur randomly throughout the day, move fecal contents farther and more rapidly than peristaltic waves do.[4,5] Giant migrating contractions commonly occur after a meal and are called the gastrocolic reflex. If giant migrating contractions diminish or are absent, constipation may result.[5]

The balance between sympathetic and parasympathetic activity establishes a neurologic influence on the colon. Parasympathetic activity enhances propulsion by increasing peristalsis and giant migrating contractions; sympathetic activity inhibits propulsion by increasing segmentation-wave activity.[6] Adrenergic function is mediated through the neural plexus of the colon from spinal and supraspinal sources.[7,8] Congenital and acquired abnormalities of the neural plexus can result in impaired colonic motility.

Hormones and metabolic factors also influence colonic motility. Hormones that increase motility include gastrin, vasoactive intestinal polypeptides, cholecystokinin, serotonin, thyroxine, estrogen, and the prostaglandins E_1 and $F_{2\alpha}$.[9] Hormones that decrease motility and promote fecal impaction include prolactin, glucagon, secretin, and the endorphins.[9] Such metabolic abnormalities as hypokalemia and hypercalcemia (which are also common in cancer and chronic renal disease) adversely affect colonic motility.[10,11]

Diet is the most important local factor in regulating co-

TABLE I
Causes of Fecal Impaction in Geriatric Cats

Category	Cause
Food and liquids	Excessive nondigestible bulk or fiber, hair impaction, foreign material, dehydration
Drugs	Agents that add to stool density (e.g., sucralfate, barium sulfate, kaolin-pectin preparations, antacids containing aluminum, calcium preparations); agents that alter colonic motility (e.g., narcotics, anticholingerics, oral iron preparations, vincristine, antihistamines, phenothiazines, diuretics, chronic laxative abuse)
Neurologic problem	Ileus, paraplegia, neurologic disorder, spinal cord or sacral nerve disease, central nervous system disease, lead intoxication, dysautonomia, pseudoobstruction, hypokalemia, intervertebral disk disease
Traumatic insult	Pelvic or spinal fracture, hematoma or contusion, laceration
Metabolic disease	Hyperthyroidism, hyperparathyroidism, pseudohyperparathyroidism, chronic renal failure, cancer
Perineal or rectal pain	Septic or nonseptic inflammation, lodged foreign object, pelvic fracture, rectal prolapse, perianal abscessation or fistula, rectal or anal growth or stricture, anal sac impaction, abscess, or infection
Colonic, rectal, or anal obstruction	Neoplasia or granulomatous inflammation, misaligned healed pelvic fracture, rectal prolapse, pseudocoprostasis, extracolonic compression, cystic uterus masculinus, sublumbar lymphadenopathy, perineal hernia
Behavioral	Elimination problems (refusal to defecate, no available litter boxes), territorial fighting, change of environment, situational depression
Miscellaneous	Idiopathic megacolon, inability to ambulate or squat, persistent inactivity, irritable bowel syndrome

lonic function. An adequate intake of dietary fiber and fluid prevents constipation.[12,13] Provision of dietary fiber has been shown to perform several functions (such as an increase in fecal output, reduction in stool density, and increase in luminal bulk) that stimulate colonic motility.[14]

The motor activity of the intrinsic smooth muscle of the colon and the striated muscles of the abdominal wall and diaphragm are important in proper defecation. Atrophy or weakness of these muscle groups hinders the act of defecation, making the passage of feces from the rectum difficult.[15]

The sensory function of the rectum and anus is also important in defecation. In some geriatric animals or animals with spinal cord lesions, abnormalities may occur in the ability to sense rectal distention. The anal canal is lined with a stratified epithelium that is very sensitive to pain. Painful lesions in this area (such as anal sacculitis or abscess, perianal fistula, and perirectal inflammation or neoplasia) therefore result in reflex inhibition of the passage of feces.[15]

Regardless of the cause of fecal retention, inhibition of the colon to absorb electrolytes and water normally leads to hardening of the feces; the peristaltic activity of the colon causes packing.[4] A mass of fecal material can become too large to pass because of the limited distensibility of the rectum. A ball-valve effect may result, allowing liquid stool to seep around the obstructing mass of harder feces during attempts at defecation, which are frequent.[16]

CAUSES OF FECAL IMPACTION

In most situations, fecal impaction is the result of a number of interacting pathophysiologic factors. Contributing causes of fecal impaction in dogs and cats are listed in Table I. A mixture of feces and nondigestible hair or bones is the most common cause of infrequent or incomplete defecation in dogs and cats.

In geriatric animals, lack of mobility plays an important role in causing fecal impaction because the ability to ambulate and exercise promotes colonic motility.[3] Neglecting the urge to defecate may contribute to constipation among demented geriatric animals. The problem is intensified if daily routines are disturbed, such as while boarding or during hospitalization. Geriatric animals are also subject to serious underlying illnesses that often contribute to constipation; cancer of the colon, hepatic disease, chronic renal disease, hyperthyroidism, and congestive heart failure are examples of such illnesses.[17,18]

Disturbances in fluid volume and electrolyte activity resulting from chronic renal failure predispose cats to fecal impaction, as do uremia and such underlying diseases as diabetes mellitus, congestive heart failure, and hyperthyroidism.[19] Calcium preparations and antacids containing aluminum used to manage renal failure also contribute to the risk of impaction.[20] Malnutrition and the use of immunosuppressive agents increase the incidence of subsequent complications.[20]

CLINICAL PRESENTATION

The presentation of fecal impaction can be subtle and nonspecific. Impaction should be considered if dogs or cats are presented with clinical deterioration, especially if the frequency or consistency of bowel movements has changed. The continual passage of stool does not rule out impaction. The incidence of constipation increases with age among healthy geriatric animals.[21] If the animal passes fewer than one stool every other day, impaction should be considered.

A gentle rectal examination combined with abdominal palpation is effective in detecting fecal impaction; this procedure is also well tolerated.[21] Abdominal palpation typically reveals fecal masses that may fill the entire length of the colon. Although impaction occurs most often in the rectal canal, the absence of palpable stool during rectal examination does not rule out fecal impaction because it can occur throughout the colon. Proximal or high impaction often suggests neoplasia or stricture of the colon. Impacted feces also can be either soft or hard and can take many forms, such as a single mass or multiple pellets.

Animals presented with fecal impaction generally are dehydrated. Cats may assume a crouched, hunched posture indicating abdominal pain. Obvious abdominal distention is occasionally observed. Although such typical signs of impaction as anorexia, depression, lethargy, nausea, vomiting, and abdominal pain may be present,[22] signs of other internal organ failure may occur. Paradoxic diarrhea and fecal incontinence may be among the most common presenting signs in geriatric animals. In humans, urinary problems (especially in children and elderly individuals), such as frequent urination, retention of urine, and incontinence, may be caused by the mechanical effects of fecal impaction.[23,24] Urinary and fecal problems that occur simultaneously in geriatric animals may imply a shared neurologic basis. Rectal prolapse may also result from severe straining associated with the impaction.

Laboratory abnormalities associated with impaction are nonspecific. Leukocytosis may occur.[25] Electrolyte abnormalities, such as hyponatremia or hypokalemia, may be associated with impaction. Although a stool that contains blood may reflect mucosal irritation from impaction, the presence of blood in stool may also indicate an underlying neoplasm of the colon.[25]

If fecal impaction is suspected but rectal examination and abdominal palpation yield no findings, abdominal radiographs should be taken in an attempt to detect accumulated feces or signs of obstruction.[21] Such signs of obstruction include colonic dilatation and unusual levels of air–fluid in the small intestine.[21] Fecal masses generally are visible in radiographs and typically appear to be bubbly or speckled.

COMPLICATIONS OF FECAL IMPACTION

Fecal incontinence is the most common serious complication of fecal impaction.[21] The continuous seepage of moist bacteria-laden mucus and fecal material fosters the development of perineal irritation and ulceration. Accompanying infections of the urinary tract may also be caused by contamination resulting from direct passage of bacteria from the perineum to the urinary bladder.[26,27] Obstruction of the colon or rectum also commonly occurs with impaction.

THE EFFECTS of pressure and ischemic necrosis on the wall of the colon may cause stercoraceous ulcerations, which generally develop into few if any clinical complications. Stercoraceous ulcers can bleed occultly, but massive bleeding is uncommon.[28-30] On rare occasions, they do perforate. Clinical findings that suggest perforation include a history of fecal impaction coupled with signs of localized or generalized peritonitis and radiographic evidence of free peritoneal air or contrast medium outside the confines of intestinal lumen.

Less common complications attributed to fecal impaction in humans include autonomic dysreflexia,[31] pneumothorax from straining,[26] hepatic encephalopathy,[32] rectal prolapse,[26] hypoxia,[33] and profound shock from massive loss of fluid into the intestinal lumen.[34] Fecal masses, termed *fecalomas*, are not only caused by neoplasia but also mimic it. Evaluations for presumed gastrointestinal or pelvic tumors may be rendered unnecessary by a rectal examination. Fecalomas generally are larger than colonic tumors, lack an annular appearance, and have greater retrograde mobility.[9]

PREVENTION OF FECAL IMPACTION

Because the success of treatment can vary, prevention is advisable. Providing adequate dietary fiber, increasing exercise, treating the underlying disease, instituting regular grooming practices, and avoiding changes in environment and medication often prevent fecal impaction. Most commercial pet foods are relatively low in dietary fiber; on a dry-matter basis, the average commercial dog food contains 2.2% to 3.8% crude fiber and the average commercial cat food 2.0% to 2.7% crude fiber. Replacing commercial dog or cat foods with a diet containing an adequate fiber content is therefore recommended in the management of recurrent fecal impaction. The crude fiber content of some higher fiber commercial foods for adult dogs and cats

TABLE II
Dietary Fiber Content of Pet Foods

Diet	Percent of Crude Fiber (on Dry-Matter Basis)	
	Dry Food	Canned Food
For adult dogs		
Prescription Diet® Canine r/d® (Hill's Pet Products)	21.8	25.2
Prescription Diet® Canine w/d® (Hill's Pet Products)	16.4	13.2
Science Diet® Canine Light® (Hill's Pet Products)	13.9	NA
Fit-N-Trim® (Ralston Purina Co.)	9.0	NA
Alpo Lite® (Alpo Pet Food, Inc.)	7.6	NA
Gaines Cycle Lite® (Quaker Oats Company)	7.0	8.0
Average commercial dog food	3.8	2.2
For adult cats		
Prescription Diet® Feline r/d® (Hill's Pet Products)	18.5	28.3
Prescription Diet® Feline w/d® (Hill's Pet Products)	10.1	12.4
Science Diet® Feline Light® (Hill's Pet Products)	7.1	NA
Average commercial cat food	2.0	2.7

are listed in Table II. Simple measures that can be taken in an attempt to prevent impaction include allowing the gastrocolic reflex sufficient time to operate shortly after eating, ensuring that indoor or outdoor facilities are easily accessible, and making litterboxes available and conducive to defecation.

The regular use of laxatives in animals with severe constipation is sometimes necessary but has associated risks. Bulk-forming laxatives generally are the safest and most effective agents in preventing impaction.[21,22] Adequate hydration and electrolyte balance must be ensured. The goal of laxative treatment is to enable the animal to pass soft, formed feces regularly. Commercial veterinary laxatives containing the active ingredient petrolatum are useful in preventing hair impaction in cats.

TREATMENT OF FECAL IMPACTION

The treatment of fecal impaction consists of gently removing impacted fecal material and, if possible, identifying and eliminating the underlying cause.[21,22] Patients with mild to moderate fecal impaction can generally be treated with oral laxatives and small-volume enemas given frequently. Patients with more severe fecal impaction are usually dehydrated and require fluid replacement therapy for dehydration and electrolyte abnormalities before correction of the impaction is attempted.

MANUAL fragmentation and removal of the fecal mass or masses should be accomplished slowly and as gently as possible. For young or debilitated patients, it is less traumatic if the impaction is softened and removed during a two- to three-day period instead of all at one time.[21,22] In patients older than four months with mild to moderate fecal impaction, fluid replacement therapy is the first goal of treatment. After fluid replacement therapy has been accomplished, oral administration of an isosmotic solution of poorly adsorbable polyethylene glycol-containing electrolyte solution (Colyte®—Reed & Carnrick; GoLytely®—Braintree Laboratories) at a dosage of about 25 ml/kg body weight every 12 hours can be used for completing the removal of residual feces.[35,36]

Laxatives

Laxatives are mild and usually eliminate formed feces; their effects depend on the dose. Therapeutic products and doses for the management of impaction are presented in Table III. Docusate sodium and docusate calcium laxatives act as detergents to alter the surface tension of liquids and also promote emulsification and softening of the feces by facilitating the mixture of water and fat. The patient must be well hydrated before agents containing these agents are administered because they decrease jejunal absorption and promote colonic secretion.[21,22] Laxatives aid in the absorption of mineral oil (liquid petrolatum) and should not be administered in conjunction with the oil.

Mineral oil and white petrolatum laxatives are nondigestible and poorly absorbed. These laxatives prevent colonic absorption of fecal water by coating the feces, thereby softening them and promoting easy evacuation. A small amount of oil absorption does occur, but the primary

TABLE III
Therapeutic Products for Management of Fecal Impaction in Cats

Therapeutic Agent	Dose Regimen	Comments
Bisacodyl	1 tablet (5 mg) daily given orally	Available in 5- and 10-mg tablets and 5-mg suppository; takes 6–12 hr to take effect; animal should be well hydrated and feces softened before its use
Bran (coarse)	1–3 tbsp mixed in 400 g of canned food daily or every 12 hr	Available in powder form; takes 12 to 24 hours to take effect
Bran cereals	3–5 tbsp mixed in food daily	Available as breakfast cereals
Canned pumpkin	1–4 tbsp mixed in food daily	Available as pie filling
Docusate sodium	1 capsule (50 mg) daily given orally	Available in 50- and 100-mg capsules, 1% liquid, 4 mg/ml syrup; takes 12–72 hr to take effect; animal should be well hydrated before its use; do not use with mineral oil
Docusate calcium	1–2 tablets (50 mg) daily given orally	Available in 50- and 240-mg tablets; similar activity and precautions as for docusate sodium
Lactose	Add to diet to effect	Available in household milk
Lactulose	0.25–1 ml daily or every 12 hr orally to start, then adjust dose to stool consistency and 2–3 bowel movements per day	Overdose can cause diarrhea, flatulence, intestinal cramping, dehydration, acidosis
Mineral oil	5–20 ml every 12 hr given orally or rectally	Available in liquid form; use with caution orally (causes lipoid aspiration pneumonia); should be given only between meals; takes 6–12 hr to take effect
Psyllium (natural)	1–3 tsp mixed with food daily or every 12 hr	Available in powder form; takes 12–24 hr to take effect
White petrolatum	1–5 ml daily given orally, then 2–3 days/wk	Available in paste form; should be given only between meals; takes 12–24 hr to take effect

danger of administering mineral oil is laryngotracheal aspiration resulting from the inability of the patient to taste the oil.[21,22] Bulk-forming laxatives, such as psyllium, canned pumpkin, and coarse bran, increase the frequency of evacuation of feces from the proximal colon by means of the stimulation that is produced by the added bulk or volume. These laxatives soften feces by causing water retention. Metamucil® (Searle Consumer Products), a laxative that contains natural psyllium and coarse bran, is best given with moistened food to ensure adequate water intake.

Another useful laxative is bisacodyl, which acts on colonic mucosa and intramural nerve plexus. Stimulation is believed to be segmental and axonal, producing a contraction of the entire colon independent of its resting tone.[21,22] Bisacodyl should only be used in well-hydrated patients older than four months of age and is contraindicated if an obstruction is present.

Lactulose (which is a synthetic disaccharide of galactose and fructose) and lactose (which is available as cows' milk) may be used as laxatives. These agents are metabolized to organic acids by intestinal bacteria and promote an osmotic catharsis of feces after oral administration. The dose is based on individual stool consistency and is titrated until the patient passes two to three semiformed soft stools per day.[37] An overdose of lactulose may induce intestinal cramping, profuse diarrhea, flatulence, dehydration, and acidosis. The taste of lactulose is generally unpalatable to cats, but milk usually is well tolerated.

Enemas

Enemas soften feces in the distal colon, thereby stimulating colonic motility and the urge to defecate. The enema should be at room temperature or tepid when given. Tap water, standard saline solution, and sodium biphosphate solution add bulk; whereas petrolatum oils soften, lubricate, and promote the evacuation of hardened fecal material.[22] Soap, hydrogen peroxide, and hot-water enemas should never be used; they irritate the colonic mucosa and may cause bleeding.[38]

STANDARD saline solution and tap water (about 5 ml/kg of body weight) are the preferred enemas for debilitated patients or those younger than six months of age. Better results are generally obtained if these enemas are repeated several times in small volumes.[22] Small volumes can be retained by the patient for longer periods, thereby softening the feces and fragmenting the impaction. Mineral oil (5 to 20 milliliters) can be instilled directly into the colon and rectum if the feces are extremely hard. Hexachlorophene should not be used because it can cause central nervous system damage.[22] Sodium phosphate retention enemas (Fleet Enema®—C.B. Fleet) are convenient preparations in relieving fecal impaction; however, the use of these enemas is generally contraindicated because they can potentially cause fatal hyperphosphatemia, hypernatremia, hyperosmolality, hypocalcemia, and acidosis.[39,40]

Surgery

If medical management with laxatives and/or enemas fails, surgery may be necessary. The goal of surgery is to remove feces and correct the underlying cause. In cases of severe or recurrent constipation or megacolon that does not respond to conservative medical management, subtotal colectomy is considered a viable option.[41]

SUMMARY

The management of fecal impaction in dogs and cats is often complicated by normal age-related changes in body systems and by spontaneous concurrent disease or traumatic insult. Thorough evaluation of the laboratory findings and of the history and clinical signs of the patient demonstrate complicating factors and permit successful treatment of fecal impaction. Prevention is the preferred approach for resolving fecal impaction. For geriatric dogs and cats, adequate dietary fiber intake and regular exercise assist in preventing fecal impaction.

About the Author

Dr. Hoskins is Professor, Department of Veterinary Clinical Sciences, School of Veterinary Medicine, Louisiana State University, Baton Rouge, Louisiana. He is a Diplomate of the American College of Veterinary Internal Medicine.

REFERENCES

1. Burrows CF: Disorders of gastrointestinal motility: More common than you think. *Proc 6th Annu ACVIM Forum* 6:573–575, 1988.
2. Meunier P, Rochas A, Lambert R: Motor activity of the sigmoid colon in chronic constipation: Comparative study with normal subjects. *Gut* 20:1095–1101, 1979.
3. Tasman-Jones C: Constipation: Pathogenesis and management. *Drugs* 5:220–226, 1973.
4. Read NW, Timms JM: Defecation and the pathophysiology of constipation. *Clin Gastroenterol* 15:937–965, 1986.
5. Karaus M, Sarna SK: Giant migrating contractions during defecation in the dog colon. *Gastroenterology* 92:925–933, 1987.
6. Mullen JP, Cartwright RC, Tisherman SE, et al: Pathogenesis and pharmacologic management of pseudo-obstruction of the bowel in pheochromocytoma. *Am J Med Sci* 290:155–158, 1985.
7. Percy JP, Neill ME, Kandiah TK, et al: A neurogenic factor in faecal incontinence in the elderly. *Age Ageing* 11:175–179, 1982.
8. Weber J, Denis P, Mihout B, et al: Effect of brain-stem lesion on colonic and anorectal motility: Study of three patients. *Dig Dis Sci* 30:419–425, 1985.
9. Wrenn K: Fecal impaction. *N Engl J Med* 321:658–662, 1989.
10. Kruger JM, Osborne CA, Polzin DJ: Treatment of hypercalcemia, in Kirk RW (ed): *Current Veterinary Therapy. IX.* Philadelphia, WB Saunders Co, 1986, pp 75–90.
11. Bell FW, Osborne CA: Treatment of hypokalemia, in Kirk RW (ed): *Current Veterinary Therapy. IX.* Philadelphia, WB Saunders Co, 1986, pp 101–107.
12. Hull C, Greco RS, Brooke DL: Alleviation of constipation in elderly by dietary fiber supplementation. *J Am Geriatri Soc* 28:410–414, 1980.
13. Iseminger M, Hardy P: Bran works! *Geriatric Nurs* Nov/Dec:402–404, 1982.
14. Burrows CF, Kronfeld DS, Banta CA, et al: Effects of fiber on digestibility and transit time in dogs. *J Nutr* 112:1726–1732, 1982.
15. Brenner BE, Simon RR: Anorectal emergencies. *Ann Emerg Med* 12:367–376, 1983.
16. Read NW, Abouzekry L: Why do patients with faecal impaction have faecal incontinence? *Gut* 27:283–287, 1986.
17. Ross LA: Healthy geriatric cats. *Compend Contin Educ Pract Vet* 11(9):1041–1046, 1989.
18. Mosier JE: Effect of aging on body systems of the dog. *Vet Clin North Am [Small Anim Pract]* 19:1–12, 1989.
19. Osborne CA, Abdullahi S, Polzin DJ, et al: Manifestations of feline renal failure. *Proc World Small Anim Cong*:55, 1985.
20. Allen TA: Management of advanced chronic renal failure, in Kirk RW, Bonagura JD (eds): *Current Veterinary Therapy. X.* Philadelphia, WB Saunders Co, 1989, pp 1195–1198.
21. Burrows CF: Medical diseases of the colon, in Jones BD, Liska WD (eds): *Canine and Feline Gastroenterology.* Philadelphia, WB Saunders Co, 1986, pp 221–256.
22. Burrows CF: Constipation, in Kirk RW (ed): *Current Veterinary Therapy. IX.* Philadelphia, WB Saunders Co, 1986, pp 904–908.
23. Kaneti J, Bar-Ziv J: Case profile: Urinary retention due to fecal impaction in a child. *Urology* 23:307, 1984.
24. Brocklehurst JC: Differential diagnosis of urinary incontinence. *Geriatrics* 33(4):36–39, 1978.
25. Gurll N, Steer M: Diagnostic and therapeutic considerations for fecal impaction. *Dis Colon Rectum* 18:507–511, 1975.
26. Young RW: The problem of fecal impaction in the aged. *J Am Geriatr Soc* 21:383, 1973.
27. Breda G, Bianchi GP, Bonomi U, et al: Faecal stasis and bacteriuria: Experimental research in rats. *Urol Res* 2:155–157, 1975.
28. Maull KI, Kinning WK, Kay S: Stercoral ulceration. *Am Surg* 48:20–24, 1982.
29. Gekas P, Schuster MM: Stercoral perforation of the colon: Case report and review of the literature. *Gastroenterology* 80:1054–1058, 1981.
30. Sutton R, Blake JR: Massive rectal bleeding following faecal impaction. *Br J Surg* 71:631, 1984.
31. McGuire TJ, Kumar VN: Autonomic dysreflexia in the spinal cord-injured: What the physician should know about this emergency. *Postgrad Med* 80:81–84, 1986.
32. Lerman BB, Levin ML, Patterson R: Hepatic encephalopathy precipitated by fecal impaction. *Arch Intern Med* 139:707–708, 1979.
33. Wright BA, Staats DO: The geriatric implications of fecal impaction. *Nurs Pract* 11:53–66, 1986.
34. McGuire T, Rothenberg MB, Tyler DC: Profound shock following intervention for chronic untreated stool retention: A case report. *Clin Pediatr [Phila]* 23:459–461, 1984.

(continues on page 45)

Canine Colitis

From the *Perspectives in Veterinary Medicine* Series
Colin F. Burrows, BVetMed, PhD, MRCVS
Diplomate, American College of Veterinary Internal Medicine
Professor of Medicine
Department of Small Animal Clinical Sciences
College of Veterinary Medicine
University of Florida
Gainesville, Florida

The canine colon is a complex and versatile organ that functions in the maintenance of fluid and electrolyte balance, as a site for nutrient absorption, as a temporary store for excreta, and as a reservoir for billions of microorganisms. Electrolyte and water absorption occur primarily in the proximal half and storage in the distal half of the organ. Colitis disrupts these functions in various ways, but the almost inevitable sequela is diarrhea.

Normal Colon

Although colonic fluid and electrolyte transport and patterns of colonic motility are relatively well understood, the complex interrelationships between the colonic mucosa and luminal contents are being increasingly scrutinized. An increasing body of knowledge suggests that short-chain fatty acids (SCFAs) produced by microbial fermentation of carbohydrate are an important energy source for the colonic mucosa and that their removal causes mucosal atrophy and increased susceptibility to damage.[1] In humans, for example, diversion of colonic flow through an ileostomy can result in colitis, which can be resolved by intracolonic infusion of short-chain fatty acids.[2] Also, rectal infusion of solutions that contain propionic and butyric acids has resolved otherwise intractable ulcerative colitis in humans.[3]

In contrast with the major nutritional role played by the colon in herbivores and some omnivores,[1] no evidence suggests that short-chain fatty acids produced by colonic microbial fermentation of luminal contents serve as an energy source for dogs. Limited intraluminal microbial fermentation of nondigestible fiber and carbohydrate to short-chain fatty acids does take place in this species, however, with the extent depending on dietary composition.[4,5] It is probable that, as in other species, short-chain fatty acids influence canine colonic mucosal health.[6]

Inflamed Colon

Colonic inflammation can result from various causes and can be acute or chronic. The cause of acute colitis is usually unknown. The disease is characterized by mucosal infiltration with a varying number of neutrophils and epithelial disruption and ulceration. Chronic colitis, by contrast, may exhibit some neutrophil infiltration but

Series Editor   Johnny D. Hoskins, DVM, PhD, Louisiana State University, Baton Rouge, Louisiana

is more often characterized by the mucosal accumulation of an increased number of plasma cells and lymphocytes.[7] In cases of acute and chronic colitis, absorption of water and electrolytes is markedly reduced and motility is disrupted. The result of these changes is production of small volumes of liquid feces, which are passed much more quickly than normal.[8-11]

Incidence

Although the prevalence of colitis in dogs is not well documented, based on the number of patients with the disorder referred to a teaching institution,[12] the disease apparently is relatively common. Approximately 30% of dogs with chronic diarrhea referred to the University of Florida Veterinary Medical Teaching Hospital have colitis. In some patients, the small and large intestines are involved in the inflammatory process, with signs of involvement of one of the two organs predominating.

Mechanisms of Disease

Regardless of the many inciting causes, the development of chronic colonic inflammation is apparently caused by a defect in mucosal immunoregulation.[13] In human inflammatory bowel disease, the data in support of a disruption of normal mucosal immunoregulation are impressive; as far as I know, there are no equivalent data that apply to dogs.

Studies in humans have implicated several products of activated immunocytes in the pathogenesis of inflammatory bowel disease, including cytokines, eicosanoids, oxygen radicals, immunoglobulins, and proteases.[14,15] It is now apparent that cytokines (protein products of activated immune cells that influence the activity, differentiation, and rate of proliferation of other cells) are key mediators in inflammatory bowel disease.[16,17]

After initial mucosal damage, submucosal lymphocytes and macrophages are exposed to various luminal antigens of dietary and bacterial origin. The antigens are taken up by macrophages, processed, and reexpressed on the cell surface; there is simultaneous secretion of a number of cytokines, including interleukin-1, which is critical in stimulating T lymphocytes. A series of multiple, complex events amplifies the number of T and B lymphocytes with concomitant accumulation of neutrophils and macrophages armed with various destructive enzymes and inflammatory mediators.

Net activation or suppression of inflammation is determined by an intricate balance of pro- and antiinflammatory forces, the nature of which is incompletely understood. The accumulation of inflammatory cytokines, however, probably initiates most of the clinical signs of colitis. Most drugs currently used to treat colitis decrease cytokine production and influence eicosanoid production and oxygen radical scavenging.[12,16]

Colonic inflammation disrupts the tight junctions between colonic epithelial cells. This reduces the transmucosal electrical potential difference and impairs the ability of the colon to absorb sodium against a strong electrochemical gradient.[18] Some of the cytokines also may stimulate colonic secretion; with the loss of mucosal integrity, protein-rich tissue fluid as well as erythrocytes and neutrophils leak into the lumen.[7,19,20] Tissue architecture is disrupted, and mucosal goblet cells are stimulated to secrete large quantities of mucus.

Colitis also disrupts motility. Experimental colitis in dogs inhibits normal segmental contractions and stimulates giant migrating contractions that sweep down the length of the organ to eliminate luminal contents rapidly and eradicate any storage function effectively.[21] Colitis also abolishes the motor response to a meal in dogs. New ingesta entering the colon stimulate an excessive number of giant migrating contractions that are probably related to postprandial discomfort and increased frequency of defecation.[22] The inflamed tissue becomes more sensitive to stretch. Stretch receptors sensitized to cytokines and distended by normal or even reduced volumes of luminal fluid stimulate peristaltic activity. The inflamed rectum also is more susceptible to stretch, and there is subsequent augmentation of the urge to defecate.[9]

Classification of Colitis

Colitis can be acute or chronic. Most patients present for evaluation of chronic disease. Colitis can be classified on a causative or a histologic basis (see Classification of Colitis). A tendency for the two to overlap has produced confusion and disagreement in the literature. Many patients with chronic colitis, for example, are said to have inflammatory bowel disease. In human medicine, *inflammatory bowel disease* refers specifically to ulcerative colitis or granulomatous ileitis and colitis (Crohn's disease), two enigmatic disorders that apparently result from a disruption in mucosal immunoregulation. The term has perhaps unfortunately been adopted and expanded in veterinary medicine to encompass any chronic disease of the small or large intestine that is characterized by mucosal inflammatory cell infiltration.

Although eosinophilic, plasmacytic–lymphocytic, histiocytic, and granulomatous colitis are the four best known types of canine inflammatory bowel disease, other systems of classification have been proposed.[23,24] These histologic classifications do not improve understanding of the disorder. They must suffice, however, until more is known about their relationships with the various mucosal immune disruptions,

Classification of Colitis

Causative	Histologic
Infectious	Plasmacytic and lymphocytic
Parasitic	Eosinophilic
Trichuris vulpis	Histiocytic
Ancylostoma caninum	Granulomatous
Entamoeba histolytica	
Balantidium coli	
Possibly *Giardia*	
Bacterial	
Salmonella species	
Clostridium species	
Campylobacter species	
Algal	
Prototheca	
Fungal	
Histoplasma capsulatum	
Phycomycosis	
Traumatic	
Uremic	
Segmental (secondary to	
chronic pancreatitis)	
Idiopathic acute	
Allergic	
Dietary protein	
Possibly bacterial protein	

Differential Diagnosis of Canine Colitis

- Tumors
  — Lymphosarcoma
  — Adenocarcinoma
  — Leiomyosarcoma
  — Colonic polyp
- Ileocolic intussusception
- Cecal inversion
- Irritable colon syndrome

sensitivities to luminal antigens, and genetic predisposition of certain breeds (e.g., boxers) to colitis.

Clinical Signs

Signs of colitis are classically those of large bowel diarrhea: increased frequency of defecation with a small volume of liquid feces passed with a sense of urgency, increased fecal mucus, and (in many patients) hematochezia and prolonged tenesmus after defecation.[25,26] Vomiting, which is reported in approximately 30% of dogs with colitis,[12] results from vagal stimulation of the emetic center from the inflamed and stretch-sensitive colonic wall.

Results of physical examination are usually normal but depend to some extent on the duration and severity of colonic disease. Loss of body weight and condition is uncommon, except in the rare cases of colonic fungal or algal infection and in histiocytic ulcerative colitis of boxers and related breeds.

The differential diagnosis includes other types of colonic disease (see Differential Diagnosis of Canine Colitis). Colonic tumors, cecal inversion, and the putative stress-induced irritable colon predominate.

Approach to Patients

A logical approach to patients with signs of large intestinal diarrhea and tenesmus must begin with the elimination of infectious agents by appropriate fecal flotation, smear, and culture techniques. If the results of these tests are negative, symptomatic dietary or antiinflammatory therapy may be attempted. Thorough endoscopic evaluation of the colon to obtain appropriate colonic mucosal biopsy specimens is preferable to symptomatic therapy. Flexible fiber-optic endoscopy allows examination of the entire organ; however, colonic preparation for flexible endoscopy is time-consuming. Because most colonic disease is diffuse, the colon can be readily examined and a representative biopsy taken via a rigid colonoscope; the investment of time, money, and effort is much lower.[26]

Results of mucosal biopsy indicate the type and severity of colitis. This allows the clinician to give an accurate prognosis and prescribe appropriate treatment. A biopsy report of normal or hyperplastic colonic mucosa in a patient with signs of large intestinal disease suggests irritable colon, which is still a diagnosis of exclusion. Before diagnosing irritable colon and committing to long-term symptomatic therapy, the clinician should be certain that all drug and dietary sensitivities have been excluded. Repeat biopsies also are indicated because there is not always a good correlation between clinical signs, the appearance of the mucosa at endoscopy, and the pathologist's interpretation of the biopsy specimen.[27]

Treatment

Treatment of colitis depends on the specific diagnosis but usually includes a combination of symptomatic, dietary, and antiinflammatory therapies.

Symptomatic Therapy

Symptomatic treatment includes the use of drugs that decrease fecal water and stimulate colonic motility. The most appropriate of these is oral loperamide (0.1 to 0.2 mg/kg every 6 to 12 hours as needed).[28] Unlike other narcotic motility modifiers, loperamide stimulates colonic segmental activity and thereby slows colonic transit. It also increases anal sphincter tone and rectal function, decreases colonic secretion, and possibly enhances salt and water absorption.[29-31]

Some clinicians recommend the use of antibiotics (e.g., metronidazole or tylosin) in the treatment of colitis; the routine use of these agents remains controversial. Metronidazole, for example, has no effect on the progress of human inflammatory bowel disease.[31] The antibiotic does, however, decrease fecal anaerobe concentration while having no effect on the metabolism of sulfasalazine.[32,33]

Because some cases of large bowel diarrhea in dogs may be associated with clostridial infection or overgrowth,[34,35] metronidazole may be warranted at least on a trial basis in some patients. Whether the drug should be prescribed before or in conjunction with antiinflammatory drugs is a matter of clinical judgment. Ideally, metronidazole is used only if an anaerobic fecal culture in a patient with large bowel diarrhea has demonstrated a high concentration of clostridia or if a test for fecal clostridial toxin is positive.

Tylosin has been recommended for the treatment of inflammatory bowel disease in dogs,[36] but the evidence of beneficial effects in colitis is unconvincing. Any positive effect is probably related to the effect of the drug on small intestinal bacterial overgrowth.

Dietary Therapy

Dietary therapy of colitis is emerging as one of the most important approaches to treatment. It can conveniently be divided into three categories: fasting, feeding a nonallergenic diet, and fiber supplementation.

Fasting

Placing the bowel in a state of physiologic rest by withholding food for 24 to 48 hours has long been advocated as part of the symptomatic therapy for acute diarrheal disease. Withholding food is apparently beneficial in diarrhea caused by acute diseases of the small intestine and should also help (at least on a theoretical and symptomatic basis) in acute colitis. I routinely fast patients with acute colitis for 24 to 48 hours until diarrhea resolves. In a controlled study in human patients, however, fasting did not affect the outcome in severe ulcerative colitis.[37]

Fasting for longer than is required for bowel preparation for colonoscopy is contraindicated in chronic disease, particularly in light of the need of patients for protein for tissue repair. In severe inflammatory bowel disease in humans, enteral feeding with refined formula diets alone or in combination with parenteral nutrition has been clearly beneficial.[38] The role of enteral and parenteral nutritional therapy is probably limited in canine colitis because of the cost and the fact that dogs with the disease (with the exception of boxers with histiocytic ulcerative colitis) apparently do not have the same degree of protein loss and catabolism as humans do.

Feeding a Nonallergenic Diet

The role of food allergy as a primary cause or at least a perpetuating factor in canine colitis is increasingly apparent. Feeding a patient a protein to which it has not been exposed thus may be a critical aspect of treatment in most dogs with colitis.

There is now distinct evidence that at least some cases of plasmacytic–lymphocytic colitis in dogs may be caused by sensitivity to dietary protein—signs improve if the diet is changed to contain a protein to which the patient has not been previously exposed.[39] Dogs with chronic idiopathic colitis were fasted for two days to allow bowel preparation for colonoscopy and biopsy and were then fed a diet of cottage cheese and rice; there was complete resolution of signs within two weeks. Challenge with the original diet resulted in recurrence of diarrhea in 80% of patients, strongly suggesting that some type of dietary sensitivity played an important role in the genesis of the disease.[39] This experience and that of others[40,41] have changed the general management of chronic colitis to include not only the use of antiinflammatory drugs but also a diet that contains, if possible, a protein to which the dog has not been exposed.

Home-prepared diets that contain cottage cheese and rice or lamb and rice are acceptable. Various commercial diets that contain rice with chicken, mutton or lamb, venison, and rabbit are now available and apparently help to reduce signs of the disease. Signs of large bowel diarrhea do not always resolve immediately with dietary therapy alone. Many clinicians, myself included, find that client satisfaction is enhanced if antiinflammatory therapy with sulfasalazine is initiated concurrently.

Fiber Supplementation

Supplementation of the diet with fiber in the form of bran or cellulose has been recommended as symptomatic therapy for large bowel diarrhea.[26] Poorly fermented fiber (e.g., α cellulose) increases fecal bulk, stretches colonic smooth muscle, and improves the muscle's contractility.[42] Such fiber also binds fecal water to produce formed feces and thus improves client satisfaction.[43] Supplementation with fiber alone is seldom sufficient to produce resolution of signs but is useful as adjunctive therapy. This approach may change as knowledge of colonic function improves.

There are many types of dietary fiber. All are fermented to various degrees by the colonic microbial flora and probably have different effects on colonic function. For example, future dietary treatment of colitis may include fermentable fibers from which colonic bacteria produce short-chain fatty acids to improve colonic mucosal nutrition and resolve signs of disease.

Immunosuppressive Therapy

Despite the knowledge of symptomatic and nutritional therapy for colitis, the basis of treatment still involves the judicious use of drugs that modulate mucosal immune function. The most important and widely used of these agents are sulfasalazine, prednisone (or prednisolone), and azathioprine. Such drugs as methotrexate, cyclosporin, and some new drugs that specifically influence individual cytokine function are now being used in the treatment of human inflammatory bowel disease.[44] It is possible that these drugs may be useful in the treatment of canine colitis.[45]

Sulfasalazine

Sulfasalazine (25 to 40 mg/kg every eight hours for three to four weeks) is the preferred drug for treating chronic plasmacytic–lymphocytic colitis, the most common type of idiopathic colitis. The mechanism of action of the drug, a combination of sulfapyridine and 5-aminosalicylate joined by an azo bond, remains controversial. The combination of the two drugs is merely a delivery mechanism, the result of a serendipitous discovery by Swedish pharmacologists in the 1940s during an experiment to find a drug for treating rheumatoid arthritis.[46]

The azo bond prevents absorption of the drug in the small intestine; the agent thus can be delivered unchanged to the colon, where colonic bacteria split it to release sulfapyridine and the active ingredient 5-aminosalicylate.[47] The exact mechanism or mechanisms of action of 5-aminosalicylate are unclear, but current evidence suggests that it has various beneficial effects. It has been demonstrated, for example, to decrease interleukin-1 production, inhibit 5-lipoxygenase, reduce platelet-activating factor, act as a free radical scavenger, and inhibit mucosal mast cell histamine release and prostaglandin production.[48-52]

Most patients respond to sulfasalazine alone or in combination with dietary change within one to four weeks of the onset of treatment. The diagnosis must be reexamined if signs fail to improve after four weeks of treatment or if they recur when the drug is withdrawn. Long-term therapy is contraindicated because sulfasalazine causes keratoconjunctivitis sicca (KCS) induced by sensitivity to sulfapyridine.[53]

A new drug, a combination of two molecules of 5-aminosalicylate (olsalazine), has recently been introduced in human medicine in an attempt to relieve some of the side effects associated with sulfasalazine therapy. Veterinary experience with the drug is limited, but dogs can apparently develop keratoconjunctivitis sicca in response to sensitivity to 5-aminosalicylate alone.[54]

Prednisone and Azathioprine

Prednisone has been widely used to treat plasmacytic–lymphocytic enteritis in dogs and cats but is apparently not as effective as sulfasalazine in the treatment of plasmacytic–lymphocytic colitis. The indication for corticosteroids in the treatment of canine colitis has not been clarified and remains empirical. Some dogs with colitis reportedly deteriorate when treated with corticosteroids; other patients apparently benefit.[12] Because chronic colitis is an inflammatory disease of unknown cause, corticosteroid use in conjunction with sulfasalazine is occasionally beneficial in patients that are unresponsive to more conventional treatment.

Eosinophilic colitis seldom responds to dietary change alone. Immunosuppressive doses of prednisone (or prednisolone, 2 to 4 mg/kg once daily for two weeks and then tapered for 6 to 10 weeks) are the preferred treatment for this disease. If mucosal changes are severe, prednisone can be combined with azathioprine (1.0 mg/kg once daily for two weeks). Occasional 7- to 14-day courses of azathioprine alone can be used to control signs in patients with plasmacytic–lymphocytic or eosinophilic colitis that are apparently resistant to other forms of treatment.

Conclusion

With appropriate therapy, the prognosis for most patients with colitis is good. The prognosis should become even better in the future, based on a better understanding of mucosal immune regulation, colonic metabolism, and the effect on colonic mucosal health by short-chain fatty acids produced by microbial fermentation of nondigestible carbohydrate. Nevertheless, there is still a long way to go in understanding this complex and enigmatic group of diseases.

REFERENCES

1. Bergman EN: Energy contribution of volatile fatty acids from the gastrointestinal tract in various species. *Phys Rev* 70:567–590, 1990.

2. Harig JM, Soergel KH, Komorowski RA, Wood GM: Treatment of diversion colitis with short chain fatty acid irrigation. *N Engl J Med* 320:23–28, 1989.

3. Breuer RI, Buto SK, Christ ML, et al: Rectal irrigation with short chain fatty acids for distal ulcerative colitis. *Dig Dis Sci* 36:185–187, 1991.

4. Banta CA, Clemens EJ, Krinsky MM, Sheffey BE: Sites of organic acid production and patterns of digesta movement in the gastrointestinal tract of dogs. *J Nutr* 109:1592–1600, 1979.

5. Meyer H, Schunemann C, Elbers H, Junker S: Precaecal and postileal protein digestion and intestinal urea conversion in dogs. *Proc Int Hanover Symp*:27–30, 1987.

6. Clemens ET, Dobesh GD: Nutritional impact of the canine colonic microstructure and function. *Nutr Res* 8:625–633, 1988.

7. Roth L, Walton AM, Leib MS, Burrows CF: A grading system for lymphocytic plasmacytic colitis in dogs. *J Vet Diagn Invest* 2:257–262, 1990.

8. Hawker PC, McKay JS, Turnberg LA: Electrolyte transport across colonic mucosa from patients with inflammatory bowel disease. *Gastroenterology* 79:508–511, 1990.

9. Rao SSG, Read NW: Gastrointestinal motility in patients with ulcerative colitis. *Scand J Gastroenterol* 25(Suppl 172):22–28, 1990.

10. Sarna SK: Physiology and pathophysiology of colonic motor activity. Part I. *Dig Dis Sci* 36:827–862, 1991.

11. Sarna SK: Physiology and pathophysiology of colonic motor activity. Part II. *Dig Dis Sci* 36:998–1018, 1991.

12. Ewing GO, Gomez JA: Canine ulcerative colitis. *JAAHA* 9:395–406, 1973.

13. Zeitz M: Immunoregulatory abnormalities in inflammatory bowel disease. *Eur J Gastroenterol Hepatol* 2:246–249, 1990.

14. MacDermott PR, Stenson WF: Alterations in the immune system in ulcerative colitis and Crohn's disease. *Adv Immunol* 42:285–328, 1988.

15. Elson CO: The immunology of inflammatory bowel disease, in Kirsner JB, Shorter RG (eds): *Inflammatory Bowel Disease*. Philadelphia, Lea & Febiger, 1988, pp 97–164.

16. Sartor RB: Cytokines in inflammatory bowel disease. *Prog Inflam Bowel Dis* 12:5–8, 1991.

17. Fiocchi C: Lymphokines and the intestinal immune response. Role in inflammatory bowel disease. *Immunol Invest* 18:91–102, 1989.

18. Edmunds CJ, Pilcher D: Electrical potential difference and sodium and potassium fluxes across rectal mucosa in ulcerative colitis. *Gut* 14:784–789, 1973.

19. Madara JL: y-IFN enhances intestinal epithelial permeability by altering tight junctions. *Gastroenterology* 94:A276, 1988.

20. Chang EW, Wang NS, Mayer LF: Lymphokines stimulate intestinal secretion. Possible role as inhibitor of arachidonic acid (AA) metabolism in IBD. *Gastroenterology* 94:A276, 1988.

21. Sethi AK, Sarna SK: Colonic motor activity in acute colitis in conscious dogs. *Gastroenterology* 100:954–963, 1991.

22. Sethi AK, Sarna SK: Colonic motor response to a meal in acute colitis. *Gastroenterology* 101:1537–1546, 1991.

23. Van der Gaag I: The histological appearance of large intestinal biopsies in dogs with clinical signs of large bowel disease. *Can J Vet Res* 52:75–82, 1988.

24. Van Kruiningen HJ: Canine colitis comparable to regional enteritis and mucosal colitis of man. *Gastroenterology* 62:1128–1142, 1972.

25. Sherding RG: Canine large bowel diarrhea. *Compend Contin Educ Pract Vet* 2(4):279–288, 1980.

26. Burrows CF: Medical diseases of the colon, in Jones B, Liska WD (eds): *Canine and Feline Gastroenterology*. Philadelphia, WB Saunders Co, 1986, pp 221–256.

27. Roth L, Leib MS, Davenport D, Monroe WE: Comparisons between endoscopic and histologic evaluation of the gastrointestinal tract in dogs and cats. *JAVMA* 196:635–638, 1990.

28. Johnson S: Loperamide: A novel antidiarrheal drug. *Compend Contin Educ Pract Vet* 11(11):1373–1375, 1989.

29. Schiller LR, Santa Ana C, Morawski SG, Fordtran JS: Mechanism of the antidiarrheal effect of loperamide. *Gastroenterology* 86:1475–1480, 1984.

30. Fioramonti J, Fargeas MJ, Bueno L: Stimulation of gastrointestinal motility by loperamide in dogs. *Dig Dis Sci* 32:641–646, 1987.

31. Read M, Read NW, Barber CD, et al: Effects of loperamide on anal sphincter function in patients complaining of chronic diarrhea with fecal incontinence and urgency. *Dig Dis Sci* 27:807–814, 1982.

32. Krook A, Danielson D, Kjellander J, Jarnerot G: The effect of metronidazole and sulfasalazine on the fecal flora in patients with Crohn's disease. *Scand J Gastroenterol* 16:183–192, 1981.

33. Shaffer JL, Kershaw A, Houston JB: Disposition of metronidazole and its effect on sulphasalazine metabolism in patients with inflammatory bowel disease. *Br J Clin Pharmacol* 21:431–435, 1986.

34. Carman RJ, Lewis JCM: Recurrent diarrhoea in a dog associated with *Clostridium perfringens* type A. *Vet Rec* 112:342–343, 1983.

35. Berry AP, Levitt PN: Chronic diarrhoea in dogs associated with *Clostridium difficile* infection. *Vet Rec* 118:102–103, 1986.

36. Van Kruiningen HJ: Clinical efficacy of tylosin in canine inflammatory bowel disease. *JAAHA* 12:498–501, 1975.

37. McIntyre PB, Powell-Tuck J, Wood SR, et al: Controlled trial of bowel rest in the treatment of severe acute colitis. *Gut* 27:481–485, 1986.

38. Teahon K, Bjarnason I, Levi AJ: The role of enteral and parenteral nutrition in Crohn's disease and ulcerative colitis. *Prog Inflam Bowel Dis* 12:1–4, 1991.

39. Nelson RW, Stookey LJ, Kazacos E: Nutritional management of idiopathic chronic colitis in the dog. *J Vet Intern Med* 2:133–137, 1988.

40. Leib MS: Dietary management of chronic large bowel diarrhea in dogs. *Proc Eastern States Vet Conf* 5:147–148, 1991.

41. Ridgeway M: Management of chronic colitis in the dog. *JAVMA* 185:804–806, 1984.

42. Burrows CF, Merritt AM: Influence of α cellulose on myoelectric activity of proximal canine colon. *Am J Physiol* 245:G301–G306, 1983.

43. Burrows CF, Kronfeld DS, Banta CA, Merritt AM: Effect of fiber on digestibility and transit time in dogs. *J Nutr* 112:1726–1732, 1982.

44. Fretland DJ, Widomski D, Bie-Shung T, et al: Effect of a leukotriene B4 receptor antagonist SC-4190 on colonic inflammation in rat, guinea pig and rabbit. *J Pharmacol Exp Ther* 255:572–576, 1990.

45. Harig JM, Soergel KH: Short chain fatty acids in inflammatory bowel disease. *Drug Anal Pharmacol Ther* 6, 1990.

46. Hoult JRS: Pharmacological and biochemical actions of sulfasalazine. *Drugs* 32(Suppl 7):18–26, 1986.

47. Goldman P, Peppercorn MA: Sulfasalazine. *N Engl J Med* 293:20–25, 1975.

48. Neilson OH, Bukhane K, Elmgreen J, Ahnfelt-Rhone I: Inhibition of 5-lipoxygenase pathway of arachidonic acid metabolism in human neutrophils by sulfasalazine and 5-aminosalicylic acid. *Dig Dis Sci* 32:577–582, 1987.

49. Eliakim R, Karmeli F, Razin E, Rachmitewitz D: Role of platelet activating factor in ulcerative colitis: Inhibition by sulphasalazine and prednisolone. *Gastroenterology* 95:1167–1173, 1988.

50. Cominelli F, Zipser RD, Dinarello CA: Sulphasalazine inhibits cytokine production in human mononuclear cells: A novel anti-inflammatory mechanism. *Gastroenterology* 96:A96, 1989.

51. Gionchetti P, Guarneri C, Campieri M, et al: Scavenger effect of sulfasalazine, 5-aminosalicylic acid, and olsalazine on superoxide radical generation. *Dig Dis Sci* 36:174–178, 1991.

52. Fox C, Moore W, Lichtenstein L: Modulating of mediator release from human intestinal mast cells by sulfasalazine and 5-aminosalicylic acid. *Dig Dis Sci* 36:179–184, 1991.

53. Sansom J, Barnett K, Long R: Keratoconjunctivitis sicca in the dog associated with the administration of salicylazosulfapyridine (sulphasalazine). *Vet Rec* 116:391–393, 1985.

54. Barnett KC: Keratoconjunctivitis sicca and the treatment of canine colitis. *Vet Rec* 117:263, 1986.

KEY FACTS

- Lymphocytic plasmacytic enteritis is a common cause of chronic intermittent vomiting and/or diarrhea in dogs and is the most common cause of the canine protein-losing enteropathy syndrome.
- Treatment involves use of single or combination immunosuppressive drug therapy and is determined by degree of clinical signs and extent of intestinal involvement.
- Lymphocytic plasmacytic enteritis in dogs may occasionally be associated with bacterial or parasitic diseases, but in the majority of cases the cause is undetermined.

Chronic Canine Lymphocytic Plasmacytic Enteritis

Todd R. Tams, DVM
Diplomate, ACVIM
Medical Director
West Los Angeles Veterinary
 Medical Group
Los Angeles, California

The term *inflammatory bowel disease* describes a group of chronic intestinal disorders characterized by a diffuse infiltration of the mucosa by various populations of inflammatory cells including lymphocytes, plasma cells, eosinophils, and neutrophils. The submucosa, muscularis, and serosa frequently are not significantly involved. Mucosal involvement can vary considerably in both severity and extent, which helps to explain the variability of the clinical manifestations of these disorders.

A variety of primary disorders can result in infiltrates of inflammatory cells in the small intestine. These include *Giardia* and *Campylobacter* infections, bacterial overgrowth, histoplasmosis, food allergy, lymphosarcoma, and others. The term *inflammatory bowel disease* is used here to describe a chronic disorder in which no definitive causative agent can be determined. By far the most common type of idiopathic inflammatory bowel disease recognized in dogs is lymphocytic plasmacytic enteritis. In my experience, the histologic diagnosis of eosinophilic enteritis is made much less commonly.

The term *malabsorption syndrome* refers to a chronic enteropathy condition that causes a generalized failure of digestion and absorption (most consistently involving fat) resulting in chronic diarrhea and weight loss. *Protein-losing enteropathy* refers to a group of chronic enteropathies, usually of a moderate to severe nature, that are characterized by an *excessive* loss of plasma proteins across the intestinal wall into the gut lumen and feces.[1] Protein-losing enteropathy and intestinal malabsorption often occur in conjunction in dogs. Moderate to severe lymphocytic plasmacytic enteritis is the most common cause of the protein-losing enteropathy syndrome in dogs. The most important physical and clinicopathologic abnormalities and recommended management of lymphocytic plasmacytic enteritis are emphasized in this article.

Clinical Course

In dogs with lymphocytic plasmacytic enteritis three general types of clinical presentations have been identified: (1) clinical course characterized primarily by vomiting, (2) clinical course characterized primarily by diarrhea, and (3) clinical course that includes both vomiting and diarrhea as the primary signs. Associated clinical signs of lymphocytic plasmacytic enteritis, as well as other categories of chronic inflammatory bowel disease, include borborygmus; halitosis; polydipsia/polyuria; changes in attitude and activity level (e.g., listlessness) that are often cyclic and seem to occur in conjunction with "flare-ups" of the primary clinical signs; intermittent or persistent inappetence; and weight loss (especially when clinical signs of vomiting or diarrhea are long-standing). Idiopathic inflammatory bowel diseases such as lymphocytic plasmacytic enteritis run a course that initially is characterized by exacerbations and spontaneous remissions, often without regard to symptomatic therapy prescribed. Abdominal cramps or pain can occur and sometimes cause the animal to assume an arched-back stance or "praying" position. The associated clinical signs, especially periodic inappetence and listlessness, occasionally are much more prominent than the primary gastrointestinal signs of vomiting and diarrhea.

When vomiting occurs in patients with lymphocytic plasmacytic enteritis, the vomitus usually consists of bile and often there is no specific time relation to eating. The vomitus occasionally includes partially digested food. When this occurs, a gastric motility disorder should be considered as a leading differential diagnosis, especially if food is vomited more than six to eight hours after a meal. Early in the course of the disease, vomiting is most often noted as an intermittent clinical sign; there is usually an increased frequency as the disorder becomes more severe. Vomiting may be reported as a problem of recent onset or can be an intermittent problem over a period of months to several years before it becomes frequent and severe enough to cause inappetence and weight loss. It is this increased frequency of vomiting that often causes client concern and leads to presentation of the patient to a veterinarian.

It is extremely important that the clinician recognize that vomiting may be the only major sign that occurs in a patient with inflammatory bowel disease. Diarrhea may occur only rarely or not at all. Gastric biopsies often are normal in these cases. Too often dogs with chronic vomiting are diagnosed and treated empirically for a gastric or pancreatic disorder when in fact the disease is in the intestine.

Chronic intermittent or chronic intractable diarrhea is the major clinical sign in some dogs with lymphocytic plasmacytic enteritis. Diarrhea is defined as an increase in the frequency, fluidity, or volume of feces. Fecal characteristics (frequency, volume, consistency, color, odor, and composition) in these patients may be consistent with either small intestinal or both small and large intestinal involvement. In some cases diarrhea does not occur until the disease is advanced. Diarrhea may range from a soft, formed consistency to intermittently watery and profuse in nature. When a moderate to severe degree of lymphocytic plasmacytic enteritis is present, intractable diarrhea, inappetence, and weight loss eventually develop. These patients often develop hypoproteinemia as well. The clinician should strongly consider lymphocytic plasmacytic enteritis as a leading differential diagnosis in cases in which adequate dietary trials, parasite elimination programs, and treatment for bacterial overgrowth have failed to resolve diarrhea.

A third category of lymphocytic plasmacytic enteritis patients exhibits *both* vomiting and diarrhea as the primary clinical signs. In these patients, appetite changes and weight loss seem to occur earlier than in patients that have only vomiting or diarrhea alone.

Incidence

Lymphocytic plasmacytic enteritis usually develops in middle-aged and older dogs; it is occasionally identified in dogs less than two years of age. No breed predilection for canine lymphocytic plasmacytic enteritis has been identified other than the immunoproliferative enteropathy syndrome in the basenji; in these cases, infiltration of the lamina propria with lymphocytes, plasma cells, and occasional neutrophils represents the most consistent histologic lesion.[2]

Physical Examination

Physical examination findings in dogs with lymphocytic plasmacytic enteritis range from unremarkable in mild cases to such significant changes as variable degrees of thickened bowel, which is often sensitive on palpation. Weight loss and dullness of the haircoat may be noted in moderate to severe cases. Hepatomegaly, splenomegaly, and lymphadenopathy suggest lymphosarcoma or histoplasmosis and are rarely associated with lymphocytic plasmacytic enteritis. Rectal examination may reveal pain or mucosal irregularity in dogs that have involvement of both the large and small intestine. Ascites, peripheral edema, and/or dyspnea resulting from hydrothorax are identified in some dogs with lymphocytic plasmacytic enteritis that have marked hypoproteinemia. Some of these dogs remain active, alert, and well fleshed, however, and these findings do not rule out a significant intestinal disorder.

Laboratory Findings

Baseline laboratory tests are often normal in mild to moderate lymphocytic plasmacytic enteritis. Abnormal findings in more involved cases can include an inflammatory leukogram (as high as 25,000 to 40,000 leukocytes/mm), eosinophilia (suggests the possibility of eosinophilic enteritis or the presence of a mixed population of lymphocytes, plasma cells, and eosinophils), anemia of chronic disease (uncommon), hypocholesterolemia, and hypoproteinemia (when identified usually indicates a moderate to severe degree of inflammatory bowel disease). The total protein level in severe cases of lymphocytic plasmacytic enteritis may drop to less than 2.5 g/dl; more commonly, the range is 3.0 to 5.0 g/dl.

A total protein level less than 6.0 g/dl is considered to be potentially significant and warrants further investigation. The initial step is to exclude the nonintestinal causes of hypoproteinemia—which include chronic liver disease with impaired synthesis of albumin and protein-losing glomerulonephropathies—through liver function testing and urine protein determinations.[1,3,4] Hypoproteinemia also can occur in dogs with congestive heart failure.[1,4] Excessive protein loss from the intestine is usually characterized by a proportional decrease of both albumin and globulin fractions, whereas in liver or renal disease it is usually only albumin that is decreased. Dogs with severe lymphocytic plasmacytic enteritis may be markedly hypoproteinemic; hypocalcemia is often identified in conjunction as a result, in part, of decreased protein-bound fractions of calcium associated with hypoalbuminemia. Total protein and albumin levels should be determined for any patient with chronic diarrhea to check for abnormalities that provide an indication of the degree of intestinal involvement. A workup should be expedited in any hypoproteinemic patient. It should be noted that a significant intestinal parasite burden, including *Giardia*, and bacterial overgrowth can cause mild hypoproteinemia (5.0 g/dl to 6.0 g/dl). These disorders should be ruled out before embarking on a more expensive, in-depth diagnostic workup.

Other tests that can be useful in the differential diagnosis of intestinal dysfunction disorders include the D-xylose absorption test and B_{12} and folate assays. A trypsin-like immunoreactivity assay is used to rule out exocrine pancreatic insufficiency in dogs with chronic diarrhea.[5,6] (The reader is referred to the article in the proceedings of this symposium in this issue by Dr. David A. Williams entitled "New Tests of Pancreatic and Small Intestinal Function" for a detailed discussion of the trypsin-like immunoreactivity, B_{12}, and folate assays.)

Survey abdominal radiographs in dogs with lymphocytic plasmacytic enteritis usually are unremarkable. Contrast examination of the stomach and small bowel (barium series) allows evaluation of the size, shape, mucosal pattern, and position of the stomach and the intestines and permits assessment of the progression of material through the gastrointestinal tract. Abnormal findings in inflammatory bowel disease include diffuse mucosal irregularities or spicular small intestinal mucosal changes and thickened bowel segments, which are evidenced by narrow dye columns.[7] Barium studies frequently demonstrate no abnormalities in dogs with chronic diarrhea, but this does not rule out infiltrative bowel disorders. In addition, positive findings do *not* afford a definitive diagnosis; rather, they confirm the need for direct examination and biopsy of the affected areas. Radiographs also can suggest false-positive findings.

Definitive Diagnosis

A presumptive diagnosis of canine idiopathic inflammatory bowel disease is made on the basis of history, physical examination, and elimination of other disorders by laboratory tests and radiographic studies. A definitive diagnosis can be made only by intestinal biopsy, the single most important diagnostic procedure in the evaluation of chronic intestinal disease. Biopsy should be done to confirm diagnosis and determine type and extent of involvement and is especially useful in determining treatment and prognosis. It is strongly suggested that biopsies be obtained from appropriate areas in gastrointestinal cases *before* clinical signs become protracted and such problems as weight loss and anorexia are allowed to develop to a significant degree. In

most cases the prognosis for satisfactory control of intestinal disorders is somewhat better the earlier a diagnosis is made.

Biopsies can be obtained under fiberoptic endoscopic control or by exploratory laparotomy. Endoscopy offers a minimally invasive means of examining the stomach and proximal small intestine. Multiple mucosal biopsies can be obtained easily; and client compliance is often greater for endoscopy, which is less invasive and less expensive, than for exploratory laparotomy. The difficulty of determining a cause in chronic canine vomiting and diarrheal disorders is lessened significantly by the availability of endoscopic equipment or referral services because biopsies can be obtained more routinely *early* in the course of a disorder. An additional major advantage of endoscopy is that it offers an alternative approach to obtaining intestinal biopsies in protein-losing enteropathy cases in which there is concern that full-thickness biopsy sites may heal slowly.

Grossly, the duodenal lumen might appear completely normal (Figure 1) in inflammatory bowel disease or there may be varying degrees of erythema or mucosal irregularity (Figures 2, 3, and 4). Multiple biopsies (four to eight) should always be obtained during endoscopy because of the small sample size that routinely is obtained. Biopsies of the small intestine and the stomach always should be done in chronically vomiting dogs that are undergoing endoscopy. As previously discussed, it is not unusual for dogs with inflammatory changes involving only the small intestine to present with signs limited to chronic intermittent vomiting. The diagnosis can be missed if only gastric biopsies are obtained.

Disadvantages of endoscopy include the limitation of visualization and biopsy to no further in the small intestine than the proximal jejunum in small dogs and the proximal duodenum in large dogs (with a standard 110-cm working-length flexible endoscope) and the collection of samples usually to no deeper than the muscularis mucosa. Most cases of canine lymphocytic plasmacytic enteritis involve the entire small intestine, and inflammatory changes always involve the mucosa. Duodenal biopsies therefore are reliably representative of the disorder present. An important disadvantage is that abdominal disorders that can cause clinical signs similar to lymphocytic plasmacytic enteritis (e.g., neoplasia involving the serosal wall of the stomach, pancreatitis) cannot be diagnosed via endoscopy. A careful review of the history, physical examination findings, and results from ancillary tests is used to determine the likelihood of an endoscopic procedure providing a definitive diagnosis. If gross and histologic changes identified at endoscopy do not correlate well with clinical impressions or if treatment does not result in improvement, then exploratory abdominal surgery may be indicated.

If endoscopic equipment is unavailable, an exploratory laparotomy to obtain biopsies is warranted in patients with chronic gastrointestinal signs. Surgery can be justified when it is clear that baseline tests as previously discussed have not elucidated a diagnosis and rational therapeutic trials have failed to control the disorder. In some cases, biop-

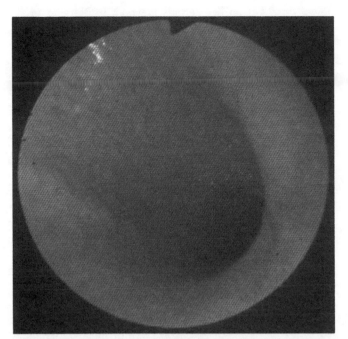

Figure 1—An endoscopic view of a normal canine duodenum.

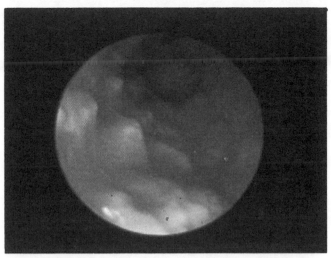

Figure 3—An endoscopic view showing a marked degree of mucosal irregularity and proliferative change in the duodenum of a six-year-old puli with vomiting, chronic diarrhea, weight loss, and hypoproteinemia. The histologic diagnosis was severe lymphocytic plasmacytic enteritis. There was chronic gastritis and chronic colitis as well.

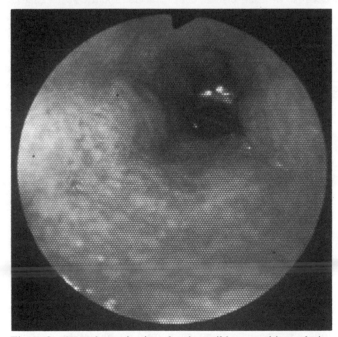

Figure 2—An endoscopic view showing mild mucosal irregularity of the duodenum. The histologic diagnosis was moderate lymphocytic, plasmacytic, and eosinophilic enteritis. There was a history of intermittent vomiting in conjunction with consistently normal stools.

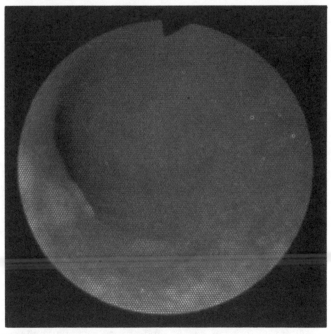

Figure 4—A 10-month endoscopic follow-up view of the duodenum from the case described in Figure 3. Grossly, there is marked improvement. There was moderate histologic improvement and clinical signs had remained under remission on continued maintenance therapy.

sies are not done until too late, when signs are severe and the patient is debilitated. Complications from anesthesia and full-thickness intestinal biopsies can be worse and treatment less successful in this situation.

At laparotomy, biopsies should be obtained from representative areas of abnormal appearance. It is actually quite common, however, for the entire small intestine to appear grossly normal in these cases because the pathologic

changes, being diffuse and confined to the mucosa, do not cause the wall of the bowel to appear abnormal.[1,3,8] If the clinical course has led to the necessity of exploratory laparotomy, biopsies must be obtained regardless of gross appearance. Biopsies should be obtained from the duodenum, jejunum, and ileum. Full-thickness intestinal biopsy complications include dehiscence secondary to poor technique or hypoproteinemia. With careful technique and the use of nonabsorbable suture, dehiscence in hypoproteinemic patients can be kept to a minimum.

Pathology

The clinician must be able to interpret the pathologist's biopsy description accurately. In lymphocytic plasmacytic enteritis, increased numbers of lymphocytes and plasma cells are present in the lamina propria; occasionally a population of eosinophils is identified as well. The disorder eosinophilic enteritis is characterized by a population of cells limited to eosinophils. Normally only a small number of inflammatory cells are found in the villous lamina propria of the duodenum. Most commonly these are mature small lymphocytes or plasma cells. Eosinophils are not observed in normal duodenal tissue.

In inflammatory bowel disease cases, histologic inflammatory changes are usually reported as mild, moderate, moderate to severe, or severe; and the percentages of inflammatory cells are noted. Changes reported as mild may simply indicate a reactive response to diarrhea, bacterial overgrowth, parasitism (e.g., *Giardia*), or other factor and usually do not support a diagnosis of inflammatory bowel disease. Moderate to severe changes are much more significant. Mucosal atrophy with villous blunting or fibrosis indicates chronic disease. Hypoproteinemia attributable to lymphocytic plasmacytic enteritis is usually associated with a moderate to severe degree of the disorder. The degree of intestinal changes noted on biopsy provides useful guidelines for both type and duration of therapy that will be needed to control the disorder.

Treatment

Corticosteroids are the initial treatment of choice for lymphocytic plasmacytic enteritis. Mild to moderate cases (as determined by clinical signs, normal protein levels, and degree of inflammatory cell infiltrate on biopsy) often respond to prednisone at a starting dose of 0.5 to 1.5 mg/kg divided twice daily for two to four weeks followed by a gradual decline in 50% increments at two-week intervals. Alternate day or every third day treatment can often be reached by two to three months. Occasionally treatment can be discontinued altogether by three to six months.

Moderate to severe cases, and any case in which the total protein is less than 5.5 g/dl, should be treated more aggressively using an initial prednisone dose of 2.2 mg/kg per day for two to four weeks before an attempt is made to decrease the dose. Dogs in this category often require long-term therapy (months to years) on an every other day or every third day basis to maintain remission. Use of combination drug therapy also may be required at the outset to control clinical signs and prevent progression of the disease. Dogs with marked hypoproteinemia (total protein less than 3.0 g/dl) caused by lymphocytic plasmacytic enteritis often respond quite well when an aggressive therapeutic course is undertaken.

Combination drug therapy is used early in severe cases or if a side effect to one drug requires that it be used at a lower dose.[9] If corticosteroids are poorly tolerated (e.g., excessive polyuria/polydipsia, listlessness, panting, inappetence associated with steroid hepatopathy) or if corticosteroids alone are unable to achieve remission, then azathioprine (Imuran®—Burroughs Wellcome) should be used. Azathioprine is an immunosuppressive drug with a nonspecific effect. Replication of rapidly dividing cells, including immunoblasts, is inhibited. Azathioprine is started *early* in the course for cases of lymphocytic plasmacytic enteritis that cause a protein-losing enteropathy with a total protein level less than 4.5 g/dl. The canine dose is 2 to 2.5 mg/kg once daily. If azathioprine is used at the outset, the prednisone dose is decreased by 50% from 2.2 mg/kg per day *after* two weeks or based on clinical improvement (i.e., remission of signs and increase in protein levels). Subsequent decreases in prednisone dose can usually be made at monthly intervals until an alternate day schedule is reached. If azathioprine is started in any type of lymphocytic plasmacytic enteritis case because of significant corticosteroid side effects, the prednisone is initially decreased by 50% to 70% but is not stopped completely unless absolutely necessary because loss of remission might result. Because of a lag effect, beneficial therapeutic results from azathioprine often are not apparent in these patients until two to three weeks after it is instituted. Azathioprine is generally used for three to nine months. Once adequate control is achieved, the daily dose is decreased by 50%, and subsequently alternate day therapy is used. Side effects are rare in dogs but may include anorexia, jaundice (hepatic damage), poor hair growth, and bone marrow suppression.[10] Azathioprine either alone or in combination with prednisone can potentially induce pancreatitis, although this is uncommon. A complete blood count should be run to monitor for evidence of anemia or leukopenia at two-week intervals for the first two months and then once monthly.

Metronidazole also plays a useful role in treatment of lymphocytic plasmacytic enteritis because of its action in suppressing cell-mediated immune reactions.[11] It is also an excellent anaerobic antibacterial drug. The initial dose of metronidazole used in treatment of lymphocytic plasmacytic enteritis is 10 to 20 mg/kg three times daily. After two to four weeks the dose often can be decreased to twice daily administration. I have successfully managed on a long-term basis patients with mild to moderate lymphocytic plasmacytic enteritis that were intolerant to corticosteroids and/or azathioprine or metronidazole alone. I use a combination of prednisone (initial dose 2.2 mg/kg divided twice daily for two to four weeks before decreasing), metronidazole, and azathioprine at the outset in patients that have lymphocytic plasmacytic enterititis and a total protein of less than 3.5 g/dl. This aggressive approach has led to control of clinical signs and return to a total protein of greater than 6.0 g/dl (by two to four months) in a number of cases. In my experience, patients with hypoproteinemia resulting from eosinophilic enteritis often respond quite well to corticosteroids alone.

Lymphocytic plasmacytic enteritis that is initially graded as moderate to severe usually can be managed quite suc-

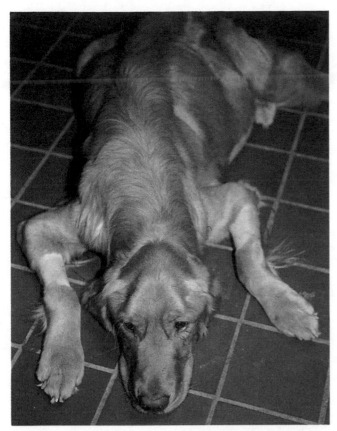

Figure 5—A three-year-old male golden retriever with chronic diarrhea, loss of muscle mass, ascites, and severe hypoproteinemia (total protein 2.6 g/dl). Intestinal biopsies revealed severe lymphocytic plasmacytic enteritis.

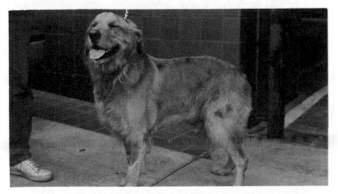

Figure 6—The same dog pictured in Figure 5 at 8½ weeks follow-up. There was significant weight gain (24 pounds), the diarrhea and ascites had resolved, and the total protein had increased to 6.2 g/dl. Treatment included prednisone, metronidazole, and azathioprine.

cessfully (Figures 5 and 6) and can be maintained in remission but not often cured. It is not unusual for follow-up biopsies in a severe case to reveal only slight to moderate histologic resolution of inflammatory infiltrates despite excellent clinical control even on lowered drug dosages. Alternatively, dramatic histologic resolution has been noted in other cases. Treatment decisions (e.g., can treatment be discontinued completely?) ideally are based on a thorough review of clinical response to date (control of clinical signs, levels of medication required, and resolution of hypoproteinemia if it was initially present) and follow-up en-

doscopic biopsy information. As a general clinical rule of thumb an attempt can be made to discontinue therapy after two to three months of successful control on twice weekly medication. If signs recur then medication is resumed on a daily basis for 7 to 14 days before a gradual reduction program is started. In some dogs with severe lymphocytic plasmacytic enteropathy and marked hypoproteinemia, therapy can be successfully discontinued as early as six months to one year. In others, lifelong treatment is required.

The two most common reasons for inadequate control of clinical signs in treatment of documented lymphocytic plasmacytic enteritis are (1) insufficiently aggressive therapy (related to dosage level or length of time) and (2) failure to recognize the presence of either concurrent gastritis, gastric motility disorder, colitis, or any combination of these disorders. Chronic gastritis is less of a problem because it is treated in much the same way as lymphocytic plasmacytic enteritis; however, lymphocytic plasmacytic colitis in dogs often does not respond well to corticosteroids alone. It is recommended that biopsies be obtained from *both* the small and large intestine in patients with chronic diarrhea so that the extent of involvement can be determined at the outset. Colitis is often managed with sulfasalazine and dietary bran supplementation and its treatment is described in detail elsewhere.[13] If vomiting persists despite adequate treatment for lymphocytic plasmacytic enteritis then a gastric motility disorder might be involved, and a course of metoclopramide to improve gastric promotility (0.3 to 0.5 mg/kg 30 minutes before each meal to a maximum of 10 mg per dose) should be administered on a trial basis.[14,15] The latter therapy is not commonly necessary in patients with lymphocytic plasmacytic enteritis.

Dietary Management

Although feeding controlled diets is an important part of long-term management of inflammatory bowel disease, dietary programs alone are rarely successful in controlling clinical signs at the time of definitive diagnosis. Dietary trials using such foods as Eukanuba Adult Maintenance® or Eukanuba Light® (The Iams Company), the Hill's Prescription Diets® i/d® and d/d®, and ANF® (Specialty Pet Products) are often successful in controlling diarrhea in dogs that are prone to dietary intolerance problems or that have early inflammatory bowel disease involvement. There is little evidence to support dietary allergy or sensitivity as a major cause of chronic diarrhea or lymphocytic plasmacytic enteritis in dogs. Clinical experience has shown that dietary management alone usually leads to only minimal or significant but temporary (weeks to several months) control of clinical signs in patients with a significant degree of inflammatory intestinal disease. When strict dietary control leads to resolution of diarrhea on a long-term basis, then a specific dietary intolerance or a motility disorder is considered to be a likely cause of the diarrhea. I have diagnosed inflammatory bowel disease in dogs that either have been fed one of the previously recommended diets as their regular lifetime diet or that have been through carefully controlled dietary trials before referral for intractable diarrhea. Referred clients often state that either the trials were only temporarily successful or not successful at all. Pharmacologic agents are used to control the disease, and high quality diets are used to help maintain remission. Diets most commonly recommended to be used in conjunction with medical management for inflammatory bowel disease include Eukanuba Adult Maintenance and Eukanuba Light, d/d, i/d, ANF, Science Diet Canine Growth or Maintenance, and Gaines® Lite® (Gaines Foods). Low fat diets, such as Eukanuba Light, should be used at least on a short-term basis if malabsorption is considered significant. Alternatively, if a client wishes to prepare home-cooked meals, a diet of four parts boiled rice or potatoes and one part cottage cheese, lean meat, or eggs can be fed.[12]

Some dogs with severe malabsorption secondary to lymphocytic plasmacytic enteritis benefit from addition of medium-chain triglycerides to the diet.[1,4,12] Dogs that have marked hypoproteinemia, weight loss, ascites, and are not eating well most commonly require supplementation. Medium-chain triglycerides provide an important source of calories when long-chain triglycerides cannot be absorbed or tolerated. Long-chain triglycerides are not readily absorbed into the intestinal mucosa without prior hydrolysis. Medium-chain triglycerides can be absorbed directly into the cell, do not require bile salts for uptake by the mucosal cell, as long-chain triglycerides do, and are more readily assimilated than long-chain triglycerides. In addition, medium-chain triglycerides are transported by the portal venous system, so their absorption does not affect the flow of lymph and they are not affected by lymphatic obstruction, as are long-chain triglycerides.[1,4] Medium-chain triglyceride supplementation is especially important in dogs that have lymphangiectasia, a disorder of the intestinal lymphatics. Many lymphangiectasia patients have lymphocytic plasmacytic enteritis as well.[4]

If anorexia is a major problem, then enteral nutrition might be required.[16] Orogastric, nasoesophageal, or gastrostomy tube feeding methods might need to be used.

Vitamin supplementation is also important in patients with chronic enteropathies that are not well controlled.[17] Any disease that results in nutrient malabsorption can decrease body stores of vitamins, especially fat-soluble vitamins. Prolonged anorexia or diarrhea can lead to marked depletion. Commercial vitamin preparations (e.g., Pet-Tabs®—Beecham Laboratories) should be used for patients with lymphocytic plasmacytic enteritis at least until clinical signs are well controlled. Folic acid should be supplemented (2.5 to 5 mg per day) if a low serum folic acid level is identified in conjunction. This usually is only necessary in dogs with severe disease that has been present for a long enough period of time to deplete body stores.

Etiology

A definitive cause for lymphocytic plasmacytic enteritis and other inflammatory bowel disorders has yet to be de-

termined. The cause of inflammatory bowel disease in people has eluded researchers as well. In 1913 Sir T. Kennedy Dalzeil described in the *British Medical Journal* a transmural inflammatory disease of the terminal ileum that later came to be known as *Crohn's disease*.[18] In concluding his report on inflammatory bowel disease Dalzeil stated, "I can only regret that the etiology of the condition remains in obscurity, but I trust that ere long further considerations will clear up the difficulty."[18] In 1987, the difficulty remains. Extensive research in the human field over the last several decades has failed to consistently implicate viruses, bacteria, prions (low molecular weight proteins), or food allergy as the cause of inflammatory bowel disease. Much of the current attention is focused on mycobacteria and immunologic phenomena.[19] There is a strong probability that lymphocytic plasmacytic enteritis is an immune-mediated disorder. The immune system may be the primary source of abnormality in some patients, and even if it is not the trigger factor, it probably mediates and perpetuates the tissue injury. A significant role for immunologic involvement is supported both by failure to consistently detect an infectious agent and by well-documented clinical responses to corticosteroids and other immunosuppressive drugs in humans and animals with inflammatory bowel disease; however, much work still needs to be done.

REFERENCES

1. Tams TR, Twedt DC: Canine protein-losing gastroenteropathy syndrome. *Compend Contin Educ Pract Vet* 3(2):105–114, 1981.
2. Breitschwerdt EB: Immunoproliferative enteropathy of basenjis. *Proc 5th Annu ACVIM Meet* 5:683–687, 1987.
3. Sherding RG: Diseases of the small bowel, in Ettinger SF (ed): *Textbook of Veterinary Internal Medicine: Diseases of the Dog and Cat*, vol 2. Philadelphia, WB Saunders Co, 1983, pp 1278–1346.
4. Sherding RG: Intestinal lymphangiectasia, in Kirk RW (ed): *Current Veterinary Therapy IX*. Philadelphia, WB Saunders Co, 1986, pp 885–888.
5. Williams DA, Batt RM: Diagnosis of canine exocrine pancreatic insufficiency by the assay of serum trypsin-like immunoreactivity. *J Small Anim Pract* 24:583–588, 1983.
6. Williams DA, Batt RM, McLean L: Bacterial overgrowth in the duodenum of dogs with exocrine pancreatic insufficiency. *JAVMA* 191:201–206, 1987.
7. O'Brien TR: Small intestine, in O'Brien TR (ed): *Radiographic Diagnosis of Abdominal Disorders in the Dog and Cat*. Philadelphia, WB Saunders Co, 1978, pp 270–351.
8. Strombeck DR: Dietary allergies, eosinophilic gastroenteritis, and gluten-induced enteropathy, in Strombeck DR (ed): *Small Animal Gastroenterology*. Davis, CA, Stonegate Publishing, 1979, pp 230–239.
9. Tams TR: Chronic inflammatory small intestinal disorders. *Proc 5th Annu ACVIM Meet* 5:123–125, 1987.
10. Finco DR, Barsanti JA: Organ transplantation in the dog: Present and future, in Kirk RW (ed): *Current Veterinary Therapy IX*. Philadelphia, WB Saunders Co, 1986, pp 114–117.
11. Grove DI, Mahmoud AF, Warren KS: Suppression of cell-mediated immunity by metronidazole. *Int Arch Allergy Appl Immunol* 54:422–427, 1977.
12. Burrows CF: The treatment of diarrhea, in Kirk RW (ed): *Current Veterinary Therapy VIII*. Philadelphia, WB Saunders Co, 1983, pp 784–790.
13. Chiapella A: Diagnosis and management of chronic colitis in the dog and cat, in Kirk RW (ed): *Current Veterinary Therapy IX*. Philadelphia, WB Saunders Co, 1986, pp 896–903.

14. Twedt DC: Disorders of gastric retention, in Kirk RW (ed): *Current Veterinary Therapy VIII.* Philadelphia, WB Saunders Co, 1983, pp 761–765.
15. Tams TR: Newer concepts in gastrointestinal therapeutics. *Proc 5th Annu ACVIM Meet* 5:126–129, 1987.
16. Crowe DT: Enteral nutrition for critically ill or injured patients—Part I. *Compend Contin Educ Pract Vet* 8(9):603–612, 1986.
17. Buffington CA: Therapeutic use of vitamins in small animals, in Kirk RW (ed): *Current Veterinary Therapy IX.* Philadelphia, WB Saunders Co, 1986, pp 40 47.
18. Dalzeil TK: Chronic interstitial enteritis. *Br Med J* 2:1068–1070, 1913.
19. Gitnick G: Evidence for infectious agents in IBD, in Gitnick G (ed): *Current Gastroenterology*, vol 7. Chicago, Year Book Medical Publishers, 1987, pp 305–313.

UPDATE

Inflammatory bowel disease (IBD) continues to be one of the most common causes of chronic vomiting and diarrhea in dogs. IBD has been identified in dogs in many countries. As veterinarians have begun to more readily recognize the various clinical manifestations of IBD, more patients are undergoing intestinal biopsies so that a definitive diagnosis can be determined and appropriate therapy instituted. The importance of evaluating gastrointestinal tissues histologically in patients whose symptoms are not readily explained by routine tests and dietary trials is (thankfully) well entrenched in our thinking. Our recognition that IBD commonly occurs in dogs (and cats) directly parallels the increased use of endoscopy in patients with symptoms of gastrointestinal disease. As we have become more proficient in advancing endoscopes into the small intestine, we have become much more capable in obtaining tissue samples from patients both more *safely* (i.e., endoscopy is less invasive than exploratory surgery with procurement of full-thickness biopsies) and more *readily* (i.e., clients are much more likely to permit their pets to undergo endoscopy than laparotomy).

Treatment for IBD is largely the same as it was in 1987. A majority of patients can be managed successfully using this protocol. Newer treatment modalities currently being investigated for IBD include cyclosporine, a potent immunosuppressive drug, and dietary supplementation with omega 3 fatty acids. Omega 3 fatty acids, which have profound anti-inflammatory effects, are a form of long-chain fatty acids. Improved dietary formulations are likely to have a significant impact as adjunctive treatment for IBD.

Feline Idiopathic Inflammatory Bowel Disease

KEY FACTS

- Inflammatory bowel disease is a common cause of chronic intermittent vomiting, diarrhea, anorexia, and weight loss in cats.
- The pathogenesis of inflammatory bowel disease may involve host hypersensitivity responses to luminal and/or mucosal antigens.
- No specific hematologic, biochemical, or radiographic findings are pathognomonic for the disorder.
- Gastrointestinal mucosal biopsy is required to confirm a diagnosis.
- Treatment involves dietary therapy and specific immunosuppressive drugs given to reduce mucosal inflammation.

Iowa State University
Albert E. Jergens, DVM

IDIOPATHIC inflammatory bowel disease (IBD) refers to a group of chronic gastrointestinal disorders characterized by infiltration of the gastrointestinal tract by inflammatory cells. The cellular infiltrate may include populations of lymphocytes, plasma cells, eosinophils, neutrophils, and histiocytes generally confined to the mucosa of the stomach, small intestine, and/or colon. This disorder encompasses at least four histologic forms of gastroenterocolitis in cats: lymphocytic–plasmacytic,[1,2] eosinophilic,[3,4] suppurative,[5] and granulomatous.[6] Inflammatory bowel disease is a common cause of persistent diarrhea, vomiting, anorexia, and weight loss in cats.[1,3,7]

Diagnosis of inflammatory bowel disease requires histologic confirmation and exclusion of other causes of gastrointestinal inflammation. There are many reports of canine inflammatory bowel disease in the veterinary literature,[7–13] but limited clinical reports and relatively sparse scientific data are available regarding the disease in cats.[1–3,14] This article describes the diagnostic evaluation and successful therapeutic management of two cats with histologically diagnosed inflammatory bowel disease. Included is a summary of the current knowledge regarding the pathogenesis, clinical features, diagnosis, and therapy of feline inflammatory bowel disease.

CASE PRESENTATIONS
Case 1

A three-year-old, castrated male, Persian cat that weighed 2.5 kilograms was examined because of intermittent vomiting, anorexia, and weight loss of two years duration. The vomitus consisted of digested food and bile. Profound lethargy and mental depression were observed during vomiting episodes. Diarrhea was not reported. Symptomatic therapy with antibiotics and parasiticides, performed by the referring veterinarian, produced slight clinical improvement. The cat was housed indoors, was currently immunized, and was fed a dry commercial feline ration. Physical examination demonstrated mental depression, thinness, and reduced muscle mass. Thickened bowel loops were detected by abdominal palpation.

A data base was developed that consisted of a complete blood count (CBC), serum biochemical profile, urinalysis, fecal examinations for parasitic ova and protozoan parasites (via zinc sulfate centrifugation), and abdominal radiography. Hematologic testing demonstrated normal red and white blood cell counts. The serum total protein concentration was high (9.4 g/dl [reference range is 5.2 to 7.0 g/dl]), and the serum albumin concentration was low (2.0 g/dl [reference range is 2.5 to 4.2 g/dl]). Serum electrophoresis demonstrated a polyclonal gammopathy indicative of chronic inflammation.

Examination of feces was negative for helminth ova, and urinalysis was normal. The cat tested negative for feline leukemia virus (FeLV) and feline immunodeficiency virus (FIV) infections by enzyme-linked immunosorbent assay (ELISA) serology. Abdominal radiographs demonstrated

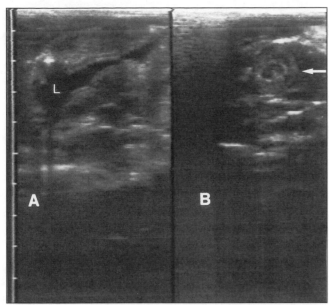

Figure 1—(*A*) Parasagittal ultrasonographic image of the stomach and (*B*) transverse image of a small intestinal loop (*arrow*). Diffuse thickening of the gastric and small intestinal walls is apparent. *L* = lumen.

numerous air-filled small intestinal loops and mild hepatomegaly. Abdominal ultrasonography confirmed mild hepatic enlargement and the presence of marked gastric and small intestinal mural thickening (Figure 1).

AFTER food was withheld overnight, upper gastrointestinal endoscopy (gastroscopy and enteroscopy) was performed. Endoscopic examination of the esophagus was normal. The gastric mucosa was markedly irregular (granular); the most severe lesions were visualized in the pyloric antrum (Figure 2). The pylorus could not be conclusively identified, and multiple attempts to enter the duodenum with the endoscope were unsuccessful. Mucosal biopsies were obtained from all regions in the stomach (fundus, body, and antrum) using pinch forceps. Histologic review of gastric biopsy specimens demonstrated diffuse lymphocytic–plasmacytic and neutrophilic infiltrates in the lamina propria as well as mucosal epithelial hyperplasia and glandular dilatation (Figure 3).

The patient was discharged, and the owner was instructed to begin frequent feeding of small amounts of a commercial controlled diet. Metronidazole (20 mg/kg three times daily) and prednisone (2 mg/kg divided twice daily) were prescribed for three weeks to reduce gastrointestinal inflammatory infiltrates. Anorexia and vomiting did not recur during this period, and the patient gained 0.5 kilograms. The metronidazole was discontinued; attempts to decrease the corticosteroid dose were accompanied by clinical relapse. A second three-week course of prednisone therapy with

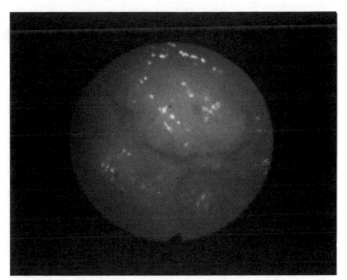

Figure 2—Endoscopic close-up demonstrating marked mucosal granularity of the pyloric antrum in a three-year-old cat.

gradual tapering of the dose alleviated the gastrointestinal signs. The patient was normal 14 months after diagnosis and treatment.

Case 2

A 10-year-old, spayed female, Domestic Shorthair cat that weighed 2.1 kilograms was presented for unthriftiness, vomiting, and weight loss of one year duration. During this period, the cat lost approximately 30% of its body weight while the appetite remained normal. The owner occasionally observed fetid, watery diarrhea in association with the vomiting episodes. The patient was current on recommended vaccinations and was housed indoors. The diet consisted of moist and dry commercial feline diets. Physical examination demonstrated reduced muscle mass and a brittle, dry haircoat. Firm, fluid- and gas-distended small intestinal bowel loops were noted during abdominal palpation.

THE ROUTINE data base that was developed comprised a complete blood count, serum biochemical profile, urinalysis, fecal examinations for parasitic ova and protozoan parasites (via zinc sulfate centrifugation), and abdominal radiography. The only hematologic abnormality noted was marked eosinophilia (1712 cells/µl). Results of urinalysis were unremarkable. Serum biochemical values were normal, with the exception of mildly elevated urea nitrogen (36 mg/dl [reference range is 15 to 34 mg/dl]). Fecal analysis was negative for parasitic ova and protozoa. Abdominal radiographs demonstrated diffuse fluid-distended small intestinal bowel loops (Figure 4). Plasma thyroxine was normal (3.5 µg/dl), and ELISA serology for feline leukemia virus was negative.

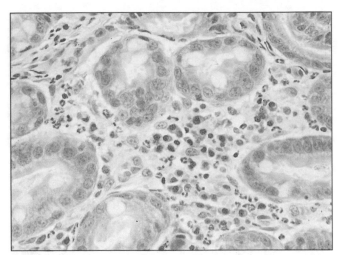

Figure 3—Photomicrograph of a gastric biopsy specimen from the patient in Figure 2. Glandular dilatation and diffuse infiltrates of lymphocytes, plasma cells, and neutrophils in the lamina propria are apparent.

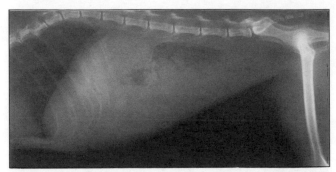

Figure 4—Lateral radiograph of the abdomen. Multiple, fluid-distended small intestinal loops fill the ventral midabdomen and produce a ropy appearance.

Upper gastrointestinal endoscopy was performed after food was withheld overnight. Mucosal abnormalities of the esophagus were not observed. Multifocal, well-circumscribed areas of gastric mucosal erythema were apparent along the greater curvature of the stomach (Figure 5). The mucosa of the descending duodenum was normal in appearance; however, light contact by the endoscope produced marked hemorrhage, indicating increased mucosal friability (Figure 6).

MULTIPLE mucosal biopsies were obtained from the descending duodenum and stomach via pinch forceps. Direct biopsy was performed on areas of gastric erythema. Review of gastric biopsy specimens did not reveal pathologic abnormalities. Histologic examination of duodenal biopsies demonstrated cryptal immaturity accompanied by diffuse lymphocytic–plasmacytic cellular infiltrate in the lamina propria (Figure 7).

The patient was discharged and treated with oral prednisone (1.5 mg/kg divided twice daily) and metronidazole (20 mg/kg three times daily) for three weeks to reduce gastrointestinal inflammation. The controlled diet was continued. Occasional vomiting was reported after the metronidazole was administered; dosing of the drug was reduced to once a day. Four weeks after discharge, the patient was free of signs of disease and had gained 0.5 kilograms. The metronidazole was discontinued, and the prednisone dose was gradually tapered during a four-week period. The cat was clinically normal eight weeks after diagnosis and therapy.

PATHOGENESIS

The cause of inflammatory bowel disease in animals and humans is not understood. The histologic features suggest an underlying immunologic mechanism.[7,8,12] According to recent theories, inflammatory bowel disease involves host hypersensitivity responses to antigens in the bowel lumen or mucosa.[15] Possible causes of antigenic exposure include alterations in the mucosal permeability barrier[16,17] and defective immunoregulation of gut-associated lymphatic tissue (GALT).[18,19] Cellular infiltration may be the response to chronic challenge as a consequence of this increased permeability or intolerance to self, diet, or bacterial antigens.

PRODUCTS of the immune and inflammatory cellular constituents include a wide variety of cytokines, eicosanoids (especially leukotriene B_4), and oxygen-free radicals that damage tissue.[20] Clinical signs in affected animals are directly attributable to gastrointestinal inflammation and its effects on gastrointestinal permeability and motility, nutrient absorption, and the vomiting center.

HISTORY AND CLINICAL SIGNS

There is no age, gender, or breed predisposition for the development of feline inflammatory bowel disease. Although most cases occur in middle-aged and old cats,[1,3,15] eight of 26 cats with histologic inflammatory bowel disease were two years of age or younger in a recent clinical study.[21] Clinical signs reflect the predominant site of gastrointestinal disease and the extent of mucosal damage. Salient clinical findings are vomiting of bile, anorexia, weight loss, signs of large bowel dysfunction (tenesmus, hematochezia, and mucoid stools), and watery diarrhea.[1,3,5,21] Clinical signs usually have a cyclic (rather than progressive) course. Affected cats often act normally and are not evaluated until clinical episodes become increasingly frequent and severe.

Physical examination findings vary. Intermittent or complete anorexia is often noted. Cats may be well fleshed with mild disease; in severe cases, they may exhibit marked cachexia and mental depression. Weight loss usually occurs

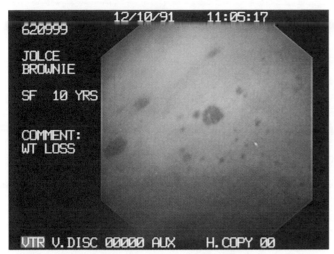

Figure 5—Endoscopic close-up of multiple circumscribed areas of mucosal erythema along the greater curvature of the stomach in a 10-year-old cat.

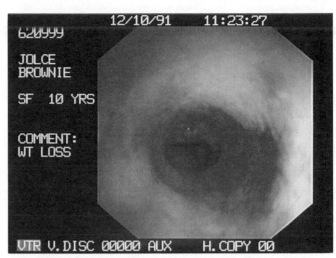

Figure 6—Endoscopic view of the descending duodenum of the patient in Figure 5. Mucosal friability (at the four o'clock position) is apparent.

in chronic cases if episodes of vomiting and/or diarrhea are protracted. In hypovolemic patients, there is clinical evidence of dehydration as a consequence of severe vomiting or watery diarrhea. In cats with eosinophilic enteritis, careful abdominal palpation might demonstrate abdominal pain or thickened small intestinal loops.[3,4] Hepatosplenomegaly may be detected in the hypereosinophilic syndrome.[4]

IN MOST CASES, history and physical examination findings facilitate localization of clinical signs to the site of organ involvement. Vomiting, anorexia, weight loss, and abdominal pain suggest gastric and/or small intestinal inflammation. Melena and hematemesis (which is rare) similarly reflect upper gastrointestinal disease. Chronic small and large bowel diarrhea can often be differentiated by combining information from the history, physical examination, and fecal characteristics (Table I). A combination of small and large bowel signs suggests diffuse intestinal disease.

DIAGNOSTIC PLAN

Differential Diagnosis. Inflammatory bowel disease is a diagnosis of exclusion and should be differentiated from other disorders that cause gastrointestinal inflammation. Giardiasis,[22] bacterial overgrowth,[23] *Campylobacter* or *Salmonella* infection,[24] dietary hypersensitivity,[25] lymphangiectasia,[26] hyperthyroidism,[1] and gastrointestinal neoplasia[3] may cause clinical signs of gastroenteritis accompanied by histologic evidence of inflammatory cellular infiltrates.

Diagnostic tests should be performed in a logical, stepwise fashion to eliminate disorders that resemble inflammatory bowel disease while minimizing patient hospitalization and owner expense. The following criteria support a diagnosis of inflammatory bowel disease: clinical signs of persistent gastrointestinal disease, failure of or inadequate clinical response to controlled diets fed exclusively, development of a thorough data base that excludes metabolic disease and other gastrointestinal causes, and histologic diagnosis of inflammatory cellular infiltrates with failure to demonstrate other causes of gastroenteritis.

Dietary Trial. All patients should undergo a trial (of at least three weeks duration) that uses a controlled diet. Remission of clinical signs in response to diet alone may occur with food intolerance, with dietary hypersensitivity, and in some cases of eosinophilic gastroenteritis.[15] Patients that fail a dietary trial warrant further diagnostic workup.

Diagnostic Tests. A routine data base (consisting of a complete blood count, serum biochemical profile, urinalysis, fecal examinations, and abdominal radiographs) should be developed for all patients with possible inflammatory bowel disease. Such a data base permits exclusion of metabolic disease and allows for anesthetic evaluation before gastrointestinal biopsy. Nonspecific hematologic and biochemical abnormalities are often observed.[21] Leukocytosis may occur in response to chronic inflammation and in patients with gastrointestinal ulceration or erosion. Peripheral eosinophilia is often present in cats with eosinophilic enteritis and hypereosinophilic syndrome.[3,4] Nonregenerative anemia is usually attributable to chronic inflammatory disease.

Disturbances of protein metabolism are common in cats.[15,21] Mild to moderate hyperproteinemia is periodically noted in association with hyperglobulinemia of chronic inflammation. Hypoalbuminemia is usually multifactorial and may be caused by reduced protein intake, malabsorption of nutrients, protein loss through exudative diarrhea, and blood loss from gastrointestinal ulceration.[27] Mild eleva-

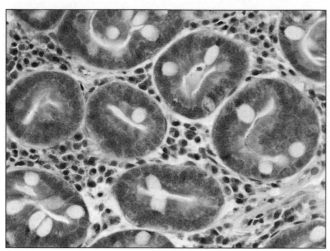

Figure 7—Photomicrograph of a duodenal biopsy specimen from the patient in Figures 5 and 6. Diffuse cryptal immaturity and lymphocytes and plasma cells are apparent in the lamina propria.

tions of hepatic enzymes (alanine transferase and alkaline phosphatase) are common and may complicate differentiation of inflammatory bowel disease, primary heptobiliary disease, and hyperthyroidism.

Parasitism must be ruled out by several fecal flotations and direct smears. Zinc sulfate centrifugation is a sensitive test for the detection of *Giardia* cysts.[28] In cases of chronic colitis in which there is reason to suspect an infectious agent, fecal cultures should be performed to rule out such bacterial enteropathogens as *Campylobacter* and *Salmonella* species.

NONSPECIFIC radiographic findings of fluid- or gas-distended small intestinal loops are common[21]; these findings do not differentiate inflammatory bowel disease from other gastrointestinal disorders. Contrast radiography may demonstrate alterations in intestinal transit time and mucosal irregularities that suggest infiltrative mucosal disease.[1,29] Cats should be screened for feline leukemia virus and feline immunodeficiency virus infections, which may be associated with inflammatory conditions of the bowel. Middle-aged and old (at least eight years of age) cats should be tested for hyperthyroidism by serum thyroxine analysis. The routine data base may be entirely normal in some cats with inflammatory bowel disease.

DEFINITIVE DIAGNOSIS

Gastrointestinal Biopsy. Definitive diagnosis requires gastrointestinal biopsy obtained via endoscope or laparotomy. Endoscopy is preferred because it is inexpensive, fast, and minimally invasive and because targeted biopsies for cytologic and histologic evaluation can be obtained. Multiple endoscopic biopsies are routinely obtained from

TABLE I
Characterization of Small and Large Bowel Diarrhea

Sign	Small Bowel	Large Bowel
Quality of stool	Soft to watery	Semisolid to solid
Stool volume	Usually increased	Usually decreased
Frequency of defecation	Mildly increased	Greatly increased
Weight loss	Common	Uncommon
Tenesmus	Absent	Present
Fecal blood	Melena	Hematochezia
Excess mucus production	Absent	Present

the stomach, duodenum, proximal jejunum, and colon using pinch forceps. Rigid colonoscopy can be performed as an alternative in patients with diffuse colonic disease.

IF ENDOSCOPY is unavailable, exploratory laparotomy should be performed to obtain full-thickness biopsies from the duodenum, jejunum, ileum, and colon. Other indications for abdominal surgery are the presence of mesenteric lymphadenopathy, focal intestinal mass lesions, or hepatosplenomegaly in association with the hypereosinophilic syndrome. Biopsy confirms a diagnosis of inflammatory bowel disease and provides prognostic information and individualization of therapy.

Endoscopic Observations. A thorough and systematic examination of mucosal structures should precede endoscopic biopsy procedures. Consistent endoscopic terminology has been proposed to aid in lesion description and in the formulation of a definitive diagnosis[30] (see Endoscopic Criteria for Mucosal Assessment). *Erythema* denotes mucosal redness, which may be pathologic or a normal physiologic response to anesthesia or alterations in blood pressure. *Friability* describes the ease with which the mucosa is damaged by contact with the endoscope or biopsy instrument. Increased *granularity* refers to alterations in mucosal texture.

Ulcers and *erosions* denote visible breaches in mucosal integrity associated with active hemorrhage. Ulcers are typically focal, crateriform, well-circumscribed lesions that penetrate deeply into the adjacent mucosa and contain central fibrinous exudate. Erosions are discrete, superficial mucosal defects that lack raised margins and necrotic centers.

Recent investigations have considered the clinical significance of endoscopic observations and their correlation to histologic findings. In one study, approximately two thirds of patients with endoscopic lesions had histologic abnormalities, including inflammatory infiltrates.[31] Excessive

Endoscopic Criteria for Mucosal Assessment

- Degree of erythema
- Tissue friability
- Increased granularity
- Erosions or ulcers
- Mass lesions
- Strictures
- Luminal distention
- Visibility of submucosal vessels

TABLE II
Histologic Grading System for Inflammatory Bowel Disease in Cats

Lesion	Mild	Moderate	Severe
Cellular infiltrate	√	√	√
Epithelial immaturity		√	√
Focal epithelial necrosis		√	√
Multifocal epithelial necrosis			√
Architectural distortion			√

mucosal granularity and friability were associated with histologic abnormalities in 82% of the cases. Another report found endoscopic lesions of granularity, friability, and erosions or ulcers in dogs and cats with histologic infiltrates of inflammatory bowel disease.[32] Mucosal biopsies should be obtained from all patients regardless of the endoscopic appearance of the mucosa.

HISTOLOGIC FINDINGS

Objective histologic criteria for differentiating inflammatory bowel disease from acute inflammatory conditions of the gastrointestinal tract have not been published. The typical histopathologic finding in inflammatory bowel disease is increased infiltration of the lamina propria by inflammatory cells, especially lymphocytes and plasma cells. Eosinophils are the predominant cell type in cats with eosinophilic gastroenteritis. Neutrophils are most numerous in focuses of mucosal necrosis and ulceration or in patients with chronic suppurative colitis. It is relatively common to find a mixed infiltrate in the mucosa of the stomach, duodenum, and/or colon.

BECAUSE of inconsistent orientation of minute specimens and extensive variation between observers, it is difficult to standardize the quantification of biopsy cellularity with routine histologic examination.[33–35] The difficulty in determining the increased cellularity in an organ that possesses a normal component of inflammatory cells has lead to the assessment of epithelial or glandular alterations as criteria for diagnosis of inflammatory bowel disease in humans.[36]

A series of endoscopic biopsy specimens from cats with gastrointestinal clinical signs was recently evaluated using epithelial or glandular alterations as criteria for severity of lesions[14,32] (Table II). Mixed populations of lymphocytes and plasma cells were observed in biopsy specimens from all subjects. Inflammatory bowel disease lesions of moderate severity (i.e., cellular infiltrate accompanied by mucosal epithelial immaturity and/or solitary epithelial necrosis) predominated in the stomach, duodenum, and colon. The diagnosis of inflammatory bowel disease requires the presence of appropriate histologic changes combined with the inability to demonstrate a specific cause.

THERAPEUTIC PLAN

Management of feline inflammatory bowel disease varies widely and includes the use of controlled diets, corticosteroids, metronidazole, sulfasalazine, and cytotoxic agents. Therapeutic protocols remain largely empirical and are influenced by the severity of clinical signs and histologic findings. No controlled studies have evaluated one or all therapies in cats. Treatment of inflammatory bowel disease should be tailored to the individual patient.

Dietary Therapy. Dietary manipulation is a rational approach to treatment because dietary antigens are often responsible for inflammatory cell infiltrates. Only commercial or homemade (baby foods or boiled chicken) controlled diets that are highly digestible, low in residue, and relatively hypoallergenic should be fed during the treatment period. Several commercial diets have been recommended for cats with inflammatory bowel disease. High-fat diets should be avoided; they are difficult to assimilate and may enhance the production of inflammation-promoting eicosanoids. Treats, preexisting medications, and dietary supplements should be excluded to minimize antigenic exposure to the alimentary tract.

CATS with colitis may benefit from fiber supplementation in the form of a commercial diet or the addition of psyllium to the regular cat food.[3,37,38] The potential benefits of added fiber include enhanced colonic motility, binding of irritating products, and increased colonic absorption of fluid and electrolytes.[39] Some patients with inflammatory bowel disease can be managed by diet alone, but most require pharmacologic intervention.

Drug Therapy. Because of their potent antiinflammatory and immunosuppressive properties, oral corticosteroids are initially the preferred drugs in many cases of inflammatory bowel disease. Prednisone is the corticosteroid used most frequently; the initial dose is 2 mg/kg/day for two to four weeks. The dose is halved every two weeks until the lowest effective maintenance dose (preferably alternate-day therapy) is reached.

Cats with hypereosinophilic syndrome require high prednisone dosages (2 to 4 mg/kg/day) and prolonged treatment.[3] Attempts should be made to avoid high-dose corticosteroids for maintenance of patients with severe inflammatory bowel disease. The salient side effects of polyuria, polydipsia, and adrenal suppression are minimized by combining prednisone with other drugs (e.g., metronidazole or azathioprine) to reduce the required prednisone dose.

Metronidazole has been used successfully to treat inflammatory bowel disease in humans[40,41] (patients with Crohn's disease), dogs,[9,13] and cats.[1] The beneficial effects of the drug include antiprotozoal action, a broad-spectrum of activity against anaerobic bacteria, and inhibition of cell-mediated immunity.[42] I have successfully used metronidazole as a single pharmaceutical agent in the management of many cases of mild to moderate enterocolitis associated with inflammatory bowel disease.

A dosage of 10 to 20 mg/kg three times daily for two to four weeks, tapering during the following one to two months, is usually effective. Metronidazole may be safely used in inflammatory bowel disease patients with gastrointestinal ulceration or erosion if corticosteroids are contraindicated. Side effects are uncommon. Vomiting and neurotoxicity have been reported with metronidazole use in dogs.[43]

SULFASALAZINE (an antibiotic combination of sulfapyridine and 5-aminosalicylate) has proven efficacy in treating colonic inflammatory bowel disease in dogs[9,13] and cats.[3] The drug is given orally and is degraded by colonic bacteria into its active component, 5-aminosalicylate. The salicylate moiety has potent topical antiinflammatory actions, which result from inhibition of lipoxygenase activity and leukotriene synthesis.[15] A dosage of 10 to 20 mg/kg one to three times daily for 7 to 10 days has been effective in treating cats with colitis.[3] The oral suspension (50 mg/ml) permits accurate dosing and minimizes the risks of salicylate toxicity. Side effects of sulfasalazine in cats include anorexia and anemia but are uncommon at the recommended dose.

Cytotoxic drugs, such as azathioprine, are required in a small percentage of patients with inflammatory bowel disease that is refractory to conventional therapy. Azathioprine is a potent immunosuppressive agent that is best used in cats as adjuvant therapy with prednisone. Azathioprine, at an alternate-day dose of 0.3 mg/kg, has benefited cats with severe inflammatory bowel disease.[3] There may be a delay of three to five weeks before beneficial clinical responses are observed. Mild myelosuppression may be associated with azathioprine use; the complete blood count thus should be monitored periodically for drug-induced neutropenia or thrombocytopenia. In my experience, azathioprine is rarely indicated in cats with inflammatory bowel disease.

PROGNOSIS

In most cases of inflammatory bowel disease, the prognosis is good for control but poor for cure. When the diagnosis is confirmed by gastrointestinal biopsy, combination therapy with controlled diets and immunosuppressive drugs is indicated to control the clinical signs of gastroenteritis.

The goal of therapy is to maintain remission by diet alone. Relapses invariably occur and are often precipitated by dietary indiscretion; short-term drug therapy (with prednisone or metronidazole) is required to facilitate recovery. A more guarded prognosis is warranted for feline patients with severe histologic lesions, mucosal fibrosis, and eosinophilic enteritis or the hypereosinophilic syndrome.

ACKNOWLEDGMENTS

The author thanks Kristina G. Miles, DVM, and Elizabeth L. Riedesel, DVM, of the Department of Veterinary Clinical Sciences, College of Veterinary Medicine, Iowa State University, for radiographic interpretation and reproductions.

About the Author
Dr. Jergens, who is a Diplomate of the American College of Veterinary Internal Medicine, is affiliated with the Department of Veterinary Clinical Sciences, College of Veterinary Medicine, Iowa State University, Ames, Iowa.

REFERENCES

1. Tams TR: Chronic feline inflammatory bowel disorders. Part I. Idiopathic inflammatory bowel disease. *Compend Contin Educ Pract Vet* 8(6):371–376, 1986.
2. Willard MD, Dalley JB, Trapp AL: Lymphocytic-plasmacytic enteritis in a cat. *JAVMA* 186:181–182, 1985.
3. Tams TR: Chronic feline inflammatory bowel disorders. Part II. Feline eosinophilic enteritis and lymphosarcoma. *Compend Contin Educ Pract Vet* 8(7):464–470, 1986.
4. Moore RP: Feline eosinophilic enteritis, in Kirk RW (ed): *Current Veterinary Therapy. VIII.* Philadelphia, WB Saunders Co, 1983, pp 791–793.
5. Leib MS, Sponenberg DP, Wilcke JR, et al: Suppurative colitis in a cat. *JAVMA* 188:739–741, 1986.
6. Van Kruiningen HJ, Ryan MJ, Snidel NM: The classification of feline colitis. *J Comp Pathol* 93:275–294, 1983.
7. Strombeck DR: Chronic inflammatory bowel disease, in Strombeck DR (ed): *Small Animal Gastroenterology.* Davis, CA, Stonegate Publishing Co, 1979, pp 240–261.
8. Sherding RG: Diseases of the small bowel, in Ettinger SJ (ed): *Textbook of Veterinary Internal Medicine.* Philadelphia, WB Saunders Co, 1982, pp 1278–1346.
9. Tams TR: Chronic canine lymphocytic plasmacytic enteritis. *Compend Contin Educ Pract Vet* 8(6):371–376, 1986.
10. Hayden DW, Van Kruiningen HJ: Lymphocytic-plasmacytic enteritis in German shepherd dogs. *JAAHA* 18:89–96, 1982.
11. Van Kruiningen HJ: Canine colitis comparable to regional enteritis and mucosal colitis of man. *Gastroenterology* 62:1128–1142, 1972.
12. Nelson RW, Stookey LJ, Kazacos E: Nutritional management of idiopathic chronic colitis in the dog. *J Vet Intern Med* 2:133–137, 1988.
13. Leib MS, Hay WH, Roth L: Plasmacytic-lymphocytic colitis in dogs, in Kirk RW (ed): *Current Veterinary Therapy. X.* Philadelphia, WB Saunders Co, 1989, pp 939–943.
14. Jergens AE, Moore FM, March P, et al: Idiopathic inflammatory bowel disease associated with gastroduodenal ulceration-erosion: A report of 9 cases in the dog and cat. *JAAHA* 28:21–26, 1992.

15. Strombeck DR, Guilford WG: Idiopathic inflammatory bowel diseases, in Strombeck DR, Guilford WG (eds): *Small Animal Gastroenterology*, ed 2. Davis, CA, Stonegate Publishing Co, 1990, pp 357–390.
16. Casellas F, Agaude S, Soriano B, et al: Intestinal permeability to ^{99m}Tc-diethylenetriaminopentaacetic acid in inflammatory bowel disease. *Am J Gastroenterol* 81:767–770, 1986.
17. Olaison G, Leandersson P, Sjodahl R, et al: Intestinal permeability to polyethyleneglycol 600 in Crohn's disease: Preoperative determination in a defined segment of the small intestine. *Gut* 29:196–199, 1988.
18. Strober W, James SP: The immunological basis of inflammatory bowel disease. *J Clin Immunol* 6:415–432, 1986.
19. Jewell DP, Patel C: Immunology of inflammatory bowel disease. *Scand J Gastroenterol [Suppl]* 114(20):120–126, 1985.
20. Podolsky DK: Inflammatory bowel disease. *N Engl J Med* 325: 928–937, 1991.
21. Jergens AE, Moore FM, Haynes JS, et al: Idiopathic inflammatory bowel disease in the dog and cat: 84 cases (1987–1990). *JAVMA*, accepted for publication.
22. Kirkpatrick CE: Feline giardiasis: A review. *J Small Anim Pract* 27:69–80, 1986.
23. Rutgers HC, Batt RM, Kelly DF: Lymphocytic-plasmacytic enteritis associated with bacterial overgrowth in a dog. *JAVMA* 192: 1739–1742, 1988.
24. Fox JG, Moore R, Ackerman JI: *Campylobacter jejuni*-associated diarrhea in dogs. *JAVMA* 183:1430–1433, 1983.
25. Finco DR, Duncan JR, Schall WD, et al: Chronic enteric disease and hypoproteinemia in 9 dogs. *JAVMA* 163:262–271, 1973.
26. Heyman MB: Food sensitivity and eosinophilic gastroenteropathies, in Sleisenger MH, Fordtran JS (eds): *Gastrointestinal Disease*, ed 4. Philadelphia, WB Saunders Co, 1989, pp 1113–1134.
27. Moon HW: Mechanisms in the pathogenesis of diarrhea: A review. *JAVMA* 172:443–448, 1978.
28. Kirkpatrick CE: Enteric protozoal infections, in Greene CE (ed): *Clinical Microbiology and Infectious Diseases of the Dog and Cat*. Philadelphia, WB Saunders Co, 1984, pp 806–823.
29. O'Brien TR: Small intestine, in O'Brien TR (ed): *Radiographic Diagnosis of Abdominal Disorders in the Dog and Cat*. Philadelphia, WB Saunders Co, 1978, pp 279–351.
30. Leib MS: Gastrointestinal endoscopy: Endoscopic and histologic correlation. *Proc 7th ACVIM Forum*:784–786, 1989.
31. Roth L, Leib MS, Davenport DJ, et al: Comparisons between endoscopic and histologic evaluation of the gastrointestinal tract in dogs and cats: 75 cases (1984–1987). *JAVMA* 196:635–638, 1990.
32. Jergens AE, Moore FM, Haynes JS, et al: Inflammatory bowel disease in the dog and cat: Histologic and endoscopic observations. *Proc Am Coll Vet Pathol*:178, 1991.
33. Lee E, Schiller LR, Fordtran JS: Quantification of colonic lamina propria cells by means of a morphometric point-counting method. *Gastroenterology* 94:409–418, 1988.
34. Salzmann JL, Peltier-Koch F, Block R, et al: Morphometric study of colonic biopsies: A new method of estimating inflammatory disease. *Lab Invest* 60:847–851, 1989.
35. Ochoa R, Breitschwerdt ED, Lincoln KL: Immunoproliferative small intestinal disease in basenji dogs. Morphologic observations. *Am J Vet Res* 45:482–490, 1984.
36. Haggit RC: The differential diagnosis of colitis. *Proc US Canad Acad Pathol*, 1988.
37. Willard MD: Dietary therapy in large intestinal diseases. *Proc 6th ACVIM Forum*:713–714, 1988.
38. Leib MS: Fiber-responsive large bowel diarrhea. *Proc 8th ACVIM Forum*:817–819, 1990.
39. Burrows CF, Merritt AM: Influence of alpha-cellulose on myoelectric activity of proximal canine colon. *Am J Physiol* 245:301–306, 1983.
40. Blichfeldt P, Blomhoff JP, Myhre E, et al: Metronidazole in Crohn's disease. *Scand J Gastroenterol* 13:123–127, 1978.
41. Ruderman WB: Newer pharmacologic agents for the therapy of inflammatory bowel disease. *Med Clin North Am* 74:133–153, 1990.
42. Miller JJ: The imidazoles as immunosuppressive agents. *Transplant Proc* 12:300–303, 1980.
43. Dow SW, LeCouteur RA, Poss ML, et al: Central nervous system toxicosis associated with metronidazole treatment of dogs: Five cases (1984–1987). *JAVMA* 195:365–368, 1989.

Fecal Impaction (*continued from page 23*)

35. Richter KP, Cleveland MB: Comparison of an orally administered gastrointestinal lavage solution with traditional enema administration as preparation for colonoscopy in dogs. *JAVMA* 195:1727–1731, 1989.
36. Burrows CF: Evaluation of a colonic lavage solution to prepare the colon of the dog for colonoscopy. *JAVMA* 195:1719–1721, 1989.
37. Center SA: Feline liver disorders and their management. *Compend Contin Educ Pract Vet* 8(12):889–903, 1986.
38. Meunier P: Physiologic study of the terminal digestive tract in chronic painful constipation. *Gut* 27:1018–1024, 1986.
39. Atkins CE, Tyler R, Greenlee P: Clinical, biochemical, acid-base and electrolyte abnormalities in cats after hypertonic sodium phosphate enema administration. *Am J Vet Res* 46:980–988, 1985.
40. Jorgenson LS, Center SA, Randolph JR, et al: Electrolyte abnormalities induced by hypertonic phosphate enemas in two cats. *JAVMA* 187:1367–1368, 1985.
41. Bright RM, Burrows CF, Goring R, et al: Subtotal colectomy for treatment of acquired megacolon in the dog and cat. *JAVMA* 188:1412–1416, 1986.

Acute Pancreatitis in Dogs

KEY FACTS

- Acute pancreatitis occurs when pancreatic proteases are prematurely activated and subsequently released into the abdominal cavity and systemic circulation.
- The condition should be suspected in any middle-aged or old dog that has a sudden onset of vomiting, anorexia, and depression.
- The history, physical findings, radiographic findings, and laboratory test results are used together to make the clinical diagnosis.
- Treatment commonly requires complete cessation of oral intake of food in addition to administration of intravenous fluids and antibiotics.
- Surgery is indicated for pancreatic phlegmon, pseudocyst, and abscess.

University of Florida
Michael Schaer, DVM

O F THE VARIOUS clinical disorders treated by veterinary practitioners, there is probably none more difficult and frustrating than acute pancreatitis. Despite the continuing acquisition of new knowledge of pancreatic physiology and pathophysiology, there is no miracle treatment to counteract the ravages of acute necrotizing pancreatitis. This article describes the pathophysiology, clinical features, and medical and surgical treatment of acute pancreatitis in dogs.

PHYSIOLOGY

The human pancreas accounts for less than 1% of the total body weight, yet it has approximately 13 times the protein-producing capacity of the liver and reticuloendothelial system combined.[1] The pancreas has endocrine and exocrine functions. Exocrine pancreatic proteases include trypsin, chymotrypsin, elastase, carboxypeptidase A and B, and phospholipase A.

In normal conditions, the following natural safeguards protect the exocrine pancreas from autodigestion by its enzymes: (1) synthesis, transport, and secretion of the enzymes in the form of inactive precursors or proenzymes; (2) enterokinase-mediated intraluminal activation of the enzymes (e.g., conversion of trypsinogen to trypsin) once they enter the duodenum; (3) membrane-bound organelles, which separate proenzymes from the acinar-cell cyto-

plasm; and (4) the presence of trypsin inhibitors (which can inactivate trace amounts of prematurely activated trypsin) in the organelles.[2] An additional safeguard against intrapancreatic proenzyme activation is provided by blood plasma, which contains several powerful antiproteases, including alpha-antitrypsin, alpha-macroglobulin, antichymotrypsin, and others.[3-7]

In humans, the determination of plasma levels of pancreatic proteases by radioimmunoassay has furthered the understanding of the pathophysiologic events in acute pancreatitis.[3] In normal conditions, proteases circulate in blood as proenzymes; in patients with acute pancreatitis, the serum levels of immunoreactive trypsin and chymotrypsin in various molecular forms increase significantly.[8] Although assays for these proteases are not yet readily available, they might have great potential for enhancing accuracy in the diagnosis of acute pancreatitis.

PATHOLOGY

Edematous pancreatitis is the mildest form and is characterized by interstitial edema with a mild inflammatory exudate composed of neutrophils or lymphocytes. Acinar tissue and duct structures remain intact. Slight interstitial fibrosis and some fat necrosis may be present (Figure 1). This inflammatory process can recur on several occasions and resolve without causing major pathologic changes.[9,10]

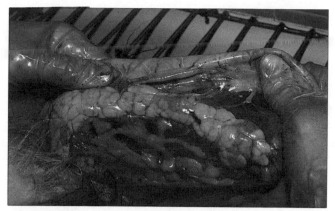

Figure 1—Edematous pancreatitis. The pancreas is swollen, whitish-pink, and glistening. Several small, white calcium-soap deposits are visible in the mesentery.

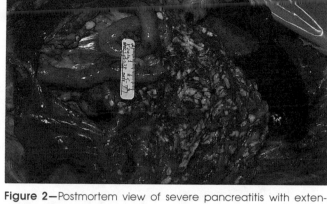

Figure 2—Postmortem view of severe pancreatitis with extensive calcium-soap deposition throughout the omentum and abdominal cavity.

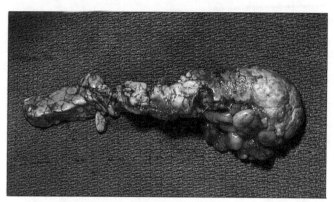

Figure 3—Hemorrhagic necrotic pancreatitis. The chalky white deposits on the surface of the thickened pancreas represent areas of necrosis.

HEMORRHAGIC pancreatitis is characterized by major pathologic changes. Pancreatic parenchyma is destroyed through coagulation necrosis. Leukocyte infiltration tends to be sparse at the onset but more plentiful later. Parenchymal blood vessels may be necrotic, thus perhaps leading to large areas of pancreatic hemorrhage. Fat necrosis can be diffuse and involve the connective tissue septae of the pancreas, the peripancreatic fat, fat in the abdominal cavity, and at times adipose deposits outside the abdominal cavity (Figure 2).

The gland may be mottled by grayish-white areas that indicate parenchymal destruction. Chalky-white deposits signify areas of fat necrosis; friable, soft, red areas indicate zones of destruction associated with bleeding (Figure 3). Areas of mild edema may merge with zones of frank necrosis with hemorrhage.[9,10]

CAUSES

Dogs are spared many of the causes of pancreatitis that affect humans (see the list on page 49); however, several general mechanisms should be considered. Such mechanisms include obstruction of the pancreatic duct, dietary factors, infectious agents, trauma, toxic drug reactions, metabolic abnormalities, and vascular alterations.

Pancreatic Duct Obstruction

Although experimental surgical ligation of the pancreatic duct along with the stimulation for hypersecretion is a common experimental model,[11] documented cases of natural-onset obstructive disease in dogs are rare. Factors that might cause pancreatic-duct occlusion include edema or spasm of the pancreatic-duct sphincter, morphine, duodenal mucosal edema, and tumors.

Once the duct is obstructed, synthesis of pancreatic enzymes and their intracellular transport to the Golgi complex remain normal but the secretion of digestive enzymes is blocked. The digestive enzymes can be found in large vacuoles containing lysosomal hydrolases that are trypsinogen activators. This colocalization might result in the activation of digestive enzymes and the release of the activated enzymes into the acinar-cell cytoplasm, thus causing autodigestion and the further release of additional activated proteases.[2]

Dietary Factors

Nutrition has been implicated as a cause of acute pancreatitis in dogs and other experimental animals. Dogs with pancreatitis are often obese.[12] The feeding of high-fat diets for extended periods can increase susceptibility to the experimental disease in dogs because such diets might cause a permeability defect in the cell membrane of pancreatic acinar cells, thus resulting in increased susceptibility to external injury and autodigestion.[10,13,14]

Infectious Agents

Although viral and parasitic infections have been associated with acute pancreatitis in humans and animals, there is no conclusive evidence that these factors play a causative role in dogs. Bacterial infection also has not been demonstrated to play a causative role in acute pancreatitis; however, it can increase the severity of the disease after the first several days of hemorrhagic necrotic pancreatitis by contributing to the formation of infected pseudocysts and pancreatic abscesses.

Trauma

Accidental or surgical trauma can cause pancreatitis in dogs. Signs of an acute abdominal syndrome after blunt abdominal trauma suggest that acute pancreatitis should be included in the differential diagnosis. Surgical manipulation (as can occur with surgery involving the duodenum, the liver and biliary tree, and the pancreas itself) are especially predisposing.

NUMEROUS drugs have been implicated as causes of pancreatitis in humans. Drugs with a strong association include azathioprine, thiazides, sulfonamides, furosemide, estrogens, and tetracycline.[15-17] Reports in the human medical literature also implicate metronidazole,[18,19] 5-aminosalicylate,[20] various chemotherapeutic agents (e.g., including cisplatin, vinblastine sulfate, bleomycin sulfate, asparaginase, and cytarabine),[21] and enalapril maleate.[22]

Considerable controversy surrounds the role of glucocorticoids as a cause of acute pancreatitis.[23] Although the validity of the older literature has been questioned, I am aware of several instances in which glucocorticoid use preceding the disorder seemed to be more than coincidental.

Metabolic Disorders

Hyperlipidemia and hypercalcemia have been associated with acute pancreatitis in dogs. The exact mechanism involving hypertriglyceridemia remains unclear[24]; perhaps free fatty acids produced by pancreatic lipase are increased to toxic concentrations (which are injurious to various tissues), thus inducing inflammatory changes.[25] There is anecdotal evidence that pancreatitis can occur in miniature schnauzers with idiopathic hyperlipoproteinemia.[26]

Hypercalcemia from any cause can lead to acute pancreatitis. In humans with hyperparathyroidism, acute pancreatitis is especially common.[3] Although the exact mechanism is obscure, the increased concentration of calcium ions in pancreatic secretion and pancreatic tissue might promote activation of trypsinogen, which not only initiates the proteolytic cascade but also stabilizes trypsin, chymotrypsinogen, prophospholipase A, and lipase.[3] Pancreatitis in dogs has been associated with hypercalcemia.[27]

Vascular Alterations

Thromboembolism, vasculitis, and severe hypotension are vascular disorders that can cause pancreatitis.[28] In a series of pathologic examinations of pancreata from humans who died of hypovolemic shock, morphologic evidence of disseminated intravascular coagulation in the pancreas supported the contention that the organ is highly sensitive to disturbances in perfusion.[29] The resulting tissue necrosis is believed to contribute to the intraparenchymal activation of the pancreatic proteases.

PATHOPHYSIOLOGY

A common denominator that can override the protective effects of the antiproteases could involve several factors that disturb cellular metabolism and increase permeability of cellular lipoprotein membranes surrounding the lysosomal hydrolases in the acinar cells, with resultant inappropriate proenzyme activation and autodigestion.[30] Table I lists the characteristics of activated pancreatic enzymes and their effects on the pancreas.

After proenzyme activation, pancreatic elastase and phospholipase A promote coagulation necrosis and vascular injury, including elastolysis, hemorrhage, and thrombosis. These vasoactive peptides (along with trypsin) may account for the glassy edema, the exudation of enzyme-rich fluids, and the severe pain in cases of acute pancreatitis.[3,10]

Phospholipase A can split a fatty acid from lecithin to form lysolecithin, which can cause pancreatic edema and necrosis. There is no known inhibitor of phospholipase A.[3]

WHEN the pancreatic proteases spill into the interstitial spaces of the pancreas and subsequently into the peritoneal fluid and serum, they can be recovered from tissue fluids in a complex with alpha$_2$-macroglobulin or alpha$_1$-antitrypsin or as proenzymes.[3,4] An imbalance of protease inhibitor has been associated with the severity of acute pancreatitis.[3,4] Furthermore, other biochemical abnormalities occur and have far-reaching systemic effects, such as the activation of the complement, kinin, coagulation, and fibrinolytic systems.[31] Finally, local ischemia attributable to impaired pancreatic microcirculation may be a critical factor for the progression from edema to pancreatic necrosis[10,29] (Figure 4).

Marked hypotension can be observed in dogs with acute pancreatitis[32] and is probably the main factor contributing to their demise.[31] Studies of the hemodynamic consequences of severe pancreatitis in humans demonstrate that the cardiac index is increased and the systemic vascular resistance is decreased; these findings are similar to those in patients with sepsis.[31,33] The mechanisms responsible for these effects are unknown, although circulating vasoactive compounds (e.g., bradykinin) and a myocardial depressant factor resulting from pancreatic necrosis remain strong possibilities.[33] Low blood pressure may be attributable to

Causes of Acute Pancreatitis in Humans[3]

- Biliary tract disease
- Ethanol abuse
- Peptic ulcer
- Trauma or surgery
- Vascular factors
- Hyperlipoproteinemia (type I, IV, or V)
- Hypercalcemia
- Drugs
- Hereditary pancreatitis, pancreas divisum
- Infectious agents (viral or bacterial)
- Methanol ingestion
- Scorpion bites (in Trinidad)
- Carcinoma of the pancreas
- Hypotensive shock
- Obstruction of the pancreatic duct by tumors

sequestration of fluid from the plasma space into the potential spaces of the peritoneal cavity and retroperitoneum.[32,34]

Experiments in dogs demonstrate that approximately 35% of the total plasma volume can be lost from the circulation four hours after the induction of acute pancreatitis.[35-37] A recent study in dogs demonstrated that the detrimental effects of acute pancreatitis on cardiovascular function are related solely to hypovolemia and reduced cardiac filling and not to humoral or reflex effects induced by the disease.[38]

DIAGNOSIS

The best way to diagnose acute pancreatitis is to suspect it in any middle-aged or old dog that has a sudden onset of depression, vomiting, and anorexia.

History and Clinical Signs

Most occurrences of acute pancreatitis involve middle-aged, obese female dogs; dogs with normal weight and male dogs can also be affected. The most common history includes a sudden onset of vomiting, anorexia, and depression. Some occurrences reportedly follow the ingestion of a fatty meal, although this event might not be necessary. The vomitus might initially contain partially digested food; later, the vomitus consists of bile and watery mucus. After the initial vomiting, dogs might exhibit regurgitative movements only. Attitude varies from mild to marked depression. Posture may be normal, upright with abdominal tucking, or lateral recumbency depending on the degree of pain and hypovolemia. Diarrhea occasionally occurs, but scant or absent feces is more common because of peritonitis-induced ileus.

The physical examination findings vary with the severity of the problem. Dogs with mild pancreatitis might exhibit only mild depression, normal vital signs, and equivocal abdominal tenderness. Signs associated with the hemorrhagic necrotic form include marked depression; fever; hypotension with accompanying tachypnea, tachycardia, and weak femoral pulse; painful abdomen; and moderate to marked dehydration.

CLINICALLY detectable icterus does not occur initially in patients with necrotic pancreatitis, but it might be evident by the third day of hospitalization and usually results from cholestasis. Bile-duct obstruction occurs rarely. Abdominal distention can result from paralytic ileus. Reddish-brown ascitic fluid sometimes accumulates in patients with hemorrhagic necrotic pancreatitis.

The initial differential diagnosis of acute pancreatitis includes the following disorders:

- Acute gastroenteritis
- Intoxication
- Blunt abdominal trauma
- Gastrointestinal obstruction
- Gastrointestinal perforation
- Intestinal volvulus
- Intestinal ischemia and infarction
- Emphysematous cholecystitis
- Ruptured organs (e.g., uterus, urinary bladder, or gallbladder)
- Acute renal failure
- Acute hepatopathy.

This list is extensive because the signs mimic many acute abdominal syndromes. Several of the differentials are surgical emergencies that require rapid diagnosis and hemodynamic stabilization.

Radiographic Findings

Abdominal radiographs of dogs with acute pancreatitis can demonstrate several abnormalities. In patients with mild edematous pancreatitis, the findings can range from normal to mild ileus involving the stomach and duodenum. The more severe forms cause the following changes as a result of peritonitis: increased fluid density with loss of visceral detail in the cranial abdomen, right-sided lateral displacement of a gas-distended duodenum, and gastric distention[39] (Figure 5). In addition to these classic findings, acute pancreatitis can cause radiographically demonstrable pleural effusion and pulmonary fluid accumulation.

Ultrasonography can be used to detect pathology associated with pancreatitis.[40,41] Although the findings associated with the edematous and hemorrhagic forms might be nonspecific, the findings associated with pancreatic pseudocyst

TABLE I
Characteristics of Pancreatic Enzymes and Their Effects on the Pancreas[a]

Enzyme	Activators	Biochemical Effect	Predominant Histologic Effect on the Pancreas
Trypsin	Enterokinase, cathepsin B, low pH	Proteolysis, activation of proenzymes	Edema, liquefaction necrosis, hemorrhage
Chymotrypsin	Trypsin	Proteolysis	Edema, hemorrhage
Elastase	Trypsin	Blood vessel elastolysis	Hemorrhage
Phospholipase A	Trypsin, bile acids	Formation of lysophosphatides	Coagulation necrosis, fat necrosis
Lipase	Bile acids	Splitting of triglycerides	Fat necrosis

[a]From Creutzfeld W, Schmidt H: Aetiology and pathogenesis of pancreatitis: Current concepts. *Scand J Gastroenterol* 5(Suppl 6):47–62, 1970. Modified with permission.

and abscess tend to be more obvious. Overlying loops of distended bowel are the major limitation of this imaging technique.[42]

Computed tomography is the preferred imaging method for human pancreatic disease.[42] Advantages can include improved abdominal detail that is not hindered by the presence of bowel gas, better definition of anatomic relationships, and a low incidence of unsatisfactory examinations.[42] This imaging technique is available in only a few veterinary hospitals.

Clinicopathologic Findings

The characteristic laboratory test abnormalities (Table II) of acute pancreatitis have been extensively described.[4,31,43-54] The choice between serum amylase or serum lipase as a diagnostic test has been needlessly controversial for several years. If serum amylase is chosen, the procedure must be done by the amyloclastic method; results for normal dogs as well as dogs with pancreatitis, renal failure, or renal failure and acute pancreatitis must be available. Knowledge of these parameters allows improved accuracy in the interpretation of the test results.[4] Increases in serum amylase levels to two to three times normal strongly suggest acute pancreatitis.[55]

The serum lipase level is reportedly more reliable than is serum amylase for diagnosing acute pancreatitis[46,48]; however, lipase as well as amylase may be elevated in patients with such serious abdominal illnesses as hepatopathy or renal or neoplastic disease.[4,44,46] I interpret serum amylase and lipase results solely in the context of the patient's presentation because in several cases laboratory values did not parallel the severity of illness.[43]

TREATMENT
Medical Therapy

Therapy involves restricting oral food intake while providing enough fluids to maintain normal hydration. The following are basic principles for treating severe pancreatitis in dogs:

- Admit to intensive care, and insert an indwelling intravenous catheter.
- Prevent oral intake of food.
- Relieve pain (if severe).
- Administer antibiotics.
- Administer replacement fluids parenterally.
- Administer insulin (if appropriate).

Patients with suspicious yet mild physical signs and history and unremarkable laboratory test results can often be treated conservatively by restricting oral intake for one to two days and periodically offering water. If vomiting continues, no oral intake should be permitted for five to seven more days; the patient's fluid requirements should be met by parenteral fluid administration. In some cases, oral intake of food is prohibited for as long as 14 days.

THE MOST important component of treatment of severe pancreatitis is the provision of adequate parenteral fluids. Marked hypotension in dogs should be treated with rapid volume expansion via lactated Ringer's solution or 0.9% saline at an initial dosage of 70 to 90 ml/kg[a] during the first one to two hours of treatment. After the vital signs are stablized and urine output is noted to be adequate, a maintenance rate of 50 to 100 ml/kg[a] can be given for the remaining 22- to 23-hour period. The intravenous maintenance solution usually consists of 2.5% to 5% dextrose in 0.45% saline supplemented with potassium chloride (3 to 5 mEq/kg/day) and soluble vitamin B complex. Any acid-base abnormalities should be recognized and appropriately treated.

Severely hypoproteinemic patients (serum albumin less

[a]When this article was originally published, more conservative dosages (i.e., 30 to 40 ml/kg loading and 15 to 25 ml/kg maintenance) were given.

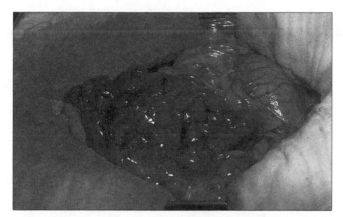

Figure 4A

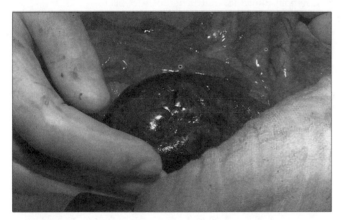

Figure 4B

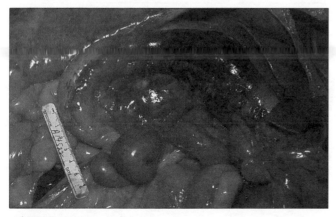

Figure 4C

Figure 4—(**A** and **B**) Surgical views of severe hemorrhagic pancreatitis with omental and pancreatic infarction. (**C**) Postmortem view of the patient; infarction and necrosis of the proximal duodenum, pancreas, and peripancreatic lymph nodes are evident.

than 2.3 g/dl) should receive fresh plasma. Plasma increases the plasma oncotic pressure and helps prevent edema, pleural effusion, pulmonary edema, and renal fail-

ure; it also might be a source of pancreatic protease inhibitors that could be of considerable therapeutic value.[1] Other colloidal solutions, such as hydroxyethyl starch or dextrans, can be used as plasma substitutes.

Urine output should be closely monitored after the volume of the patient's plasma space is adequately expanded. Oliguria or anuria should prompt furosemide-induced diuresis after rehydration is completed. The induction of osmotic diuresis should be avoided if the patient's plasma is already hyperosmotic. During the oliguric period, maintenance volumes of parenteral fluid should equal the volume of urine produced plus insensible fluid losses (10 ml/kg per day). Unsuccessful forced attempts at fluid diuresis during anuria can cause potentially fatal pulmonary edema.

Various gastrointestinal drugs, such as atropine and propantheline bromide, were once commonly used in the management of acute pancreatitis[12]; however, the adverse parasympatholytic side effects often exceeded the benefits.[56] The current recommendation is to withhold these drugs as long as restriction of food and water suppresses vomiting. The antiemetic drug metoclopramide hydrochloride can be used without the parasympatholytic effects typical of many antiemetics. The recommended dosage is 0.2 to 0.4 mg/kg subcutaneously every six to eight hours or 1 mg/kg/day by continuous intravenous infusion.

Cimetidine has been recommended because it inhibits gastric secretion of acid. Although there are theoretical justifications for cimetidine use, no well-controlled clinical trials have substantiated benefit in the treatment of acute pancreatitis.[3,4,56]

Antibiotics are usually reserved for moderately and severely ill patients. Such animals are prone to various conditions, including septicemia, urinary tract infection (especially when an indwelling urethral catheter is used), pneumonia, and pancreatic abscess. Because some of these infections are polymicrobial, broad-spectrum antimicrobial coverage for aerobic and anaerobic bacteria is recommended.[3,40,41] Bacterial infection of the pancreas can result from spread of bacteria from the portal lymph nodes, the biliary tree, the colon, or other body sites.[3] Ampicillin, chloramphenicol, and cephalothin sodium can be safely used. Aminoglycoside antibiotics should be used with caution because of potential nephrotoxicity; the patient's renal function might already be impaired.

PROVIDING adequate nourishment is probably the most difficult aspect of treatment. Although 5% dextrose solution provides some calories that might suffice for the first few days of treatment, it falls far short of the patient's caloric needs for one to two weeks of complete cessation of oral intake; such fasting is sometimes required to inhibit pancreatic secretion of proteolytic enzymes. Most patients are able to resume intake of liquids and then solids after

TABLE II
Clinicopathologic Abnormalities Accompanying Acute Pancreatitis in Dogs

Abnormality	Proposed Mechanism
Leukocytosis	Inflammation, stress, hemoconcentration, secondary infection
Hemoconcentration	Dehydration, translocation of plasma into abdominal cavity
Anemia	Hemorrhagic abdominal effusion, iatrogenic crystalloid fluid effusion
Azotemia	Prerenal from dehydration,[30] renal from hypovolemia or disseminated intravascular coagulation; idiopathic renal failure[52]
Liver enzymes and bilirubin	Focal hepatic necrosis, hepatic lipidosis, cholangiohepatitis, cholangiostasis
Hyperglycemia	Elevated stress hormones (growth hormones, glucocorticoids, glucagon, epinephrine), hypoinsulinemia, destruction of islet beta cells
Hypocalcemia	Calcium-soap formation (the most widely accepted mechanism)[48,53]
Hyperlipidemia	Might preexist as a separate entity; can occur with pancreatitis, but exact mechanism is unknown; possibly related to release of stress hormones (growth hormones, glucocorticoids, glucagon, epinephrine)
Hypernatremia	Dehydration
Hyponatremia	Vomiting, pseudohyponatremia from hyperlipidemia
Hypokalemia	Vomiting, failure to supplement parenteral fluids, osmotic diuresis from hyperglycemia
Hyperamylasemia and hyperlipasemia	Direct venous absorption of enzymes from the inflamed pancreas and absorption via transperitoneal lymphatics and lymphatic drainage from the pancreas and surrounding tissue[70,71]

the first five to seven days of no oral intake.

Intravenous parenteral nutrition should be considered if the patient resumes vomiting after oral feedings commence.[56-60] This therapy is controversial because intravenous infusion of amino acid and lipid solutions can evidently stimulate pancreatic secretion in dogs.[57] Problems associated with intravenous hyperalimentation include catheter-induced phlebitis, septicemia, plasma hyperosmolarity, meticulous preparation requirements, and expense. This feeding technique is thus usually reserved for large medical facilities that can afford the expense and the personnel requirements.

Tube jejunostomy and infusion of elemental nutrients might be an alternative way of nourishing a patient with protracted acute pancreatitis.[58] Hyperalimentation probably has minimal effect on the pathophysiology of acute pancreatitis in humans, but it is a useful adjunct for protracted nutritional support.

Analgesic treatment should be reserved for patients with severe and intractable pain. Phenothiazine drugs are contraindicated initially because they might worsen hypotension. Small doses of meperidine hydrochloride (5 to 10 mg/kg) are the preferred treatment.

Insulin treatment is indicated if blood glucose exceeds 300 mg/dl. Regular crystalline zinc insulin (0.5 U/kg) is preferred because of its short duration of action, especially if the hyperglycemia is transient. If the patient exhibits a continued need for insulin, it should be managed as other diabetics are.

Surgical Therapy

According to one surgeon, "a 10-minute surgical discussion on acute pancreatitis should probably include 9 minutes of silence."[61] This physician was referring to the fact that patients with edematous pancreatitis usually respond well to conservative medical treatment but those with the hemorrhagic form are too moribund to withstand the stress of a major surgical procedure.

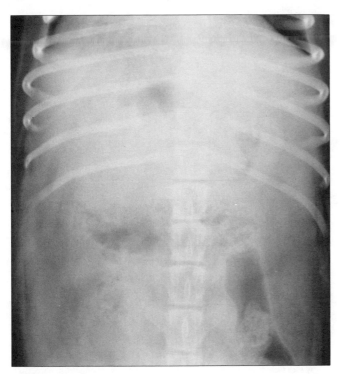

Figure 5—Ventrodorsal radiograph of the upper abdomen of a patient with acute pancreatitis. A hazy fluid accumulation in the upper right quadrant and gastric ileus are apparent.

TABLE III
Complications of Acute Pancreatitis

Complication	Phase of Disease
Diabetes mellitus	Early[a] or late
Pancreatic abscess and pseudocyst	Early
Bowel infarction	Early
Bowel obstruction	Early
Bile-duct obstruction	Early
Renal failure	Early
Septicemia	Early
Consumption coagulopathy	Early
Relapsing pancreatitis	Late
Pancreatic exocrine insufficiency	Late

[a]Within the first 14 days.

There are several major indications for surgery in patients with acute pancreatitis: (1) to rule out surgically correctable disease, such as pancreatic pseudocyst or abscess; (2) to eliminate diseases initiating pancreatic inflammation; (3) to remove necrotic or infected foci during the septic phase of hemorrhagic necrotizing pancreatitis; and (4) to correct complicating problems, such as bile-duct obstruction.[62,63] In a study of pancreatic abscess in six dogs, surgery was performed on four of the patients; three of the four recovered.[41] In another report describing surgical necrosectomy in six dogs with extensive hemorrhagic necrotic pancreatitis, the fatality rate was 100%.[40]

THERE is no easy way to decide whether to perform surgery during the initial stages of acute pancreatitis. In veterinary patients that have an acute abdominal syndrome, the surgeon usually performs a laparotomy in anticipation of finding a perforated viscus. When the surgeon has opened the abdomen, the diagnosis should be readily apparent and the surgeon must decide what to do next. If the patient has edematous pancreatitis, the surgeon should avoid injuring the organ and restrict efforts to peritoneal lavage.

Surgical peritoneal lavage was recommended in the 1970s for humans with severe pancreatitis. The rationale is threefold: (1) it may help establish a diagnosis if hemor-rhagic peritoneal fluid with a high amylase content is aspirated (although this finding is not necessarily confirmatory), (2) it may help determine the severity of the attack (if the aspirate is brownish red), and (3) it may remove the activated proteases and vasoactive substances that are released from the pancreas and that are believed to be responsible for the systemic complications.[64] One major study of humans with alcoholic pancreatitis found no appreciable improvement in morbidity or mortality in patients treated with peritoneal lavage[65]; however, many patients have benefited from this procedure.

I recommend laparotomy and peritoneal lavage for moderately to severely sick patients that fail to respond to medical treatment after the first five to seven days or that are in the early stages of severe hemorrhagic necrotic pancreatitis. Lavage-induced hypoproteinemia and serum electrolyte deficiencies should be corrected with plasma and balanced electrolyte solutions, respectively. At surgery, a jejunostomy tube can be inserted to allow for postoperative enteral feeding.

Although surgery is not routinely recommended initially for most patients with acute pancreatitis, it should be chosen if (1) pancreatic abscess or pseudocyst are suspected; (2) the patient with hemorrhagic necrotic pancreatitis does not adequately respond to medical management, possibly because of extensive phlegmon formation (Figure 6); or (3) bile-duct obstruction or bowel ischemia are suspected. The surgical procedures vary according to the pathology and include peritoneal lavage, necrosectomy,[40] and various pancreatic drainage procedures (e.g., Whipple or Roux-en-Y pancreaticojejunostomy).[66] The prognosis for all patients undergoing such major procedures is guarded to grave.[67]

COMPLICATIONS AND LONG-TERM MANAGEMENT

Table III outlines the complications that can occur during the early and late phases of pancreatitis. Long-term medical management involves a commercial low-fat diet that is divided into two or three feedings per day. Diabetes

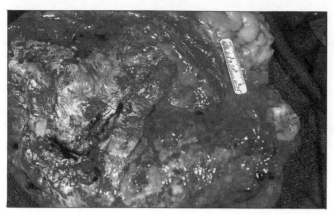

Figure 6—Postmortem view of pancreatic phlegmon. Note the extensive necrosis and calcium-soap formation.

mellitus and exocrine pancreatic insufficiency should be treated according to established protocols.[68,69]

About the Author

Dr. Schaer is affiliated with the Department of Small Animal Clinical Sciences, College of Veterinary Medicine, University of Florida, Gainesville, Florida.

REFERENCES

1. Kukral JC, Adams AP, Preston FW: Protein producing capacity of the human exocrine pancreas: Incorporation of ^{35}S-ethionine in serum and pancreatic juice protein. *Am Surg* 162:63–73, 1965.
2. Steer ML, Meldolesi J: The cell biology of experimental pancreatitis. *N Engl J Med* 316:144–150, 1987.
3. Geokas MC: Acute pancreatitis. *Ann Intern Med* 103:86–100, 1985.
4. Williams DA: Exocrine pancreatic disease, in Ettinger SJ (ed): *Textbook of Veterinary Internal Medicine: Diseases of the Dog and Cat.* Philadelphia, WB Saunders Co, 1989, pp 1528–1554.
5. Satake K, Reichman J, Carballo J, et al: Plasma levels of elastase, trypsin and their inhibitors in bile-induced pancreatitis in the dog. *Ann Surg* 179:58–62, 1974.
6. Ohlsson K, Eddeland A: Release of proteolytic enzymes in bile-induced pancreatitis in dogs. *Gastroenterology* 69:668–675, 1975.
7. Go VLW, Dimagno EP: Normal pancreas, in Gambill EE (ed): *Pancreatitis.* St Louis, CV Mosby Co, 1973, p 14.
8. Geokas MC, Yalow RS, Straus EW, Gold EM: Peptide radioimmunoassays in clinical medicine. *Ann Intern Med* 97:389–407, 1982.
9. Banks PA: *Pancreatitis.* New York, Plenum Medical Book Co, 1979, pp 53–59.
10. Baggenstoss AH: Pathology of pancreatitis, in Gambill EE (ed): *Pancreatitis.* St Louis, CV Mosby Co, 1973, pp 179–212.
11. Estourgie RJA, Yap SH, Van Haelst UJG, DeBoer HHM: The clinical and histopathological effects of pancreatic duct occlusion in experimental acute pancreatitis in dogs. *J Surg Res* 34:164–170, 1983.
12. Anderson NV: Pancreatitis in dogs. *Vet Clin North Am [Small Anim Pract]* 2:79–97, 1972.
13. Haig TH: Cellular membranes in the etiology of acute pancreatitis. *Surg Forum* 20:380–382, 1969.
14. Haig TH: Pancreatic digestive enzymes: Influence of a diet that augments pancreatitis. *J Surg Res* 10:601–607, 1970.
15. Mallory A, Kern F: Drug-induced pancreatitis: A critical review. *Gastroenterology* 78:813–820, 1980.
16. Broe PJ, Cameron JL: Azathioprine and acute pancreatitis: Studies with an isolated perfused canine pancreas. *J Surg Res* 34:159–163, 1983.
17. Moriello KA, Bowen D, Meyer DJ: Acute pancreatitis in two dogs given azathioprine and prednisone. *JAVMA* 191:695–696, 1987.
18. Pltonick BH, Cohen I, Tsang T, Cullinane T: Metronidazole-induced pancreatitis. *Ann Intern Med* 103:891–892, 1985.
19. Sanford KA, Mayle JE, Dean HA: Metronidazole-associated pancreatitis. *Ann Intern Med* 109:756–757, 1988.
20. Sachedina B, Saibil F, Cohen LB, Whittey J: Acute pancreatitis due to 5-aminosalicylate. *Ann Intern Med* 110:490–492, 1989.
21. Socinski MA, Garnick MB: Acute pancreatitis associated with chemotherapy for germ cell tumors in two patients. *Ann Intern Med* 108:567–568, 1988.
22. Tilkemeier P, Thompson PD: Acute pancreatitis possibly related to enalapril. *N Engl J Med* 318:1275–1276, 1988.
23. Steinberg WM, Lewis JH: Steroid-induced pancreatitis: Does it really exist? *Gastroenterology* 81:799–808, 1981.
24. Toskes PP: Hyperlipidemic pancreatitis. *Med Clin North Am* 19:783–792, 1990.
25. Havel RJ: Pathogenesis, differentiation, and management of hypertriglyceridemia. *Adv Intern Med* 15:117–154, 1969.
26. Rogers WA, Donovan EF, Kociba GJ: Idiopathic hyperlipoproteinemia in dogs. *JAVMA* 166:1087–1091, 1975.
27. Neuman NB: Acute hemorrhagic pancreatitis associated with hypercalcemia in a dog. *JAVMA* 166:381–383, 1975.
28. Banks PA: *Pancreatitis.* New York, Plenum Medical Book Co, 1979, pp 34–35.
29. Nikulin EG, Nikulin A, Plamenac P, et al: Pancreatic lesions in shock and their significance. *J Pathol* 135:223–236, 1981.
30. Renner IG, Rinderknecht H, Douglas AP: Profiles of pure pancreatic secretions in patients with acute pancreatitis: The possible role of proteolytic enzymes in pathogenesis. *Gastroenterology* 75:1090–1098, 1978.
31. Pitchumoni CS, Agarwal N, Jain NK: Systemic complications of acute pancreatitis. *Am J Gastroenterol* 83:597–606, 1988.
32. Amundsen E, Ofstad E, Hagen PO: Experimental acute pancreatitis in dogs. I. Hypotensive effect induced by pancreatic exudate. *Scand J Gastroenterol* 3:659–664, 1968.
33. Bradley EL, Hall JR, Lutz J, et al: Hemodynamic consequences of acute pancreatitis. *Ann Surg* 198:130–133, 1983.
34. Takada Y, Appert HE, Howard JM: Vascular permeability induced by pancreatic exudate formed during acute pancreatitis in dogs. *Surg Gynecol Obstet* 143:779–783, 1976.
35. Anderson MC, Schoenfeld FB, Iams WB, Suwa A: Circulatory changes in acute pancreatitis. *Surg Clin North Am* 47:127–140, 1967.
36. Carey LC, Rogers RE: Pathophysiologic alterations in experimental pancreatitis. *Surgery* 60:171–178, 1966.
37. Rylan JW, Moffat JC, Thompson AG: Role of bradykinin system in acute hemorrhagic pancreatitis. *Arch Surg* 91:14–24, 1965.
38. Horton JW, Burnweit CA: Hemodynamic function in acute pancreatitis. *Surgery* 93:538–546, 1988.
39. Klein LJ, Hornbuckle WE: Acute pancreatitis: The radiographic findings in 182 dogs. *J Am Vet Radiol Soc* 19:102–115, 1978.
40. Edwards DF, Bauer MS, Walker MA, et al: Pancreatic masses in seven dogs following acute pancreatitis. *JAAHA* 26:189–198, 1990.
41. Salisbury SK, Lantz GC, Nelson RW, Kazacos EA: Pancreatic abscesses in dogs: Six cases (1978–1986). *JAVMA* 193:1104–1108, 1988.
42. Van Dyke JA, Stanley RJ, Berland LL: Pancreatic imaging. *Ann Intern Med* 102:212–217, 1985.
43. Schaer M: A clinicopathologic survey of acute pancreatitis in 30 dogs and 5 cats. *JAAHA* 15:681–687, 1979.
44. Mulvany MH, Feinberg CK, Tilson DL: Clinical characterization of acute necrotizing pancreatitis. *Compend Contin Educ Pract Vet* 4(5):394–405, 1982.
45. Drew SI, Jaffe B, Vinik A, et al: The first 24 hours of acute pancreatitis—Changes in biochemical and endocrine homeostasis in patients with pancreatitis compared with those in control subjects undergoing stress for reasons other than pancreatitis. *Am J Med* 64:795–803, 1978.
46. Strombeck DR, Farver T, Kaneko JJ: Serum amylase and lipase activities in the diagnosis of pancreatitis in dogs. *Am J Vet Res* 42:1966–1970, 1981.
47. Moosa AR: Diagnostic tests and procedures in acute pancreatitis. *N Engl J Med* 311:639–643, 1984.
48. Steinberg WM, Goldstein SS, Davis ND, et al: Diagnostic assays in acute pancreatitis—A study of sensitivity and specificity. *Ann Intern Med* 102:576–580, 1985.

49. Weir GC, Lesser PB, Drop LJ, et al: The hypocalcemia of acute pancreatitis. *Ann Intern Med* 83:185–189, 1975.
50. Geokas MC, Rinderknecht H, Walberg CB, Weissman R: Methemalbumin in the diagnosis of acute hemorrhagic pancreatitis. *Ann Intern Med* 81:483–486, 1974.
51. Banks PA: *Pancreatitis*. New York, Plenum Medical Book Co, 1979, pp 65–79.
52. Gambill EE: Laboratory tests in pancreatitis, in Gambill EE (ed): *Pancreatitis*. St Louis, CV Mosby Co, 1973, pp 115–128.
53. Goldstein DA, Llach F, Massry SG: Acute renal failure in patients with acute pancreatitis. *Arch Intern Med* 136:1363–1365, 1976.
54. Stewart AF, Longo W, Kreutter D, et al: Hypocalcemia associated with calcium-soap formation in a patient with a pancreatic fistula. *N Engl J Med* 315:496–498, 1986.
55. Polzin DJ, Osborne CA, Stevens JB, Hayden DW: Serum amylase and lipase activities in dogs with chronic primary renal failure. *Am J Vet Res* 44:404–410, 1983.
56. Lankisch PG: Acute and chronic pancreatitis—An update on management. *Drugs* 28:554–564, 1984.
57. Kirby DF, Craig RM: The value of intensive nutritional support in pancreatitis. *J Parenter Enteral Nutr* 9:353–357, 1985.
58. Goodgame JT, Fischer JE: Parenteral nutrition in the treatment of acute pancreatitis. *Ann Surg* 186:651–658, 1977.
59. Blackburn GL, Williams LF, Bistrian BR, et al: New approaches to the management of severe acute pancreatitis. *Am J Surg* 131:114–124, 1976.
60. Armstrong PJ, Lippert AC: Selected aspects of enteral and parenteral nutritional support. *Semin Vet Med Surg [Small Anim]* 3:216–226, 1988.
61. Machleder HI: Surgical management. *Ann Intern Med* 76:111–114, 1972.
62. Frey CF: Surgery for acute pancreatitis. *Ann Intern Med* 103:95–96, 1985.
63. Rosato EF: Aid for the ailing pancreas—Surgery when it's needed. *Emerg Med Clin North Am* 14(4):108–115, 1982.
64. Pellegrini CA: The treatment of acute pancreatitis: A continuing challenge. *N Engl J Med* 312:436–438, 1985.
65. Mayer AD, MacMahon MJ, Corfield AP, et al: Controlled clinical trial of peritoneal lavage for the treatment of severe acute pancreatitis. *N Engl J Med* 312:399–404, 1985.
66. ReMine WH: Surgical treatment, in Gambill EE (ed): *Pancreatitis*. St Louis, CV Mosby Co, 1973, pp 235–259.
67. Gambill EE: Prognosis of pancreatitis, in Gambill EE (ed): *Pancreatitis*. St Louis, CV Mosby Co, 1973, pp 260–281.
68. Schaer M: A review of insulin treatment for the diabetic dog and cat. *Compend Contin Educ Pract Vet* 5(7):579–588, 1983.
69. Williams DA: Exocrine pancreatic insufficiency, in Kirk RW (ed): *Current Veterinary Therapy. X. Small Animal Practice*. Philadelphia, WB Saunders Co, 1989, pp 927–932.
70. Sugimoto Y, Hayakawa T, Kondo T, et al: Alimentary tract and pancreas-peritoneal absorption of pancreatic enzymes in bile-induced acute pancreatitis in dogs. *J Gastroenterol Hepatol* 5:493–498, 1990.
71. Bigelow CP, Strocchi A, Levitt MD: Where does serum amylase come from and where does it go? *Gastroenterol Clin North Am* 19:793–810, 1990.

Current Concepts of the Pathogenesis and Pathophysiology of Acute Pancreatitis in the Dog and Cat*

The Royal Veterinary College
University of London
Kenneth W. Simpson, BVM&S, PhD, MRCVS

KEY FACTS

❏ Acute pancreatitis should always be viewed as a potentially life-threatening condition with a guarded prognosis.

❏ Dietary imbalances, hyperlipidaemia, hypercalcaemia, drugs, and genetic predisposition are considered clinically important risk factors for acute pancreatitis.

❏ Experimental studies suggest that dietary imbalances and hyperstimulation can cause premature activation of digestive enzymes within the pancreatic acinar cell.

❏ The release of active pancreatic enzymes and inflammatory mediators into the circulation is associated with multi-organ dysfunction.

It is now almost a century since pancreatitis and pancreatic acinar atrophy were first recognised in the dog.[1,2] Despite this long time span, the diagnosis of pancreatitis is still difficult to confirm, its treatment is non-specific, and prognosis is always guarded because there are no accurate criteria for predicting response or survival.[3,4] In contrast, pancreatic acinar atrophy, the most common cause of exocrine pancreatic insufficiency (EPI) in the dog,[5,6] can now be reliably diagnosed and treated specifically.[7] The difference in our ability to diagnose and treat these diseases can be attributed to a more complete understanding of the pathophysiology of exocrine pancreatic insufficiency, which has enabled the development of better diagnostic tests and more specific treatment.

The aim of this article is to review current concepts of the pathophysiology of pancreatitis in the dog and cat, with specific emphasis placed on the aetiopathogenesis.

CLASSIFICATION OF PANCREATITIS

Pancreatitis can be broadly categorized as acute, recurrent acute, or chronic. Acute and recurrent acute pancreatitis are characterised by sudden episodes of inflammation of the pancreas and appear to be the most frequent form of pancreatitis in the dog.[6,8] Chronic pancreatitis is associated with progressive, often subclinical, chronic inflammation and seems to be the most common form of pancreatitis in the cat,[9,10] though acute pancreati-

*Editor's Note: The integrity of British English has been preserved in this review article.

TABLE I
Evidence for Involvement

Potential Aetiology	Clinical	Experimental
Hyperlipidaemia or diet	Lipaemia[13–15] Abnormal lipid profiles[18,19] Diet indiscretion[23] Obesity[15,23]	High-fat diet[16,17,22] Intravenous free fatty acids[20] High-fat, low-protein diet[17] Ethionine-supplemented diet[24]
Hypercalcaemia	Calcium infusion[26] Hyperparathyroidism[25]	Calcium infusion[28]

Corticosteroids	Hyperadrenocorticism?
	Steroids in association with
	   disc surgery[27]
		Increased cholecystokinin
		   sensitivity[29]
		Pancreatic ductal hyperplasia[30]

Drug related	L-asparaginase[31] Azathioprine,[32] various[36]	Organophosphates[33]
Ischaemia or reperfusion	Post-gastric dilatation volvulus?	Ex-vivo pancreas[34]
Hereditary	Miniature Schnauzers?[14]	
Bile reflux	Concomitant biliary disease in cats[9,10]	Bile infusion[21]

tis does appear to be emerging as a clinically significant disease in the cat.[11,12]

FACTORS ASSOCIATED WITH THE DEVELOPMENT OF PANCREATITIS

The major factors which have been implicated (by association) as causes of acute pancreatitis in the dog and cat and the experimental evidence to support their involvement are listed in Table I.

The frequent association of obesity and lipaemia with acute pancreatitis in dogs has led to speculation that diet or disturbances in lipid metabolism cause pancreatitis.[13–15,23] The development of pancreatitis and fatty liver in 11 of 13 animals fed a high-fat low-protein diet[17] and an increased severity of pancreatitis in dogs on a high-fat diet[16,22] provide experimental support. Further evidence that diet influences the development of pancreatitis was provided by Lopes de Almeida and Grossman,[24] who clearly demonstrated that ethionine supplementation results in pancreatitis. Therefore it seems highly likely that diet has a significant role in the development of pancreatitis. Analysis of plasma lipids from dogs with naturally occurring and experimental pancreatitis has not established a clear-cut abnormality of lipid metabolism predisposing dogs to the development of pancreatitis.[14,18,19]

Pancreatitis has been associated with hypercalcaemia in several dogs with hyperparathyroidism and a dog receiving a calcium infusion.[25,26] Pancreatitis in the cat has been induced experimentally by ionised calcium concentrations greater than 1.8 mM.[28] How-

ever, as pancreatitis does not appear to be a common abnormality in animals with hypercalcaemia,[35] the clinical significance of hypercalcaemia as a cause of pancreatitis is unclear.

While many drugs have been associated with the development of pancreatitis in humans,[36] reports of drug-induced pancreatitis in dogs and cats are scant. Azathioprine, L-asparaginase, and corticosteroids in association with spinal surgery have been associated with pancreatitis in dogs.[27,31,32] Anecdotal reports suggest that pancreatitis is common in dogs with hyperadrenocorticism and that dogs given glucocorticoids are more likely to develop pancreatitis. Experimentally, corticosteroids increase the sensitivity of dispersed acinar cells to cholecystokinin (CCK) and stimulate proliferation of the pancreatic ductular epithelium.[29,30] However, firm evidence which clearly establishes a link between pancreatitis and hyperadrenocorticism or administration of glucocorticoids is not available.

Ischaemia and reperfusion injury have been demonstrated to cause pancreatitis experimentally[34] and may be involved in pancreatitis observed in dogs with gastric dilatation volvulus syndrome.

Hereditary factors may influence the development of pancreatitis.[37] These factors may be associated with the high prevalence of pancreatitis in miniature Schnauzers.

As a cause-and-effect relationship has not been clearly established for factors associated with naturally occurring pancreatitis (hyperlipidaemia, diet, excessive circulating glucocorticoids, hypercalcaemia)

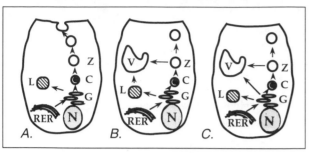

Figure 1—Intracellular trafficking of digestive and lysosomal enzymes. Digestive and lysosomal enzymes are synthesised in the rough endoplasmic reticulum (*RER*) and transported to the Golgi apparatus (*G*) next to the nucleus (*N*). *A.* Normal separation of lysosomal and digestive enzymes. Digestive enzymes are concentrated in condensing vacuoles (*C*) and zymogen granules (*Z*) that fuse with the luminal plasma membrane and release their contents into the luminal space by exocytosis. *B.* A choline-deficient ethionine-supplemented diet blocks exocytosis and zymogen granules accumulate. The zymogen granules fuse with lysosomes to form large vacuoles (*V*) which contain digestive and lysosomal enzymes. *C.* Hyperstimulation with caerulein results in co-segregation of lysosomal and digestive enzymes in large vacuoles. Mature zymogen granules also fuse with these vacuoles. Exocytosis at the luminal plasma membrane is blocked.(Adapted from Steer ML, Meldolesi J: The cell biology of experimental pancreatitis. *N Engl J Med* 316:144–150, 1987.)

and as most animals with these factors do not develop pancreatitis, it is perhaps wise to consider them as risk factors rather than direct causes.

INITIATING MECHANISMS

Irrespective of the underlying aetiology, pancreatitis is considered to occur when pancreatic enzymes are activated within the pancreas.[38] In the normal pancreas, safeguards are present to ensure that harmful pancreatic enzymes are not activated until they reach the intestinal lumen.[39] Pancreatic enzymes are synthesised in the endoplasmic reticulum, modified in the Golgi apparatus, and stored in zymogen granules within the acinar cell in the presence of pancreatic secretory trypsin inhibitor (PSTI) (Figure 1A). Enzymes are released at the apical surface directly into the duct system and are activated in the intestine by trypsin, following the cleavage of trypsin activation peptide from trypsinogen by enterokinase. Potential sites for the intrapancreatic activation of pancreatic enzymes can therefore logically be divided into interstitial (within the duct system and interstitium) and intracellular (within the acinar cell). Experimental studies suggest that bile and enteric reflux and intravenous free fatty acid (FFA) infusion initiate pancreatitis by an interstitial mechanism[40,41]; whereas hyper-

stimulation with caerulein (cerulein), pancreatic duct obstruction, and a choline-deficient ethionine-supplemented diet (CDE diet)[38,42,43] result in intracellular activation.

INTERSTITIAL ACTIVATION

Enteric reflux introduces enterokinase, trypsin, bile salts, and lecithin (phosphatidylcholine) into the pancreatic duct system. Enterokinase catalyses the conversion of trypsinogen to trypsin with subsequent activation of proelastase, prophospholipase A_2, chymotrypsinogen, and procarboxypeptidase to their active forms. Lecithin in bile is converted by phospholipase A_2 to lysolecithin and in concert with bile salts damages ductal and acinar cell membranes.[41] The net result is massive destruction of pancreatic acinar tissue and haemorrhagic pancreatitis.

Intravenous free fatty acid infusion in the ex-vivo perfused pancreas results in edematous pancreatitis.[20] Pancreatitis is largely prevented by pre-treatment with allopurinol, catalase, and superoxide dismutase, suggesting that free fatty acid infusion results in the generation of excessive amounts of free radicals (superoxide, hydroxyl, and peroxide) by activation of xanthine oxidase.[40] White blood cell depletion has no effect on the development of the lesion, suggesting an alternate site of free radical generation.[44]

In-vitro free fatty acids, generated by the action of lipase on triglycerides, damage the acinar cell membrane, releasing lecithin, which when converted to lysolecithin by phospholipase A_2 causes marked necrosis of acinar cells.[45,46]

Intracellular Activation

It is widely recognized that cholecystokinin and acetylcholine (ACh) are the principal physiologic mediators of pancreatic enzyme secretion. They are thought to initiate fusion of zymogen granules with the apical acinar cell membrane via the second messengers inositol 1,4,5-triphosphate and diacylglycerol[47] (Figure 2). Hyperstimulation of the pancreas with supraphysiologic doses of caerulein (a cholecystokinin analogue) appears to cause pancreatitis in experimental animals by interfering with the intracellular trafficking of proteins leading to co-segregation of pancreatic zymogens and lysosomal enzymes (Figure 1C).[38,42,48] The lysosomal enzyme cathepsin B is then thought to activate trypsinogen (pancreatic secretary trypsin inhibitor appears to be inactive in the lysosomal compartment) and precipitate pancreatitis. Feeding a choline-deficient ethionine-supplemented diet and stimulating pancreatic secretion in the face of ductal obstruction also appear to initiate pancreatitis intracellularly.[49,50] This diet results in the accumulation

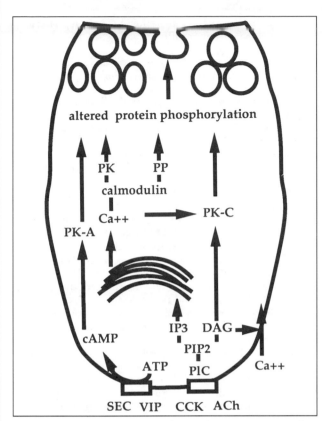

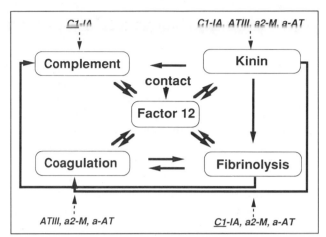

Figure 2—Summary diagram of stimulus-secretion coupling of pancreatic acinar cell protein secretion. Cholecystokinin (*CCK*) and acetylcholine (*ACh*) act via the second messengers inositol triphosphate and diacylglycerol while secretin (*SEC*) and vasoactive intestinal peptide (*VIP*) act via cyclic AMP (*cAMP*) to cause increases in intracellular calcium and protein kinases which result in altered phosphorylation of structural and regulatory proteins and acinar cell protein secretion. *PIP2* = phosphatidylinositol 4,5-bisphosphate; *IP3* = inositol 1,4,5-triphosphate; *DAG* = diacylglycerol; *PK-A* = cyclic AMP activated protein kinase; *PK* = protein kinase; *PP* = protein phosphatase; *PK-C* = phospholipid-dependent protein kinase; *Ca++* = calcium ion.

Figure 3—Schematic diagram of the complex interactions of the complement, kinin, fibrinolytic, and coagulation pathways following activation of factor 12 (Hageman factor) by contact or trypsin. Inhibitors are shown in italics. *ATIII* = antithrombin III; *a2M* = alpha₂-macroglobulin; *a-AT* = alpha₁-antitrypsin; *C1-1A* = complement fragment C1̄,1Ā. (Adapted with permission from Lasson A: Acute pancreatitis in man. A clinical and biochemical study of pathophysiology and treatment. *Scand J Gastroenterol [Suppl]* 99:1–57, 1984.)

of zymogen granules within the acinar cell and fusion with lysosomes (Figure 1B) and is considered a consequence of uncoupling the formation of inositol triphosphate from phosphatidylinositol 4,5-bisphosphate (Figure 2).[51] Pancreatic duct obstruction also appears to cause co-segregation of zymogens and lysosomal enzymes.[43,49] Organophosphates and intravenous calcium could also potentially cause pancreatitis by hyperstimulation. However, despite the apparent similarities of the ultrastructural findings in these models, it is still not known why caerulein hyperstimulation results in oedematous pancreatitis and choline-deficient ethionine-supplemented diet in haemorrhagic pancreatitis. In addition, it has become clear that lysosomal co-segregation with zymogen granules does not automatically

result in pancreatitis; therefore some trigger mechanism may be involved.[43]

Although it is premature to ascribe sites of activation for naturally occurring pancreatitis, it is interesting to speculate about its potential aetiopathogenesis. One example is that long-term ingestion of a high-fat diet could result in pancreatitis following chronic hyperstimulation of the pancreas by cholecystokinin released in response to intraluminal fat. A high-fat meal could also damage acinar cells and blood vessels as a result of free fatty acids and lecithin generated by the action of lipase on excessive amounts of circulating triglycerides. The threshold for hyperstimulation could be decreased in dogs with hyperadrenocorticism. Abuse of organophosphate flea products or hypercalcaemia could potentially induce pancreatitis by hyperstimulation. The development of chronic pancreatitis in the cat may be due to interstitial activation by bile reflux secondary to biliary disease.

PATHOPHYSIOLOGY

Regardless of initiating cause, active pancreatic enzymes (trypsin, phospholipase, collagenase, and elastase)[52-54] and inflammatory mediators (kallikreins, kinins, free radicals, complement factors, and thromboplastins)[55,57,65] are released into the pancreatic tissues and blood vessels. Activated factor 12 (Hageman factor) and trypsin appear to be largely responsible for the activation of the coagulation, fibrinolytic, kinin, and complement cascades[57] (Figure 3). Circulating defence mechanisms in the form of alpha$_1$-antitrypsin and alpha$_2$-macroglobulin bind to active enzymes to contain local and prevent systemic damage.[52,57,63] When these defences are overwhelmed, increased pancreatic capillary permeability leads to fluid loss into the pancreas and the abdomen, a decline in pancreatic blood flow, and an increase in the local concentrations of pancreatic enzymes and inflammatory mediators. Large numbers of leukocytes migrate to the inflamed pancreas and serve as a continued source of free radicals, inflammatory mediators, and enzymes.[58] This viscious, self-perpetuating cycle can ultimately lead to thrombosis of pancreatic blood vessels and pancreatic necrosis. Systemic complications can develop, such as impaired cardiovascular function (hypovolaemic shock, myocardial damage[55,56,66]), haematological function (disseminated intravascular coagulation[57,59,66]), respiratory function (pleural effusion[25,66]), hepatic function (parenchymal damage, biliary stasis[60,66]), renal function (glomerular, tubular damage[61,66]), and metabolic function (lipaemia, hypocalcaemia, diabetes mellitus, hypoproteinaemia[14,25,62,64,67]). In experimental pancreatitis, death ensues when alpha$_2$-macroglobulin is depleted.[57]

CONCLUSIONS

It is hoped that continued advances in pancreatic physiology and pathophysiology will enable the identification of mechanisms which cause pancreatitis and enable the development of diagnostic tests and therapeutics specific for acute pancreatitis.

About the Author

Dr. Simpson is affiliated with the Department of Small Animal Medicine and Surgery, The Royal Veterinary College, University of London in Hatfield, Herts, England. He is a Diplomate of the American College of Veterinary Internal Medicine.

REFERENCES

1. Prettner M: Haemorrhagia pancreatitis beim hund. *Tierartzl Zentbl* 17:342–343, 1894.
2. Ball V: Aplasie du Pancreas. *J Med Vet* 62:200-204, 1911.
3. Murtaugh RJ: Acute pancreatitis: Diagnostic dilemmas. *Seminars in Veterinary Medicine and Surgery (Small Animal)* 2:282–295, 1987.
4. Williams DA: Exocrine pancreatic disease, in Ettinger SJ (ed): *Textbook of Veterinary Internal Medicine*, ed 3, vol 2. Philadelphia, WB Saunders Co, 1989, pp 1528–1554.
5. Holroyd JB: Canine exocrine pancreatic disease. *J Small Anim Pract* 9:269–281, 1968.
6. Rimaila-Parnanen E, Westermarck E: Pancreatic degenerative atrophy and chronic pancreatitis in dogs; a comparative study of 60 cases. *Acta Vet Scand* 23:400–406, 1982.
7. Williams DA, Batt RM: Sensitivity and specificity of serum trypsin-like immunoreactivity for the diagnosis of canine exocrine pancreatic insufficiency. *JAVMA* 192:195–201, 1988.
8. Anderson NV, Low DC: Diseases of the canine pancreas: A comparative study of 103 cases. *Anim Hosp* 1:189–194, 1965.
9. Duffel SJ: Some aspects of pancreatic disease in the cat. *J Small Anim Pract* 16:365-374, 1975.
10. Owens JM, Drazner FH, Gilbertson SR: Pancreatic disease in the cat. *JAAHA* 11:83–89, 1975.
11. Macy DW: Feline pancreatitis, in Kirk RW (ed): *Current Veterinary Therapy. Small Animal Practice. X.* Philadelphia, WB Saunders Co, 1989, pp 893–896.
12. Hill R, Van Winkle TJ: Acute pancreatitis in the cat. *Proc Eighth Annu Vet Med Forum ACVIM*:329-331, 1990.
13. Rogers WA, Donovan EF, Kociba GJ: Idiopathic hyperlipoproteinemia in dogs. *JAVMA* 166:1087–1091, 1975.
14. Rogers WA, Donovan EF, Kociba GJ: Lipids and lipoproteins in normal dogs and dogs with secondary hyperlipoproteinemia. *JAVMA* 166:1092–1100, 1975.
15. Thordal-Christensen A, Coffin DL: Pancreatic disease in the dog. *Nord Vet Med* 8:89–114, 1956.
16. Goodhead B: Importance of nutrition in the pathogenesis of experimental pancreatitis in the dog. *Arch Surg* 103:724–728, 1971.
17. Lindsay S, Entenmann C, Chaikoff IL: Pancreatitis accompanying hepatic disease in dogs fed a high fat, low protein diet. *Arch Pathol* 45:635–638, 1948.
18. Whitney MS, Boon GD, Rebar AH, Ford RB: Effects of acute pancreatitis on circulating lipids in dogs. *Am J Vet Res* 48:1492–1497, 1987.
19. Bass VD, Hoffman WE, Dorner JL: Normal canine lipid profiles and effects of experimentally induced pancreatitis and hepatic necrosis on lipids. *Am J Vet Res* 37:1355–1357, 1976.
20. Saharia P, Margolis S, Zuidema GD, Cameron JL: Acute pancreatitis with hyperlipemia: Studies with an isolated perfused canine pancreas. *Surgery* 82:60–67, 1977.
21. Reber HA: Pancreatic duct and microvascular permeability to macromolecules: The relation to acute pancreatitis. *Scand J Gastroenterol* 20(Suppl 112):96–100, 1985.
22. Haig TH: Pancreatic digestive enzymes: Influence of a diet that augments pancreatitis. *J Surg Res* 10:601–608, 1970.
23. Anderson NV: Pancreatitis in dogs. *Vet Clin North Am* 2:79–96, 1972.
24. Lopes de Almeida A, Grossman MI: Experimental production of pancreatitis with ethionine. *Gastroenterology* 20:554–577, 1952.
25. Schaer M: A clinicopathologic survey of acute pancreatitis in 30 dogs and 5 cats. *JAAHA* 15:681–687, 1979.
26. Neuman NB: Acute hemmorrhagic pancreatitis associated with iatrogenic hypercalcemia in a dog. *JAVMA* 166:381–382, 1975.
27. Moore RW, Withrow SJ: Gastrointestinal hemorrhage and pancreatitis associated with intervertebral disk disease in the dog. *JAVMA* 180:1443–1447, 1982.
28. Frick TW, Hailemariam S, Heitz PU, et al: Acute hypercalcemia induces acinar cell necrosis and intraductal protein precipitates in the pancreas of cats and guinea pigs. *Gastroenterology* 98:1675–1681, 1990.
29. Otsuki M, Okabayashi Y, Nakamura T, et al: Hydrocortisone treatment increases the sensitivity and responsiveness to cholecystokinin in rat pancreas. *Am J Physiol* 257:G364–G370, 1989.
30. Bourry J, Sarles H: Secretory pattern and pathological study of the pancreas of steroid-treated rats. *Dig Dis Sci* 23:423–428, 1978.

31. Hansen JF, Carpenter RH: Fatal acute systemic anaphylaxis and hemorrhagic pancreatitis following asparaginase treatment in a dog. *JAAHA* 19:977–980, 1983.

32. Moriello KA, Bowen D, Meyer DJ: Acute pancreatitis in two dogs given azathioprine and prednisone. *JAVMA* 191:695–696, 1987.

33. Dressel TD, Goodale RL, Arneson MA, et al: Pancreatitis as a complication of anticholinesterase insectiside intoxication. *Ann Surg* 189:199–204, 1979.

34. Broe PI, Zuidema GD, Cameron JL: The role of ischemia in acute pancreatitis: Studies with the isolated perfused canine pancreas. *Surgery* 91:377–382, 1982.

35. Chew DJ, Carothers M: Hypercalcemia. *Vet Clin North Am [Small Anim Pract]* 19(2):265–287, 1989.

36. Mallory A, Kern F: Drug-induced pancreatitis: A critical review. *Gastroenterology* 78:813–818, 1980.

37. Gross JB: Hereditary pancreatitis, in Go VLW, et al (eds): *The Exocrine Pancreas: Biology, Pathology and Diseases.* New York, Raven Press 1986, p 829.

38. Steer ML, Meldolesi J: Pathogeneis of acute pancreatitis. *Ann Rev Med* 39:95–105, 1988.

39. Rindernecht H: Activation of pancreatic zymogens. Normal activation, premature intrapancreatic activation, protective mechanisms against inappropriate activation. *Dig Dis Sci* 31:314–321, 1986.

40. Sanfey H, Bulkley GB, Cameron JL: The pathogenesis of acute pancreatitis; the source and role of oxygen-derived free radicals in three different experimental models. *Ann Surg* 201:633–639, 1985.

41. Adler G: Experimental models and concepts in acute pancreatitis, in Go VLW, et al (eds): *The Exocrine Pancreas: Biology, Pathology and Diseases.* New York, Raven Press 1986, p 407.

42. Steer ML, Meldolesi J: The cell biology of experimental pancreatitis. *N Engl J Med* 316:144–150, 1987.

43. Ohshio G, Saluja I, Steer ML: Effects of short-term pancreatic duct obstruction in rats. *Gastroenterology* 100:196–202, 1991.

44. Sarr MG, Bulkley GB, Cameron JL: The role of leukocytes in the production of oxygen-derived free radicals in acute experimental pancreatitis. *Surgery* 101:292–296, 1987.

45. Mossner J, Boedeker H, Kimura W, et al: Role of lipolytic enzymes and their substrates in the pathogenesis of acute pancreatitis. Part 2: Phospholipase A_2. *Gastroenterology* 100:A279, 1991.

46. Kimura W, Mossner JW, Boedeker H, et al: Role of lipolytic enzymes and their substrates in the pathogenesis of acute pancreatitis. Part 1: Lipase. *Gastroenterology* 100:A290, 1991.

47. Hootman SR, Williams JA: Stimulus secretion coupling in the pancreatic acinus, in Johnson LR (ed): *Physiology of the Gastrointestinal Tract.* New York, Raven Press, p 1129–1146.

48. Saluja AK, Hashimoto S, Saluja M, et al: Subcellular redistribution of lysosomal enzymes during cerulin-induced pancreatitis. *Am J Physiol* 251:G508–G516, 1987.

49. Saluja A, Saluja M, Villa A, et al: Pancreatic duct obstruction in rabbits causes digestive zymogen and lysosomal enzyme colocalization. *J Clin Invest* 84:1260–1266, 1989.

50. Koike H, Steer ML, Meldolesi J: Pancreatic effects of ethionine: Blockade of exocytosis and appearance of crinophagy and autophagy precede cellular necrosis. *Am J Physiol* 242:G297–G307, 1982.

51. Powers RE, Saluja AK, Houlihan MJ, et al: Diminished agonist-stimulated inositol triphosphate generation blocks stimulus-secretion coupling in mouse pancreatic acini during diet-induced experimental pancreatitis. *J Clin Invest* 77:1668–1674, 1986.

52. Ohlsson K: Experimental pancreatitis in the dog: Appearance of complexes between proteases and trypsin inhibitors in ascitic fluid, lymph and plasma. *Scand J Gastroenterol* 6:645–652, 1971.

53. Westermarck E, Rimaila-Parnanen E: Serum phospholipase A_2 in acute pancreatitis. *Acta Vet Scand* 24:477–487, 1983.

54. Borgstrom A, Ohlsson K: Immunoreactive trypsins in the sera from dogs before and after induction of experimental pancreatitis. *Hoppe-Seyelers Z Physiol Chem* 361:625–631, 1980.

55. Satake K, Rozmanith JS, Appert HE, et al: Hemodynamic change and bradykinin levels in plasma and lymph during experimental acute pancreatitis in dogs. *Ann Surg* 178:659–662, 1973.

56. Satake K, Rozmanith JS, Appert HE, et al: Hypotension and release of kinin-forming enzyme into ascitic fluid exudate during experimental pancreatitis in dogs. *Ann Surg* 177:497–502, 1973.

57. Lasson A: Acute pancreatitis in man. A clinical and biochemical study of pathophysiology and treatment. *Scand J Gastroenterol [Suppl]* 99:1–57, 1984.

58. Rindernecht H: Fatal pancreatitis, a consequence of excessive leukocyte stimulation? *Int J Pancreatology* 3:105–112, 1988.

59. Feldman BF, Attix EA, Strombeck DR, et al: Biochemical and coagulation changes in a canine model of acute necrotizing pancreatitis. *Am J Vet Res* 42:805–809, 1981.

60. Andrzejewska A, Dlugosz J, Kurasz S: The ultrastructure of the liver in acute experimental pancreatitis in dogs. *Exp Pathol* 18:167–176, 1985.

61. Giacobino JP, Simon GT: Experimental glomerulonephritis induced by minimal doses of trypsin. *Arch Pathol* 91:193–200, 1971.

62. Jacobs RM, Murtaugh RJ, DeHoff WD: Review of the clinicopathological findings of acute pancreatitis in the dog: Use of an experimental model. *JAAHA* 21:795–780, 1985.

63. Murtaugh RJ, Jacobs RM: Serum antiprotease concentrations in dogs with spontaneous and experimentally induced acute pancreatitis. *Am J Vet Res* 46:80–83, 1985.

64. Ling GV, Lowenstine LJ, Pulley LT, et al: Diabetes mellitus in dogs: A review of initial evaluation, immediate and long term management, and outcome. *JAVMA* 170:521–530, 1977.

65. Glazer G, Bennett A: Prostaglandin release in canine acute hemorrhagic pancreatitis. *Gut* 17:22–26, 1976.

66. Pitchumoni CS, Agarwal N, Jain NK: Systemic complications of acute pancreatitis. *Gastroenterology* 83:597–606, 1988.

67. Kitchell B, Strombeck DR, Cullen J, et al: Clinical and pathologic changes in experimentally induced acute pancreatitis in cats. *Am J Vet Res* 47:1170–1173, 1986.

New Tests of Pancreatic and Small Intestinal Function

Purdue University
David A. Williams, MA, Vet MB, PhD, MRCVS

KEY FACTS

- ❏ **Trypsinogen is synthesized only by pancreatic acinar cells.**

- ❏ **Trypsinogen normally leaks from the pancreas and can be measured in serum using a radioimmunoassay for trypsin-like immunoreactivity.**

- ❏ **Assay of serum trypsin-like immunoreactivity is a sensitive and specific test for canine exocrine pancreatic insufficiency.**

- ❏ **Folate is absorbed only in the upper small intestine, cobalamin only in the lower small intestine.**

- ❏ **Small intestinal bacterial overgrowth may increase folate absorption but decrease cobalamin absorption.**

- ❏ **Assay of serum cobalamin and folate and of fecal proteolytic activity can be used to investigate suspected malabsorption in cats.**

Clinical signs of weight loss and diarrhea are common with diseases in which digestion of food or subsequent absorption of nutrients or both are defective. These disorders are traditionally classified as either primary failure to digest the food (maldigestion) or primary failure to absorb the constituent nutrients (malabsorption). The principal cause of maldigestion is exocrine pancreatic insufficiency, while most cases of malabsorption are caused by small intestinal disease.[1] This manner of classification is somewhat misleading because failure of absorption is an inevitable consequence of defective digestion. Furthermore, most diseases affecting the small intestine inevitably impair the terminal processes of digestion that take place at the luminal surface of the intestinal mucosa. This division does nonetheless emphasize that the most useful application of tests of pancreatic and intestinal function is to distinguish patients with exocrine pancreatic insufficiency from those with small intestinal disease.

Established tests for evaluation of possible maldigestion or malabsorption in dogs include microscopic examination of feces for the presence of undigested food, several methods that indirectly assess fat absorption, assay of pancreatic enzyme activities in feces, and bentiromide (N-benzoyl-L-tyrosyl-p-aminobenzoic acid, BT-PABA) and xylose absorption tests.[1,2] Many of these tests have found limited application because of their unreliability (lack of sensitivity or specificity),[3] practical constraints, or expense. Several new tests are now available to the veterinary practitioner and are the focus of this article.

TESTS FOR EXOCRINE PANCREATIC INSUFFICIENCY

Previously available tests of pancreatic function include the oral fat absorption test (plasma turbidity test),[4] starch tolerance test,[5] assay of pancreatic proteolytic enzyme activity in feces,[5–12] and the bentiromide test.[13–17] Unfortunately, the more easily employed of these tests are frequently misleading or unhelpful because they yield a high proportion of equivocal results.

Measurement of fecal proteolytic activity is a reliable indicator of pancreatic function provided that a reproducible assay method (such as measuring digestion of casein-based substrates) is used.[11] At least three fecal samples collected on different days, a three-day pooled collection of feces, or (in

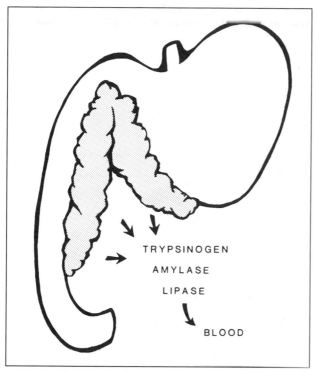

Figure 1—The source of pancreatic zymogens (trypsinogen) and enzymes (amylase, lipase) in the bloodstream. These proteins leak either directly from pancreatic cells into venous blood or indirectly via lymphatic vessels. Enzymes are not absorbed intact into the portal blood following secretion into the intestinal lumen.

dogs) feces collected after feeding a soybean meal supplement for two days must be examined.[12] The bentiromide test also identifies most dogs affected with exocrine insufficiency, although some dogs with small intestinal disease also have abnormal bentiromide test results. Neither of these tests has found wide application in general practice, largely because of practical constraints. The results of the bentiromide test in normal cats vary widely, and fecal proteolytic assay by a reproducible method remains the test of choice for exocrine pancreatic function in this species.[12] In dogs, however, it has been shown that radioimmunoassay of serum trypsin-like immunoreactivity in a single serum sample is a convenient, sensitive, and specific test for identification of dogs with exocrine pancreatic insufficiency.

Serum Trypsin-like Immunoreactivity

Serum trypsin-like immunoreactivity (TLI) refers to the concentration of proteins recognized by antibodies raised against the pancreatic digestive enzyme trypsin. In healthy animals, serum TLI results from the presence of trypsinogen, the inactive zymogen form of the enzyme, which leaks out of the pancreas in trace amounts (Figure 1). There are two immuno-

logically distinct isoenzymes of trypsinogen (anionic and cationic) in most species. The cationic isoenzyme has been assayed in most clinical studies. Serum TLI can be detected in all normal dogs provided that a species-specific assay[a] is used.[18] Assays for human TLI do not detect canine TLI. Serum TLI concentrations in 100 normal dogs, determined using an assay developed by the author, ranged from 5.0 to 35.0 μg/L (mean 14.0 μg/L). Another laboratory, using a different assay, reported values from 7.0 to 19.0 μg/L in a group of 10 normal dogs.[19]

The total daily flow of cationic trypsinogen into the blood accounts for 0.01% to 0.1% of the total daily production.[20] The half-life of circulating trypsinogen is short (less than 30 minutes) because its low molecular weight (approximately 24,000) and the fact that it does not bind to other serum proteins allow it to pass readily through the glomerular filter. Filtered trypsinogen is subsequently catabolized by renal tubular cells.[20] Preliminary clinical observations indicate that serum TLI concentrations are sometimes above normal in dogs with naturally occurring renal failure; these findings are consistent with experimental findings in nephrectomized dogs.[21]

Trypsin-like immunoreactivity is a pancreas-specific marker because trypsinogen is synthesized and stored only in pancreatic acinar cells. Evidence that serum TLI is a clinical marker for exocrine pancreatic function comes from the observation that concentrations in humans with chronic pancreatitis decline in parallel to the progressive decrease in bicarbonate and enzyme secretion. Steatorrhea does not develop in such patients until the concentration of serum TLI falls below normal.[22–24] In contrast with serum TLI, canine amylase and lipase activities are not exclusively pancreatic in their origins. Quantitation of a putative pancreas-specific isoenzyme of amylase, using either electrophoresis or selective inhibition, has not yet proved reliable in the identification of dogs with exocrine pancreatic insufficiency.[25–28]

Pancreatic acinar atrophy, the most common cause of canine exocrine pancreatic insufficiency, is characterized by almost total absence of pancreatic acinar cells. It is, therefore, not surprising that serum TLI concentrations are dramatically reduced (<2.5 μg/L) in affected dogs (Figure 2).[18] In contrast, serum TLI concentrations in dogs with small intestinal disease are not significantly different from those in healthy control dogs (Figure 2). Intestinal disease does not affect serum TLI because pancreatic enzymes enter the blood directly from the pancreas and are not absorbed intact from the intestinal lumen.[29–31]

[a]Canine TLI Assay, Diagnostic Products Corporation, 5700 West 96th Street, Los Angeles, CA 90045. Telephone (213) 776-0180; FAX (213) 642-0192.

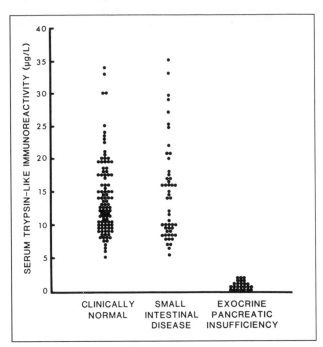

Figure 2—Serum trypsin-like immunoreactivity in normal dogs, dogs with small intestinal disease, and dogs with exocrine pancreatic insufficiency. (From Williams DA, Batt RM: Sensitivity and specificity of radioimmunoassay of serum trypsin-like immunoreactivity for the diagnosis of canine exocrine pancreatic insufficiency. *JAVMA* 192:195–201, 1988. Reproduced with permission.)

Serum TLI is stable under normal circumstances, and specimens can be shipped without special packing precautions for analysis at an appropriate laboratory. Dogs that are already being treated with pancreatic enzymes can be tested without undergoing a withdrawal period.

A very small portion of samples submitted to the author's laboratory for assay of TLI has borderline subnormal concentrations in the range 3.0 to 5.0 μg/L. The dogs involved have been unavailable for further investigation using alternative tests, but on repeat assay of serum TLI results have usually been either clearly normal or diagnostically subnormal. A few dogs with exocrine pancreatic insufficiency exhibit a transient rise in serum TLI following a meal (Figure 3). Failure to obtain serum after withholding food for at least three hours may explain the initial equivocal results in dogs that clearly have exocrine pancreatic insufficiency on retesting.

Prolonged exposure of serum to excessive heat during shipping with resultant deterioration of TLI might explain the variation of results between tests done in dogs that are normal on retesting. Alternatively, the return to normal in some dogs may reflect regeneration of acinar cell function following an episode of pancreatic disease.

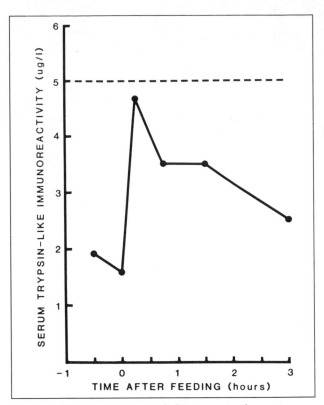

Figure 3—Transient postprandial increase in the concentration of serum trypsin-like immunoreactivity in a dog with exocrine pancreatic insufficiency. This response is uncommon in affected dogs; but, to avoid equivocal test results, blood should be taken no sooner than 3 hours, and preferably at least 12 hours, after feeding.

Rarely, serum TLI values are consistently subnormal but above the 2.5 μg/L value considered diagnostic for exocrine pancreatic insufficiency. On followup of the few pertinent cases seen to date, those dogs have not shown signs of weight loss or diarrhea. In such cases, functional exocrine tissue has probably decreased but not enough to cause clinical signs of exocrine pancreatic insufficiency. I examined the pancreas of one such animal and found severe chronic pancreatitis. This animal had clinical signs resulting from severe eosinophilic colitis that responded to treatment with sulfasalazine and prednisolone. For a two-year period following resolution of the colitis, the dog was clinically normal but serum TLI values were consistently subnormal and ranged from 2.8 to 4.6 μg/L. The dog was eventually euthanatized because of problems unrelated to gastrointestinal disease. Although such a case suggests that results consistently in the "gray zone" reflect chronic pancreatic disease, further studies are needed to substantiate that conclusion.

While none have been reported, assay of serum TLI probably has some limitations. For example, serum TLI might be normal in dogs with exocrine pancreatic insufficiency secondary to obstruction of the pancreatic ducts. Bentiromide test results and fecal proteolytic activity should be abnormal in such dogs, however, because chymotrypsin and other proteases are not secreted into the gut lumen. For similar reasons, serum TLI concentrations should be normal in dogs with congenital deficiencies of intestinal enteropeptidase (enterokinase) or pancreatic digestive enzymes other than trypsinogen. Finally, serum TLI concentrations may not always be as low in dogs with exocrine pancreatic insufficiency caused by chronic pancreatitis as in dogs with pancreatic acinar atrophy. Inflammation in residual pancreatic tissue might lead to slightly greater serum TLI concentrations than would be expected from the mass of acinar tissue remaining.

Immunoassay of serum TLI in cats has recently been reported.[32] Concentrations in the serum of normal cats are greater than in normal dogs, and the assays for canine and feline TLI show no cross-reactivity. Serum concentrations of TLI in a group of cats with EPI were lower than in healthy control cats. This assay is presently only available from the author's laboratory at Purdue University.[b]

TESTS FOR SMALL INTESTINAL DISEASE

Theoretically, results of intestinal function tests should be normal in dogs and cats with exocrine pancreatic insufficiency because the primary defect is of pancreatic and not intestinal function. Several studies have shown, however, that fatty acid or xylose absorption is often abnormal in these dogs.[14,15,33-36] The abnormalities might reflect either intestinal mucosal changes that arise secondary to exocrine pancreatic insufficiency per se or the high prevalence of bacterial overgrowth associated with that disease in dogs.[37] Regardless, it is clear that intestinal function tests only provide useful information after pancreatic function has been assessed. Function tests are not always helpful even then, because results can be normal in patients with small intestinal disease. For example, fat and xylose absorption can be normal in Irish setters with wheat-sensitive enteropathy.[38] Thus, it is impossible to eliminate a diagnosis of small intestinal disease on the basis of function tests alone.

Serum concentrations of the water-soluble vitamins cobalamin and folate are useful alternative markers of intestinal function.[39] Like xylose absorption and fat-balance studies, tests for serum vitamin concentrations are not particularly sensitive or specific for small intestinal disease. Results may be normal in patients

with small intestinal disease and abnormal in patients with exocrine pancreatic insufficiency. These tests only require assay of a single serum sample, however; and abnormal results do support a diagnosis of small intestinal disease when pancreatic function is normal.

Serum Cobalamin (Vitamin B$_{12}$)

Cobalamin is a water-soluble vitamin that is plentiful in canine and feline diets. Dietary deficiency is highly improbable; indeed, it is very difficult to induce cobalamin deficiency in most species.[40] In humans with gastrointestinal diseases, severe cobalamin deficiency that results from malabsorption causes megaloblastic anemia and neurologic disease. Cobalamin malabsorption also occurs in some dogs with gastrointestinal disease, although there are no reports of clinical signs in conjunction with vitamin deficiency.[39]

Studies of cobalamin absorption in normal dogs show that the mechanisms involved are similar to those in humans.[41,42] Acid and pepsins (proteolytic enzymes) in gastric juice release cobalamin from dietary protein. At the acid pH in the stomach, the free vitamin is bound by proteins called *R proteins* that are probably secreted in saliva and perhaps gastric juice. R-protein-bound cobalamin then passes into the duodenum where pancreatic proteolytic enzymes degrade the R protein and thereby release cobalamin.[43] At neutral pH in the small intestine, the free cobalamin binds to *intrinsic factor*, a protein secreted in the gastric juice of most species and, in dogs and cats, also in pancreatic juice.[44-47] Absorption of cobalamin bound to intrinsic factor finally occurs via specific receptors located exclusively in the distal small intestine (Figure 4).

Cobalamin malabsorption results in a subnormal serum concentration of the vitamin when malabsorption is severe and has been present for a sufficiently long period of time to deplete body reserves. In humans, cobalamin malabsorption occurs in association with atrophic gastritis or gastric resection, chronic exocrine pancreatic insufficiency, duodenal bacterial overgrowth, and ileal disease or ileal resection.[48] Rare causes of malabsorption in humans include failure to synthesize intrinsic factor, synthesis of nonfunctional intrinsic factor, and selective defects in ileal absorption.[48] In dogs and cats, both small intestinal disease and exocrine pancreatic insufficiency can cause subnormal serum cobalamin concentrations.[38,39] Pancreatic intrinsic factor may maintain cobalamin absorption following gastric disease in dogs and cats.[44-47]

Cobalamin malabsorption associated with small intestinal disease sometimes develops as a result of disorders affecting the intrinsic factor-cobalamin receptors in the distal small intestine. Disease localized exclusively in the ileum is uncommon. Ileal dysfunc-

[b]GI Lab, Purdue University, 1248 Lynn Hall, West Lafayette, IN 47907. Telephone (317) 494-0331; FAX (317) 449-8640.

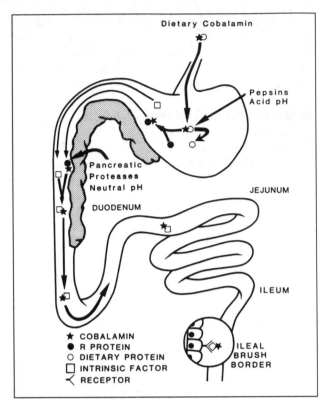

Figure 4—Normal absorption of dietary cobalamin. Cobalamin is liberated from dietary protein by acid and pepsins in the stomach, where it is bound by R proteins. Subsequent degradation of R protein by pancreatic proteases at neutral pH in the small intestine allows cobalamin to be bound by intrinsic factor. Cobalamin is absorbed only in the ileum where specific receptors for the intrinsic factor–cobalamin complex are located.

tion is more frequently associated with generalized disease affecting additional segments of the intestinal tract. Ileal resection causes cobalamin malabsorption in humans and probably does so in dogs too.

Another cause of cobalamin malabsorption is competition for the vitamin by abnormally high numbers of bacteria (bacterial overgrowth) proximal to the ileum.[48,49] While bacteria are the ultimate source of all naturally available cobalamin, many species of bacteria present in the intestine, particularly obligate anaerobes, are dependent on exogenous cobalamin.[49] Uptake of cobalamin by large numbers of bacteria can therefore lead to a reduction in serum concentrations.[50]

Cobalamin malabsorption associated with exocrine pancreatic insufficiency can develop by several mechanisms: (1) failure of pancreatic enzymes to liberate cobalamin from binding by R protein, (2) failure to secrete pancreatic intrinsic factor, (3) abnormally acidic pH in the intestine secondary to reduced pancreatic bicarbonate secretion resulting in failure of intrinsic factor to bind cobalamin, and (4) competition

for available cobalamin by intestinal microflora in those dogs with coexisting bacterial overgrowth. Whatever the mechanism, serum cobalamin concentrations can be subnormal in dogs with exocrine pancreatic insufficiency, even following otherwise effective treatment.

Serum cobalamin can be assayed by a variety of bioassay or competitive-binding assay methods. Bioassays are more technically demanding, however, and therefore less readily available. Assay results, thus normal ranges, can vary considerably among laboratories because different test methods are used. It should also be noted that some radioassay methods employed by many laboratories to assay cobalamin and folate in human patients do not give reliable results in dogs; in the author's experience, so-called charcoal boil assay methods are reliable in dogs and cats.[51,52] Reported normal-serum and whole-blood cobalamin concentrations determined by *Euglena viridis* and protozoa bioassays, respectively, are 200 to 400 ng/L[38] and 135 to 950 ng/L.[53] Normal canine serum concentrations determined by a charcoal boil competitive-binding radioassay in the author's laboratory range from 225 to 860 ng/L. Serum cobalamin in healthy control cats ranges from 200 to 1680 µg/L.

Serum Folate

Folate is a water-soluble vitamin plentiful in canine and feline diets, and therefore nutritional deficiency is unlikely. Dietary folate is usually present in a poorly absorbed form because of conjugation with several glutamate residues (folate polyglutamates). Folate deconjugase, an enzyme located in the brush border of the jejunal mucosa, removes all but one residue before mucosal uptake.[48,54] Specific folate carriers located only in the proximal small intestine then transport folate monoglutamate into mucosal cells (Figure 5). The canine distal small intestine has little ability to absorb folate.[55,56]

As with cobalamin, malabsorption results in a subnormal serum concentration of folate only when the defect in absorption is severe and has been present for a long enough time to deplete body reserves. Canine small intestinal disease is sometimes associated with subnormal serum folate concentrations.[39] It is likely that in dogs and cats, as in humans, subnormal serum folate concentration in the face of normal dietary intake reflects disease involving the proximal small intestine. Disease restricted to the middle and/or distal segments of the small intestine does not impair folate absorption. Various drugs, including phenytoin and sulfasalazine, impair folate absorption in humans and might also do so in dogs.[48,57]

Serum folate concentrations can increase in dogs

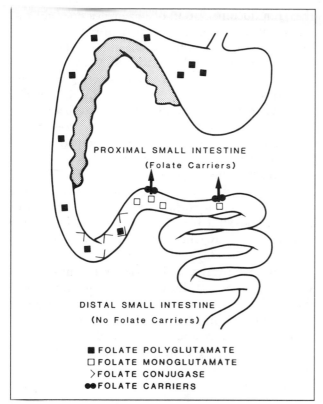

PROXIMAL SMALL INTESTINE
(Folate Carriers)

DISTAL SMALL INTESTINE
(No Folate Carriers)

■ FOLATE POLYGLUTAMATE
□ FOLATE MONOGLUTAMATE
> FOLATE CONJUGASE
●● FOLATE CARRIERS

Figure 5—Normal absorption of dietary folate. Folate polyglutamates are converted to monoglutamates by the intestinal brush border enzyme folate conjugase. Folate monoglutamate is then absorbed by a carrier-mediated mechanism located only in the proximal segments of the small intestine.

with bacterial overgrowth as a result of folate synthesis by the abnormal microflora.[38,50,55,56] Overgrowth must be in the proximal small bowel for serum folate concentrations to increase; changes in the microflora distal to the site of absorption have no effect.[55,56]

Dogs with exocrine pancreatic insufficiency often have elevated serum folate concentrations, which could reflect associated bacterial overgrowth.[37] Alternatively, impaired pancreatic bicarbonate secretion can enhance folate absorption by decreasing the pH in the proximal small intestine. Folate absorption is optimal at a mildly acidic pH, and even minimal reductions in intraluminal pH promote uptake.[58]

Folate can be assayed by a variety of bioassays and competitive-binding assays. As with cobalamin, normal values vary with different methods and laboratories. Published normal canine serum and plasma concentrations determined by *Lactobacillus casei* bioassay are 4.8 to 13.0 µg/L[39] and 4.0 to 26.0 µg/L,[53] respectively. Normal canine serum concentrations determined by competitive-binding assay in the author's laboratory range from 6.7 to 17.4 µg/L. The author is not aware of studies of folate absorption in cats,

but serum concentrations of this vitamin are greater in normal cats than in normal dogs. Reported control plasma concentrations determined by bioassay are 3.2 to 34 ng/L,[53] while normal serum concentrations determined by charcoal boil competitive-binding radioassay in the author's laboratory range from 13.4 to 38.0 ng/L. Folate concentrations inside erythrocytes are much greater than in serum, and hemolyzed samples may show falsely increased values.

CLINICAL APPLICATION OF SERUM COBALAMIN AND FOLATE ASSAYS

Serum cobalamin and folate concentrations are indicative of dysfunction of the small intestine only if pancreatic function is normal. It is also important to consider whether prolonged anorexia or inappetence might have led to decreased vitamin intake, although in the author's experience, even complete anorexia for several weeks does not cause significant reductions in serum cobalamin or folate concentrations in dogs. Oral or parenteral vitamin supplements may also affect serum concentrations.

It is preferable to assay both cobalamin and folate because interpretation is most useful if results for both are available. Markedly increased concentrations of both vitamins, for example, suggest supplementation before sampling, because no diseases increase cobalamin absorption. Interpretation of folate concentration alone in such instances could mistakenly indicate bacterial overgrowth.

Decreased serum concentrations of both cobalamin and folate are relatively uncommon findings and suggest severe, long-standing disease affecting the entire small intestine. This pattern of changes has been observed in association with a canine enteropathy resembling chronic tropical sprue in humans.[38]

Reductions in serum folate accompanied by normal cobalamin concentrations are consistent with dysfunction localized predominantly in the upper small intestine. These changes often accompany wheat-sensitive enteropathy in Irish setters, but they are not a consistent finding with the disease.[38]

Perhaps the most useful information provided by assay of serum folate and cobalamin is evidence of possible bacterial overgrowth.[59] Decreased serum cobalamin and increased serum folate in dogs with normal exocrine pancreatic function are highly suggestive of bacterial overgrowth (Figure 6). These characteristic changes have led to the identification of an antibiotic-responsive enteropathy associated with bacterial overgrowth in German shepherds.[38] Bacterial overgrowth can also occur in other breeds, either as a primary enteropathy or as a secondary complication of other gastrointestinal disorders.[37,60–63]

The prevalence of bacterial overgrowth in dogs is

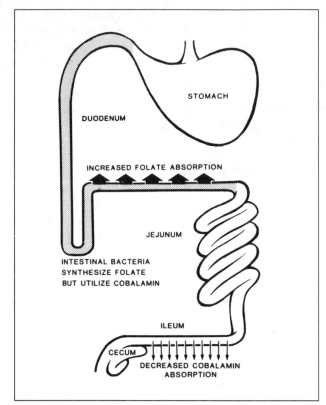

Figure 6—Effects of small intestinal bacterial overgrowth on the absorption of cobalamin and folate in the proximal small intestine. Bacteria in the upper segments of the small intestine may synthesize folate that is subsequently absorbed; in contrast, microbial competition for dietary cobalamin may inhibit absorption in the ileum.

unknown, but it has probably been underdiagnosed in the past. Diagnosis is difficult because histologic examination of intestinal biopsies reveals minimal, if any, morphologic change. Furthermore, documentation of overgrowth by quantitative bacteriologic culture of intestinal aspirates is both technically demanding and expensive.[37,38,59] While serum cobalamin and folate concentrations are sometimes normal in dogs with bacterial overgrowth, characteristic serum concentrations of folate and cobalamin provide strong evidence that overgrowth is present.

TESTS OF FELINE PANCREATIC AND INTESTINAL FUNCTION

Pancreatic dysfunction in the few reported cases of feline exocrine pancreatic insufficiency has been a result of either chronic pancreatitis or surgical disruption of the normal flow of pancreatic juice into the gut lumen.[64-66] Pancreatic acinar atrophy as described in dogs has not been reported in cats.

Many tests used to diagnose canine exocrine pancreatic insufficiency are of questionable validity and usefulness in cats. Affected cats would have steator-

rhea, but documentation of steatorrhea does not rule out small intestinal diseases.[67] Bentiromide absorption test results are quite variable in normal cats, limiting the diagnostic value of the test.[68,69] Assays for feline TLI are not routinely available.[32] Quantitative assay of fecal proteolytic enzyme activity is probably the most reliable approach presently available.[11,12,64] Analysis of at least three fecal samples is necessary because normal cats, like normal dogs, sometimes produce feces with negligible activity.[11,12,64]

Although feline small intestinal disease is relatively common, no laboratory tests are of proven diagnostic value.[70,71] Documentation of steatorrhea confirms malabsorption but is of little practical value because the condition may reflect pancreatic or intestinal dysfunction.[64] The range of normal values for xylose absorption in healthy cats is wide, and results in cats with small intestinal disease usually fall within those limits.[68,69,72] The value of serum cobalamin, folate, or fat-soluble vitamin concentrations in the investigation of feline pancreatic and intestinal disease has not been reported. In the author's experience, however, serum cobalamin is usually markedly subnormal in cats with EPI, and examination of intestinal biopsies from cats with subnormal serum cobalamin or folate concentrations but with normal pancreatic function, reveals disease of the small intestine.

CONCLUSION

Accurate identification of dogs with exocrine pancreatic insufficiency has been simplified by the development of an assay for canine TLI. If pancreatic function is normal, assay of serum cobalamin and folate concentrations can provide information about intestinal function. Abnormal serum vitamin concentrations are consistent with a diagnosis of small intestinal disease and may also provide clues about the location and severity of the enteropathy. Serum cobalamin and folate concentrations are particularly useful in identifying dogs with bacterial overgrowth. It is important to remember that normal levels do not rule out the possibility of disease of the small intestine. There is evidence to support the validity of a similar approach to interpretation of test results in cats.

Presently available tests of intestinal function clearly lack sensitivity or specificity, or both, in dogs and cats. Recent reports of a breath hydrogen excretion test to detect carbohydrate malabsorption[36] and a [51]chromium-labeled ethylenediaminetetraacetate (^{51}Cr-EDTA) absorption test to assess intestinal permeability[73] offer encouraging prospects for improvements in the assessment of intestinal function. Technical constraints will probably restrict these tests to research centers, but they may facilitate the development of alternative tests that will be available to the veterinary practitioner.

REFERENCES

1. Lorenz MD: Canine malabsorption syndromes. *Compend Contin Educ Pract Vet* 2:885–893, 1980.
2. Burrows CF: The assessment of canine gastrointestinal function: Recent advances and future needs, in *31st Gaines Veterinary Symposium*. Lawrenceville, NJ, Veterinary Learning Systems, Co, Inc, 1981, pp 1–9.
3. Handelman CT, Blue J: Laboratory data: Read beyond the numbers. *Compend Contin Educ Pract Vet* 5:687–694, 1983.
4. Simpson JW, Doxey DL: Quantitative assessment of fat absorption and its diagnostic value in exocrine pancreatic insufficiency. *Res Vet Sci* 35:249–251, 1983.
5. Hill FWG: Malabsorption syndrome in the dog: A study of thirty-eight cases. *J Small Anim Pract* 13:575–594, 1972.
6. Burrows CF, Merritt AM, Chiapella AM: Determination of fecal fat and trypsin output in the evaluation of chronic canine diarrhea. *JAVMA* 174:62–66, 1979.
7. Westermarck E, Sandholm M: Fecal hydrolase activity as determined by radial enzyme diffusion: A new method for detecting pancreatic dysfunction in the dog. *Res Vet Sci* 28:341–346, 1980.
8. Westermarck E: The diagnosis of pancreatic degenerative atrophy in dogs—A practical method. *Acta Vet Scand* 23:197–203, 1982.
9. Canfield PJ, Fairburn AJ, Church DB: Effect of various diets on fecal analysis in normal dogs. *Res Vet Sci* 34:24–27, 1983.
10. Canfield PJ, Fairburn AJ, Church DB: Fecal analysis for maldigestion in pancreatectomised dogs. *Res Vet Sci* 34:28–30, 1983.
11. Williams DA, Reed SD: Comparison of methods for assay of fecal proteolytic activity. *Vet Clin Path* 19:20–24, 1990.
12. Williams DA, Reed SD, Perry L: Fecal proteolytic activity in clinically normal cats and in a cat with exocrine pancreatic insufficiency. *JAVMA* 197:210–212, 1990.
13. Freudiger U, Bigler E: The diagnosis of chronic exocrine pancreatic insufficiency by the PABA test. *Kleintier-Praxis* 22:73–79, 1977.
14. Batt RM, Mann LC: Specificity of the BT PABA test for the diagnosis of exocrine pancreatic insufficiency in the dog. *Vet Rec* 108:303–307, 1981.
15. Rogers WA, Stradley RP, Sherding RG, et al: Simultaneous evaluation of pancreatic exocrine function and intestinal absorptive function in dogs with chronic diarrhea. *JAVMA* 177:1128–1131, 1980.
16. Strombeck DR, Harrold D: Evaluation of 60-minute blood p-aminobenzoic acid concentration in pancreatic function testing of dogs. *JAVMA* 180:419–421, 1982.
17. Zimmer JF, Todd SE: Further evaluation of bentiromide in the diagnosis of canine exocrine pancreatic insufficiency. *Cornell Vet* 75:426–440, 1985.
18. Williams DA, Batt RM: Diagnosis of canine exocrine pancreatic insufficiency by the assay of serum trypsin-like immunoreactivity. *J Small Anim Pract* 24:583–588, 1983.
19. Borgstrom A, Ohlsson K: Immunoreactive trypsins in sera from dogs before and after induction of experimental pancreatitis. *Hoppe-Seyler's Z Physiol Chem* 361:625–631, 1980.
20. Borgstrom A: The fate of intravenously injected trypsinogens in dogs. *Scand J Gastroenterol* 16:281–287, 1981.
21. Geokas MC, Reidelberger R, O'Rourke M, et al: Plasma pancreatic trypsinogens in chronic renal failure and after nephrectomy. *Am J Physiol* 242:177–182, 1982.
22. Andriulli A, Masoero G, Felder M, et al: Circulating trypsin-like immunoreactivity in chronic pancreatitis. *Dig Dis Sci* 26:532–537, 1981.
23. Andriulli A, Masoero G, Benitti V, et al: Relation between serum cathodic trypsinogen levels and exocrine pancreatic function. *J Clin Gastroenterol* 6:239–244, 1984.
24. Jacobson DG, Curington C, Connery K, et al: Trypsin-like immunoreactivity as a test for pancreatic insufficiency. *N Engl J Med* 310:1307–1309, 1984.
25. Blum AL, Linscheer WG: Lipase in canine gastric juice. *Proc Soc Exp Biol Med* 135:565–568, 1970.
26. Stickle JE, Carlton WW, Boon GD: Isoamylases in clinically normal dogs. *Am J Vet Res* 41:506–509, 1980.
27. Jacobs RM, Hall RL, Rogers WJ: Isoamylases in clinically normal and diseased dogs. *Vet Clin Path* 11:26–32, 1982.
28. Simpson JW, Doxey DL, Brown R: Serum isoamylase in normal dogs and dogs with exocrine pancreatic insufficiency. *Vet Res Commun* 8:303–308, 1984.
29. Geokas MC, Largman C, Brodrick JW, et al: Molecular forms of immunoreactive pancreatic elastase in canine pancreatic and peripheral blood. *Am J Physiol* 238:G238–G246, 1980.
30. Levitt MD, Ellis CJ, Murphy SM, et al: Study of the possible enteropancreatic circulation of pancreatic amylase in the dog. *Am J Physiol* 241:G54–G58, 1981.
31. Williams DA, Batt RM: Sensitivity and specificity of radioimmunoassay of serum trypsin-like immunoreactivity for the diagnosis of canine exocrine pancreatic insufficiency. *JAVMA* 192:195–201, 1988.
32. Medinger TM, Burchfield T, Williams DA: Assay of trypsin-like immunoreactivity (TLI) in feline serum. *J Vet Int Med* 7:133, 1993.
33. Clark CH: Pancreatic atrophy and absorption failure in a boxer. *JAVMA* 136:174–177, 1960.
34. Kallfelz FA, Norrdin RW, Neal TM: Intestinal absorption of oleic acid ^{131}I and triolein ^{131}I in the differential diagnosis of malabsorption syndrome and pancreatic dysfunction in the dog. *JAVMA* 153:43–46, 1968.
35. Sateri H: Investigations on the exocrine pancreatic function in dogs suffering from chronic exocrine pancreatic insufficiency. *Acta Vet Scand (Suppl)* 53:1–86, 1975.
36. Washabau RJ, Strombeck DR, Buffington CA, et al: Use of pulmonary hydrogen gas excretion to detect carbohydrate malabsorption in dogs. *JAVMA* 189:674–679, 1986.
37. Williams DA, Batt RM, McLean L: Bacterial overgrowth in the duodenum of dogs with exocrine pancreatic insufficiency. *JAVMA* 191:201–206, 1987.
38. Batt RM: New approaches to malabsorption in dogs. *Compend Contin Educ Pract Vet* 8:783–795, 1986.
39. Batt RM, Morgan JO: Role of serum folate and vitamin B_{12} concentrations in the differentiation of small intestinal abnormalities in the dog. *Res Vet Sci* 32:17–22, 1982.
40. Kark JA, Victor M, Hines JD, et al: Nutritional vitamin B_{12} deficiency in rhesus monkeys. *Am J Clin Nutr* 27:470–478, 1974.
41. Marcoullis G, Rothenberg SP: Intrinsic factor-mediated intestinal absorption of cobalamin in the dog. *Am J Physiol* 241:G294–G299, 1981.
42. Levine JS, Allen RH, Alpers DH, et al: Immunocytochemical localization of the intrinsic factor–cobalamin receptor in dog ileum. Distribution of intracellular receptor during cell maturation. *J Cell Biol* 98:1111–1118, 1984.
43. Herzlich B, Herbert V: The role of the pancreas in cobalamin (vitamin B_{12}) absorption. *Am J Gastroenterol* 79:489–493, 1984.
44. Abels J, Muckerheide MM: Absorption of vitamin B_{12} in dogs. *Clin Res* 18:530, 1970.

(continues on page 150)

Functional Tumors of the Pancreatic Beta Cells

James W. Wilson, DVM, MS
Diplomate, ACVS
South Shore Veterinary Associates
South Weymouth, Massachusetts

Dennis D. Caywood, DVM, MS
Assistant Professor
Department of Small Animal
Clinical Sciences
College of Veterinary Medicine
University of Minnesota
St. Paul, Minnesota

Functional pancreatic beta cell tumors, or islet cell tumors or insulinomas, are infrequently observed but well-recognized entities in animals; they have been reported in several species.[1] In the dog, the tumor has a high incidence of malignancy with metastasis to regional lymph nodes and the liver.[1-3] Although the rate and severity of metastasis are extremely variable, several long-term survivors have been reported.[3,4] Since metastasis may become widespread, early diagnosis is extremely important for successful surgical management.

Clinical Features

All reported tumors have occurred in dogs older than four years of age. Boxers, poodles, and terriers have the highest reported incidence. There is no sex predilection.

Clinical signs are all attributable to hypoglycemia and include muscle weakness, muscle tremors, ataxia, collapse, and convulsions. Onset is usually precipitated by exercise or a stressful situation. Signs become more frequent and severe as the disease progresses. Although muscle weakness, muscle tremors, and ataxia are more common, most dogs have seizures during the course of the disease. Owners often remain unconcerned until convulsions occur; therefore, signs may exist for several months before initial examination. Many owners report that, following an abnormal episode, their dog has a ravenous appetite or recovers more quickly if it is fed. Dogs also appear to partially adapt to chronic hypoglycemia: The authors observed dogs late in the course of the disease that appear clinically normal with blood glucose concentrations of 20 to 30 mg/dl.

Unfortunately, the disease is often initially misdiagnosed. It is not uncommon for dogs with functional beta cell tumors to have been put on anticonvulsant therapy sometime during the course of the disease. Diseases and conditions with signs similar to those of a functional beta cell tumor include viral encephalitis, hydrocephalus, cryptococcosis, toxoplasmosis, hepatic encephalopathy, brain tumor, trauma, idiopathic epilepsy, tetanus, hypocalcemia, and drug toxicosis. Thus, blood glucose concentrations should always be examined when signs include muscle weakness, muscle tremors, ataxia, or convulsions.

Originally published in Volume 3, Number 5, May 1981

Laboratory Tests

Tentative diagnosis of a functional pancreatic beta cell tumor is traditionally based on demonstration of Whipple's triad (i.e., neurologic disturbances associated with hypoglycemia, fasting plasma glucose concentration ≤40 mg/dl, and relief of neurologic disturbances by feeding or administration of glucose). However, Whipple's triad is, in fact, characteristic of hypoglycemia, regardless of cause. Although pancreatic beta cell tumors may be the most common cause of hypoglycemia in the dog, other possible causes of fasting hypoglycemia include inadequate glucose supply, hepatic disorders, hormone deficiencies, drug induction, and increased secretion of insulin.[5] Thus, additional laboratory data is needed to confirm a diagnosis of hyperinsulinism.

There are several tests whose results may support the diagnosis of functional pancreatic beta cell tumor in a dog that demonstrates Whipple's triad. The high-dose intravenous glucose tolerance test is useful for evaluating the ability of an animal to shift glucose out of the plasma space. After a 24-hour fast, a zero-time blood sample is collected and 1 g glucose/kg body weight is rapidly given intravenously (within 30 to 45 seconds). Blood samples are obtained 5, 15, 30, 45, and 60 minutes after infusion and analyzed for glucose concentration. In normal dogs, plasma glucose concentration should return to normal in 30 to 60 minutes. In addition, a K value can be obtained from a semilogarithmic plot of glucose values (Figure 1). The K value reveals the percentage rate of glucose disappearance per minute. Normal dogs have a K value that is > 2.5 and <3.0. Diabetic dogs, which have a low population of islet cells or unreactive cells, have

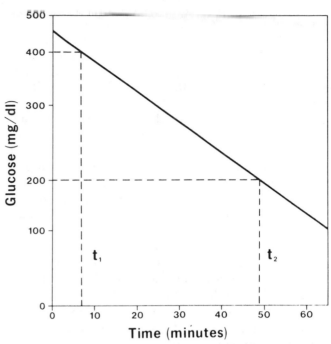

High Dose Intravenous Glucose Tolerance Test

Time (minutes)

Figure 1—Plasma glucose response to intravenous glucose administration. Calculation of the K value is done according to the formula $K = \dfrac{69.3}{T_2 - T_1}$, where T_1 and T_2 are times arbitrarily chosen to correspond with a pair of glucose values that represents a 50% decrease in blood glucose concentration. (From Caywood DD, Wilson JW: Functional pancreatic islet cell adenocarcinoma in the dog, in Kirk RW (ed): *Current Veterinary Therapy VII*. Philadelphia, WB Saunders Co, 1980. Reprinted with permission.)

a K value < 2.0. All but one of the authors' cases had K values in the "prediabetic" range (<2.5 but >2.0) (Table I). This suggests that beta cell tumors

TABLE I

LABORATORY VALUES AND CALCULATED INDICES FOR SIX FASTED DOGS WITH PANCREATIC BETA CELL ADENOCARCINOMA*

Case No.	Plasma Glucose (mg/dl)	Serum Insulin (mμ/ml)	Glucose: Insulin Ratio	Insulin: Glucose Ratio	Amended Insulin: Glucose Ratio	K value
1	32	13	2.46	0.40	658	2.5
2	40	14	2.85	0.35	140	2.1
3	36	200	0.18	5.55	3333	–
4	52	8	6.5	0.15	36.3	2.1
5	40	–	–	–	–	2.1
6	40	14	2.86	0.35	240	2.04
Values diagnostic of beta cell tumor	<40	>20	<2.5	>0.3	>30	>3

*From Caywood DD, Wilson JW: Functional pancreatic islet cell adenocarcinoma in the dog, in Kirk RW (ed): *Current Veterinary Therapy VII*. Philadelphia, WB Saunders Co, 1980. Reprinted with permission.

are generally unresponsive to glucose overload and that the existing nonneoplastic beta cells are also unresponsive as a result of constant negative feedback from insulin released by the tumor.[3,4]

The glucagon tolerance test evaluates insulin release through direct tumor stimulation and insulinogenesis and indirectly through glycogenolysis.[6] The test is performed following a 24-hour fast by giving 0.03 mg of glucagon USP/kg body weight intravenously. Plasma glucose concentrations are determined 0, 1, 5, 15, 30, 45, 60, and 120 minutes after administration of glucagon. In dogs with pancreatic beta cell tumors, the blood glucose concentration should not exceed 150 mg/dl and returns to the hypoglycemic state within 60 minutes (Figure 2). However, false-negative test results have been obtained by the authors and others using this test regime.[7]

Other tests that have been used are the oral glucose tolerance test, the L-leucine tolerance test, and the tolbutamide tolerance test. All give variable results and are of less value than the following test.

Assay for serum insulin is now widely available through commercial and research laboratories. Results are reported as μU/ml of immunoreactive insulin (IRI). The authors' normal range of IRI in the dog is 9.8 to 20 μU/ml. With this test, direct confirmation of the presence of a functional beta cell tumor, through identification of abnormally high concentrations of serum insulin, is possible. Increased insulin concentrations have been re-

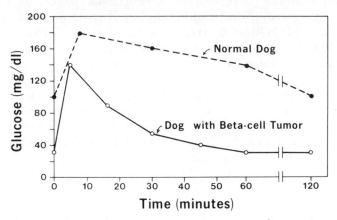

Glucagon Tolerance Test

Figure 2—Plasma glucose response to intravenous glucagon in a normal dog and in a dog with a functional beta cell neoplasm. (From Caywood DD, Wilson JW: Functional pancreatic islet cell adenocarcinoma in the dog, in Kirk RW (ed): *Current Veterinary Therapy VII.* Philadelphia, WB Saunders Co, 1980. Reprinted with permission.)

ported with beta cell tumors; however, insulin values within normal range have also been noted. Therefore, insulin concentrations alone are not sufficient for a diagnosis.

If the circulating insulin concentration is compared with the corresponding circulating glucose concentration, a ratio can be derived. Three ratios have been developed and utilized in humans. The first was the glucose:insulin ratio. Values <2.5 were considered diagnostic of an insulinoma;[5,8] however, false-negative ratios began to be recognized.[8] Thus,

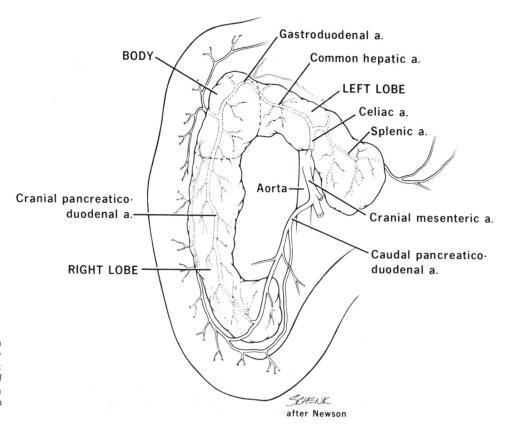

Figure 3—Anatomy of the pancreas in the dog. (From Caywood DD: Surgery of the pancreas, in Bojrab MJ (ed): *Current Techniques in Small Animal Surgery II.* Philadelphia, Lea & Febiger, in press. Reprinted with permission.)

a second ratio, the insulin:glucose ratio, was formulated. Values >0.3 were considered diagnostic, but once again false-negative results were identified.[8] The third and most recent ratio was created following reports of ethanol-induced hypoglycemia.[9,10] Serum IRI concentrations were found to be near zero when plasma glucose concentrations were ≤30 mg/dl.[10,11] A discriminant based on this observation has been used in humans and dogs.[7,11,12] An *amended insulin:glucose ratio* is obtained by evaluating the formula

$$\frac{\text{Serum insulin } (\mu\text{U/ml}) \times 100}{\text{Plasma glucose } (\text{mg/dl}) - 30}$$

It has been suggested that normal ratios for the dog are <30.[11,12]

The authors have compared all three ratios (Table I). The glucose:insulin ratio resulted in the highest percentage of false-negative results. The insulin:glucose ratio was more accurate, but one false-negative was observed. The amended insulin:glucose ratio was calculated in five out of six cases and was elevated in all five cases. Rather than suggesting hyperinsulinism, as the high-dose intravenous glucose tolerance and glucagon tolerance tests do, the amended insulin-glucose ratio confirms abnormal circulating insulin concentrations for the amount of circulating glucose.

Surgical Management
Pancreatic Anatomy

The pancreas is a coarsely lobulated, elongated gland with a nodular surface. It is located caudal to the liver in the dorsal part of the epigastrium. The pancreas consists of three parts: the right lobe, left lobe, and body (Figure 3). The right lobe lies in the mesoduodenum near the dorsal portion of the right flank. It extends from the ninth intercostal space to the fourth lumbar vertebra. The left lobe lies in the greater omentum near the caudate process of the liver, portal vein, caudal vena cava, and aorta. Much of the left lobe is hidden behind the stomach. The right and left lobes unite at a 45° angle to form the body.

The cranial and caudal pancreaticoduodenal arteries are the main vessels to the right lobe of the pancreas (Figure 3). They anastomose within the gland and supply the duodenum as well as the pancreas. Loss of these vessels markedly impairs duodenal blood supply, often leading to ischemic necrosis of the duodenum. The left lobe is primarily supplied by a branch of the splenic artery, but it may also receive small branches from the common hepatic and celiac arteries. The caudal pancreaticoduodenal vein drains the right lobe, while branches to the splenic vein drain the left.

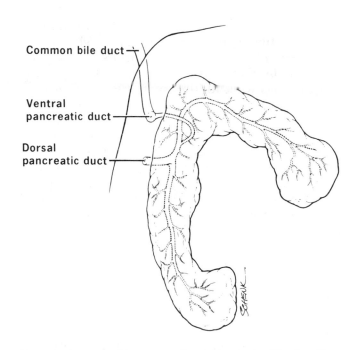

Figure 4—Anatomy of the pancreatic exocrine ducts of the dog. (From Caywood DD: Surgery of the pancreas, in Bojrab MJ (ed): *Current Techniques in Small Animal Surgery II*. Philadelphia, Lea & Febiger, in press. Reprinted with permission.)

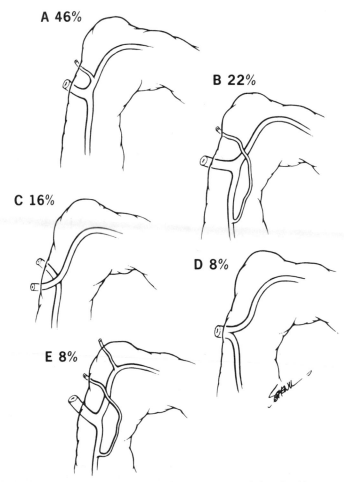

Figure 5—Pancreatic exocrine duct variation of the dog.[11] (From Caywood DD: Surgery of the pancreas, in Bojrab MJ (ed): *Current Techniques in Small Animal Surgery II*. Philadelphia, Lea & Febiger, in press. Reprinted with permission.)

The pancreas has two excretory ducts resulting from the dual origin of the gland. The ducts usually communicate and lie within the parenchyma of the pancreas (Figure 4). There are numerous variations in the anatomic relationship between the excretory ducts as they enter the duodenum (Figure 5). At one extreme (Figure 5[A]) each duct may terminate in the duodenum at entirely separate papillae; at the other extreme (Figure 5[D]) the two ducts may join and enter the duodenum at a single papilla. Careful surgical discretion is mandatory when working at the pancreatic angle; inadvertent damage to these excretory ducts could result in severe postoperative exocrine dysfunction.

Lymph drainage of the pancreas is via the duodenal, hepatic, splenic, and mesenteric group of lymph nodes.

Surgical Features

Unfortunately, no laboratory test will predict widespread metastasis, nor does any test suggest a favorable prognosis. Exploratory celiotomy is the best prognostic tool available and the ideal choice of therapy. Animals should be prepared for surgery as for any other exploratory celiotomy. Some surgeons have suggested that postoperative pancreatitis is a frequent complication of pancreatic surgery. Although the authors suggest monitoring serum amylase and lipase activity, they have not observed postoperative pancreatitis in a single case. They conclude that, unlike in humans, pancreatitis is extremely uncommon following pancreatic surgery in the dog. Consequently, the authors do not recommend prophylactic therapy for pancreatitis.

Many clinicians have also urged aggressive glucose administration during surgery to prevent possible hypoglycemic crises caused by insulin release following tumor manipulation. In the authors' experience, intraoperative plasma glucose rises to greater than normal values without glucose administration. Apparently, stress gluconeogenesis induced by anesthesia and surgery more than counteracts possible insulin release from the tumor resulting from manipulation. Glucose administration may still be advisable, but it certainly is not mandatory.

Since generalized abdominal inspection may be necessary, the authors recommend the ventral midline incision. The incision should extend from the xiphoid process caudally for a sufficient length to allow adequate exposure. The pancreas is exposed

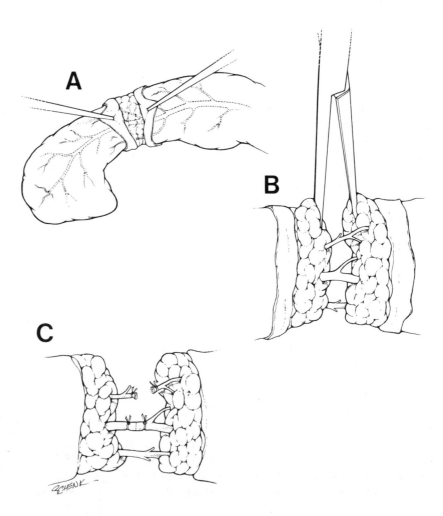

Figure 6—Partial pancreatectomy technique. Duct and vessel isolation. (From Caywood DD: Surgery of the pancreas, in Bojrab MJ (ed): *Current Techniques in Small Animal Surgery II*. Philadelphia, Lea & Febiger, in press. Reprinted with permission.)

by isolating and exteriorizing the duodenum and by anteriorly reflecting the stomach. The remainder of the abdominal contents are reflected caudally and to the left with moistened laparotomy sponges. The entire pancreas, mesentery, associated lymph nodes, and liver should be carefully inspected and palpated. If the neoplastic mass is confined to the pancreas and regional lymph nodes, it should be excised. The portion of the pancreas to be excised is isolated by incising the mesentery along the border of the gland and ligating blood vessels in the mesentery. The exposed pancreatic parenchyma can then be gently separated, and ducts and small vessels can be ligated (Figure 6). If the tumor is in the right lobe near the duodenum, pancreatic tissue adhering to the duodenum should be carefully peeled free from the intestine and pancreaticoduodenal vessels using a gauze sponge (Figure 7). Resulting hemorrhage is easily controlled by tamponade with gauze. Great care should be taken to ensure adequate duodenal blood supply. When operating at the pancreatic body, exocrine duct location and preservation should be considered. Involved regional lymph nodes can be excised as individual nodes or by mass resection, depending on particular involvement and location.

Plasma glucose content may be monitored during surgery. An increase in plasma glucose content occurring one-half to one hour after removal of the neoplastic mass is sufficient evidence that a functional beta cell tumor has been removed and that others have not been left behind. The glucose and amylase activity should then be monitored closely for the first 12 to 24 hours postoperatively and thereafter daily for a four- to five-day period.

If there is liver or widespread abdominal metastasis, the condition should be considered operatively uncorrectable.

Results and Prognosis

Surgery should be considered palliative. Several investigators have reported that removal of the neoplasm does not extend life. However, the authors have treated three dogs with tumors involving both the pancreas and the mesenteric lymph nodes in which surgical excision was possible. As a result, the dogs were asymptomatic for 270, 575, and 875

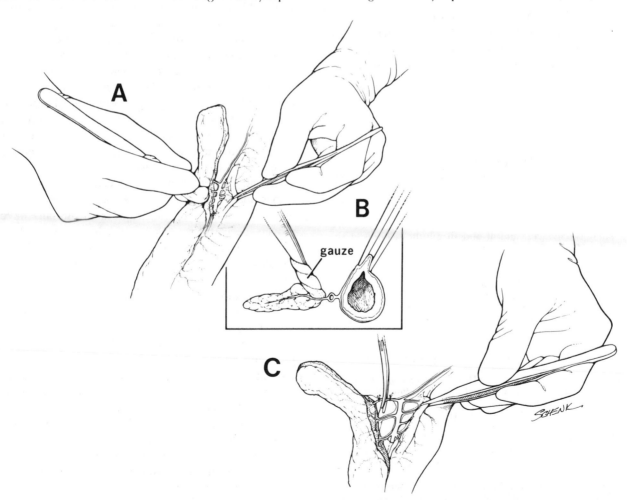

Figure 7—Partial pancreatectomy technique: isolation of the pancreaticoduodenal vessels and separation of pancreas from the duodenum. (From Caywood DD: Surgery of the pancreas, in Bojrab MJ (ed): *Current Techniques in Small Animal Surgery II.* Philadelphia, Lea & Febiger, in press. Reprinted with permission.)

days, respectively. One dog had additional surgery after recurrence of signs caused by lymph node metastasis at 270 days, which extended its asymptomatic life to 600 days. Life was thus prolonged for at least 575 days in each animal.

The mesenteric lymph nodes appear to be the first target organ for metastasis, and their ability to prevent further metastasis seems to be considerable. Only after overwhelming the lymph nodes does widespread, surgically unresectable metastasis occur. If exploratory celiotomy indicates no hepatic or widespread metastasis and if the dog is not hypoglycemic following surgical excision of the tumor, a good, immediate postoperative recovery can be expected.

Temporary diabetes mellitus may be encountered postoperatively as a result of feedback inhibition caused by high levels of insulin or proinsulin produced by the tumor. The authors have observed persisting diabetes in one dog. In this case, although the pancreatic islets appeared histologically normal, suppression of normal beta cells by tumor insulin may have resulted in irreversible loss of insulin production.

Temporary remission of hypoglycemia by treatment with streptozotocin has been reported in a dog with a beta cell tumor. The drug is associated with hepato- and nephrotoxicity and should be used with caution.

REFERENCES

1. Njoku CO, Strafuss AC, Dennis SM: Canine islet cell neoplasia: A review. *JAAHA* 8:284-290, 1972.
2. Johnson RK: Insulinoma in the dog. *Vet Clin North Am* 7:629-635, 1977.
3. Caywood DD, Wilson JW, Hardy RM, Shull RM: Pancreatic islet cell adenocarcinoma: Clinical and diagnostic features of six cases. *JAVMA* 174:714-717, 1979.
4. Wilson JW, Hulse DA: Surgical correction of islet cell adenocarcinoma in a dog. *JAVMA* 164:603-606, 1974.
5. Shatney CH, Grage TB: Diagnostic and surgical aspects of insulinoma. *Am J Surg* 127:174-184, 1974.
6. Johnson RK: Insulinoma in the dog, in Kirk RW (ed): *Current Veterinary Therapy V*. Philadelphia, WB Saunders Co, 1974, pp 818-822.
7. Kaneko JJ: Personal communication, 1974.
8. Service FJ, Dale AJD, Elveback LR, Jiang NS: Insulinoma. *Mayo Clin Proc* 51:417-429, 1976.
9. Bleicher SJ, Freinkel N, Byrne JJ, et al: Effect of ethanol on plasma glucose and insulin in the fasted dog. *Proc Soc Exp Biol Med* 115:369-373, 1965.
10. Turner RC, Oakley NW, Nabarro JDN: Changes in plasma insulin during ethanol-induced hypoglycemia. *Metabolism* 22:111-121, 1973.
11. Turner RC, Oakley NW, Nabarro JDN: Control of basal insulin secretion, with special reference to diagnosis of insulinomas. *Br Med J* 2:132-135, 1971.
12. Mattheeuws D, Rottiers R, DeRijcke J, et al: Hyperinsulinism in the dog due to pancreatic islet cell tumor: A report of three cases. *J Small Anim Pract* 7:313-318, 1976.
13. Nielson SW, Bishop EJ: The duct system of the canine pancreas. *Am J Vet Res* 15:266-271, 1954.

UPDATE

No breed or sex predilection has been noted in several reports concerning insulin-secreting tumors in a large number of animals. Almost all of these cases occurred in animals older than five years of age.[1-4]

Criteria for diagnosing insulin-secreting tumors and for related diagnostic testing continue to be debated. Because many dogs with confirmed cases of insulin-secreting tumors have normal plasma insulin concentrations, evaluation of plasma insulin values alone can result in an incorrect diagnosis. Severe hypoglycemia is not diagnostic. It is possible in dogs with severely debilitating conditions and has been documented in 4 dogs with sepsis[5] and 13 dogs with nonislet cell tumors.[6] Some of these animals also had abnormal insulin/glucose ratios. Fortunately, the laboratory test results for and the clinical signs of most of these animals suggested a condition other than that caused by a beta cell tumor.

Many authors have reported that the amended insulin glucose ratio (AIGR) provides the least false-negative diagnostic data. Nonetheless, considering the aforementioned animals that did not have beta cell tumors, an abnormal ratio should not be deemed diagnostic. An abnormal AIGR only documents a mismatch of insulin and glucose. When blood glucose is below 35 mg/dl, the ratio will be high, even with low plasma insulin concentrations. Therefore, ratio values must be interpreted with caution in cases of extreme hypoglycemia. If other features of these cases point to an insulin-secreting tumor, however, an abnormal AIGR and elevated insulin concentrations are the most reliable diagnostic tools that would support this diagnosis. Further work is needed to define insulin/glucose ratios and provide more definitive diagnostic testing.

Recently, much attention has been given to the medical management of beta cell tumors. Many of the drugs used to manage insulin-secreting tumors in humans have not proven successful nor has their use been adequately evaluated in dogs. Potentially serious side effects have been commonly associated with many of these pharmaceuticals. Medical management with or without surgical excision does not appear to be any better than surgical excision alone for long-term abeyance of hypoglycemic episodes. Long-term survival of individuals is markedly affected by the owner's willingness and ability to manage hypoglycemic episodes. Several excellent reviews should be consulted before contemplating medical management.[7,8]

Beta cell tumors are considered malignant and have a high likelihood of metastasis. In several reports, metastasis was not identified at necropsy in dogs that had died or been euthanatized for unrelated conditions several years after initial excision.[2,3] Although the long-term, symptom-free prognosis for insulin-secreting tumors remains very poor, surgical cures appear remotely possible.

REFERENCES

1. Kruth SA, Feldman EC, Kennedy PC: Insulin-secreting islet cell tu-

mors: Establishing a diagnosis and clinical course for 25 dogs. *JAVMA* 181:54–58, 1982.

2. Mehlhaff CJ, Peterson ME, Patnaik AK, Carrillo JM: Insulin-secreting islet cell neoplasms: Surgical considerations and general management in 35 dogs. *JAAHA* 21:607–612, 1985.

3. Leifer CE, Peterson ME, Matus RE: Insulin-secreting tumor. Diagnosis and medical and surgical management in 55 dogs. *JAVMA* 188:60–64, 1986.

4. Caywood DD, Klausner JS, O'Leary TP, et al: Pancreatic insulin-secreting neoplasms: Clinical, diagnostic, and prognostic features in 73 dogs. *JAAHA* 24:577–583, 1988.

5. Breitschwerdt EB, Loar AS, Hribernik TN, McGrath RK: Hypoglycemia in four dogs with sepsis. *JAVMA* 178:1072–1076, 1981.

6. Leifer CE, Peterson ME, Matus RE, Patnaik AK: Hypoglycemia associated with nonislet cell tumors in 13 dogs. *JAVMA* 186:53–55, 1985.

7. Nelson RW, Foodman MS: Medical management of canine hyperinsulinism. *JAVMA* 187:78–82, 1985.

8. Nelson RW: Disorders of the endocrine pancreas, in Ettinger SJ (ed): *Textbook of Veterinary Internal Medicine*, ed 3. Philadelphia, WB Saunders Co, 1989, pp 1707–1720.

Medical Management of Canine Chronic Hepatitis

M. L. Magne, DVM, MS
Diplomate, ACVIM
Santa Cruz Veterinary Hospital
Santa Cruz, California

A. M. Chiapella, DVM
Diplomate, ACVIM
Beltway Internal Medicine Referral Service
Glenn Dale, Maryland

Chronic hepatitis in dogs encompasses a diverse group of inflammatory liver disorders resulting from multiple causes. Chronic *active* hepatitis is a specific form of chronic hepatitis that is characterized histologically by the presence of piecemeal necrosis, bridging necrosis, and a portal-to-periportal inflammatory infiltrate consisting of lymphocytes, plasma cells, macrophages, and lesser numbers of neutrophils.[1,2] Many liver biopsy samples, however, demonstrate inflammatory histopathologic changes that do not meet the histologic criteria for chronic active hepatitis. In these cases, the severity, anatomic localization, and inflammatory cell type can vary widely. Such inflammatory changes can result from viral infections, drug or chemical exposure, immunologic processes, or chronic gastrointestinal inflammatory disorders.[3-7] Regardless of the cause, if hepatic inflammation is not treated it can lead to hepatocellular necrosis, fibrosis, and eventually progress to cirrhosis.[8]

The aims of appropriate therapy in chronic hepatitis are to arrest inflammation, minimize fibrosis, prevent secondary bacterial invasion, and control ascites or hepatoencephalopathy. Problems encountered by the clinician in determining the appropriate therapy include establishing the correct diagnosis, determining chronicity of the disease, and deciding when to initiate and stop therapy. Drug action and pharmacokinetics, therapeutic sequelae, and optimum treatment regimens for canine chronic hepatitis have been poorly defined. It must be stressed that controlled clinicopharmacologic trials in dogs with chronic hepatitis are lacking, and that specific therapeutic recommendations often are speculative and empiric.

Antiinflammatory and Antifibrotic Therapy

Corticosteroids are advocated in the therapy of chronic hepatitis because of their antiinflammatory and antifibrotic effects[9-16]; however, published clinical data documenting the efficacy of corticosteroids in the management of canine chronic hepatitis are lacking. Prednisolone is the corticosteroid usually recommended, at a dosage of 1 to 2 mg/kg orally once daily until clinical remission. The dosage then is tapered slowly to reach a maintenance level of 0.5 mg/kg daily or on alternate days. If biochemical and histopathologic data indicate that complete remission has been achieved, corticosteroid therapy can be discontinued; however, patients must be evaluated periodically for evidence of relapse. Because corticosteroids can induce elevations in both serum alkaline phosphatase and alanine aminotransferase levels, hepatic histopathology is the only truly objective means of determining resolution of inflammation. It is recommended, therefore, that hepatic biopsy be repeated during therapy to assess the degree of histologic improvement. Because of the immunosuppressive, catabolic, and fluid-retaining effects of corticosteroids, their use theoretically is contraindicated in cases of hepatoencephalopathy, severe ascites, or infectious hepatitis.[17-19] Morbidity and mortality both increase when corticosteroids are administered to humans or animals with viral hepatitis.[14,20-23]

Other more potent immunosuppressive agents have been recommended for use in patients that fail to respond to corticosteroid therapy alone. The combination of azathioprine and a corticosteroid has been shown to be efficacious in inducing remissions in human patients with chronic active hepatitis,[9,10,16,24] and, in our experience, in cases of canine chronic hepatitis. In humans, the frequency of side effects is lower with this combination therapy than with high-dose corticosteroid therapy alone. Pretreatment cytopenia precludes use of azathioprine because of its potentially suppressive effect on bone marrow. Early signs of azathioprine toxicity include leukopenia, thrombocytopenia, gastrointestinal upset, dermatologic reactions, and hepatotoxicity. These effects usually resolve with reduced dosage or discontinuation. Because azathioprine inhibits nucleic acid synthesis, teratogenicity and oncogenicity are theoretically possible complications.[25,26] We recommend combination therapy with prednisolone at a dosage of 0.5 to 1.0 mg/kg per day and azathioprine at a dosage of 1.0 mg/kg per day. Once clinical remission is achieved, both drugs may be administered on an alternate-day basis.

Hepatic conversion of prednisone to prednisolone and azathioprine to 6-mercaptopurine is required for optimal immunosuppressive and antiinflammatory activity. Because of this requirement, administration of active rather than precursor compounds may be justified theoretically. The conversion of prednisone to prednisolone, however, is adequate in severe cases of human chronic active hepatitis, although these two drugs have not been compared with regard to clinical effectiveness.[17,27] Likewise, a clinical comparison of azathioprine and 6-mercaptopurine has not been performed.

Specific antifibrotic agents that have been used in the therapy of human chronic liver disease include colchicine, zinc gluconate, and polyunsaturated phosphatidylcholine. These are experimental drugs, and no data exist proving their efficacy in the prevention or resolution of hepatic fibrosis in dogs.

Colchicine is an antimitotic agent that acts by inhibiting the microtubular apparatus and the transcellular movement of collagen. It also may function as an antifibrotic agent by inducing the production of collagenase. Controlled studies in human cirrhotic patients have shown that long-term colchicine therapy results in improvement in ascites, hyperbilirubinemia, hepatoencephalopathy, and survival rate.[28] Numerous side effects have been noted with colchicine and include hemorrhagic gastroenteritis, bone marrow suppression, renal damage, and peripheral neuropathies.[11,29] We recommend a dosage of 0.03 mg/kg given intravenously.

Zinc gluconate has been shown to inhibit the accumulation of hepatic collagen in carbon tetrachloride–induced liver disease in rats. Additionally, human patients with cirrhosis have been shown to have reduced serum zinc levels. Polyunsaturated phosphatidylcholine is a highly unsaturated phospholipid extract of soy beans which, when used experimentally in human chronic hepatitis, was shown to reduce the severity of hepatic inflammation.[30] We have no personal experience with use of these drugs in dogs.

Dietary Management

Dietary management is primarily indicated to minimize abnormalities in protein metabolism that result in hyperammonemia and abnormal plasma amino acid ratios. This is accomplished by feeding a diet with a low—but high biologic value—protein level. Essentially, the patient should be fed as much protein as can be tolerated without developing hyperammonemia. The regeneration of hepatic tissue requires adequate dietary protein, and excessive restriction of dietary protein can lead to hypoproteinemia and deterioration of the liver condition. On the other hand, excessive dietary protein can lead to hyperammonemia and hepatoencephalopathy. The minimum amount of protein required in the dog's diet is 2.0 g/kg per day, while the normal maintenance requirement in adult dogs is 4.8 g/kg per day.[11,14,31,32]

Appropriate protein-restricted commercial diets are available or a homemade diet based on rice and cottage cheese can be used. Approximately 2.0 g/kg per day of high biologic value protein are provided in the commercially available kidney diet[a] if adequate amounts are eaten to meet caloric needs. An ultra-low protein diet is also available[b] but should be reserved for those patients with severe or refractory hepatoencephalopathy. Formulations for balanced, homemade diets for dogs with hepatic insufficiency have been published.[31,32] With these diets, daily caloric requirements are met by providing a carbohydrate, such as rice, in the diet. If inadequate calories are provided, energy needs will be supplied by metabolizing proteins in the diet and body tissues, with ammonia as a by-product. Beneficial properties of cottage cheese as a protein source include its high biologic value, high digestibility, lack of chemical additives, and good ratio of branched-chain to aromatic amino acids.[14,31,32] Multiple daily feedings of small amounts are recommended to maximize digestion and assimilation in the small intestine, thus decreasing the amount of protein that enters the colon to serve as a substrate for ammonia production. Low residue diets are also beneficial because intestinal epithelial cell desquamation is decreased, thereby reducing the amount of protein entering the colon.

The amount of fat in the diet should also be limited because certain short-chain fatty acids can contribute to the development of hepatoencephalopathy.[11,14,33] Fats should make up approximately 6% of the diet on a dry weight ba-

---

[a]Prescription Diet k/d®—Hill's Pet Products.
[b]Prescription Diet u/d®—Hill's Pet Products.

sis to provide the minimum requirement of 1.32 g/kg per day.[11]

A balanced vitamin and mineral supplement is recommended, especially in cases in which patients are fed homemade diets. Humans with chronic hepatitis are deficient in vitamin B_6, vitamin B_{12}, thiamine, vitamin A, vitamin E, riboflavin, nicotinic acid, pantothenic acid, folic acid, zinc, and cobalt.[11]

Management of Ascites

The development of ascites in individuals with chronic liver disease is a complex, multifactorial process. Viewed simplistically, ascites results from an interplay of three factors: portal hypertension resulting from hepatic fibrosis and cirrhosis, renal sodium and water retention, and decreased plasma oncotic pressure resulting from hypoalbuminemia.[34-37]

Therapeutic alternatives helpful in the management of ascites include cage rest, dietary sodium restriction, and the administration of diuretics. Ascites often tends to be regarded as an emergency condition, and thus overtreatment is not uncommon. The presence of ascites does not necessarily dictate the use of diuretics, and many animals with mild ascites may improve with cage rest and sodium restriction alone. The low protein diets discussed earlier also are moderately sodium restricted, and a severely sodium-restricted commercial diet also is available.[c] Formulas for homemade, sodium-restricted diets have been published in the veterinary literature.[31]

Diuretics are indicated when ascites is impairing vital organ function (dyspnea, reduced renal perfusion), limiting the patient's activity, or when cage rest and sodium restriction have been unsuccessful in controlling ascites formation. Initially, diuretics with a moderate natriuretic potency and minimal toxicity are recommended. Aldosterone antagonists, such as spironolactone, or thiazide diuretics are representative of this group. If the ascites is unresponsive, or becomes refractory to these agents, therapy with more potent loop diuretics, such as furosemide, is recommended. When administering loop diuretics, routine evaluation of serum electrolyte levels, especially potassium, is recommended. Fortunately, hypokalemia appears to be an uncommon complication of loop diuretic usage in dogs as long as the animal is neither anorectic nor vomiting.

A recommended protocol for diuretic therapy in chronic hepatitis-associated ascites in dogs is as follows. Initially, spironolactone is given at a dosage of 1.0 mg/kg twice daily. If diuresis has not occurred after four days (decreased body weight and abdominal girth), the dosage of spironolactone is increased to 2.0 mg/kg twice daily. If diuresis is achieved and ascites controlled, the dosage of spironolactone is tapered gradually to the lowest amount necessary to maintain the ascites in remission. If the ascites remains refractory, furosemide is added at a dosage of 1.0 mg/kg twice daily. This dosage can be doubled if ascites remains or becomes refractory. In patients that are severely

hypoalbuminemic, the administration of plasma followed by intravenous furosemide may be more effective.[34]

In humans with ascites, a rate of diuresis is established in which weight loss is not greater than 1.0 kg per day or 1.5% of body weight.[38] Extrapolating this figure to the dog would represent a weight loss not greater than 0.45 kg per day in a 30-kg animal.

Abdominal paracentesis rarely is indicated in the management of ascites except for diagnostic reasons. Reasonable indications for paracentesis include the relief of abdominal discomfort or respiratory distress resulting from massive ascites, a "tense" ascites in which renal perfusion may be compromised, or to facilitate physical examination and radiographic, laparoscopic, or surgical procedures. The potential complications of paracentesis include perforation of abdominal viscera, hypotensive shock resulting from rapid fluid removal, peritonitis, protein depletion, and hyponatremia.[8,34]

Fluid, Electrolyte, and Acid–Base Disturbances

Polyuria, polydipsia, and impaired renal function may accompany chronic liver disease. The pathogenesis of polyuria/polydipsia is multifactorial and is probably related to abnormal neurotransmitters, reduced renal medullary concentrating ability, hypokalemia, or altered function of portal vein osmoreceptors.[34,39,40] Renal function may be impaired primarily by the causative agent involved in the liver disease, such as in leptospirosis, or renal dysfunction may occur secondary to advanced liver disease. The hepatorenal syndrome, i.e., spontaneous deterioration in renal function secondary to advanced liver disease, has not been documented in veterinary medicine. In humans, this syndrome is characterized by progressive oliguria and azotemia occurring in patients with ascites and cirrhosis. The kidneys in these patients are normal histologically, and renal shutdown probably results from alterations in renal blood flow and glomerular filtration.[14,41] It is our opinion that this syndrome does occur in canine patients with advanced chronic liver disease, and thus manipulation of these patients must be undertaken cautiously. The hepatorenal syndrome is poorly responsive to therapy and merits a grave prognosis.

The treatment for polyuria/polydipsia of hepatic origin involves treatment of the underlying liver disorder. Salt supplementation to increase renal medullary concentrating ability should be avoided because of the tendency for sodium and fluid retention in patients with chronic liver disease. Prerenal azotemia should be corrected by the judicious administration of intravenous fluids, plasma, or albumin. As previously discussed, paracentesis to decrease intraabdominal pressure and improve renal perfusion may be helpful in patients with "tense" ascites.

Electrolyte and acid–base disturbances are variable in patients with chronic liver disease. Sodium retention and potassium depletion are the most common electrolyte imbalances seen,[34,42] while acid–base disturbances may be characterized by respiratory alkalosis, metabolic alkalosis, or metabolic acidosis.[34,43] Respiratory alkalosis is felt to

---

[c]Prescription Diet h/d® —Hill's Pet Products.

result from stimulation of either the medullary respiratory center or peripheral pulmonary stretch receptors. This stimulation is mediated by hypoxemia caused by pulmonary shunting, abnormal neurotransmitters, hyperammonemia, hyponatremia, increased plasma progesterone levels, or reduced thoracic expansion because of ascites.[44-46] Because of renal compensatory mechanisms, the predominant electrolyte pattern seen with respiratory alkalosis consists of hyperchloremia, hypokalemia, and reduced serum bicarbonate. Metabolic alkalosis is most commonly associated with overzealous diuretic usage, which results in extracellular volume contraction, potassium depletion, and increased aldosterone secretion.[34,43,47] These abnormalities lead to renal retention of sodium, chloride, and bicarbonate, whereas potassium and hydrogen loss in the urine is excessive. Metabolic acidosis results from lactic acidosis, which is most severe in patients with severe liver dysfunction, renal failure, or sepsis.[48] Lactic acid normally is metabolized by the liver. Thus, liver dysfunction accompanied by increased lactate production, as in sepsis or renal failure, can lead rapidly to hyperlactacidemia.

Because of the complexity of the acid–base and electrolyte disturbances that occur in chronic, advanced liver disease, mixed acid–base disturbances are common and therapy must be individually tailored based on measurement of electrolyte, bicarbonate, pH, and pCO_2 levels. Correction of hypokalemia, dehydration, renal dysfunction, infection, or overzealous diuretic usage will often lead to improvement in the acid–base status of these patients. Specific acid–base therapy usually is not indicated unless the blood pH is greater than 7.55 or less than 7.10, or if a base deficit greater than 10 mEq/L exists. When patients are symptomatic for acid–base disturbances (mental depression, cardiac arrhythmias), specific therapy may be indicated. Therapy for alkalosis includes the administration of 0.45% saline/2.5% dextrose, potassium supplementation, and adjustment of diuretic dosage. Therapy for acidosis includes fluid therapy to correct tissue and renal perfusion in addition to sodium bicarbonate administration. Fluids containing sodium must be used cautiously because of the tendency for sodium and fluid retention. To reiterate, therapy for acid–base disturbances in these patients is best determined by serial measurement of serum electrolyte, pH, pCO_2, and bicarbonate levels.

Antibiotic Therapy

Hepatic reticuloendothelial function is reduced in chronic hepatitis; thus, gut-origin bacteria are not cleared from the portal circulation, and bacterial invasion and septicemia may result. Antibiotic therapy, therefore, is directed against intestinal aerobic and anaerobic organisms. Penicillins, ampicillins, cephalosporins, and aminoglycosides can be used safely in patients with liver disease, and routine pharmacologic doses are recommended. Penicillin, ampicillin, or cephalosporins can be used in combination with aminoglycosides to yield very broad-spectrum coverage. When possible, specific isolation and identification of infectious organisms should be made. Antibiotics that should be avoided in patients with chronic liver disease include chloramphenicol, erythromycin, hetacillin, lincomycin, and sulfonamides. These agents either depend on hepatic metabolism for activation or clearance, or are capable of causing liver damage.[14,33,49]

Copper-Chelating Agents

Elevated hepatic copper levels occur in various types of chronic liver disease in dogs. Copper accumulation may be a primary event, as occurs in copper storage disease of Bedlington terriers, or secondary to reduced biliary copper excretion, as suggested in chronic active hepatitis of Doberman pinschers.[11,40,50,51]

D-Penicillamine promotes a reduction in hepatic copper content by forming a chelate with serum copper that is subsequently excreted in the urine. Other possible beneficial actions of D-penicillamine include inhibition of tropocollagen cross-linking and suppression of T-cell immunologic function. Clinical evidence suggests that D-penicillamine may actually be more effective than corticosteroids in preventing or reversing hepatic fibrosis.[52,53] Vomiting and anorexia are common side effects with this drug. The recommended dosage is 10 to 15 mg/kg twice daily.

Recently, in a limited number of dogs, a chelating agent known as 2,3,2-tetramine was shown to be superior to D-penicillamine in its ability to reduce hepatic copper content. No side effects of this drug were observed in this study.[54]

Management of Hepatoencephalopathy

Hepatoencephalopathy is a complex, multifactorial disorder characterized by abnormalities of ammonia and amino acid metabolism, false or inhibitory neurotransmitter synthesis, and increased blood levels of mercaptans and short-chain fatty acids. A complete discussion of the pathogenesis and management of hepatoencephalopathy is beyond the scope of this article. For a more detailed discussion, the reader is referred to several excellent reviews in the veterinary literature.[33,55-57]

One of the first considerations in management of the patient with hepatoencephalopathy is the identification and correction of factors that may precipitate or exacerbate the encephalopathy. Patients with chronic liver disease have an increased susceptibility to infection because of decreased hepatic reticuloendothelial function. The presence of infection, therefore, especially of the urinary, respiratory, and gastrointestinal systems, should be determined and therapy with appropriate antibiotics instituted. Concurrent drug therapy that may precipitate encephalopathy should be discontinued. Sedatives, tranquilizers, and analgesics have a depressant effect on the central nervous system. In addition, many of these agents are metabolized in the liver; thus prolonged effects may occur in the patient with compromised liver function. Organophosphate drugs also are metabolized in the liver and are contraindicated in these patients because of potential toxicity. Methionine-containing preparations, such as many of the lipotropic drugs, should not be administered to patients with chronic liver disease or hepatoencephalopathy as they can lead to elevated blood mercaptan levels and thus exacerbate encephalopathy. Excessive diuretic usage can lead to azotemia and hypokalemia, especially in patients that are anorectic or vomiting. Appropriate therapy includes discontinuation of diuretic use, intravenous fluid administration, and potassium supplementation.

Gastrointestinal bleeding can precipitate hepatoencephalopathy because blood in the gastrointestinal tract serves as a source of ammonia production. Potential sources of gastrointestinal hemorrhage include ulcers, hemorrhagic gastroenteritis, parasite infestation, or coagulopathies, and these disorders should be diagnosed and treated appropriately. Nonsteroidal antiinflammatory agents can potentiate gastrointestinal hemorrhage and ulceration, and they should not be administered to patients with chronic liver disease.

A primary goal in the treatment of hepatoencephalopathy is to reduce the formation and absorption of toxic substances from the gastrointestinal tract. Food should be withheld for several days to minimize the amount of protein entering the gut to act as a substrate for ammonia production. Enemas also are beneficial and act by reducing the number of urease-producing bacteria in the colon, thus decreasing ammonia production. In addition, enemas with acidic solutions serve to "ion-trap" ammonia within the colon as ammonium ion, thereby decreasing its absorption. We recommend an enema consisting of povidone-iodine solution (Betadine®—Purdue Frederick) diluted 1:10 with warm water. Enemas may be repeated at four- to six-hour intervals, depending on the animal's clinical response. Lactulose and neomycin may also be added to enema solutions. Repeated enemas can cause electrolyte depletion, and Fleet® enemas (C. B. Fleet) are contraindicated in small dogs, cats, or debilitated animals because of possible electrolyte and osmolality disturbances which can result from their use in such patients.

Intravenous fluid therapy is of critical importance in the proper management of hepatic coma. Appropriate fluid therapy serves to correct hypovolemia and maintain normal fluid, electrolyte, and acid–base balance. Maintenance of normovolemia optimizes hepatic and renal blood flow, as well as correcting or preventing the development of azotemia. Azotemia causes an increase in endogenous ammonia production and must be avoided in patients with chronic liver disease. The type of fluid used is also important. Lactate-containing solutions such as lactated Ringer's solution should be avoided because lactate must be metabolized to bicarbonate in the liver. Hyperaldosteronism and sodium retention occur in chronic liver disease, thus solutions with high sodium content should be avoided. We routinely use 0.45% saline with 2.5% dextrose in patients with chronic liver disease. Glucose serves as a source of calories (minimal), minimizes gluconeogenesis, and is important in preventing sepsis-related hypoglycemia.[33,57] Glucose is thought to decrease central nervous system ammonia levels by stimulating the combination of ammonia with glutamic acid to form glutamine.[57] As discussed previously, hypoka-

lemia frequently occurs in chronic liver disease, and appropriate supplementation is indicated. If renal and cardiovascular function are normal, 20 to 30 mEq of potassium chloride may be added safely to each liter of fluids administered.[33] Continued potassium supplementation should be dictated by measurement of serum levels.

Lactulose therapy can be extremely beneficial in the treatment of hepatoencephalopathy. Lactulose is a synthetic disaccharide which is hydrolyzed by colonic bacteria to acidic by-products. The by-products serve to acidify colonic contents, thus reducing ammonia absorption, and also act as an osmotic laxative, which reduces the numbers of colonic bacteria. In comatose patients, lactulose may be given via stomach tube (20 to 60 ml every 4 to 6 hours), or as an enema solution (300 to 450 g diluted in warm water to 200 to 300 ml).[33,58] For maintenance therapy, lactulose is given at a dosage of 1 ml to 2 ml per 5 kg to 10 kg three times daily. The daily dose is adjusted to achieve a therapeutic end point of two to three soft stools per day. Diarrhea and flatulence are the most common side effects.

H_2 receptor blockers, such as cimetidine or ranitidine, are indicated in patients with evidence of gastrointestinal bleeding (hematemesis, melena, positive occult blood). Recommended dosages are: cimetidine, 5 mg/kg orally, intravenously, or intramuscularly three to four times a day; ranitidine, 0.5 mg/kg orally twice a day. Therapy should be continued for several weeks beyond resolution of the gastrointestinal hemorrhage.

Oral nonabsorbable antibiotics, such as neomycin, are helpful in treating hyperammonemia. Neomycin may act synergistically with lactulose, and both drugs can be given by enema in critical patients. Recently, metronidazole has been shown to be efficacious in the management of hepatoencephalopathy.[59] This drug is very effective against *Bacteroides* and other colonic anaerobes, and it is felt that such organisms may be important in the colonic production of ammonia.[33,55] We recommend a dosage for metronidazole of 7.5 mg/kg three times a day.

Seizures may occur in patients with hepatoencephalopathy and should be controlled; however, caution is necessary when using anticonvulsants in patients with liver disease. Initially, glucose (0.5 g/kg) as a 25% solution is given intravenously because seizures in these patients may be caused by hypoglycemia. If seizures persist, diazepam is given intravenously at a reduced dosage (2.5 mg). Barbiturate anticonvulsants should be avoided.

Newer therapies in human hepatoencephalopathy patients include infusion of branched-chain amino acid solutions and the use of dopamine agonists such as L-dopa and bromocriptine.[55,60,61] Branched-chain amino acid solutions are available commercially; however, they are extremely expensive. We have no personal experience with the use of these drugs in dogs.

Conclusion

Chronic hepatitis in dogs is a complex clinical syndrome that presents a challenge in medical management. Appropriate therapeutic modalities include antiinflammatory therapy; dietary manipulation; management of ascites; fluid, electrolyte, and acid–base balance; and the control or prevention of hepatoencephalopathy. Therapy must be individualized to the abnormalities present in a particular patient, and constant monitoring is essential in assessing the need for ongoing therapy. The ideal goal is earlier diagnosis and therapeutic intervention so that the sequelae of chronic liver disease are avoided.

REFERENCES

1. Meyer DJ, Iverson WO, Terrell TG: Obstructive jaundice associated with chronic active hepatitis. *JAVMA* 176:41–44, 1980.
2. Zawie DA, Gilbertson SR: Interpretation of liver biopsy: A clinician's perspective. *Vet Clin North Am [Small Anim Pract]* 15:67–76, 1985.
3. Dew MJ, Thompson H, Allan RN: The spectrum of hepatic dysfunction in inflammatory bowel disease. *Q J Med* 48:113–135, 1979.
4. Dillon R: The liver in systemic disease: An innocent bystander. *Vet Clin North Am [Small Anim Pract]* 15:97–117, 1985.
5. Gocke DJ, Morris TQ, Bradley SE: Chronic hepatitis in the dog: The role of immune factors. *JAVMA* 156:1700–1708, 1970.
6. Thornburg LP: Diseases of the liver in the dog and cat. *Compend Contin Educ Pract Vet* 4(7):538–546, 1982.
7. Whitcomb FF: Chronic active liver disease: Definition, diagnosis, and management. *Med Clin North Am* 63:413–421, 1979.
8. Twedt DC: Cirrhosis: A consequence of chronic liver disease. *Vet Clin North Am [Small Anim Pract]* 15:151–176, 1985.
9. Cook GC, Mulligan R, Sherlock S: Controlled prospective trial of corticosteroid therapy in active chronic hepatitis. *Q J Med* 40:159–185, 1971.
10. Czaja AJ: Current problems in the diagnosis and management of chronic active hepatitis. *Mayo Clin Proc* 56:311–323, 1981.
11. Hardy RM: Chronic hepatitis: An emerging syndrome in dogs. *Vet Clin North Am [Small Anim Pract]* 15:135–150, 1985.
12. Schalm SW: Treatment of chronic active hepatitis. *Liver* 2:69–76, 1982.
13. Seef LB, Koff RS: Therapy for chronic active hepatitis. *Adv Intern Med* 29:109–145, 1984.
14. Strombeck DR: Management of canine chronic active hepatitis, in Kirk RW (ed): *Current Veterinary Therapy VII.* Philadelphia, WB Saunders Co, 1980, pp 885–891.
15. Strombeck DR, Gribble DG: Chronic active hepatitis in the dog. *JAVMA* 173:380–386, 1978.
16. Wright EC, Seef LB, Berk PD, et al: Treatment of chronic active hepatitis: An analysis of three controlled trials. *Gastroenterology* 73:1422–1430, 1977.
17. Uribe M, Summerskill WHJ, Go VLW: Comparative serum prednisone and prednisolone concentrations following administration to patients with chronic active liver disease. *Clin Pharmacokinet* 7:452–459, 1982.
18. Uribe M, Summerskill WHJ, Go VLW: Why hyperbilirubinemia and hypoalbuminemia predispose to steroid side effects during treatment of chronic active liver disease (CALD). *Gastroenterology* 72:1143, 1977.
19. Uribe M, Wolf AM, Summerskill WHJ: Steroid side effects during therapy of chronic active liver disease (CALD): What to expect. *Gastroenterology* 71:932, 1976.
20. Conn HO, Maddrey WC, Soloway RD: The detrimental effects of adrenocorticosteroid therapy in HBsAg-positive chronic active hepatitis. Fact or fallacy? *Hepatology* 2:885–887, 1982.
21. Lam KC, Lai CL, Trepo C, et al: Deleterious effect of prednisolone in HBsAg-positive chronic hepatitis. *N Engl J Med* 304:380–386, 1981.
22. Redeker AJ: Treatment of chronic active hepatitis: Good news and bad news. *N Engl J Med* 304:420–421, 1981.
23. Wu PC, Lai CL, Lam KC, et al: Prednisolone in HBsAg-positive chronic active hepatitis: Histologic evaluation in a controlled prospective study. *Hepatology* 2:777–783, 1982.
24. Summerskill WHJ, Korman MG, Ammon HV, et al: Prednisone for chronic active liver disease: Dose titration, standard dose, and combination with azathioprine compared. *Gut* 16:876–883, 1975.
25. Elion GB: Action of purine analogs: Enzyme specificity studies as a basis for interpretation and design. *Cancer Res* 29:2448–2453, 1969.
26. Speck WT, Rosenkranz HS: Mutagenicity of azathioprine. *Cancer Res* 36:108–109, 1976.
27. Powell LW, Axelsen E: Corticosteroids in liver disease: Studies on the biological conversion of prednisone to prednisolone and plasma protein binding. *Gut* 13:690–696, 1972.
28. Rojkind M, Kershenobich D: Hepatic fibrosis, in Popper H, Schaffner F (eds): *Progress in Liver Diseases.* New York, Grune & Stratton, 1976, pp 294–310.
29. Kershonobich D, Uribe M, Suares GI, et al: Treatment of cirrhosis with colchicine: A double-blind, randomized trial. *Gastroenterology* 77:532, 1979.
30. Jenkins PJ, Portmann ALW, Eddleston F, et al: Use of polyunsaturated phosphatidylcholine in HBsAg-negative chronic active hepatitis: Results of a prospective double-blind controlled trial. *Liver* 2:77, 1982.
31. Lewis LD, Morris UL: Gastrointestinal, pancreatic and hepatic diseases, in *Small Animal Clinical Nutrition.* Topeka, KS, Mark Morris Associates, 1983, pp 6-1–6-32.
32. Strombeck DR, Schaffer ML, Rogers QR: Dietary therapy for dogs with chronic hepatic insufficiency, in Kirk RW (ed): *Current Veterinary Therapy VIII.* Philadelphia, WB Saunders Co, 1983, pp 817–821.
33. Tamms TR: Hepatic encephalopathy. *Vet Clin North Am [Small Anim Pract]* 15:177–195, 1985.
34. Grauer GF, Nichols CER: Ascites, renal abnormalities, and electrolyte and acid-base disorders associated with liver disease. *Vet Clin North Am [Small Anim Pract]* 15:197–214, 1985.
35. Lieberman FL, Denison EK, Reynolds TB: The relationship of plasma volume, portal hypertension, ascites, and renal sodium retention in cirrhosis: The overflow theory of ascites formation. *Ann NY Acad Sci* 170:202–212, 1970.
36. Schilling JA, McCoord AB, Clausen SW, et al: Experimental ascites. Studies of electrolyte balance in dogs with partial and complete occlusion of the portal vein and of the vena cava above and below the liver. *J Clin Invest* 31:702–710, 1952.
37. Wyllie R, Arasu TS, Fitzgerald JF: Ascites: Pathophysiology and management. *J Pediatr* 97:167–176, 1980.
38. Beck LH: Edema states and the use of diuretics. *Med Clin North Am* 65:291–301, 1981.
39. Berl T, Linas SL, Aisenbrey GA, et al: On the mechanism of polyuria in potassium depletion: The role of polydipsia. *J Clin Invest* 60:620–625, 1977.
40. Hardy RM: Diseases of the liver, in Ettinger SJ (ed): *Textbook of Veterinary Internal Medicine,* ed 2. Philadelphia, WB Saunders Co, 1983, pp 1372–1434.
41. Conn HO: A rational approach to the hepatorenal syndrome. *Gastroenterology* 65:021–210, 1973.
42. Reynolds TB: Water, electrolyte, and acid-base disorders in liver disease, in Maxwell MH, Kleeman CR (eds): *Clinical Disorders of Fluid and Electrolyte Metabolism.* New York, McGraw-Hill Book Co, 1980, pp 1251–1265.
43. Sabatini S, Arruda JA, Kurtzman DA: Disorders of acid-base balance. *Med Clin North Am* 62:1223–1255, 1978.
44. Wichner J, Kazenii H: Ammonia and ventilation: Site and mechanism of action. *Resp Physiol* 20:393–396, 1974.
45. Wilder CE, Morrison RS, Tyler JM: Relationship between serum sodium and hyperventilation in cirrhosis. *Am Rev Resp Dis* 96:971–975, 1967.
46. Wolfe JD, Tashkin DP, Holly FE, et al: Hypoxemia or cirrhosis. Detection of small pulmonary vascular channels by a quantitative radionuclide method. *Ann Intern Med* 63:746–750, 1977.
47. Cogan MG, Fu-Ying L, Berger BE, et al: Metabolic alkalosis. *Med Clin North Am* 67:903–914, 1983.
48. Frommer JP: Lactic acidosis. *Med Clin North Am [Small Anim Pract]* 67:815–828, 1983.
49. Papich MG, Davis LE: Drugs and the liver. *Vet Clin North Am [Small Anim Pract]* 15:77–95, 1985.
50. Johnson GF, Zawie DA, Gilbertson SR, et al: Chronic active hepatitis in Doberman Pinschers. *JAVMA* 180:1435–1442, 1982.
51. Twedt DC, Sternlieb I, Gilbertson SR: Clinical, morphologic, and chemical studies on copper toxicosis of Bedlington Terriers. *JAVMA* 175:269–275, 1979.

52. Chen TS, Zaki GF, Levy CM: Studies of nucleic acid and collagen synthesis: Current status in assessing liver repair. *Med Clin North Am* 63:583, 1979.
53. Popper H: Hepatic fibrosis and collagen metabolism in the liver, in Popper H, Becker K (eds): *Collagen Metabolism in the Liver*. New York, Stratton Intercontinental Medical Book Corp, 1975, pp 1–14.
54. Twedt DC, Allen KD, Magne ML: The use of 2,3,2-tetramine as a hepatic copper chelator in the therapy of Bedlington terrier dogs with copper toxicosis. *Proc Am Gastroenterol Soc* 88:1701, 1985.
55. Drazner FH: Hepatic encephalopathy in the dog, in Kirk RW (ed): *Current Veterinary Therapy VIII*. Philadelphia, WB Saunders Co, 1983, pp 829–834.
56. Sherding RG: Hepatic encephalopathy in the dog. *Compend Contin Educ Pract Vet* 1(1):55–63, 1979.
57. Twedt DC: Jaundice, hepatic trauma, and hepatic encephalopathy. *Vet Clin North Am [Small Anim Pract]* 11:121–146, 1981.
58. Vince AJ, Burridge SM: Ammonia production by intestinal bacteria: The effects of lactose, lactulose, glucose. *J Med Microbiol* 13:177–191, 1980.
59. Morgan MH, Read AE: Treatment of hepatic encephalopathy with metronidazole. *Gut* 23:1–7, 1982.
60. Cerra FB, Cheung NK, Fischer JE, et al: A multicenter trial of branched chain enriched amino acid infusion (F080) in hepatic encephalopathy. *Hepatology* 5:699, 1982.
61. Freund F, Dienstag J, Lehrich J, et al: Infusion of branched-chain enriched amino acid solutions in patients with hepatic encephalopathy. *Ann Surg* 196:209–220, 1982.

UPDATE

Since this article was published in 1986, there have been few advancements in the therapeutic manipulation of chronic hepatitis in dogs. Ursodeoxycholic acid (ursodiol), a bile acid originally used for cholecystolith dissolution in humans, has shown promise in the treatment of other chronic inflammatory liver disorders. The mechanisms by which ursodiol exerts its beneficial effects are not completely understood, although this drug is thought to act primarily by displacing other toxic, detergent bile acids from the enterohepatic circulation and hepatocyte membranes. Ursodiol comes in 300-mg capsules (Actigall®—Summit Pharmaceuticals, Summit, New Jersey), and the suggested dosage for dogs is 10 to 15 mg/kg daily. No side effects have been observed in dogs undergoing long-term therapy at this dosage. Colchicine, an antifibrotic agent, is now available in tablet form for oral use. (Colchicine is typically combined with probenecid, a uricosuric agent.) The recommended dosage for dogs is 0.03 mg/kg daily. Gastrointestinal side effects, which have been seen in some patients, may be alleviated by reducing the dosage.

Hepatoencephalopathy. Part I. Clinical Signs and Diagnosis

KEY FACTS

- Animals with hepatoencephalopathy can present with a wide variety of signs involving the central nervous system, and these signs often occur intermittently.
- Specific liver function tests that are used to document functional liver impairment include ammonia tolerance, preprandial and postprandial serum bile acid levels, and sulfobromophthalein clearance.
- After the diagnosis of hepatoencephalopathy, the underlying liver disease is identified by liver biopsy or radiographic contrast study of the portal vascular system.

Veterinary Medical Referral Service
Riverwoods, Illinois
John W. Tyler, DVM

HEPATOENCEPHALOPATHY (HE) is a neurophysiologic disorder of the central nervous system (CNS) that occurs secondary to hepatic malfunction or an abnormality in the portal blood supply of the liver.[1,2] The disorder is associated with very few anatomic lesions, gross or microscopic, of the central nervous system. Clinical signs vary from intermittent behavioral changes to episodic seizures. Signs that indicate involvement of other body systems are often present but are not specific to the underlying liver disease. A key diagnostic feature is that clinical signs are intermittent. Except in some long-standing cases, hepatoencephalopathy is a reversible condition.

The first part of this two-part presentation discusses the clinical signs and diagnosis of hepatoencephalopathy. Part II will consider the development of a rational therapeutic plan based on a thorough understanding of the pathophysiology of the condition.

SIGNALMENT AND PRESENTING CLINICAL SIGNS

Signalment depends on the cause of hepatic dysfunction. Although most dogs and cats with congenital portosystemic shunts (PSS) present at younger than one year of age, the condition has been diagnosed in dogs as old as eight years of age.[3,4] Congenital portosystemic shunts are reported more frequently in purebred dogs; the significance of this fact is debatable. Acquired portosystemic shunts tend to occur in middle-aged and old dogs and cats.

Most dogs and cats with portosystemic shunts demonstrate signs of hepatoencephalopathy.[1,3-9] Patients with liver failure secondary to toxic or infectious processes can also exhibit signs of hepatoencephalopathy. There is no age or breed predisposition for animals with toxic or infectious liver disease.

Chronic liver failure with or without hepatoencephalopathy occurs in Bedlington terriers secondary to copper storage disease. Female Doberman pinschers are predisposed to hepatic failure secondary to a disease entity with a clinical course best described as chronic active hepatitis. These dogs often have hepatoencephalopathy.

Patients with hepatoencephalopathy usually have a history of chronic, intermittent, relapsing central nervous system signs. An exception is hepatoencephalopathy secondary to acute hepatic failure. Central nervous system signs often consist of changes in behavior or attitude. Dogs and cats can become depressed and lethargic and/or hysterical and vicious. Some animals become stuporous or comatose, and intermittent seizure activity is occasionally present.

Other central nervous system signs that have been observed are ataxia, circling, compulsive pacing, head pressing, disorientation, and amaurosis. Owners might report that pets seem to pant excessively or inappropriately. Ptyalism is a common presenting sign in cats with portosystemic shunts; it has also been noted in dogs.[3,4,10] Central nervous system signs can occur or intensify three to four hours after meals, especially high-protein meals. An intolerance to anesthetic agents or organophosphates might be reported.

IN DOGS with hepatoencephalopathy, intermittent and sometimes vague gastrointestinal signs can be concurrent with central nervous system signs.[1,3-9,11] Vomiting, diarrhea, anorexia, and weight loss are common problems. Stunting is often present in dogs with hepatoencephalopathy secondary to congenital portosystemic shunts. Ascites can also occur.

Polyuria and polydipsia are often present in addition to central nervous system signs.[1,3,6] Less frequently, pollakiuria and dysuria occur secondary to urate or ammonium biurate calculi in the bladder.[1,9]

Occasionally, patients with hepatoencephalopathy have a history of recurrent systemic infections or unexplained fevers that tend to aggravate or induce central nervous system signs. The fevers and infections respond to antibiotic therapy but tend to recur after therapy is discontinued.[1,6,8]

DIAGNOSIS
Differential Diagnosis and Laboratory Evaluation

The first step in diagnosing patients with signs referable to the central nervous system is to determine whether the disease process is a primary central nervous system problem or a systemic disease that secondarily affects the central nervous system. Idiopathic epilepsy usually occurs in dogs that are one to three years of age; this age range overlaps the period during which dogs with hepatoencephalopathy caused by congenital portosystemic shunts are usually diagnosed. In dogs younger than one year of age, canine distemper is a primary ruleout in the differential diagnosis; this is particularly true if respiratory signs are mild or inapparent.

Distemper encephalitis is also included in the differential diagnosis of old dogs with central nervous system signs. Hypoglycemia should be an element in the differential diagnosis of intermittent central nervous system signs. In old patients, various metabolic and endocrine abnormalities can produce clinical signs similar to those of hepatoencephalopathy. Uremia, diabetes mellitus, and hypoadrenocorticism are prime examples.

Evaluation of patients with central nervous system signs that might be secondary to liver failure and/or portosystemic shunts should include complete blood count (CBC), determination of serum total protein, albumin, serum urea nitrogen (SUN), serum creatinine, serum alkaline phosphatase (SAP), serum alanine transferase (SALT), serum electrolytes (especially potassium), blood glucose, fasting blood ammonia levels, blood gases, and a complete urinalysis. Abdominal radiographs should also be taken.

In patients with hepatoencephalopathy, abnormalities in the complete blood count or serum chemical analysis are consistent with or indicative of liver disease. The complete blood count can demonstrate a normal or slightly decreased packed cell volume (PCV). Microcytosis, with normochromia and a normal or mildly decreased packed cell volume, is a common finding in dogs with portosystemic shunts.[9,12] In a retrospective study of cats with congenital portosystemic shunts, poikilocytosis was frequently noted[13]; the researchers stressed that the finding was not specific for liver disease.

The white blood cell count (WBC) can be normal, or mature neutrophilia can be present. Neutrophilia with a significant left shift is often present in patients with concurrent infections. The serum total protein is usually decreased; most of the decrease results from markedly reduced albumin levels.[9,12]

In patients with congenital portosystemic shunts or portosystemic shunts secondary to liver cirrhosis, serum alkaline phosphatase and serum alanine transferase levels are normal or mildly elevated (three to five times).[3] As might be expected from the serum alkaline phosphatase levels, bilirubin levels are often not markedly elevated in patients with portosystemic shunts or cirrhosis.[13,14] Acute fulminant hepatic disease or acute exacerbations of chronic liver disease usually lead to marked increases in serum alkaline phosphatase and serum alanine transferase levels.

DECREASED conversion of ammonia to urea by the liver can lead to abnormally low serum urea nitrogen levels.[3] Interestingly, dogs with urea cycle enzyme deficiencies have normal serum urea nitrogen concentrations. It is believed that enzyme activity is adequate to keep the serum urea nitrogen level normal but not to maintain normal blood ammonia levels.[15] Decreased functional liver tissue might also lead to decreased glycogen stores and decreased gluconeogenesis, which in turn might result in fasting hypoglycemia.[9]

Patients with liver disease are often hypovolemic and can have a wide variety of acid-base and electrolyte abnormalities. Metabolic or respiratory alkalosis and hypokalemia are common problems. Hypokalemia, hypovolemia, and alkalosis and can play significant roles in the pathogenesis of hepatoencephalopathy. Hypokalemia is caused by decreased oral intake, gastrointestinal losses (vomiting or diarrhea), renal losses, and overuse of diuretics to reduce ascites secondary to liver disease.[12] Hypokalemia can be aggravated by hypovolemia secondary to gastrointestinal fluid losses. Hypovolemia causes increased plasma aldosterone levels, which enhance renal potassium excretion.

Respiratory alkalosis and metabolic alkalosis are common blood gas abnormalities in patients with liver disease.[16] Respiratory alkalosis is secondary to hyperventilation caused by (1) a direct stimulatory effect of toxins on the respiratory center[16,17] or (2) decreased magnitude of diaphragmatic excursions because of abdominal ascites.

Metabolic alkalosis is caused by excessive vomiting and volume depletion. Metabolic alkalosis can be enhanced by hypokalemia. Hypokalemia causes increased proximal renal tubular hydrogen secretion and subsequently increased bicarbonate (HCO_3^-) absorption. Distal renal tubular hydrogen excretion is enhanced secondary to increased ammonia formation by the distal renal tubular cells. Subsequently, hydrogen is trapped in the tubular lumen as ammonium (NH_4^+). Increased bicarbonate absorption and increased ammonia production are secondary to hypokalemia-induced intracellular acidosis.[18,19]

Patients with liver failure can have hematuria and proteinuria secondary to lower urinary tract inflammation caused by ammonium biurate or urate crystals or calculi.[1,3] Because uric acid is normally converted by the liver to allantoin, liver failure leads to increased concentrations of uric acid in the serum and urine. These concentrations can result in the formation of ammonium biurate or urate calculi.[3]

Patients with hepatoencephalopathy can exhibit clotting problems caused by the inability of the liver to manufacture adequate amounts of clotting factors. Because factor VII has the shortest half-life of the clotting factors, the activity of this factor is the most sensitive indicator of the ability of the liver to produce clotting factors.[20] Factor VII plays an integral role in the extrinsic clotting pathway. One-stage prothrombin time (OSPT) is the preferred method for evaluating factor VII deficiency because the method examines the extrinsic and common pathways of the coagulation cascade.

SURVEY abdominal radiographs are important diagnostic tools in evaluating patients with possible hepatoencephalopathy.[3,6,11] The vast majority of animals with portosystemic shunts have markedly small livers. Renomegaly often is a concurrent finding.[3,11] In many patients with portosystemic shunts, ascites or lack of intraabdominal fat results in poor abdominal detail; evaluation of liver and kidney size is thus difficult.[3] An enlarged liver silhouette can be evident on plain abdominal radiographs of patients with hepatoencephalopathy secondary to acute hepatitis, hepatic tumors, or other infiltrative liver diseases.

Dogs and cats with hepatoencephalopathy that present with an acute onset of profound neurologic signs might be initially evaluated for primary central nervous system disease. During the workup, a cerebrospinal fluid (CSF) tap or an electroencephalogram (EEG) might be performed. Analysis of cerebrospinal fluid from patients with hepatoencephalopathy usually does not demonstrate abnormalities.[11] The electroencephalogram can be normal or can demonstrate increased slow-wave activity, which is not specific for hepatoencephalopathy but is consistent with metabolic encephalopathy.[11]

If the results of these diagnostic tests are compatible with or suggestive of liver disease, tests designed specifically to evaluate the portal blood supply and/or the functional capabilities of the liver should be performed. These tests include sulfobromophthalein (BSP) clearance, ammonia tolerance, and preprandial and postprandial serum bile acid levels. Depending on the results of these tests, a liver biopsy via laparoscopy or an exploratory laparotomy might be indicated. A radiographic contrast study of the portal vascular system might also be justified.

Specific Liver Function Tests

The ammonia tolerance test can be used to evaluate the integrity of the portal blood supply and the functional mass of the liver.[20,21] The test does not evaluate the hepatobiliary system and is not affected by derangements in bilirubin metabolism or excretion. The ammonia tolerance test is performed by administering via stomach tube 100 mg/kg (a maximum of 3 g) of ammonium chloride (NH_4Cl) diluted in 30 to 50 cc of water. A (12-hour) fasting baseline sample is taken before the test, and another sample is taken 30 minutes after the ammonium chloride is given.

It has been suggested that the most accurate interpretation of an ammonia tolerance test is obtained by comparing absolute baseline and postchallenge blood ammonia levels with laboratory values for normal animals.[20] High postchallenge blood ammonia levels indicate decreased functional hepatic tissue and/or portosystemic shunts.

The most common side effect of ammonium chloride administration is vomiting, but this usually does not interfere with accurate testing.[14] If vomiting is a problem, protocols can be followed for performing the test via ammonium chloride enema.[3] Signs of hepatoencephalopathy are rarely induced or enhanced after ammonium chloride is administered.[1] Falsely elevated ammonia values can occur if the blood sample is hemolyzed.[21] To obtain accurate values, samples must be processed immediately[20,21]; the test is thus impractical for most private practices.

Increased retention of sulfobromophthalein in the blood after intravenous injection indicates decreased hepatic functional mass and/or abnormalities in bilirubin metabolism or excretion.[21] The test is performed by giving 5 mg/kg of sulfobromophthalein intravenously and measuring blood levels 30 minutes later. Normal retention values are less than 5% in dogs.[20,21] Some researchers suggest that retention values of less than 3% are normal in cats.[4] Sulfobromophthalein levels can be falsely elevated secondary to decreased hepatic blood supply caused by cardiac insufficiency or hypovolemia.[20,21]

HYPOALBUMINEMIA can enhance the clearance rate of sulfobromophthalein.[21] High-protein effusions increase the volume of distribution of sulfobromophthalein and falsely lower retention values; transudates and other low-protein effusions should not affect sulfobromophthalein clearance.[21] In hyperbilirubinemic patients, the sulfobromophthalein test does not provide new information and should not be performed.

The measurement of fasting and postprandial serum bile

acid levels is the most practical liver function test available to private practitioners. The necessary samples are easy to obtain and do not require special handling.

The liver has a large reserve capacity for the production of bile acids. The acids are secreted into the duodenum after gallbladder contraction induced by cholecystokinin (CCK). Ninety-five percent of the bile acids that are released into the gut are resorbed from the ileum into the portal blood and are subsequently removed by the liver.[20] After a normal meal, the total bile acid pool recycles through the liver three to five times.[20] After a 12-hour fast, there should be minimal amounts of bile acids in the blood: less than 5 μmol/L in dogs and less than 2 μmol/L in cats.[20]

FASTING SERUM bile acid levels can increase as a result of decreased hepatic uptake (decreased functional mass), cholestasis, and decreased hepatic portal blood flow. After a 12-hour fast, blood levels can be nearly normal in patients with portosystemic shunts or decreased hepatic functional mass. Fasting serum bile acid levels remain higher in patients with cholestatic disease.[20]

In dogs, there is a 90% chance of liver disease if fasting serum bile acid levels are greater than 30 μmol/L. If levels exceed 50 μmol/L, liver disease is present.[14] In cats, there is a 90% chance of liver disease if fasting levels exceed 5 μmol/L; levels greater than 15 μmol/L are associated with a 100% incidence of liver disease.[13] One researcher suggests obtaining a liver biopsy if the fasting bile acid level exceeds 30 μmol/L in dogs or 20 μmol/L in cats.[20]

Endogenous challenge testing can be performed in individuals that have fasting bile acid concentrations in or near the normal range but that are still believed to have liver disease. Such a patient is fed; two hours later, a postprandial serum sample is obtained. The meal stimulates the release of cholecystokinin from the duodenum; the hormone causes bile acids to be released into the duodenum. These acids act as an endogenous challenge to the failing liver. Animals that have liver failure or portosystemic shunts cannot adequately remove recycling bile acids from the blood. Serum bile acid levels increase to greater than 15.5 μmol/L in dogs and greater than 10.0 μmol/L in cats.[20] Animals with cholestatic disease also exhibit an increase in serum bile acids after endogenous challenge, but the level and the slope of the increase are less than in animals with portosystemic shunts or liver failure.[20] This lesser response occurs because the enterohepatic cycle is interrupted and the endogenous challenge is reduced in cholestatic disease.

Problems in interpreting the endogenous challenge test arise from the inconsistent release of bile acids into the duodenum. A standardized amount and type of food is essential because various foods have various effects on gastric emptying, cholecystokinin release, gallbladder contraction, and intestinal transit time.[20] These factors can affect postprandial serum concentrations of bile acids as well as the time of peak concentration.[20,22]

Prescription Diet® Canine p/d® (Hill's Pet Products) has been used to determine normal postprandial serum bile acid concentrations in dogs.[22] Dogs that were fed a low-fat meal (Prescription Diet® Canine r/d®—Hill's Pet Products) to induce bile acid secretion into the duodenum had postprandial serum bile acid levels that were lower and that peaked later than did those of dogs fed Prescription Diet® Canine p/d®.[22] In cats, normal postprandial serum bile acid levels were determined after meals of Prescription Diet® Feline c/d® (Hill's Pet Products).[22]

In patients that might have hepatoencephalopathy, low-protein meals (Prescription Diet® Canine k/d® or Feline k/d®—Hill's Pet Products) mixed with one or two tablespoons of corn oil have been recommended.[20] It is believed that the low-protein meal will not cause or aggravate central nervous system signs and that corn oil will facilitate gallbladder contraction.

Definitive Diagnosis of the Underlying Liver Disease

After a diagnosis of hepatoencephalopathy, the underlying liver disease must be identified. A specific diagnosis is necessary so that an accurate prognosis can be given and definitive treatment instituted. The type of liver disease can be determined by obtaining liver biopsy specimens or by contrast radiographic studies of the portal blood supply of the liver.

Liver biopsy specimens can be obtained by various methods. Percutaneous biopsy (blind biopsy or finger-hole technique) is most appropriate and easiest to perform if the liver is enlarged or normal in size.[23] Blind biopsy is contraindicated if the liver is smaller than normal. Both percutaneous methods can yield nondiagnostic samples if liver disease is localized.

The dangers associated with percutaneous liver biopsy include puncture of the gallbladder, penetration or biopsy of other organs, and excessive hemorrhage. Excessive bleeding might not be identified until the patient has lost a large amount of blood. Ultrasonographically guided percutaneous biopsy procedures avoid most of these complications. Alternative methods of obtaining a sample involve laparoscopy or laparotomy. These methods permit direct visualization of the liver and thus circumvent many of the complications inherent to percutaneous methods.

Regardless of the biopsy method used, patients should be evaluated for clotting problems before liver biopsy is performed. Activated partial thromboplastin time (APTT), one-stage prothrombin time, and platelet count should be determined; if possible, hemostatic abnormalities should be corrected before biopsy.

Portosystemic shunts are best identified by contrast angiography of the portal vascular system. Techniques include cranial mesenteric or celiac arterial portography, transabdominal splenoportography, and operative mesenteric portography.[24]

SUMMARY

Patients with hepatoencephalopathy can be presented

with numerous central nervous system signs; clinical signs often occur intermittently. Signs that involve other body systems are frequently present and help to identify liver disease as the underlying cause of the neurologic signs. A complete blood count and routine serum chemistry analysis provide additional information to support a diagnosis of hepatoencephalopathy. Specific liver function tests are indicated to evaluate the functional status of the liver.

After diagnosis of hepatoencephalopathy, the underlying liver disease is identified by obtaining liver biopsy samples or by radiographic contrast study of the portal vascular system. Prognosis and definitive treatment vary depending on the underlying liver disease.

About the Author

Dr. Tyler is affiliated with the Veterinary Specialty Clinic, Veterinary Medical Referral Service, Riverwoods, Illinois.

REFERENCES

1. Tams TR: Hepatic encephalopathy. *Vet Clin North Am [Small Anim Pract]* 15(1):177–195, 1985.
2. Fraser CL, Arieff AI: Hepatic encephalopathy. *N Engl J Med* 313(14):865–873, 1985.
3. Vulgamott JC: Portosystemic shunts. *Vet Clin North Am [Small Anim Pract]* 15(1):229–242, 1985.
4. Scavelli TD, Hornbuckle WE, Roth L, et al: Portosystemic shunts in cats: Seven cases (1976–1984). *JAVMA* 189(3):317–325, 1986.
5. Levesque DC, Oliver JE, Cornelius LM, et al: Congenital portacaval shunts in two cats: Diagnosis and surgical correction. *JAVMA* 181(2):143–145, 1982.
6. Ewing GO, Suter PF, Bailey CS: Hepatic insufficiency associated with congenital anomalies of the portal vein in dogs. *JAAHA* 10:463–476, 1974.
7. Strombeck DR, Weiser MG, Kaneko JJ: Hyperammonemia and hepatic encephalopathy in the dog. *JAVMA* 166(11):1105–1109, 1975.
8. Cornelius LM, Thrall DE, Halliwell WH, et al: Anomalous portosystemic anastomoses associated with chronic hepatic insufficiency in six young dogs. *JAVMA* 167(3):220–228, 1975.
9. Johnson CA, Armstrong PJ, Hauptman JG: Congenital portosystemic shunts in dogs: 46 cases (1976–1986). *JAVMA* 191(11):1478–1483, 1987.
10. Gandolfi RC: Hepatoencephalopathy associated with patent ductus venosus in a cat. *JAVMA* 185(3):301–302, 1984.
11. Sherding RG: Hepatic encephalopathy in the dog. *Compend Contin Educ Pract Vet* I(1):55–63, 1979.
12. Griffiths GL, Lumsden JH, Valli VEO: Hematological and biochemical changes in dogs with portosystemic shunts. *JAAHA* 17:705–710, 1981.
13. Center SA, Baldwin BH, Erb HN, et al: Bile acid concentrations in the diagnosis of hepatobiliary disease in the cat. *JAVMA* 189(8):891–896, 1986.
14. Center SA, Baldwin BH, Erb HN, et al: Bile acid concentrations in the diagnosis of hepatobiliary disease in the dog. *JAVMA* 187(9):935–940, 1985.
15. Strombeck DR, Meyer DJ, Freedland RA: Hyperammonemia due to a urea cycle/enzyme deficiency in two dogs. *JAVMA* 166(11):1109–1111, 1975.
16. Grauer GF, Nichols CER: Ascites, renal abnormalities, and electrolyte and acid-base disorders associated with liver disease. *Vet Clin North Am [Small Anim Pract]* 15(1):197–214, 1985.
17. Reynolds TB: Water, electrolyte and acid-base disorders in liver disease, in Maxwell MH, Kleeman CR (eds): *Clinical Disorders of Fluid and Electrolyte Metabolism.* New York, McGraw-Hill Book Co, 1980, pp 1251–1265.
18. Rose BD: Regulation of acid-base balance, in Rose BD (ed): *Clinical Physiology of Acid-Base and Electrolyte Disorders*, ed 2. New York, McGraw-Hill Book Co, 1984, pp 225–247.
19. Hardy RM, Robinson EP: Treatment of alkalosis, in Kirk RW (ed): *Current Veterinary Therapy. IX.* Philadelphia, WB Saunders Co, 1986, pp 67–75.
20. Center SA: Biochemical evaluation of hepatic function in the dog and cat, in Kirk RW (ed): *Current Veterinary Therapy. IX.* Philadelphia, WB Saunders Co, 1986, pp 924–936.
21. Duncan JR, Prasse KW: Liver, in *Veterinary Laboratory Medicine: Clinical Pathology*, ed 2. Ames, IA, Iowa State University Press, 1986, pp 121–144.
22. Center SA, Leveille CR, Baldwin BH, et al: Direct spectrometric determination of serum bile acids in the dog and cat. *Am J Vet Res* 45(10):2043–2050, 1984.
23. Godshalk CP: Liver biopsy in the dog. *Mod Vet Pract* 63(10):805–809, 1982.
24. Suter PF: Portal vein anomalies in the dog: Their angiographic diagnosis. *J Am Vet Rad Soc* 16:84–97, 1975.

Hepatoencephalopathy. Part II. Pathophysiology and Treatment

KEY FACTS

- Hepatoencephalopathy is caused by marked alteration of neurotransmission in the central nervous system; changes in central nervous system transmission are secondary to toxic agents that have been absorbed from the gut into the portal circulation.
- Prevention of hepatoencephalopathy in chronic liver failure involves the avoidance of factors that may precipitate hepatoencephalopathy; prevention also requires administration of a high-quality, low-protein diet.
- Goals of treatment of hepatoencephalopathy are to stop the formation and subsequent absorption of toxic substances from the gut, to correct any acid-base electrolyte or fluid abnormality, to control concurrent infection, and to normalize blood glucose levels.
- The use of benzodiazepine or γ-aminobutyric acid antagonists, which have proven to be useful in human medicine, may provide an innovative breakthrough in the treatment of hepatoencephalopathy in veterinary medicine.

Veterinary Medical Referral Service
Riverwoods, Illinois
John W. Tyler, DVM

Hepatoencephalopathy (HE) is believed to be caused by toxic products released from the gut that are normally detoxified by the liver. Among these toxic products are short-chain fatty acids (SCFA), mercaptans, ammonia (NH_3), and γ-aminobutyric acid (GABA).[1-4] Systemic metabolic-endocrine abnormalities, which are present in liver failure, enhance the toxicity of these agents.[5-7] Toxic agents accumulate in the systemic circulation as a result of decreased functional hepatic mass that may or may not be accompanied by portosystemic shunting of blood. A rare cause of hepatoencephalopathy is a urea cycle enzyme deficiency.[8] The final toxic mechanism for all of these agents is a disturbance in neurotransmission in the central nervous system (CNS). Neurotransmission can be altered by direct toxic effects on neurons, changes in neurotransmitter levels and metabolism, and changes in neurotransmitter receptor densities and affinities.[1,2,9-12]

The first part of this two-part presentation discussed the clinical signs and diagnosis of hepatoencephalopathy. This part discusses the development of a rational therapeutic plan based on a thorough understanding of the physiology of the condition.

PATHOPHYSIOLOGY
Abnormalities in Neurotransmitter Balance, Receptor Densities, and Affinities

One of the primary inhibitory neurotransmitters in the mammalian brain is γ-aminobutyric acid (GABA).[4,13,14] This neurotransmitter binds to receptors that are part of a chloride ionophore on postsynaptic neuronal membranes. Binding of γ-aminobutyric acid to this receptor induces chloride conductance into the neuron, resulting in hyperpolarization of it.[13,14] Benzodiazepines and barbiturates bind to the same chloride ionophore but at distinctly different receptor sites.[13,16]

The number of high- and low-affinity brain receptors for γ-aminobutyric acid increased in rats[17] and rabbits[18,19] with hepatoencephalopathy secondary to experimentally induced liver failure. In hepatoencephalopathy, there is also an increased number of brain binding sites for diazepines.[20] If the chloride ionophore receptor complex is regulated as a single unit, this observation provides additional evidence for increased numbers of γ-aminobutyric acid receptors. An increased number of receptors for diazepines would also explain the clinical observation that patients with hepatoencephalopathy have an increased sensitivity to diazepines.

In hepatic failure, there are increased levels of γ-aminobutyric acid in the blood.[13,14,21] The intestines are believed to be the primary source of increased blood γ-aminobutyric acid levels seen in hepatic failure.[13,14] Enteric bacteria (*Escherichia coli* and *Bacteroides fragilis*) have been shown to produce γ-aminobutyric acid, and, in rabbits, γ-aminobutyric acid has been shown to be present in higher levels in portal blood than in arterial blood.[22] Gamma-aminobutyric acid is normally degraded by γ-aminobutyric acid transaminase in the liver.[13,14] Blood γ-aminobutyric acid normally does not cross the blood-brain barrier; however, in hepatoencephalopathy, the blood brain-barrier is damaged, thus providing γ-aminobutyric acid with access to the central nervous system.[23] This increased passage is by diffusion, not transport. (See update at the end of this article.)

INSTILLATION of γ-aminobutyric acid into the brains of rabbits resulted in coma with electroencephalogram patterns similar to those obtained from animals in hepatic coma.[13] Gamma-aminobutyric acid receptors are not increased in rats in uremic or hypoglycemic coma,[17] thereby supporting the assertion that the increase in γ-aminobutyric acid receptors is not a nonspecific change found in other metabolic disorders but is instead a unique finding in animals with hepatoencephalopathy.

Glycine is another inhibitory central nervous system neurotransmitter. Most glycine receptors are located in the spinal cord but are also present in the brain. An increase in both high- and low-affinity glycine receptors was present in the brains of rabbits with experimentally induced hepatoencephalopathy.[12]

Receptor densities for the brain and absolute levels of excitatory neurotransmitters in the brain are altered in animals with hepatoencephalopathy. Receptors for the excitatory amino acid (AA) neurotransmitters glutamate, aspartate, and kainic acid are reduced in rabbit or rat experimental models of hepatoencephalopathy.[9,12] In contrast, normal rabbits with experimentally induced hyperammonemia (not secondary to liver disease) had increased numbers of glutamate receptors with no decrease in receptor affinity for glutamate.[9] In a rabbit model of hepatoencephalopathy, brain receptors for dopamine had reduced affinity for that excitatory neurotransmitter.[12] Reduced brain dopamine levels also have been noted by some investigators. Brain norepinephrine levels have been shown to be reduced by as much as 50% in some experimental models of hepatoencephalopathy.[24-26] Brain levels of norepinephrine and dopamine are affected greatly by the levels of their precursor aromatic amino acids (AAA), tyrosine, and phenylalanine, in the central nervous system (Figure 1).[27,31]

The concentration of serotonin, an inhibitory neurotransmitter, is increased in the brains of animals with hepatoencephalopathy. Serotonin, in addition to being an inhibitory transmitter, can replace both norepinephrine and dopamine in presynaptic synaptosomes. Brain serotonin levels depend on the amount of tryptophan in the brain; tryptophan levels in the brain are also elevated in animals with hepatoencephalopathy.[10,31-33]

Concentrations of false neurotransmitters, such as octopamine, tyramine, phenylethylamine, and phenylethanolamine, are elevated in animals with hepatoencephalopathy.[1,2,5,11,27,28,33] False neurotransmitters replace norepinephrine and dopamine from the synaptasomes in the presynaptic neuron. False neurotransmitters have decreased neural excitatory activity; for example, octopamine has 1/50 the activity of norepinephrine. Brain levels of false neurotransmitters are determined by the levels of their precursors, the aromatic amino acids, tyrosine, and phenylalanine.[5,11,27-29,33] Phenylalanine is the precursor of phenylethylamine and phenylethanolamine, and it can also be converted to tyrosine by the enzyme tyrosine hydroxylase (Figure 1).[29] Tyrosine is the initial substrate for enzymatic conversion to tyramine and octopamine, as well as dopamine and norepinephrine (Figure 1).[27,29]

Tyrosine hydroxylase (rate-limiting enzyme in catecholamine synthesis) is working at near-peak efficiency when brain tyrosine levels are at normal physiologic levels. As tyrosine levels increase in hepatoencephalopathy,[34] the ability of tyrosine hydroxylase to convert tyrosine to L-dopa (precursor of dopamine and subsequently norepinephrine) is overwhelmed (Figure 1).[27,28] Aromatic amino acid decarboxylase converts excess tyrosine to tyramine and then to octopamine.[27,28,33] An increased proportion of tyrosine is shunted toward production of octopamine because increased levels of phenylalanine are present in the brains of animals with hepatoencephalopathy. Phenylalanine has an affinity for tyrosine hydroxylase equal to that of tyrosine; increased levels of phenylalanine therefore lead to decreased conversion of tyrosine to L-dopa by tyrosine hydroxylase.[29] A proportion of the phenylalanine is converted by tyrosine hydroxylase to tyrosine, and the rest is converted to phenylethylamine and subsequently to phenylethanolamine by aromatic amino acid decarboxylases.[27,28,33]

INFUSION of phenylalanine and tryptophan into the carotid artery of normal dogs leads to increases in cerebrospinal fluid levels of phenylalanine, tyrosine, octopamine, and phenylethanolamine to levels in naturally occurring hepatoencephalopathy. Tryptophan cerebrospinal fluid levels were higher than those in naturally occurring hepatoencephalopathy. The resulting neurologic signs resembled those of hepatoencephalopathy. The dogs became comatose but returned to normal when cerebrospinal fluid levels of the aforementioned substances returned to normal.[35]

PATHOPHYSIOLOGY
Peripheral Toxins and Metabolic-Endocrine Derangements that Cause or Enhance Hepatoencephalopathy

Animals with liver failure are in a catabolic state. They

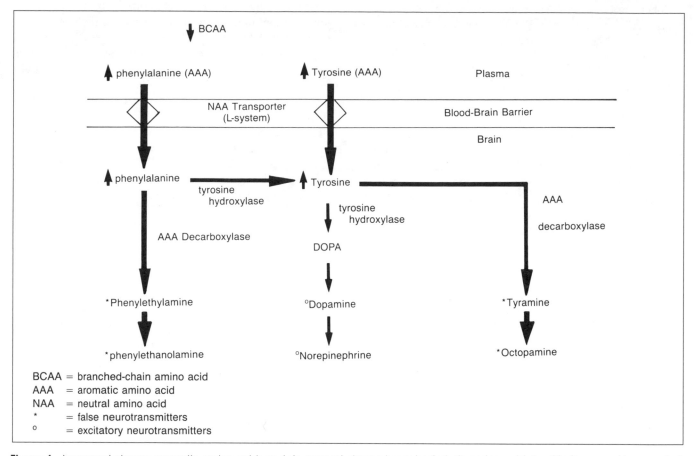

Figure 1—Increased plasma aromatic amino acids and decreased plasma branched-chain amino acids lead to increased transport of aromatic amino acids into the brain by a neutral amino acid transport system. Increased levels of phenylalanine and tyrosine in the brain lead to increased levels of false neurotransmitters. The majority of the increased tyrosine is shunted toward the formation of tyramine because of saturation of tyrosine hydroxylase.

have a negative nitrogen balance and a decreased serum ratio of insulin to glucagon.[6,7,36-39] The changes in respective levels of insulin to glucagon and the alteration of the insulin and glucagon ratios lead to marked abnormalities in amino acid metabolism.[2,6,7,36] Insulin is believed to enhance the entrance of branched-chain amino acids (BCAA), such as valine, isoleucine, and leucine, into muscle cells.[5] Glucagon induces glycogenolysis, gluconeogenesis, and possibly increases skeletal muscle catabolism with increased release of aromatic amino acids into the blood.[5,40] Decreased serum levels of branched-chain amino acids and increased serum levels of aromatic amino acids accompany many catabolic states, including liver disease.[5,34,41]

Patients with portosystemic shunts (and possibly those with cirrhosis and no portosystemic shunts) have increased blood glucagon and insulin levels, but the ratio of insulin to glucagon is decreased.[2,6,7,36-39] Increased glucagon levels in animals with hepatoencephalopathy are caused by increased pancreatic secretion.[42] Ammonia has been shown to cause increased glucagon secretion,[43] but other researchers have not noted this response.[40,42] Increased insulin levels in patients with hepatoencephalopathy are caused by decreased hepatic degradation. Normally, 40% to 50% of insulin is degraded on its first pass through the liver.[6]

Fifty percent of branched-chain amino acids taken up by skeletal muscle are oxidized for energy, instead of being incorporated in muscle proteins.[44,45] In comparison, none of the aromatic amino acids are oxidized by skeletal muscle for energy.[44,45] The kidneys, brain, and fat cells also have the ability to oxidize branched-chain amino acids for energy. Branched-chain amino acid oxidation by skeletal muscle increased three to five times in starved rats; there was no increase in skeletal muscle oxidation of aromatic amino acids. The uptake of branched-chain amino acids by skeletal muscle was also increased in starved rats when compared with controls.[44,45] No increase in the uptake of other amino acids by skeletal muscle occurred; in fact, most other amino acids are released by skeletal muscle during starvation for utilization by the liver for gluconeogenesis. Branched-chain amino acids, however, are not utilized by the liver.

In chronic liver disease, concentrations of branched-chain amino acids are decreased, whereas those of aromatic amino acids are increased. In acute hepatic failure, concentrations of aromatic amino acids are markedly increased while those of branched-chain amino acids remain at normal levels. The normal ratio of branched-chain amino acids to aromatic amino acids is approximately three or four to one; in hepatic failure, this ratio approaches one to one.[1,34,41] Aromatic amino acids (phenylalanine, tyrosine, and tryptophan) are normally removed from the blood by the liver.[5,40] Phenylalanine and tyrosine blood levels are increased in hepatic failure, but total tryptophan levels remain normal.[34-39,41] Free tryptophan levels are increased, however, because of decreased serum albumin and increased serum levels of free fatty acids, which compete with tryptophan for attachment to albumin.[5,32,34,43] Albumin levels are typically decreased in liver disease and free fatty acids are often increased.[1,5]

THE SIGNIFICANCE of altered branched-chain amino acid and aromatic amino acid metabolism in liver failure is that both are neutral amino acids (NAA) that must be transported across the blood-brain barrier by a common transport system; they do not diffuse. They compete for uptake by the neutral amino acid transporter (L-system).[47-49] The altered ratio of serum branched-chain amino acids to aromatic amino acids leads to increased central nervous system levels of aromatic amino acids (tyrosine, phenylalanine, and tryptophan). The increased central nervous system levels of aromatic amino acids lead to altered neurotransmitter levels and metabolism (Figure 1).

Infusion of branched-chain amino acids into dogs with hepatoencephalopathy secondary to portacaval anastomosis (PCA) restored plasma and cerebrospinal fluid levels of aromatic amino acids, octopamine, phenylethanolamine, and cerebrospinal fluid 5-hydroxyindolacetic acid (serotonin) to normal. Dogs recovered from comatose states subsequent to normalization. This effect was thought to be because of a decreased uptake of aromatic amino acids by the L-system secondary to increased competition for uptake with branched-chain amino acids.[34]

In hepatic disease, the increased concentrations of aromatic amino acids in the brain are greater than can be explained by the elevated levels of these amino acids in the plasma. Brain levels of branched-chain amino acids are also normal (although their plasma levels are decreased)[34]; it thus becomes apparent that competition for the carrier system is not the only mechanism involved in the altered aromatic amino acid levels in the brain. One postulated mechanism is that the increased influx of neutral amino acids results from increased activity of the L-system.[40] This increased activity is believed to result from increased glutamine (a neutral amino acid) efflux from the brain secondary to increased brain glutamine levels.[5,40,48,50] The increased glutamine efflux is believed to be joined with the increased uptake of other neutral amino acids from blood in proportion to their blood concentrations.[50]

In support of this theory, increased brain and cerebrospinal fluid glutamine levels occur in animals with hepatic failure and the levels seem to correlate strongly with the severity of hepatoencephalopathy.[5,51] Glutamine efflux from the central nervous system also increases in animals with hepatoencephalopathy.[40] Inhibition of glutamine synthetase results in decreased uptake of aromatic amino acids

and branched-chain amino acids by the brain and has been shown to obviate the signs of ammonia intoxication.[52-54]

Increased levels of central nervous system glutamine are secondary to increased ammonia influx into the brain. Astrocytes detoxify ammonia by forming glutamine from glutamate. Blood ammonia levels are often elevated in animals with hepatoencephalopathy, but the levels may also be normal. Most of the ammonia present in the blood of animals is generally believed to originate from bacterial breakdown of dietary protein, blood, urea, and shed cellular and bacterial debris in the colon. Gram-negative anaerobes are considered to be the major source of ammonia production in the gut[55]; however, germ-free dogs with surgically created portosystemic shunts developed hyperammonemia.[56] Possible endogenous sources of ammonia are skeletal muscle, brain, kidneys, heart, and gastrointestinal tissue.

IN FASTING DOGS, the jejunum and ileum produced an amount of ammonia equal to that produced by the colon.[57] A large majority of the ammonia was derived from the conversion of glutamine to glutamate by enterocytes. The other aforementioned tissues also produce ammonia secondary to the deamination of various amino acids, especially glutamine and glutamate. In addition, the liver is able to produce ammonia secondary to gluconeogenesis. The majority of ammonia is detoxified by the liver, although one report has suggested that as much as 50% of ammonia is metabolized by skeletal muscle in normal human subjects.[58]

After absorption into the circulation, ammonia enters the liver where it is metabolized to urea through the Krebs-Henseleit cycle. A majority of blood urea is excreted by the kidneys, but 25% to 50% diffuses back into the colon and is reconverted to ammonia. Decreased ammonia detoxification by the liver occurs secondary to decreased functional mass and/or portosystemic shunts. A third possibility for an increase in blood ammonia levels is through a urea cycle enzyme deficiency, two cases of which have been reported in veterinary literature.[8]

The toxic effect of ammonia on the brain and the significance of ammonia in the pathogenesis of hepatoencephalopathy is a much-debated subject.[5,14,59,60] Proposed mechanisms for the toxic action of ammonia include the following: disturbances of cerebral energy metabolism, interference with neuronal membrane sodium-potassium adenosinetriphosphatase, interference with movement of chloride out of neurons (may be synergistic with γ-aminobutyric acid),[14,60] disruption of the blood-brain barrier, alteration of amino acid transfer across the blood-brain barrier,[5,41] and reduced levels of the excitatory amino acid neurotransmitters, glutamate and aspartate.[14,59]

Mercaptans and short-chain fatty acids (valeric, hexanoic, and octanoic) are elevated in animals with hepatoencephalopathy and are considered to be synergistic with ammonia in producing hepatoencephalopathy.[2,61-63] Mercaptans and short-chain amino acids have both been shown to interfere with microsomal sodium-potassium adenosine-triphosphatase activity in the brains of rats.[2] It is speculated,[63] although debated,[61] that mercaptans may inhibit detoxification of ammonia by the liver. Mercaptans are derived from bacterial metabolism of methionine in the gut and are usually degraded to dimethyl sulfide by the liver.[63] Methionine is a component of some lipotrophic drugs purported to be of value in the treatment of hepatic disease. Hepatoencephalopathy has resulted from the oral administration of methionine or methionine-containing drugs to dogs with naturally occurring or experimental portosystemic shunts.[62-64]

In general, short-chain fatty acids and free fatty acids, which are normally cleared from plasma by the liver, are increased in liver failure.[1,2] One possible mechanism for the toxic effect of these acids is their ability to displace tryptophan from albumin, thus increasing free-serum tryptophan levels that eventually increase the uptake of tryptophan by the brain.[46] Another possible mechanism is by the increased production of ammonia from glutamine by the kidneys. In rats given sodium valproate (a branched-chain fatty acid antiepileptic drug), increased levels of ammonia in the blood occurred[65]; however, no increase in the levels of ammonia in the blood of bilaterally nephrectomized rats occurred.[65] The mode of action and significance of the involvement of mercaptans and short-chain fatty acid in the development of hepatoencephalopathy is largely undetermined.

TREATMENT

The goals of treatment of severe hepatoencephalopathy are to (1) stop the formation and subsequent absorption of toxic substances from the gut (e.g., ammonia, mercaptans, short-chain fatty acids, and γ-aminobutyric acid); (2) correct any acid-base, electrolyte, or fluid abnormality; (3) control concurrent infection; and (4) normalize blood glucose levels.

To control production and absorption of toxic products from the gut, it is necessary to reduce the numbers of colonic bacteria and decrease dietary precursors of toxic agents. Food intake should be stopped until the neurologic status of the patient stabilizes, at which point a high-quality, low-protein diet should be instituted (i.e., Prescription Diet Canine® k/d®—Hill's Pet Products). To decrease colonic bacteria, various methods have been suggested. Enemas cleanse the bowel and reduce substrates available for toxin formation by bacteria. To reduce colonic bacteria, an enema containing a 1:10 dilution of povidone-iodine solution can be instilled into the colon and subsequently drained 10 to 15 minutes later; this procedure may be repeated every four to six hours, as needed.[66,67] Povidone-iodine enemas not only reduce colonic bacteria, they also acidify the contents of the colon as well.[66,67]

Lactulose, a synthetic disaccharide that is not digested or absorbed in the small intestine, is degraded in the colon by the resident bacterial population.[1,67,68] This causes acidification of the colon and also induces osmotic diarrhea.

Acidification of colonic contents results in the conversion of ammonia to ammonium (NH_4^+), which is a charged molecule. Ammonium, therefore, cannot be absorbed through the colonic mucosa. Osmotic diarrhea reduces colonic bacteria and shortens the time that colonic contents remain in the bowel. In comatose or stuporous patients, lactulose can be administered by means of a stomach tube or as an enema. If administered by stomach tube, 20 to 60 milliliters of lactulose can be given every four to six hours, or, if given as an enema, 300 to 450 grams can be diluted in 200 to 300 milliliters of water.[1] In less severely depressed patients, lactulose can be given orally at a dosage of 5 ml/5 to 10 kg divided three times a day. This administration of lactulose is also used for long-term management of patients with chronic hepatic failure. The dosage is adjusted, however, so that two to three soft stools are passed each day.

ORAL ANTIBIOTICS may be used to reduce colonic bacteria further. Metronidazole has an excellent level of activity against gram-negative anaerobes, which are the primary source of ammonia production in the colon.[1,69] The drug is administered at a dosage of 7.5 mg/kg three times a day for two to four weeks as needed.[1] An additional source of ammonia could be from bacterial degradation of blood following gastrointestinal hemorrhage.[1,67] Gastrointestinal bleeding can result from hookworms in young dogs, renal failure in older dogs, or coagulation abnormalities secondary to liver failure. If transfusion becomes necessary, fresh blood should be used; ammonia concentrations in stored blood increase with storage to levels that are toxic to patients with hepatic failure.[1,67]

Animals with liver failure are often hypovolemic and they present with a wide variety of acid-base and electrolyte abnormalities.[70,71] Hypovolemia may lead to prerenal azotemia and increased delivery of urea to the colon and thus to increased blood ammonia levels.[72] Hypokalemia induces increased formation of ammonia by the kidneys, possibly through the intracellular acidosis that it creates.[73] When serum potassium levels drop, potassium leaves the cell and electroneutrality is maintained by hydrogen entering the cell. The resulting acidic intracellular environment enhances the breakdown of glutamine to glutamate thus increasing the subsequent production of ammonia by the kidneys.[73]

Alkalosis enhances ammonia toxicity by increasing ammonia in the blood relative to blood ammonium concentration. Ammonia is nonionic and it can, therefore, diffuse across lipid membranes into cells. The intracellular pH is more acidotic than extracellular fluid, and ammonia is thereby converted to ammonium and trapped in the cell. Hypokalemia can enhance this process by lowering intracellular pH.

For initial volume expansion in patients with hepatoencephalopathy, Ringer's solution or half-strength saline and 2.5% dextrose are the fluids of choice. The latter must be

TABLE I
Precipitating Causes of Hepatoencephalopathy in Liver Disease Patients[1,76]

Causes	Presumed Mechanism	Prevention/Treatment
Azotemia (spontaneous or iatrogenic)	Decreased renal clearance of urea leads to increased urea excretion into the colon. Colonic bacteria degrade urea. Ammonia is subsequently absorbed into portal blood.	Avoid excessive use of diuretics. Correct any fluid deficits with intravenous fluid administration. Ringer's solution or .45% saline and 2.5% dextrose.
Hypokalemia (spontaneous or iatrogenic)	Hypokalemia can induce intracellular acidosis with increased trapping of ammonia as ammonium intracellularly.	Use potassium sparing diuretics (aldosterone inhibitors).
	Hypokalemia aggravates alkalotic conditions thus leading to increased blood ammonia levels.	Correct potassium deficits.
	Hypokalemia causes increased ammonia production by kidneys and subsequently increased renal vein ammonia.	Supplement potassium-poor IV solutions with KC l.
Alkalosis	Increases levels of ammonia in blood ($NH_4^+ \rightarrow NH_3 + H^+$). Ammonia can cross biologic membranes and is subsequently trapped intracellularly as ammonium.	Correct any potassium deficits.
		Metabolic alkalosis in liver failure should be treated with half-strength (.45%) saline.
		Control vomiting.
		If ascites is causing tachypnea with resultant respiratory alkalosis, then the ascitic fluid should be drained.
Sedatives, tranquilizers, analgesics	Increased sensitivity subsequent to enhanced GABAergic neurotransmission and decreased metabolism by liver.	Use these agents cautiously; ideally only those drugs which are metabolized normally in the presence of liver disease or that have a very short half-life should be used.
Gastrointestinal hemorrhage	Colonic bacteria break down blood proteins leading to increased production of ammonia.	Treat any gastrointestinal parasites which may be causing gastrointestinal hemorrhage.
	Hypovolemia leading to prerenal azotemia.	Avoid use of gastrointestinal irritants (i.e., nonsteroidal anti-inflammatory drugs).
		Use antibiotics (metronidazole) and/or lactulose to reduce the colonic bacterial population and reduce ammonia absorption.
Infection	Sepsis is associated with decreased ratio of branched-chain amino acids to aromatic amino acids in the blood.	Infections should be pursued aggressively, both diagnostically and therapeutically.
	Bacterial infections are associated with increased tissue catabolism leading to an increased endogenous nitrogen load and increased blood ammonia.	
Excess dietary protein	Excess protein provides substrate for ammonia production by colonic bacteria.	Administer a low-protein diet. Protein that is fed should be high in branched-chain amino acids and low in aromatic amino acids.
Constipation	Slow transit time increases bacterial production of toxic products and subsequent intestinal absorption.	Administer lactulose, enemas.

supplemented with potassium, 20 to 30 mEq KCl/liter, assuming renal function is normal.

Animals with hepatic failure or portosystemic shunts are particularly susceptible to infection, septicemia, and/or endotoxemia. This is secondary to the increasing inability of the liver to filter portal blood adequately or portal blood being shunted around the liver. Without the intervention of the liver, the bacteria- and toxin-ladened portal blood gains access to the systemic circulation. The resulting infection and/or septicemia can precipitate hepatoencephalopathy.[1] Septicemia leads to a catabolic state that may have an amino acid profile similar to hepatoencephalopathy[36] and can, therefore, cause signs of hepatoencephalopathy in liver failure patients. Infections in liver failure patients must be pursued vigorously, both diagnostically and therapeutically.

HYPOGLYCEMIA is a common problem in chronic liver failure.[74] If a dog with liver failure has neurologic signs, the blood glucose level should be checked and low levels corrected. If the patient is seizuring, then an intravenous bolus of .5 gm/kg of 25% glucose should be given.[1] Seizures other than those resulting from hypoglycemia can be controlled with valium. The dosage should be the minimum amount necessary to control the seizures. Patients with liver failure have an increased sensitivity to benzodiazepam, in addition to decreased hepatic clearance.

Patients that fail to respond to conventional therapeutic regimens designed to reverse hepatoencephalopathy may be helped by a correction of the plasma amino acid imbalance that exists in animals with chronic liver disease or portosystemic shunts. In one study, intravenous infusion of a branched-chain-amino-acid-enriched parenteral solution resulted in reversal of hepatic coma in dogs with surgically created portacaval shunts within one to eight hours.[34] Improvement in clinical status was accompanied by a normalization of the plasma amino acid pattern. Simultaneously, cerebrospinal fluid levels of the aromatic amino acids octopamine and phenylethanolamine (false neurotransmitters) and 5-hydroxyindolacetic acid (a metabolite of serotonin) returned to normal levels. Continued infusion of the branched-chain-amino-acid-enriched parenteral solution prevented recurrence of hepatoencephalopathy; when the infusion was stopped, the biochemical alterations and clinical hepatoencephalopathy returned.[34]

An innovative development in the treatment of chronic and/or nonresponsive hepatoencephalopathy is the use of a benzodiazepine antagonist and/or a γ-aminobutyric acid antagonist. A recent case report in human medical literature[75] describes a patient with chronic hepatoencephalopathy who was nonresponsive to traditional therapeutic measures. The patient responded dramatically to treatment with a benzodiazepine antagonist (flumazenil). The patient remained free of clinical signs of hepatoencephalopathy while on flumazenil. Future developments in this area need to be monitored by veterinarians.

PREVENTION of hepatoencephalopathy in chronic liver failure patients involves the avoidance of factors that may precipitate hepatoencephalopathy (Table I).[1,76] Prevention also requires the administration of a high-quality, low-protein diet. Chronic administration of lactulose may be used if dietary therapy is not sufficient to control development of neurologic signs. Intermittent use of metronidazole also may be warranted to decrease colonic ammonia formation. The chronic use of enteral formulas with high levels of branched-chain amino acids to control or ameliorate the catabolic state associated with chronic liver failure has not been investigated in veterinary medicine.

Human medical literature suggests that chronic branched-chain amino acid supplementation may be beneficial in the management of chronic liver failure and in the prevention of hepatoencephalopathy.[34,35] As mentioned previously, intravenous infusion of branched-chain amino acids not only reversed hepatoencephalopathy, chronic intravenous administration prevented recurrence.[34] Chronic enteral administration of branched-chain amino acids to patients with chronic liver failure should be evaluated by the veterinary profession.

Long-term therapy for patients with hepatoencephalopathy secondary to congenital portosystemic shunts should include surgical correction of the shunt.[74] Medical management is warranted preoperatively and for a variable postoperative length of time as the reperfused liver function increases. Animals with congenital portosystemic shunts that cannot be completely corrected surgically often require some level of ongoing medical management to prevent hepatoencephalopathy.[74] Acquired portosystemic shunts, in contrast, should be managed medically instead of being corrected surgically.

SUMMARY

Hepatoencephalopathy is caused by marked alteration of neurotransmission in the central nervous system. Changes in central nervous system neurotransmission are secondary to toxic agents that have been absorbed from the gut into the portal circulation. Normally, the liver removes or modifies most of these toxins before they reach the systemic circulation. The goal of medical treatment of hepatoencephalopathy is to stop the formation and the absorption of these toxins from the gut. Proper medical management of patients with chronic liver failure can ameliorate or prevent hepatoencephalopathy. The nature of the underlying liver diseases determines the long-term prognosis.

About the Author
Dr. Tyler is affiliated with the Veterinary Specialty Clinic, Veterinary Referral Service, Riverwoods, Illinois.

REFERENCES
1. Tams TR: Hepatic encephalopathy. *Vet Clin North Am [Small Anim Pract]* 15(7):177–195, 1985.
2. Fraser CL, Arieff AI: Hepatic encephalopathy. *N Engl J Med* 313(14):865–873, 1985.

3. Sherding RG: Hepatic encephalopathy in the dog. *Compend Contin Educ Pract Vet* 1(1):55–63, 1979.

4. Roberts E: The gamma-aminobutyric acid (GABA) system and hepatic encephalopathy. *Hepatology* 4(2):342–345, 1984.

5. Bernardini P, Fischer JE: Amino acid imbalance and hepatic encephalopathy. *Ann Rev Nutr* 2:419–454, 1982.

6. Munro HN, Fernstrom JD, Wurtman RJ: Insulin, plasma amino acid imbalance and hepatic coma. *Lancet* 1:722–724, March, 1975.

7. Marchesini G, Zoli M, Angiolini A, et al: Muscle protein breakdown in liver cirrhosis and the role of altered carbohydrate metabolism. *Hepatology* 1(4):294–299, 1981.

8. Strombeck DR, Meyer DJ, Freedland RA: Hyperammonemia due to a urea cycle/enzyme deficiency in two dogs. *JAVMA* 166(11):1109–1111, 1975.

9. Ferenci P, Pappas SC, Munson PJ, et al: Changes in glutamate receptors on synaptic membranes associated with hepatic encephalopathy or hyperammonemia in the rabbit. *Hepatology* 4(1):25–32, 1984.

10. Cummings MG, Soeters PB, James JH, et al: Regional brain indoleamine metabolism following chronic portacaval anastomosis in the rat. *J Neurochem* 27:501–509, 1976.

11. Fischer JE, Baldessarini RJ: False neurotransmitters and hepatic failure. *Lancet* 2:75–80, July, 1971.

12. Ferenci P, Pappas SC, Munson PJ, et al: Changes in the status of neurotransmitter receptors in a rabbit model of hepatic encephalopathy. *Hepatology* 4(2):186–191, 1984.

13. Schafer DF, Jones EA: Hepatic encephalopathy and the gamma-aminobutyric acid neurotransmitter system. *Lancet* 1:18–20, Jan, 1982.

14. Schafer DF, Jones EA: Potential neural mechanisms in the pathogenesis of hepatic encephalopathy, in Popper H, Schaffner F (eds): *Progress in Liver Disease*, vol VII. New York, Grune & Stratton, 1982, pp 615–627.

15. Tallman JF, Paul SM, Skolnick P, et al: Receptors for the age of anxiety: Pharmacology of the benzodiazepines. *Science* 207:274–278, 1980.

16. Skolnick P, Moncada V, Barker JL, et al: Phenobarbital: Dual actions to increase brain benzodiazepine receptor affinity. *Science* 211:1448–1450, 1981.

17. Baraldi M, Zeneroli Milliliters: Experimental hepatic encephalopathy: Changes in the binding of gamma-aminobutyric acid. *Science* 216(2):427–429, April, 1982.

18. Schafer DF, Thakur AK, Jones EA: Increased gamma-aminobutyric acid receptors associated with acute hepatic encephalopathy in rabbits. *Clin Res* 28:485A, 1980.

19. Schafer DF, Thakur AK, Jones EA: Acute hepatitis coma and inhibitory neurotransmission: Increase in gamma-aminobutyric acid levels in plasma and receptors in brain. *Gastroenterol* 79:1123, 1980.

20. Fowler JM, Schafer OF: A mechanism for the increased sensitivity to benzodiazepines in hepatocellular failure: Evidence from an animal model. *Gastroenterol* 80:1359, 1981.

21. Schafer DF, Ferenci P, Kleinberger G, et al: Elevated serum concentrations of the inhibitory neurotransmitter gamma-aminobutyric acid in patients with hepatocellular disease. *Hepatology* 1:543, 1981.

22. Schafer DF, Fowler JM, Jones EA: Colonic bacteria: A source of gamma-aminobutyric acid in blood. *Proc Soc Exp Bio Med* 167(3):301–303, 1981.

23. Horowitz ME, Schafer DF, Molnar P, et al: Increased blood-brain transfer in a rabbit model of acute liver failure. *Gastroenterol* 84:5, Part 1, 1003–1011, 1983.

24. Dodsworth JM, James JH, Cummings MG, et al: Depletion of brain norepinephrine in acute hepatic coma. *Surgery* 75:811–820, 1974.

25. Faraj BA, Camp VM, Ansley JD, et al: Evidence of central hypertyraminemia in hepatic encephalopathy. *J Clin Invest* 67:395–402, 1981.

26. Tyce GM, Owen CA: Dopamine and norepinephrine in the brains of hepatectomized rats. *Life Sci* 22:781–786, 1978.

27. James JH, Hodgman JM, Funovics JM, et al: Alteration in brain octopamine and brain tyrosine following portocaval anastomosis in rats. *J Neurochem* 27:223–227, 1976.

28. Fischer JE, Rosen HM, Ebeid AM, et al: The effect of normalization of plasma amino acids on hepatic encephalopathy in man. *Surgery* 80(1):77–91, 1976.

29. Karobath M, Baldessarini RJ: Formation of catechol compounds from phenylalanine and tyrosine with isolated nerve endings. *Nature New Biol* 236:206–208, 1972.

30. Kamata S, Okada A, Watanabe T, et al: Effects of dietary amino acids on brain amino acids and transmitter amines in rats with a por-

tacaval shunt. *J Neurochem* 35(5):1190–1199, 1980.

31. Curzon G, Kantamaneni BD, Winch J, et al: Plasma and brain tryptophan changes in experimental acute hepatic failure. *J Neurochem* 21:137–145, 1973.

32. Cummings MG, James JH, Soeters PB, et al: Regional brain study of indoleamine metabolism in the rat in acute hepatic failure. *J Neurochem* 27:741–746, 1976

33. Ono J, Hutson OG, Dombro RS, et al: Tryptophan and hepatic coma. *Gastroenterol* 74:2, Part 1, 196–200, 1978.

34. Smith AR, Rossi-Faneli F, Ziparo V, et al: Alterations in plasma and cerebrospinal fluid amino acids, amines and metabolites in hepatic coma. *Ann Surg* 187(3):343–350, March, 1978.

35. Rossi-Fanelli F, Freund H, Krause R, et al: Induction of coma in normal dogs by the infusion of aromatic amino acids and its prevention by the addition of branched-chain amino acids. *Gastroenterol* 83(3):664–671, 1982.

36. Mizock BA: Branched-chain amino acids in sepsis and hepatic failure. *Arch Inter Med* 145:1284–1288, 1985.

37. Marchesini G, Forlani G, Zoli M, et al: Insulin and glucagon levels in liver cirrhosis: Relationship with plasma amino acid imbalance of chronic hepatic encephalopathy. *Dig Dis Sci* 24(8):594–601, 1979.

38. Soeters PB, Weir G, Ebeid AM, et al: Insulin, glucagon: Portal systemic shunting and hepatic failure in the dog. *J Surg Res* 23:183–188, 1977.

39. Sherwin R, Joshi P, Hendler R, et al: Hyperglucagonemia in Laennec's cirrhosis: The role of portal-systemic shunting. *N Engl J Med* 290(5):239–243, 1974.

40. James JH, Ziparo V, Jeppsson B, et al: Hyperammonemia, plasma amino acid imbalance and blood-brain amino acid transport: A unified theory of portal-systemic encephalopathy. *Lancet* 2:772–775, Oct, 1979.

41. Strombeck DR, Rogers Q: Plasma amino acid concentrations in dogs with hepatic disease. *JAVMA* 173(1):93–96, 1978.

42. Sherwin RS, Fisher M, Bessoff J, et al: Hyperglucagonemia in cirrhosis: Altered secretion and sensitivity to glucagon. *Gastroenterol* 74:1224–1228, 1978.

43. Strombeck DR, Roger Q, Stern JS: Effects of intravenous ammonia infusion on plasma levels of amino acids, glucagon, and insulin in dogs. *Gastroenterol* 74:1165, 1978.

44. Odessey R, Goldberg AL: Oxidation of leucine by rat skeletal muscle. *Am J Physiol* 223(6):1376–1383, 1972.

45. Goldberg AL, Odessey R: Oxidation of amino acids by diaphragms from fed and fasted rats. *Am J Physiol* 223(6):1384–1391, 1972.

46. Knott PJ, Curzon G: Free tryptophan in plasma and brain tryptophan metabolism. *Nature* 239:452–453, Oct, 1972.

47. Oldendorf WH, Szabo J: Amino acid assignment to one of three blood-brain barrier amino acid carriers. *Am J Physiol* 230(1):94–98, 1976.

48. James JH, Fischer JE: Transport of neutral amino acids at the blood-brain barrier. *Pharmacol* 22:1–7, 1981.

49. James JH, Escourrou J, Fischer JE: Blood-brain neutral amino acid transport activity is increased after portacaval anastomosis. *Science* 200:1395–1397, June, 1978.

50. James JH, Cangiano C, Cardelli-Cangiano P, et al: Glutamine links hyperammonimia and neurotransmitter derangements in portal systemic shunting. *Gastroenterol* 78:5 Part 2, 1308, 1980.

51. Hourani BT, Hamillilitersin EM, Reynolds TB: Cerebrospinal fluid glutamine as a measure of hepatic encephalopathy. *Arch Int Med* 127:1033–1036, 1971.

52. Warren KS, Schenker S: Effect of an inhibitor of glutamine synthesis (methione sulfoximine) on ammonia toxicity and metabolism. *J Lab Clin Med* 64:442–449, 1964.

53. Cangiano C, Cardelli-Cangiano P, James JH, et al: Ammonia stimulates amino acid uptake by isolated bovine brain microvessels. *Gastroenterol* 78:1302, 1980.

54. Samuels S, Fish I, Freedman LS: Effect of gamma glutamyl cycle inhibitors on brain amino acid transport and utilization. *Neurochem Res* 3:619–631, 1978.

55. Vince AJ, Burridge SM: Ammonia production by intestinal bacteria: The effects of lactose, lactulose and glucose. *J Med Microbiol* 13(2):177–191, 1980.

56. Nance FC, Kline DG: Eck's fistula encephalopathy in germ-free dogs. *Surgery* 70(2):169–174, 1971.

57. Weber FL, Veach GL: The importance of the small intestine in gut ammonium production in the fasting dog. *Gastroenterol* 77(2):235–240, 1979.

58. Lockwood AH, McDonald JM, Reiman RE: The dynamics of hy-

perammonemia metabolism in man: Effects of liver disease and hyperanemia. *J Clin Invest* 63:449–460, 1979.

59. Cooper AJL, Plum F: Biochemistry and physiology of brain ammonia. *Physiol Rev* 67(2):440–519, 1987.
60. Crossley IR, Wardle EN, Williams R: Biochemical mechanisms of hepatic encephalopathy. *Clin Sci* 64:247–252, 1983.
61. Merino GE, Jetzer T, Doizaki WMD, et al: Methionine-induced hepatic coma in dogs. *Am J Surg* 130:41–46, 1975.
62. Zieve FJ, Zieve L, Doizaki WM, et al: Synergism between ammonia and fatty acids in the production of coma: Implications for hepatic coma. *J Pharmacol Exp Ther* 191(1):10–16, 1974.
63. Zieve L, Doizaki WM, Zieve FJ: Synergism between mercaptans and ammonia or fatty acids in the production of coma: A possible role for mercaptans in the pathogenesis of hepatic coma. *J Lab Clin Med* 83(1):16–28, 1974.
64. Branam JE: Suspected methionine toxicosis associated with a portacaval shunt in a dog. *JAVMA* 181(9):929–931, 1982.
65. Imler M, Warter JM, Chabrier G, et al: Hyperammonemia of renal origin: New aspects, in *Advances in Hepatic Encephalopathy and Urea Cycle Diseases.* Karger, Basel, 1984, 169–177.
66. Jones FE, DeCosse JJ, Condon RE: Experimental evaluation of "instant" preparation of the colon with povidone-iodine. *Surg Clin North Am* 55(6):1343–1348, 1975.
67. Twedt DC: Jaundice, hepatic trauma and hepatic encephalopathy. *Vet Clin North Am [Small Anim Pract]* 11(1):121–145, 1981.
68. Drazner FH: Hepatic encephalopathy in the dog, in Kirk RW (ed): *Current Veterinary Therapy. VIII.* Philadelphia, WB Saunders Co, 1983, pp 829–834.
69. Morgan MH, Read AE, Speller DCE: Treatment of hepatic encephalopathy with metronidazole. *Gut* 23:1–7, 1982.
70. Grauer GF, Nichols CER: Ascites, renal abnormalities, and electrolyte and acid-base disorders associated with liver disease. *Vet Clin North Am [Small Anim Pract]* 15(1):197–214, 1985.
71. Reynolds TB: Water, electrolyte and acid-base disorders in liver disease, in Maxwell NH, Kleeman CR (ed): *Clinical Disorders of Fluid and Electrolyte Metabolism.* New York, McGraw-Hill Inc, 1980, pp 1251–1265.
72. Shear L, Gabuzda GJ: Potassium deficiency and endogenous ammonium overload from kidney. *Am J Clin Nutr* 23(5):614–618, 1970.
73. Rose BD: Regulation of acid-base balance, in Rose BD: *Clinical Physiology of Acid-Base and Electrolyte Disorders, ed 2.* New York, McGraw-Hill Inc, 1984, pp 225–247.
74. Johnson CA, Armstrong PJ, Hauptman JG: Congenital portosystemic shunts in dogs: 46 cases (1976–1986). *JAVMA* 191(11):1478–1483, 1987.
75. Ferenci P, Grimm G, Meryn S, et al: Successful long-term treatment of portal-systemic encephalopathy by the benzodiazepine antagonist flumazenil. *Gastroenterol* 6(1):240–243, 1989.
76. Hoyumpa AM, Desmond PV, Avant GR, et al: Hepatic encephalopathy. *Gastroenterol* 76(1):184–195, 1979.

UPDATE

Recent research into the pathogenesis of hepatoencephalopathy (HE) has centered on abnormalities in GABAergic neurotransmission. Therefore, understanding how the GABA/benzodiazepine receptor chloride ionophore complex (GABA/BZR) functions is essential to understanding the current theories pertaining to the pathogenesis of HE. The GABA/BZR has separate and distinct binding sites for GABA and benzodiazepines. When GABA binds to its receptor, the chloride ionophore opens and chloride moves into the postsynaptic neuron, thus hyperpolarizing it. Binding of GABA to its receptor also increases the affinity of the benzodiazepine receptor (BZR) for its ligands. Agonists for BZR have no direct effect on the function of the chloride ionophore; however, these agonists increase the frequency/duration of GABA-initiated chloride channel openings. Antagonists for BZR have no effect on chloride conductance into a neuron unless an antagonist displaces a BZR agonist from its receptor. The GABA-initiated chloride movement into a neuron will then decrease because of the removal of the positive influence of the BZR agonist. The chloride ionophore also contains a receptor for barbiturates; however, the barbiturate receptor is not thought to play a role in the pathogenesis of HE.

Research concerning the postulated perturbation in GABAergic neurotransmission has focused on changes in brain GABA concentrations and changes in the density and affinity of brain GABA receptors. In contrast with earlier studies, recent studies have demonstrated that even though plasma levels of GABA are elevated in humans and laboratory animals with HE, CSF and brain levels are not elevated in these groups. Furthermore, the density and affinity of brain GABA receptors are unchanged in most experimental models of hepatic failure. Numerous studies have demonstrated that the uptake of GABA into the brain, either by specific transport or by a generalized increase in the permeability of the blood-brain barrier, is not increased. This is particularly true in experimental models of chronic liver failure. The significance of increased plasma GABA levels in humans with liver failure has been further questioned because of a poor correlation between plasma GABA levels and the severity of encephalopathy. Currently, changes in brain GABA concentrations or brain GABA receptor density or affinities are not thought to play a significant role in the pathogenesis of HE.

Increased levels of an endogenous benzodiazepine-like compound in the central nervous system (CNS) has provided an alternative method by which GABAergic neurotransmission may be altered in animals with HE. Investigation in this area was triggered by the observation that flumazenil (a BZR antagonist) ameliorated the clinical signs associated with HE in some humans with liver failure. Because BZR antagonists have no direct effect on the function of the GABA/BZR, it was hypothesized that the antagonist was displacing an unidentified BZR agonist from BZR, thus decreasing chloride conductance into the postsynaptic neuron. Subsequently, benzodiazepine-like compounds were shown to be elevated in the plasma, cerebrospinal fluid (CSF), and brain tissue of humans and experimental animals with acute or chronic liver failure. Ultraviolet and mass spectroscopic analysis confirmed that a variable percentage of these compounds were part of the family 1,4 benzodiazepines, particularly diazepam and N-desmethyldiazepam. In one study of humans with HE, plasma levels of the benzodiazepine-like compounds correlated well with the severity of encephalopathy. Elevated levels of these compounds were not identified in the plasma or CSF of humans without HE that had liver disease nor in humans with encephalopathy that was unrelated to liver disease. Not all patients with HE, however, have elevated levels of benzo-

(continues on page 138)

Feline Liver Disorders and Their Management

Cornell University
Sharon A. Center, DVM

LIVER DISORDERS commonly encountered clinically in cats can be grouped into general categories on the basis of histopathologic findings (Table I). The most important physical and clinicopathologic abnormalities and management of each of these disorders are emphasized in this discussion. The typical biochemical findings associated with each category are shown in Figure 1.

EXTRAHEPATIC BILE DUCT OBSTRUCTION

The biochemical and pathologic consequences of experimentally induced complete obstruction of the common bile duct have been described in detail.[1,2] The experimental work has allowed the characterization of the clinical, biochemical, and histopathologic signs that are expected in acute total extrahepatic impairment of bile flow. Clinically, extra hepatic bile duct obstruction (EHBDO) usually is recognized after several days or a week of bile duct occlusion. Complete EHBDO causes bilirubinemia within 36 hours and jaundice within 3 days. Urine urobilinogen values decrease to trace levels or are undetectable after 7 days. Acholic stools can occur as early as 4 days, at which time fat malabsorption is evident on the basis of Sudan III fecal stains. Nonpainful gallbladder enlargement can be palpable as early as 12 days. Within 2 weeks cats can develop bleeding tendencies that are responsive to vitamin K_1 administration.

Biochemical abnormalities associated with EHBDO include hyperbilirubinemia and marked increases in alkaline phosphatase (ALP), gamma glutamyl transferase (GGT), alanine aminotransferase (ALT), and aspartate aminotransferase (AST) activities. Serum bile acid values increase up to 100-fold over normal and often there is little difference between fasting and postprandial bile acid concentrations. Cats become anemic after several weeks of EHBDO and may develop a marked neutrophilic leukocytosis.

Grossly, the liver is enlarged and dark brown/green, and the common bile duct is dilated and tortuous. Histologically, bile duct proliferation and luminal dilatation associated with a multicellular inflammatory infiltrate is observed (Figure 2). Chronic EHBDO is associated with periportal deposition of fibrous connective tissue, which may evolve into biliary cirrhosis. A percutaneous liver biopsy should be avoided if an extrahepatic obstructive lesion is suspected as the result of palpation of an enlarged gallbladder or ultrasonographic findings because of the potential for bile leakage from engorged intrahepatic bile ducts or inadvertent laceration of an enlarged common bile duct or gallbladder.

A cholecystoduodenostomy or cholecystojejunostomy can be performed for biliary diversion if the common bile duct is the site of biliary occlusion. Chronic cholangitis may be a sequela to the surgery but long-term survival in an acceptable condition can result if antibiotics are used intermittently if lethargy and fever develop. If a resectable gallbladder lesion is identified, cholecystectomy can be performed. Surgical resection is less rewarding when used to treat obstructing neoplasia—most commonly adenocarcinoma involving the common bile duct, pancreas, or duodenum—because of the likelihood of metastasis or local recurrence.

Inflammation and fibrosis of the common bile duct and cholangitis may be associated with pancreatitis in cats.[3–5] The high frequency of interstitial pancreatitis and pancreatic fibrosis as an incidental finding in cats necropsied for a variety of reasons suggests that pancreatitis is a more common problem than is recognized clinically.[3,4] Because the major pancreatic duct of the cat joins the common bile duct before entering the duodenum, reflux of the enzyme- and bile-rich fluid from the intestinal lumen could invoke an inflammatory response in either system. Spontaneous reflux of intestinal contents into the pancreatic duct has been shown experimentally to occur postprandially in dogs[6]; similar work, however, has not been reported in cats. If

TABLE I
Liver Diseases Commonly Encountered in Cats

Extrahepatic Bile Duct Obstruction
Common bile duct stricture
  Pancreatic inflammation/fibrosis
  Duodenal inflammation
  Neoplasia (bile duct adenocarcinoma)
  Cholangitis
Common bile duct obstruction
  Cholelithiasis
  Sludged bile
  Parasitic (liver flukes)

Cholangitis–Cholangiohepatitis Syndrome
Ascending inflammation up biliary tree
  Pancreatitis
  Duodenal inflammation
  Spontaneous reflux pancreatic enzymes,
    ingesta, microorganisms
Cholelithiasis
Sludged bile (cause or effect)
Parasitic (liver flukes)
Copper accumulation (?)
Immunologically mediated

Biliary Cirrhosis
Chronic extrahepatic bile duct obstruction
Chronic cholangitis–cholangiohepatitis syndrome

Hepatic Necrosis
Toxins
  Bacterial
  Fungal
  Drugs (acetaminophen)
  Organophosphates
  Heavy metals
  Plants
Hypoxia
  Anemia
  Shock
  Congestive heart failure
  Thromboembolism

Infectious disease
  Feline infectious peritonitis
  Calicivirus
  Toxoplasmosis
  Septicemia
  Endotoxemia

Hepatic Lipidosis
Obesity
Prolonged overnutrition
Chronic anorexia
Protein malnutrition
Endocrine disorders (diabetes mellitus)
Hypoxia
Toxins
  Bacterial
  Drugs (tetracycline)
  Chemicals (carbon tetrachloride, alcohol)
  Plants
Idiopathic

Neoplasia
Primary (rare)
  Hepatocellular carcinoma
  Bile duct carcinoma
  Hemangiosarcoma
Secondary
  Lymphosarcoma
  Myeloproliferative disease
  Systemic mastocytosis

Portosystemic Vascular Anastomosis
Congenital
  Left gastric vein
  Porto-azygous
  Portal-vena cava
  Multiple portal-vena cava
  Patent ductus venosus
Secondary (rare)

ductal reflux occurs in cats, the consequent bile duct inflammation and fibrosis may be an important cause of cholangitis. Major duct occlusion for even a few days can cause histologic liver changes similar to those of the cholangitis–cholangiohepatitis syndrome.

Cholelithiasis is an uncommon[7–10] cause of EHBDO and is difficult to diagnose because of the radiolucent composition of the choleliths (gallstones). Pigment stones, which are friable dark green stones, are the most common type of cholelith in cats. Although pigment stones are often radiolucent, they can be detected using ultrasonography. Infection and impaired bile flow are predisposing factors for cholelith formation. Surgical removal of choleliths provides at least temporary improvement but recurrence is possible if predisposing conditions remain uncorrected. The biliary concretions and bile should be cultured at the time of surgery and

the liver should be biopsied. Postoperative therapy with antibiotics and a hydrocholeretic may be advisable.

Inspissated bile (dehydrated sludged biliary secretions) can form "casts" within the lumen of intrahepatic and extrahepatic bile ducts in association with cholestasis of any origin or as a seemingly isolated event.[5,11] It is possible that abnormal bile flow resulting from an associated hepatobiliary disease and continued resorption of the water component of bile by the gallbladder as a consequence of the patient's dehydrated condition results in the formation of the rubbery, tenacious plugging material. Surgical treatment for a firm, noncompressible gallbladder includes cholecystotomy, removal of any inspissated biliary material, and biopsy of the gallbladder. Flushing of the major ducts is advised; care should be taken to avoid peritoneal contamination with bile. Inspissated or sludged bile necessitating surgical inter-

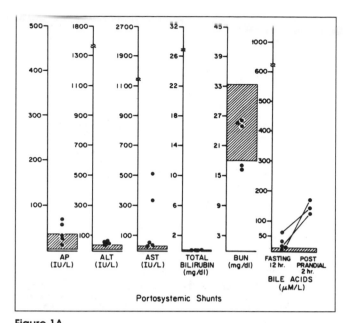

Figure 1A

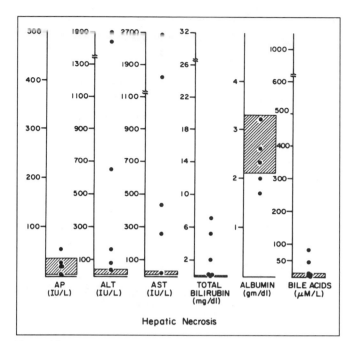

Figure 1C

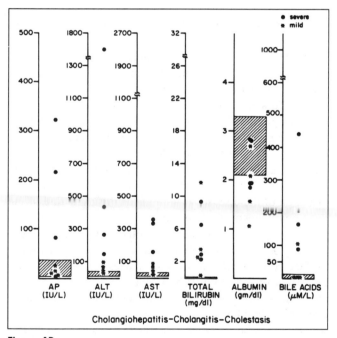

Figure 1B

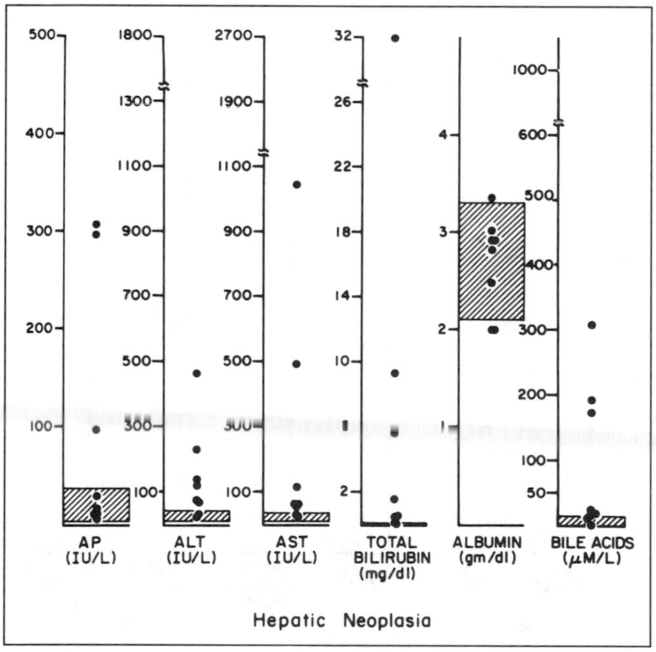

Figure 1D

Figure 1—(**A** through **G**)—Biochemical features of different hepatobiliary diseases in cats (*n*=65, New York State College of Veterinary Medicine, 1985). EHBDO, extrahepatic bile duct obstruction; AP, alkaline phosphatase; ALT, alanine aminotransaminase; AST, aspartate aminotransaminase. Bile acids represent 12-hour fasting values. (Figures 1**E**, 1**F**, and 1**G** appear on the next page.)

vention generally warrants a poor prognosis. A liver biopsy should be performed at the time of surgery in order to identify a possible predisposing disease. Fluid and electrolyte therapy, with or without the use of a hydrocholeretic agent such as dehydrocholic acid, and treatment of any underlying disease are important in postsurgical management.

CHOLANGITIS–CHOLANGIOHEPATITIS SYNDROME

Cholangitis, inflammation of the bile ducts, and cholangiohepatitis, inflammation of the bile ducts and surrounding hepatic parenchyma, most commonly present as an intrahepatic cholestasis syndrome. Mild cholangitis is a com-

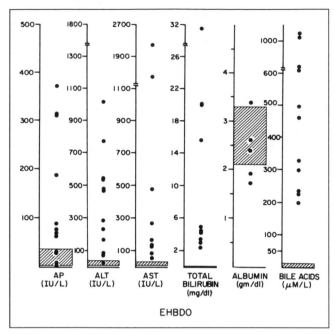

Figure 1E

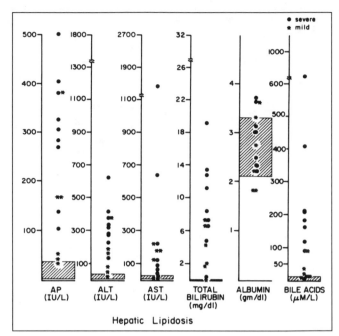

Figure 1G

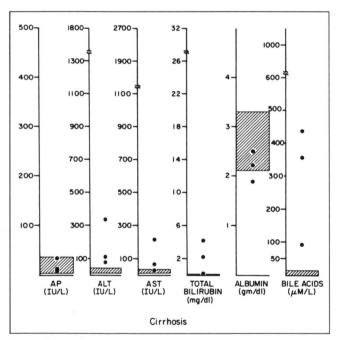

Figure 1F

mon histologic observation in the liver of cats that do not have clinical evidence of liver disease. Clinical signs of the cholangitis–cholangiohepatitis syndrome (CCHS) are vague and recurrent; in many cases jaundice has developed by the time the liver disorder is suspected. Cats may be affected at any age but are usually older than 4 years. Persian-type cats (long-haired cats) were overrepresented in one report of 21 cats with lymphocytic cholangitis and 67% of those cats were less than 4 years of age.[12] A review of

cases of CCHS ($n = 41$) in my hospital shows no breed predilection.

Laboratory findings include increased ALP and GGT activities, conjugated hyperbilirubinemia, hyperglobulinemia, and mild hypoalbuminemia. In the anicteric cat, the fasting serum bile acid concentration may be normal but the two-hour postprandial bile acid concentration is usually abnormal. There may be a mild nonregenerative anemia noted on the hemogram and a neutrophilia with a mild left shift.

Percutaneous needle biopsy can be used as successfully as a wedge biopsy taken at laparotomy for histologic confirmation of the disease because of the diffuse nature of the liver involvement. Grossly, the liver may appear swollen, pale in suppurative cholangiohepatitis, and soft or firm depending on the amount of connective tissue proliferation. Surface contour may be smooth or irregular depending on the extent of regenerative hyperplasia and fibrosis. Thickened dilated bile ducts with accentuation of the portal areas may be observed on cut section. A similar gross hepatic appearance may be observed subsequent to infection with liver flukes.

Histologically, the CCHS can be grouped according to the predominant type of inflammatory cell in the portal triad and the degree of periductal hepatocyte involvement. The inflammatory cell component may be suppurative (neutrophils) or nonsuppurative (lymphocytes or plasma cells or both); the latter form is more common.[5,7,11] Touch imprints made from the biopsy tissue before formalin fixation may differentiate expediently the type of CCHS present. If neutrophils are the primary cell type observed, liver tissue and bile should be cultured for aerobic and anaerobic bacteria. Chronic cholangiohepatitis usually is characterized by nonsuppurative inflammation and variable degrees of portal triad fibrosis, bile duct proliferation, and centrilobular accumulation of bile with bile casts in canalicular areas.[5]

It has been suggested that suppurative CCHS may, for unexplained reasons, not resolve but progress to the lymphocytic form.[11] While this pathogenesis may occur, it is probable that more than one pathogenic mechanism is involved (cholelithiasis, pancreatitis, infection, toxins, immune-mediated disorders). In some cats with CCHS, bile duct changes have been likened to those developing in sclerosing cholangitis and primary biliary cirrhosis, immune-mediated diseases described in humans that involve inflammation of the bile ducts.[12,13]

If a laparotomy is performed to obtain the liver biopsy, the major bile ducts should be evaluated for patency and the gallbladder expressed and palpated for mass lesions, choleliths, and inspissated bile. The duodenum and pancreas should be inspected for evidence of inflammation. The bile and liver tissue should be collected for histologic examination and touch print cytology and cultured for aerobic and anaerobic bacteria and for antibiotic sensitivity testing. Antibiotics are indicated initially for all forms of CCHS, with protracted use (three to five weeks) if the suppurative form is identified. An immunosuppressive regimen of corticosteroids is recommended for the lymphocytic form. It is speculated that the chronic form of CCHS involves self-perpetuation of the injury by immune-mediated mechanisms. This can involve the release of antigens from injured liver tissue that activate immunocompetent cells, which perpetuate the inflammatory process. In my experience, the signs of CCHS may be controlled with glucocorticoids but cure should not be anticipated. Intermittent therapy may be needed as the disease waxes and wanes in activity. In one report, some cats with lymphocytic cholangitis had continued remission following discontinuation of glucocorticoid treatment.[12]

BILIARY CIRRHOSIS

Cirrhosis is uncommon in cats and appears to develop as the sequela of chronic cholangitis–cholangiohepatitis or major bile duct occlusion. Biochemically, liver enzyme tests may be normal except for the serum GGT activity, which may be increased 12-fold over normal values.[14] Even in anicteric patients, fasting and two-hour postprandial serum bile acids are increased and ammonia tolerance is abnormal. The liver may not be difficult to palpate or appear small radiographically.

Histologically, severe bridging portal fibrosis, bile duct proliferation and hyperplasia, and nodular regeneration are observed. Nonsuppurative inflammatory cells may be evident. Medical management for an end-stage liver is at best palliative regardless of the initiating cause. Glucocorticoids can be used if there is a prominent lymphocyte infiltrate. Prudent use is stressed because of the associated catabolic effects, which may hasten loss of body condition and predispose to encephalopathy.

HEPATIC NECROSIS

Acute hepatic necrosis, focal or diffuse, results predominantly in increased serum aminotransferase activities. Serum ALP and GGT activities are normal or only slightly increased. Diffuse necrosis may cause hyperbilirubinemia as well as abnormal coagulation tests, which will not correct with vitamin K_1 administration. In some cats, hepatic necrosis is so extensive that they die before the development of hyperbilirubinemia.

Histologically, hepatocellular necrosis or degeneration can occur with minimal inflammatory cell infiltrates. Patterns described as zonal or focal may be referred to as toxin induced, but this rarely is proved.[11] The liver serves as an important protective mediator between the systemic and the portal circulation, thereby limiting the systemic exposure to enteric bacteria and toxins. Because of this "guardian" role, the liver may be injured preferentially by toxins of enteric origin. The central role the liver plays in the biotransformation, metabolism, and excretion of endogenous and exogenous substances heightens its susceptibility to noxious insults. Acute gastroenteritis clinically manifested by vomiting and bloody diarrhea may be associated with so-called toxic hepatopathy in cats. Recognized causes of hepatic necrosis in cats include: feline infectious peritonitis; toxoplasmosis; calicivirus; *Bacillus piliformis*; endotoxemia; septicemia; toxicities from certain drugs (acetaminophen), chemicals, or plants; and hypoxemia from anemia, circulatory failure, shock, or thromboembolism.[11,15–17] The initiating agent or event usually remains unidentified, necessitating symptomatic treatment.

Supportive care should include intravenous fluid therapy with balanced electrolyte fluids supplemented with glucose, B vitamins, and potassium. Parenteral antibiotics also are recommended. Oral alimentation with foods containing limited amounts of high biologic value proteins and ample carbohydrates should be accomplished. If toxic substances are suspected to remain within the alimentary canal, warm saline enemas can be useful to hasten their elimination. The use of activated charcoal given by stomach tube or per rectum and oral cholestyramine can be beneficial in binding toxic substances.[18]

HEPATIC LIPIDOSIS

Hepatic lipidosis is a common hepatobiliary disorder that probably has multiple causes.[19–23] In humans and laboratory animals, a diverse range of abnormalities, including endocrine, metabolic, and nutritional abnormalities and reactions to drugs and toxins, is associated with the accumulation of excessive lipid in the liver.[22,23] Many cats have no discernible underlying disease and therefore are considered to have idiopathic hepatic lipidosis,[20,21] which has a poor prognosis. In a few cases, disrupted lipid metabolism appears to be associated with overt diabetes mellitus.[11,20,21]

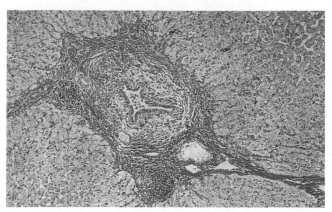

Figure 2—Photomicrograph of liver tissue from a cat with extrahepatic bile duct occlusion of 49 days' duration. Tissue stained pink represents connective tissue. Bridging portal fibrosis, bile duct hyperplasia, and aggregates of lymphocytes are evident. (Van Gieson's, ×100)

Affected cats frequently are presented with jaundice following prolonged anorexia (weeks). Obesity followed by recent weight loss is a common history. Liver insufficiency may develop resulting in encephalopathic signs. A mild nonregenerative anemia and stress leukogram may be observed. In addition to the biochemical abnormalities illustrated in Figure 1, the cholesterol and glucose concentrations may be mildly to moderately increased. Notably, the serum ALP activity may be as high or higher than that associated with extrahepatic bile duct obstruction. The disproportionate increase in the magnitudes of the serum ALP and GGT activities may be suggestive of hepatic lipidosis when used in association with the history and clinical features.[14]

Grossly, the liver appears enlarged with rounded margins and a yellow, greasy, friable texture with a prominent reticulated pattern. Definitive diagnosis requires histologic examination of liver tissue. Because of the diffuse hepatic involvement, a percutaneous needle biopsy is adequate. The tissue should float when placed in formalin. A touch imprint of the biopsied tissue will demonstrate vacuolated hepatocytes. Although routine tissue processing extracts fat, histologic examination reveals varying degrees of hepatocyte vacuolation. Two histologic forms of hepatic vacuolation occur: macrovesicular and microvesicular (Figure 3).[11,20–23] In some cases a combination of macro- and microvesicular vacuolation is present. The diagnostic importance or pathophysiologic implications of these patterns is uncertain at this time. Usually, few inflammatory infiltrates or areas of necrosis are identified. Oil red O, a lipid stain, applied to sectioned frozen liver tissue confirms the presence of fat within the vacuoles (Figure 4).

Initial treatment focuses on restoring normal hydration, electrolyte deficits, B vitamin supplementation, and forcing oral alimentation. A nasogastric or pharyngostomy tube usually is required to provide a positive calorie and protein balance. Although glucose intolerance and diabetes mellitus have been reported to be associated with hepatic lipido-

sis in cats, in a review of the case records of 150 cats with histologically diagnosed hepatic lipidosis, only 8 cats had diabetes mellitus and only one of these had a severe form of lipidosis.[21] Low-dose insulin therapy is only appropriate if a cat is overtly diabetic. Exquisite responsiveness to small doses of insulin (1/4 to 1 unit per cat NPH insulin subcutaneously once daily) given inappropriately may result in life-threatening hypoglycemia. If insulin therapy is given to a cat that is believed to have glucose intolerance but is not convincingly diabetic, the patient should be hospitalized and the serum glucose frequently monitored.

Lipotropic compounds containing methionine and choline do not appear to assist in resolution of hepatic lipidosis and, in fact, may be contraindicated because of the potential for augmenting the development of encephalopathy. Experimentally, feeding laboratory animals diets deficient in methionine or choline or both does result in the formation of hepatic lipidosis, which resolves following the replacement of the deficient nutrients.[24] A similar pathogenesis, however, has not been demonstrated in clinical cases.

HEPATIC NEOPLASIA

Primary hepatic neoplasia is uncommon in cats. The most common metastatic neoplasms are lymphosarcoma and myeloproliferative disorders, but mast cell tumors also can occur. Clinical signs may include chronic debilitation, anemia, hepatomegaly, splenomegaly, palpable abdominal masses, and jaundice. Increases in serum enzyme activities and total bilirubin are inconsistent. Abdominal radiography and ultrasonography may disclose irregular lobular involvement or discrete hepatic masses. Examination of a buffy coat blood smear may be diagnostic for mastocytosis, myeloproliferative disease, or lymphosarcoma.

A needle biopsy may miss focal lesions. When marked hepatomegaly is present, however, needle biopsy usually is successful. Touch imprints of the biopsied tissue often will provide a rapid diagnosis.

Once the diagnosis is confirmed, appropriate chemotherapy can be considered. Although some chemotherapeutic agents are hepatotoxic (methotrexate, L-asparaginase), they can be used with caution.[11] Chemotherapeutic agents requiring hepatic biotransformation or excretion or both (cyclophosphamide) should be avoided if substantial hepatobiliary functional impairment is evident.

PORTOSYSTEMIC VENOUS ANOMALIES

Congenital anomalies of the portal venous system are being recognized with increasing frequency.[25–28] Most cats with portosystemic venous anomalies (PSVAs) demonstrate neurobehavioral signs at a young age. In addition to the encephalopathic signs, anorexia, polyphagia, diarrhea, vomiting, ptyalism, and polydipsia may be noted in the history. Neurologic signs reflect diffuse symmetrical central nervous system aberration and may include depression, aggression, head pressing, blindness, mydriasis, and seizures.

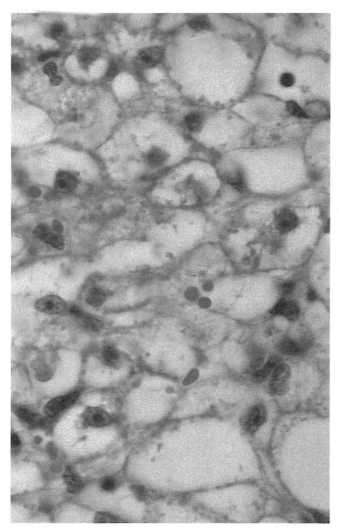

Figure 3—Photomicrograph of liver tissue from a cat with diffuse hepatic lipidosis of the macrovesicular form. Hepatocytes are swollen, the cytoplasm is displaced by vacuoles and in some cells the nucleus is displaced to the cell periphery. (H&E, ×1000)

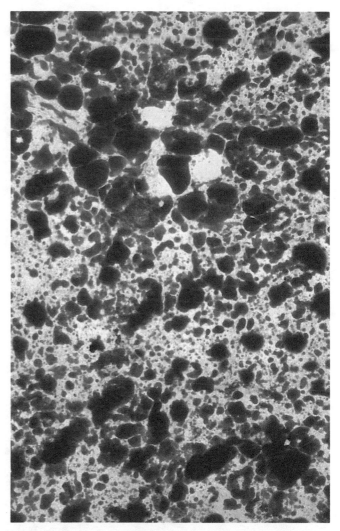

Figure 4—Photomicrograph of liver tissue from a cat with diffuse hepatic lipidosis. The positive uptake of the fat stain confirms the presence of diffuse lipidosis dominating the hepatocyte architecture. (Oil red O, ×100)

Signs may or may not be associated with protein-rich meals. Unexpected prolonged recovery from general anesthesia or an exaggerated response to tranquilizers has been noted. There does not appear to be a gender or breed predisposition for this disorder.

Findings on physical examination are often unremarkable. Occasionally, the body stature is inappropriately small. Some affected cats also have systolic cardiac murmurs and slightly enlarged kidneys.[27] Some cats have radiolucent renal or cystic calculi that are detected easily by abdominal ultrasonography.

The most consistent hematologic abnormality has been excessive erythrocyte shape variation (poikilocytosis).[27] On the biochemical profile, liver enzymes frequently are normal. Mild decreases in blood urea nitrogen (BUN) and blood glucose may occur. Ammonium biurate crystalluria develops inconsistently. The most important tests for recog-

nition of the hepatic insufficiency in cats with PSVA are serum bile acid and blood ammonia values.[29]

The presence of a PSVA is confirmed by ultrasonography or contrast portal venography or both (Figures 5 and 6). Surgical occlusion of the anomalous vessel is the preferred treatment. Prior to and immediately following surgical correction, medical therapy is aimed at controlling or minimizing episodes of hepatic encephalopathy. Medical therapy consists of the feeding of diets restricted in protein content, providing vitamin supplementation, and oral administration of lactulose and antibiotics capable of reducing intestinal ammonia production and absorption. The serum bile acid concentrations have been used to monitor the resolution of hepatic insufficiency. A gradual discontinuation of medical management and return to a regular diet is advised if hepatic function tests indicate a normalization of the patient's condition. In some cats, serum bile acid values

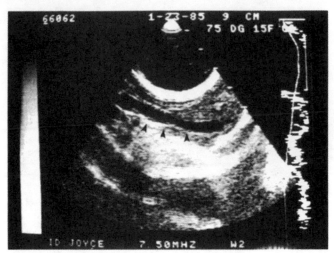

Figure 5—Ultrasonogram of the aberrant portal vascular communication (*arrows*) in a cat with a portosystemic vascular anomaly. (Photograph courtesy of Dr. Amy Dietze, New York State College of Veterinary Medicine)

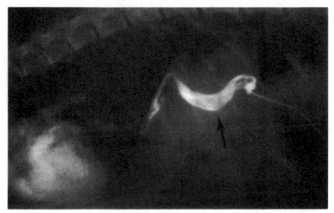

Figure 6—Abdominal radiograph taken after the injection of radiocontrast into a cannulated mesenteric vessel of a cat with a portosystemic vascular anomaly. An aberrant portal vascular communication with the vena cava is indicated (*arrow*). (Photograph courtesy of Dr. Amy Dietze, New York State College of Veterinary Medicine)

have decreased to normal levels within four weeks of shunt ligation and a gradual changeover to a normal diet has been possible.

GENERAL RECOMMENDATIONS FOR THE MANAGEMENT OF FELINE LIVER DISORDERS

The medical management of liver disease is dependent on the type and severity of the pathologic process. Histologic findings may focus on treatment but often an empirical approach is used. A summary of the therapeutic products discussed in this article is given in Table II.

Fluid and Electrolyte Therapy

Fluid therapy plays a central role in the management of the anorexic cat. Balanced electrolyte solutions supplemented with dextrose to 2.5% or 5.0% and potassium chloride (20 mEq/L) are used to correct the hypovolemia and to replace contemporary fluid losses. Hypoglycemia can develop as a result of severe liver insufficiency[30]; patients with PSVA are predisposed to hypoglycemia.[31] In dogs with portosystemic vascular anastomosis, abnormal responsiveness to glucagon, deficient glycogen stores, and possible abnormal insulin metabolism have been shown.[32,33] Neuroglycopenia can be difficult to recognize and if left untreated can result in permanent neurologic impairment. Low blood glucose levels intensify the encephalopathic signs of hyperammonemia.[34] The addition of glucose to fluids given to encephalopathic patients can be beneficial therapeutically because glucose can increase the metabolic removal of ammonia by enhancing glutamine formation.[32]

Hypokalemia should be avoided because it potentiates the development of encephalopathy and impairs intestinal smooth muscle function.[34,35] Potassium supplementation should be guided by repeated serum measurements and the sliding scale provided in Table III.

A metabolic alkalosis must be avoided in hyperammonemic patients because it enhances the diffusion of ammonia across the blood–brain barrier. If hypoalbuminemia and edema or ascites or both are a problem, solutions low in sodium should be used preferentially. The long-term management of ascites may require sodium restriction, loop diuretics (furosemide), and repeated abdominocentesis. Some cats are exquisitely sensitive to diuretic therapy and may become dehydrated, azotemic, and hypokalemic following routine dosages of furosemide (5 mg orally once or twice a day given daily or on alternate days). Repeated abdominocentesis is not advised in a hypoalbuminemic patient as it may worsen the protein depletion and can occasionally lead to hypovolemia, hepatic encephalopathy, and acute renal failure.[36]

Diet

Cats that have liver disease but are not clinically encephalopathic should be fed balanced feline diets with a goal of achieving 80 to 100 kcal/kg body weight per day.[37,38] Cats require a diet with a high protein content; 12% to 20% of their caloric needs are in the form of protein.[38–40] Tissue catabolism is rapid subsequent to feeding a diet deficient in protein or during times of anorexia. Arginine, a critical component of the urea cycle, is an essential amino acid for cats.[41,42] Experimental restriction of the dietary intake of arginine in normal cats results in encephalopathic signs, presumably the consequence of hyperammonemia and insufficient ornithine synthesis.[42]

A diet high in carbohydrates and low in fat, with restricted protein of a high biologic value, is beneficial for cats that develop encephalopathic signs on regular rations. Dairy- or plant-derived protein as opposed to meat-derived protein is recommended because the latter type is ammoni-

TABLE II
Therapeutic Products Available for the Management of Hepatobiliary Disorders in Cats

Therapeutic Agent	Dose	Route	Frequency	Indications and Comments
Antibiotics				
Ampicillin	22 mg/kg	PO, SQ, IV	tid	Broad-spectrum antibacterial; well concentrated in bile; renal excretion
Amoxicillin	11–22 mg/kg	PO, IV	bid	Broad-spectrum antibacterial; well concentrated in bile; renal excretion
Cefazolin	11–33 mg/kg	IM, IV	tid-qid	Broad-spectrum antibacterial; well concentrated in bile compared with other cephalosporins; renal excretion
Enrofloxacin	2.5–5 mg/kg	PO	sid-bid	Broad-spectrum antimicrobial; good absorption and tissue penetration; avoid use in very young animals or those with epilepsy
Chloramphenicol	50 mg/cat	PO, IV	bid	Empiric dose reduction; broad-spectrum antibacterial; enterohepatic circulation; can cause anorexia and erythroid hypoplasia; use of this drug in liver disease is controversial and restricted to situations where culture sensitivities direct its use; relatively poor bile concentration
Doxycycline	5 mg/kg	PO	loading dose once	Broad spectrum, good absorption, and availability; good concentration in bile; fecal elimination; sensitivity testing should
	2.5 mg/kg	PO	sid	direct its use because of the danger of inducing lipidosis with tetracyclines
Metronidazole	7.5 mg/kg	PO, IV	bid-tid	Empiric dose reduction because clearance depends on hepatobiliary function; good enteric absorption; useful against anaerobic organisms; used to modify flora responsible for encephalopathic toxins
Neomycin	22 mg/kg	PO	bid-tid	Used to modify intestinal flora responsible for encephalopathic toxin production; inhibits ammonia producers; synergistic with lactulose; is not systemically absorbed

Antibiotics to avoid: tetracyclines, lincomycin, erythromycin, streptomycin, sulfonamides, trimethoprim-sulfa preparations. These drugs are either dependent on hepatobiliary processing for activation or elimination or are associated with idiosyncratic hepatobiliary reactions. Tetracyclines can induce hepatic lipidosis in other species, warranting concern in cats particularly susceptible to lipidosis.

Therapeutic Agent	Dose	Route	Frequency	Indications and Comments
Hydrochloeretic				
Dehydrocholic acid	10–15 mg/kg	PO	tid	No documented proof of efficacy; is contraindicated in complete bile duct obstruction and in hepatic insufficiency; may be metabolized to lithocholic acid, a highly toxic bile acid capable of producing cholestasis
Appetite Stimulants				
Diazepam	0.2 mg/kg	PO, IV	sid-bid	Contraindicated in severe hepatic dysfunction because benzodiazepines are involved in the genesis of hepatic
Oxazepam	0.2 mg/kg	PO	sid	encephalopathy; short-lived response, side effects of ataxia and sedation; depends on liver for plasma clearance; oxazepam is longer acting: effects seen in 1 hour may last 6 to 12 hours
Glucocorticoids				
Prednisolone	2.2 mg/kg	PO, SQ, IV	sid	Indicated for nonseptic, active nonsuppurative inflammation suspected to be immune-mediated; also used to curtail developing
	taper dose to 0.5–1.5 mg/kg	PO	sid alternate day sid	fibrosis; catabolic; ↑ protein deamination, ↑ ammonia production; side effects: polyuria, polydipsia, immune suppression, appetite stimulation, disturbed sodium and water balance; may induce diabetes mellitus if high dose used chronically; contraindicated in hepatic lipidosis as it promotes lipolysis
Treatment for Gastro-Duodenal Ulceration				
H₂ Blockers				
Famotidine	1–2 mg/cat	PO	sid	Used to limit gastric acidity, new generation H₂ blocker; does not
		IV	bid	impede drug metabolizing enzymes like cimetidine or ranitidine; the preferred H₂ blocker
Cimetidine	5 mg/kg	PO, IV	bid-tid	Impedes hepatic p450 cytochrome oxidases, which could lead to adverse drug interactions
Ranitidine	0.5 mg/kg	PO, IV	bid	Impedes hepatic p450 cytochrome oxidases less so than cimetidine

TABLE II (continued)
Therapeutic Products Available for the Management of Hepatobiliary Disorders in Cats

Therapeutic Agent	Dose	Route	Frequency	Indications and Comments
Gastric Cytoprotection				
Sucralfate	0.25 gm/cat	PO	tid-qid	Locally stimulates prostaglandin production, which assists with mucosal blood flow, production of mucin, and ulcer healing; not systemically absorbed
Antiemetic				
Metoclopramide	1-2 mg/kg	IV	slow 24 hr drip	Strong centrally acting antiemetic; also facilitates gastric emptying in cats with gastrostomy tubes
	0.5–1 mg/kg 20 minutes before feeding	PO or in gastric tube		
Vitamins				
Vitamin K_1	5 mg/cat	IM, SQ	sid	Bleeding tendencies caused by vitamin K depletion (anorexia and antibiotic treatment derange vitamin K-producing flora) and vitamin K malabsorption caused by the absence of bile acids in intestines (complete bile duct occlusion at 14 days); corrects coagulation times by > 30% within 12 hours; begin therapy at least 12 hours before hepatic biopsy; chronic use, once weekly, recommended in acquired hepatic insufficiency; overdosage with vitamin K can result in Heinz-body anemia
	never administer IV → anaphylaxis			
Thiamine (B_1)	50 mg/cat	PO, IM	sid	Chronic anorexia in cats is believed to lead to thiamine deficiency associated with neck ventroflexion and neurologic signs (fixed dilated pupils, weakness, lethargy, tucked or curled posture); thiamine is a safe prophylactic treatment
Water-soluble vitamins	double daily dose		sid	Abundant co-factors necessary for optimal intermediary metabolism; water-soluble vitamins are believed to be easily depleted in severe hepatobiliary disease, especially in those patients with anorexia
Alteration of Intestinal Flora **Ammonium Ion Trapping**				
Lactulose	0.25 ml/cat	PO	sid-tid	Used in hepatic encephalopathy to decrease intestinal ammonia production and absorption and to promote fecal elimination (cathartic effect); lactulose is a nondigestible synthetic disaccharide broken down by gut flora to yield an acidic product; too high a dose can produce severe diarrhea, flatulence, and cramping, which are associated with gas production, dehydration, and metabolic acidosis; the dose is titrated to stool consistency and 2 to 3 soft-stool bowel movements per day are desirable
Binding of Toxins				
Cholestyramine	0.25–0.5 gm in 15 ml H_2O	PO	sid	Empiric dose approximated from human dose; a basic anion-exchange resin capable of binding bile acids and endotoxins in the GI tract forms insoluble complexes that are excreted in feces; short-term use only because chronic use can lead to fat-soluble vitamin depletion (malabsorption)
Activated charcoal	mix with water		sid	Bind toxins in GI tract; Super Char-Vet® (Gulf Biosystems, Inc., Dallas, Texas) liquid or powder is more miscible with water and has greater toxin binding capacity than generic activated charcoal
Retention Enemas				
Lactulose	15–20 ml diluted 1:3 retain for 20–30 minutes if fecal pH > 6.0, repeat enema		tid-qid	Enemas may be used to acutely modify colonic contents in encephalopathic patients; warm saline cleansing enemas are initially used to mechanically flush the contents from the intestinal lumen; retention enemas, comprised of agents capable of altering bacterial flora responsible for toxin production or of impeding the absorption of ammonia, are given after the colon is cleansed
Neomycin	15–20 ml of 1% solution		tid-qid	
Dietary Supplements (appropriate for cats with hepatic lipidosis, *unproved* efficacy)				
l-Carnitine	150–250 mg/cat	PO in food		Important cofactor promoting mitochondrial fatty-acid oxidation; use l-carnitine *not* d-l carnitine; clinical impression is that l-carnitine hastens recovery from lipidosis but this remains unproven

TABLE II (continued)
Therapeutic Products Available for the Management of Hepatobiliary Disorders in Cats

Therapeutic Agent	Dose	Route	Frequency	Indications and Comments
Taurine	250–500 mg/cat	PO in food		Important for bile acid conjugation; assists in detoxification of bile acid effects; cats with lipidosis have very low serum taurine concentrations
Arginine	1000 mg/cat	PO in food		Necessary only if human enteral diets are fed because well-balanced feline rations have adequate arginine concentrations; serum arginine is severely low in cats with lipidosis; arginine is an essential amino acid in the urea cycle
Zinc	7–8 mg/cat	PO in food		Important intermediary metabolism cofactor known to be deficient in humans with severe liver diseases; deficiency can also cause disordered taste perception, which may invoke anorexia; consider using zinc if home-formulated diets are used

agenic and contains small amounts of methionine and aromatic amino acids.[43–45] Boiled white rice is a good carbohydrate source because it is highly digestible, resulting in low colonic residue and leaving minimal ingesta for the production of toxic substances in the lower bowel.[43] Excessive dietary fat should be avoided because short-chain fatty acids may contribute to encephalopathic signs.[46] Meals should be small and fed three to four times per day to maximize digestion and absorption. A protein-restricted diet formulated for cats with renal disease is suitable for patients with hepatic encephalopathy. Unfortunately, most cats with advanced liver disease are inappetent and diet modifications are not well accepted. The recommendations must be individualized for each patient, taking advantage of the dietary recommendations when possible. We have seen a few cats with PSVA accept a diet containing corn meal and molasses that is formulated for dogs with liver insufficiency.[43] Although cats show good short-term improvement on this diet it is not adequately balanced for their nutritional needs on a long-term basis.

Vitamin Supplements

Thiamine deficiency can produce clinical signs that mimic those associated with hepatic encephalopathy.[47,48] Because this vitamin is not extensively stored, deficiency may develop following chronic anorexia.[47,48] Thiamine deficiency is responsive to oral thiamine supplementation and it can be effectively avoided in cats prophylactically treated. We recommend giving chronically anorexic cats oral thiamine routinely on a prophylactic basis.

General vitamin supplementation is justified because hypovitaminosis may result from reduced intake, insufficient hepatic activation of certain vitamins, and increased metabolic needs.[49] The B complex and fat-soluble vitamins can be given orally; however, in the patient with cholestasis, fat-soluble vitamins should be given parenterally because of the possibility of inadequate bile salts in the intestinal lumen for fat emulsification and absorption. The role of copper in the genesis or perpetuation of liver injury

in cholestatic disorders is unclear. Because copper is excreted in bile, it is probably prudent to avoid supplements containing copper in patients with liver disease.

As mentioned earlier, drugs containing methionine should not be given because of the possibility of potentiating encephalopathy.

Vitamin K₁

Coagulation deficiencies may be associated with liver insufficiency. If bleeding tendencies are evident or coagulation times are prolonged, subcutaneous administration of vitamin K_1 should be given. A dose of 5 mg of vitamin K_1 is recommended once or twice a day for one week in an attempt to activate the vitamin K–dependent procoagulants (Factors II, VII, IX, and X). Oral administration can be used in nonjaundiced patients. If bleeding tendencies persist or abnormal coagulation times fail to correct with vitamin K_1 therapy, a fresh blood or plasma transfusion is indicated, especially if a liver biopsy is anticipated. Transfused blood should be fresh because stored blood may contain large amounts of ammonia.[50]

Amino Acid Supplements

Amino acid imbalances have been described in patients with severe hepatic dysfunction.[51–53] An increased aromatic to branched-chain amino acid ratio occurs subsequent to chronic liver insufficiency. The intravenous administration of a specially formulated solution (HepatAmine®—American McGaw) high in branched-chain amino acids and low in aromatic amino acids and methionine has been therapeutically effective in the management of human patients with hepatic encephalopathy.[54,55] The product has not been evaluated in veterinary patients. Ordinary amino acid–rich solutions should not be used in patients with liver insufficiency because the increased nonspecific protein burden may invoke encephalopathic signs.

Benzodiazepines

Chronic anorexia is a common, frustrating problem in

TABLE III
Recommended Potassium Supplementation for Fluids Administered Intravenously

Serum Potassium (mEq/L)	Potassium Chloride[a] (mEq added per 250 ml)
3.0–3.5	7
2.5–2.9	10
2.0–2.4	15
< 2.0	20

[a]Rate of KCl infusion should not exceed 0.5 mEq/kg/hour.

cats with liver disease. Certain benzodiazepine compounds have been used with variable response as central-acting appetite stimulants.[11,37] A rapid but transient response (seconds to minutes) may occur following the intravenous administration of diazepam. Sedation and ataxia may impair an initially positive response. Orally administered oxazepam may stimulate the appetite within an hour and persist for up to 12 hours with fewer depressive side effects. Oxazepam may be a more suitable drug to use than diazepam because the latter drug requires more extensive hepatic metabolism.[56] The appetite modulators usually are not as successful in ensuring adequate nutritional intake as is force feeding. The insertion of a nasogastric or pharyngostomy tube is recommended in cats requiring prolonged nutritional support.

Glucocorticoids

Glucocorticoids are indicated when active nonseptic nonsuppurative (lymphocytic) inflammation is demonstrated histologically. In addition to the benefit derived from suppression of inflammation, glucocorticoids may stimulate the appetite and promote gluconeogenesis and bile flow. Long-term use should be avoided when possible because of the predisposition to infection and the catabolic effects that may increase protein deamination and endogenous ammonia generation. Prednisolone is recommended at an initial immunosuppressive dosage of 2.2 mg/kg orally given once daily in the evening; this dosage is tapered gradually over several weeks to 1.0 mg/kg orally to be given once daily on alternate days for chronic therapy.

Anabolic Steroids

The use of anabolic steroids in cats with liver disease remains controversial. They are used for the promotion of anabolism, stimulation of erythropoiesis, and appetite enhancement. There must be adequate caloric and protein intake to realize a beneficial effect. In human patients, methyltestosterone derivatives can induce hepatocellular cholestasis.[57,58]

Antibiotics

Antibiotics are recommended when the hepatobiliary disease is associated with sepsis, suppurative inflammation, enteropathies, endotoxemia, or when the hepatic macrophage function is suspected to be compromised. [36,59–61] Antibiotics not reliant on hepatic biotransformation or excretion are preferable. Ampicillin, amoxicillin, and cephalosporins are broad-spectrum antibiotics that are concentrated in bile. These antibiotics have minimal side effects in patients with impaired liver function and may be used orally or parenterally. The oral administration of ampicillin and amoxicillin has been observed to have therapeutic value in controlling episodes of encephalopathy in some cats with PSVA. Metronidazole is a bactericidal antibiotic that has been shown to suppress the ammonia-producing enteric anaerobic flora.[62] This drug is well absorbed systemically after oral administration and does not require hepatic biotransformation. The aminoglycosides neomycin and kanamycin may be used safely orally to suppress the intestinal microflora involved in ammonia production because they are absorbed poorly from the intestinal tract. Parenteral gentamicin may be used in conjunction with penicillins, cephalosporins, or metronidazole when systemic infection with intestinal aerobes is suspected.

The use of chloramphenicol is controversial in cats with liver disease. It has been recommended for the treatment of infectious processes associated with the biliary system because it has an enterohepatic circulation.[11] Chloramphenicol inhibits hepatic microsomal enzymes and may cause anorexia and reversible erythroid hypoplasia in cats. The base form of chloramphenicol is preferred over the succinate form because it does not require hepatic metabolism to yield active drug. A dosage of 50 mg twice daily has been suggested.[11]

I do not recommend chlortetracycline, oxytetracycline, erythromycin, hetacillin, lincomycin, streptomycin, or sulfonamides in the management of hepatobiliary disease in cats because of undesirable side effects or reliance on hepatic metabolism for drug activation or elimination.

Lactulose

Lactulose, a semisynthetic disaccharide, is metabolized to organic acids by intestinal bacteria. The resulting decrease in luminal pH "traps" the ammonium ion and the increase in osmolality causes an osmotic catharsis which evacuates potentially encephalopathic substances.[63–65] Lactulose also reduces the number of ammonia-producing intestinal bacteria.[64] The dose of lactulose is adjusted on the basis of stool softness. Two to three soft bowel movements per day indicate a desirable effect. Overdosage may induce intestinal cramping, profuse diarrhea, flatulence, dehydration, and acidosis. It has been reported that neomycin and lactulose act synergistically in lowering the blood ammonia concentrations in encephalopathic patients.[66]

Cleansing or Retention Enemas

Cleansing colonic enemas with warm isotonic saline solution may be used to evacuate toxic substances from the colon during an encephalopathic episode. Neomycin, lactulose, or povidone-iodine can be used as retention enemas to decrease ammonia absorption and suppress the intestinal flora decreasing ammonia production[50]; 15 to 20 ml of a 1% solution of neomycin, 5 to 10 ml of lactulose diluted 1:3 with warm water, and 5 to 10 ml of a 10% solution of povidone-iodine are administered rectally.[50] The latter solution should be removed after 10 minutes. Enemas can be repeated once or twice if necessary but serum electrolytes must be monitored. Hypertonic high-phosphate enema solutions must not be used in cats because of life-threatening electrolyte imbalances that develop.[67]

Dehydrocholic Acid

Dehydrocholic acid is a synthetic bile acid that stimulates the canalicular addition of water to bile. Although this substance, along with fluid therapy, may improve the flow of bile it does not hasten the clearance of jaundice and is contraindicated if there is severe hepatobiliary disease or complete bile duct obstruction or if inspissated bile has not been surgically removed.[68] There is limited evidence of the efficacy of hydrocholeresis in the treatment of cholestatic disorders in cats and prolonged therapy with dehydrocholic acid cannot be advised. This drug has been used empirically along with fluid therapy in cats with CCHS.

Cholestyramine

Endotoxins of enteric origin may be involved in the pathogenesis of certain forms of intrahepatic cholestasis and hepatic lipidosis. The ingestion of endotoxins by macrophages in the liver can block temporarily further phagocytic activity predisposing to endotoxemia of enteric origin.[69] Cholestyramine may be used in treatment of endotoxemia of enteric origin.[69] Orally administered cholestyramine has been reported to decrease intestinal endotoxin toxicity and portal circulatory endotoxin absorption.[70] The use of cholestyramine in cats has not been studied adequately.

Cimetidine, Ranitidine, Sucralfate

Gastric ulceration can develop secondary to hepatobiliary disease. Because the pathogenesis of gastric ulceration involves gastric hydrochloric acid production, drugs modifying acid release, such as the H_2 receptor antagonists cimetidine and ranitidine, are beneficial.[71,72] Care should be taken to anticipate drug interactions during cimetidine use. Cimetidine alters hepatic metabolic capabilities and therefore may influence the active serum concentrations of many drugs requiring hepatic biotransformation or excretion. In addition to the H_2 receptor antagonists, the oral administration of sucralfate will facilitate the healing of ulcerated or inflamed mucosal surfaces.[73] This drug is activated in an acidic environment and binds to denuded mucosal surfaces, providing a protective barrier against further acid-associated injury. Sucralfate can also bind to bile salts, which can effect mucosal irritation when they are refluxed into the stomach. Thirty to 45 minutes should elapse after sucralfate administration before the H_2 blockers are given to allow for proper acid activation. There is limited experience with ranitidine or sucralfate in cats; suggested dosages are given in Table III. At this time, ranitidine is only available in a 150-mg unscored tablet, which is difficult to break, and is therefore impractical for use in cats. Toxic side effects of sucralfate are not expected because it is not absorbed from the intestines. It may prohibit expected absorption of certain drugs given concurrently.

REFERENCES

1. Center SA, Baldwin BH, King JM, et al: Hematologic and biochemical abnormalities associated with induced extrahepatic bile duct obstruction in the cat. *Am J Vet Res* 44:1822–1828, 1983.
2. Cantarow A, Stewart HL: Alteration in serum bilirubin and bromosulphalein retention in relation to morphological changes in the liver and bile passages in cats with total biliary stasis. *Am J Pathol* 11:561–581, 1935.
3. Owens JM, Drazner FH, Gilbertson SR: Pancreatic disease in the cat. *JAAHA* 11:83–89, 1975.
4. Kelly DF, Baggot DG, Gaskell CJ: Jaundice in the cat associated with inflammation of the biliary tract and pancreas. *J Small Anim Pract* 16:163–172, 1975.
5. Prasse KW, Mahaffey EA, DeNovo R, et al: Chronic lymphocytic cholangitis in three cats. *Vet Pathol* 19:99–108, 1982.
6. Hendricks JD, DiMagno EP, Go VLW, et al: Reflux of duodenal contents into the pancreatic duct of dogs. *J Lab Clin Med* 96:912–921, 1980.
7. Hirsch VM, Doige CE: Suppurative cholangitis in cats. *JAVMA* 183:1223–1226, 1983.
8. O'Brien JR, Mitchum GD: Cholelithiasis in a cat. *JAVMA* 156:1015–1017, 1970.
9. Wolf AM: Obstructive jaundice in a cat resulting from choledocholithiasis. *JAVMA* 185:85–87, 1984.
10. Heidner GL, Campbell KL: Cholelithiasis in a cat. *JAVMA* 186:176–177, 1985.
11. Zawie DA, Garvey MS: Feline hepatic disease. *Vet Clin North Am [Small Anim Pract]* 14:1201–1230, 1984.
12. Lucke VM, Davies JD: Progressive lymphocytic cholangitis in the cat. *J Small Anim Pract* 25:249–260, 1984.
13. Edwards DF, McCracken MD, Richardson DC: Sclerosing cholangitis in a cat. *JAVMA* 182:710–712, 1983.
14. Center SA, Dillingham S, Baldwin BH, et al: Serum gamma glutamyl transferase and alkaline phosphatase in cats with hepatobiliary disease. *JAVMA* 188:507–510, 1986.
15. Jones TC, Hunt RD: *Veterinary Pathology*, ed 5. Philadelphia, Lea & Febiger, 1983, pp 1411–1442.
16. Jubb KVF, Kennedy PC: *Pathology of Domestic Animals*, vol 2, ed 2. New York, Academic Press, 1970, pp 201–240.
17. Sherding RG: Acute hepatic failure. *Vet Clin North Am [Small Anim Pract]* 15:119–132, 1985.
18. Eder H: Chronic toxicity studies on phenacetin, *n*-acetyl-*p*-aminophenol (NAPA) and acetylsalicylic acid on cats. *Acta Pharmacol Toxicol* 21:197–204, 1964.
19. Barsanti JA, Jones BD, Spano JS, et al: Prolonged anorexia associated with hepatic lipidosis in three cats. *Feline Pract* 7:52–55, 1977.
20. Burrows CF, Chiapella AM, Jezyk P: Idiopathic feline hepatic lipidosis: The syndrome and speculations on its pathogenesis. *Florida Vet J* Winter:18–20, 1981.
21. Center SA: Hepatic lipidosis in the cat. *Proc 4th Annu Vet Med Forum* 2:13-71–13-79, 1986.
22. Hoyumpa AM, Greene HL, Dunn D, et al: Fatty liver: Biochemical and clinical considerations. *Dig Dis Sci* 20:1142–1170, 1975.
23. Alpers DH, Isselbacher KJ: Fatty liver: Biochemical and clinical aspects, in Schiff L (ed): *Diseases of the Liver*. Philadelphia, JB Lippincott Co, 1975, pp 815–832.
24. Lucas CL, Ridout JH: Fatty liver and lipotropic phenomena. *Prog Chem Fats Other Lipids* 10:1, 1967.
25. Vulgamott JC, Turnwald GH, King GK, et al: Congenital portacaval anomalies in the cat: Two case reports. *JAAHA* 16:916–919, 1980.

26. Levesque DC, Oliver JE, Cornelius LM, et al: Congenital portacaval shunts in two cats: Diagnosis and surgical correction. *JAVMA* 181:143–145, 1982.
27. Scavelli TD, Hornbuckle WE, Roth L, et al: Portosystemic shunts in cats: Seven cases (1976–1984). *JAVMA* 189:317–325, 1986.
28. Berger BS, Whiting PG, Breznock EM, et al: Congenital feline portosystemic shunts. *JAVMA* 188:117–121, 1986.
29. Center SA, Baldwin BH, de Lahunta A, et al: Evaluation of serum bile acid concentrations for the diagnosis of portosystemic anomalies in the dog and cat. *JAVMA* 186:1090–1094, 1985.
30. Feingold KR, Siperstein MD: Abnormalities of glucose metabolism in liver disease, in Zakim D, Boyer TD (eds): *Hepatology—A Textbook of Liver Disease*. Philadelphia, WB Saunders Co, 1982, pp 499–508.
31. Magne ML, Macy DW: Intravenous glucagon challenge test in the diagnosis and assessment of therapeutic efficacy in dogs with congenital portosystemic shunts. *Proc 12th Annu Sci Prog ACVIM*:36, 1984.
32. Lickley HLA, Chisholm DJ, Rabinovitch A, et al: Effects of portacaval anastomosis on glucose tolerance in the dog: Evidence of an interaction between the gut and the liver in oral glucose disposal. *Metabolism* 24:1157–1162, 1975.
33. Holdsworth CD, Nye L, King E: The effect of portacaval anastomosis on oral carbohydrate tolerance and on plasma insulin levels. *Gut* 13:58–63, 1972.
34. Schenker S, Breen KJ, Hoyumpa AM: Hepatic encephalopathy: Current status. *Gastroenterology* 66:121–151, 1974.
35. Sherding RG: Hepatic encephalopathy in the dog. *Compend Contin Educ Pract Vet* 1(1):55–63, 1979.
36. Twedt DC: Cirrhosis: A consequence of chronic liver disease. *Vet Clin North Am [Small Anim Pract]* 15:151–176, 1985.
37. Rogers KS, Cornelius LM: Feline icterus. *Compend Contin Educ Pract Vet* 7(5):391– 399, 1985.
38. Lewis LD, Morris ML: *Small Animal Clinical Nutrition*. Topeka, KS, Mark Morris Associates, 1983, pp 4–12.
39. Kronfeld DS: Feeding cats and feline nutrition. *Compend Contin Educ Pract Vet* 5(5):419–423, 1983.
40. Rogers QR, Morris JG: Protein and amino acid nutrition of the cat. *AAHA 50th Annu Meet Proc*:333–336, 1983.
41. Morris JG, Rogers QR: Arginine: An essential amino acid for the cat. *J Nutr* 108:1944–1953, 1978.
42. Morris JG, Rogers QR: Ammonia intoxication in the near-adult cat as a result of a dietary deficiency of arginine. *Science* 199:431–432, 1978.
43. Strombeck DR, Schaffer ML, Rogers QR: Dietary therapy for dogs with chronic hepatic insufficiency, in Kirk RW (ed): *Current Veterinary Therapy VIII*. Philadelphia, WB Saunders Co, 1983, pp 817–821.
44. Hoyumpa AM, Schenker S: Perspectives in hepatic encephalopathy. *J Lab Clin Med* 100:477–487, 1982.
45. Uribe M, Marquez MA, Ramos GG, et al: Treatment of chronic portal-systemic encephalopathy with vegetable and animal protein diets: A controlled crossover study. *Dig Dis Sci* 27:1109–1116, 1982.
46. Gabuzda GJ: Hepatic coma, in Schiff L (ed): *Diseases of the Liver*, ed 4. Philadelphia, JB Lippincott Co, 1975, pp 466–499.
47. de LaHunta A: *Veterinary Neuroanatomy and Clinical Neurology*, ed 2. Philadelphia, WB Saunders Co, 1983, pp 385–386.
48. Russell RM: Vitamin and mineral supplements in the management of liver disease. *Med Clin North Am* 63:537–544, 1979.
49. Herman RH: Metabolism of vitamins by the liver in normal and pathologic conditions, in Zakim D, Boyer TD (eds): *Hepatology—A Textbook of Liver Disease*. Philadelphia, WB Saunders Co, 1982, pp 152–196.
50. Twedt DC: Jaundice, hepatic trauma and hepatic encephalopathy. *Vet Clin North Am* 11:121–146, 1981.
51. Strombeck DR: Introduction to diseases of the liver, in *Small Animal Gastroenterology*. Davis, CA, Stonegate Publishing, 1979, pp 363–405.
52. Aquirre A, Yoshimura N, Westman T, et al: Plasma amino acids in dogs with two experimental forms of liver damage. *J Surg Res* 16:339–345, 1974.
53. Fischer JE, Funovics JM, Aquirre A, et al: The role of plasma amino acids in hepatic encephalopathy. *Surgery* 78:276–290, 1975.
54. Fischer JE, Rosen HM, Ebeid AM, et al: The effect of normalization of plasma amino acids on hepatic encephalopathy in man. *Surgery* 80:77–91, 1976.
55. Rossi-Fanelli F, Riggio O, Cangiano C, et al: Branched-chain amino acids vs. lactulose in the treatment of hepatic coma: A controlled study. *Dig Dis Sci* 27:929–935, 1982.
56. Baldessarini RJ: Drugs and the treatment of psychiatric disorders, in Gilman AG, Goodman LS, Rall TW, et al (eds): *The Pharmacological Basis of Therapeutics*, ed 7. New York, MacMillan Publishing Co, 1980, pp 387–445.
57. Kastrup EK, Boyd JR, Olin BR, et al (eds): *Facts and Comparisons*. St. Louis, JB Lippincott Co, 1985, pp 111b–111c.
58. Fratta W, Merev G, Chessa P, et al: Benzodiazepine-induced voraciousness in cats and inhibition of amphetamine-anorexia. *Life Sci* 18:1157–1166, 1976.
59. Canalese J, Grove C, Gimson A, et al: Reticuloendothelial system and hepatocyte function in fulminant hepatic failure. *Gut* 23:265–269, 1982.
60. Rimola A, Soto R, Bory F, et al: Reticuloendothelial system phagocyte activity in cirrhosis and its relation to bacterial infections and prognosis. *Hepatology* 1:53–58, 1984.
61. Liehr H, Grun M: Endotoxins in liver disease, in Popper H, Schaffner F (eds): *Progress in Liver Disease*. New York, Grune & Stratton, 1979, pp 313–326.
62. Morgan MH, Read AE: Treatment of hepatic encephalopathy with metronidazole. *Gut* 23:1–7, 1982.
63. Conn HO, Leevy CM, Vlahceviac ZR, et al: Comparison of lactulose and neomycin in the treatment of chronic portal systemic encephalopathy. *Gastroenterology* 72:573–583, 1977.
64. Vince AJ, Burridge SM: Ammonia production by intestinal bacteria: The effects of lactose, lactulose, glucose. *J Med Microbiol* 13:177–191, 1980.
65. Drazner FH: Hepatic encephalopathy in the dog, in Kirk RW (ed): *Current Veterinary Therapy VIII*. Philadelphia, WB Saunders Co, 1983, pp 829–832.
66. Pirotte J, Guffens JM, Devo SJ: Comparative study of basal arterial ammonemia in chronic portal systemic encephalopathy treated with neomycin, lactulose and an association of neomycin and lactulose. *Digestion* 10:435–444, 1974.
67. Atkins CE, Tyler R, Greenlee P: Clinical, biochemical, acid-base, and electrolyte abnormalities in cats after hypertonic sodium phosphate enema administration. *Am J Vet Res* 46:980–988, 1985.
68. Kastrup EK, Boyd JR, Olin BR, et al (eds): *Facts and Comparisons*. St. Louis, JB Lippincott Co, 1985, pp 314–315.
69. Nolan JP, Ali MV: Effect of cholestyramine on endotoxin toxicity and absorption. *Am J Dig Dis* 17: 161–166, 1979.
70. Kastrup EK, Boyd JR, Olin BR, et al (eds): *Facts and Comparisons*. St. Louis, JB Lippincott Co, 1985, pp 171h–171i.
71. Finkelstein W, Isselbacher KJ: Drug therapy—cimetidine. *N Engl J Med* 299:992–996, 1978.
72. Zeldis JB, Friedman LS, Isselbacher KJ: Drug therapy—Ranitidine: A new H₂-receptor antagonist. *N Engl J Med* 309:1368–1373, 1983.
73. Richardson CT: Sucralfate. *Ann Intern Med* 97:269–272, 1982.

UPDATE

HEPATIC LIPIDOSIS

Severe hepatic lipidosis is a common hepatobiliary disorder seen in cats in the United States. Affected cats are usually presented with dehydration, weakness, jaundice, and prolonged anorexia (1 week or longer). Obesity followed by recent weight loss is common.[1] Many cats have a history of vomiting. Overt encephalopathic signs are uncommon. Physical examination usually reveals nonpainful hepatomegaly. Severe hepatic lipidosis can occur as an idiopathic syndrome or develop secondary to disease in another major organ system or in association with another primary hepatobiliary disorder.[1,2]

Hematologic features include a mild nonregenerative

anemia, poikilocytes, and, sometimes, a mild neutrophilic leukocytosis. The serum enzyme activities in cases of lipidosis have a unique pattern compared with other feline liver diseases.[3] While the serum ALP activity may be as high or higher than that associated with EHBDO, GGT activity will remain within the normal range or increase only slightly. In all other feline liver diseases, the magnitude of the increase in GGT equals or exceeds that of ALP. The disproportionate increase in the magnitudes of serum ALP and GGT activities can be used as a predictive indicator of lipidosis. When this feature is observed with ultrasonographic evidence of a diffusely hyperechoic liver,[4] aspiration or biopsy of the liver is warranted. Other clinicopathologic features of lipidosis include mild hyperglycemia, hypokalemia, marked hyperbilirubinemia, and coagulation abnormalities.

Grossly, the liver appears enlarged with rounded margins and a yellow, greasy, friable texture with a prominent reticulated pattern. Definitive diagnosis requires examination of the liver tissue taken by aspiration or biopsy. Because there is diffuse liver involvement, needle procedures are recommended. Tissue samples placed in formalin frequently will float because of their increased lipid composition. Wright's or Giemsa stains used on cytologic preparations will demonstrate obvious hepatocellular cytosolic vacuolation (Figure 3). The routine tissue processing for histopathology includes paraffin embedment of tissues for sectioning and results in the loss of the vacuole lipid moieties. Frozen liver sections can be prepared for staining with Oil red O or Sudan black to confirm the presence of fat within vacuoles (Figure 4). Two histologic forms of hepatic vacuolation occur: macrovesicular and microvesicular. In some cats, macro- and microvesicular vacuolation coexist. It is speculated that small vacuoles represent a transition stage in the formation of lipid vacuoles and that these small vacuoles coalesce, which causes them to have a macrovesicular appearance.

Initial treatment should focus on establishing normal hydration, correcting electrolyte abnormalities, and providing sufficient nutritional support. Polyionic fluids, judiciously supplemented with water soluble vitamins and with potassium chloride based on the serum or plasma electrolyte concentration and a commonly used sliding scale, should be administered intravenously. Parenteral (subcutaneous or intramuscular) vitamin K_1 should be given at a dose of 5 mg once or twice daily for 2 days and then once or twice weekly until full recovery is realized. Vitamin K is recommended because of the dependency on derivation from gut microorganisms or ingested foods and because of the central role of the liver in rejuvenating vitamin K to its active form following activation of factors II, VII, IX and X. Abnormal coagulation test results have been demonstrated in 50% of cats with hepatic lipidosis.[1]

Administration of benzodiazepines as an appetite stimulant is contraindicated. Benzodiazepines are known to be involved in the genesis of hepatic encephalopathy, are dependent on hepatic metabolism for elimination, and do not ensure adequate caloric intake.[5] Nutritional support should initially be done via hand feeding or nasogastric intubation. For nasogastric intubation, a 3 to 5 French soft-rubber feeding tube is passed through the nose and positioned with the end just cranial to the gastric cardia. The tube is sutured and glued to the face and an Elizabethan collar is placed on the patient to prevent removal of the tube.

A liquid diet such as CliniCare® Feline Liquid Diet (PetAg, Inc.) has been used successfully via oral and nasogastric tube routes. When the condition of the cat has stabilized, a gastrostomy tube is inserted using either a percutaneous endoscopic placement or via laparotomy.[6,7] Mushroom-tip catheters are preferable to balloon-tipped urethral catheters for this purpose.

A gastrostomy tube is the optimal mechanism of support for cats with hepatic lipidosis. These tubes appear to be more comfortable for the patient than nasogastric tubes and can be easily managed by most owners. Commercially prepared "prescription" feline maintenance diets can be mixed with water, put in a blender, and processed with a fine-gauge (i.e., food) grinder to facilitate feeding through the gastrostomy tube. The tube must be flushed with a small quantity of warm water before and after feeding. Prior to feeding, the tube is aspirated to appraise the rate of gastric emptying. If food remains in the stomach 6 hours after feeding or if vomiting is a persistent problem, metoclopramide can be used (1 to 2 mg/kg, given as a slow intravenous infusion over 24 hours, or 0.5 to 1.0 mg/kg via gastrostomy tube, 15 to 20 minutes prior to feeding). If the position of the tube is questionable, its exact location can be determined by radiography following injection of iodinated contrast media (commonly used for urography) into the feeding tube. If a tube becomes occluded with food, injecting a small amount of cola will usually dissolve the obstruction after a 10-minute dwell time.

The unique nutritional requirements of cats affected with the lipidosis syndrome are poorly understood. Our use of routine maintenance diets at a caloric intake equal or exceeding 60 kcal/kg/day has been successful in treating these cats. In some cats, however, encephalopathic signs should be treated with oral lactulose and neomycin. Dietary protein should be restricted in these cats.

We have also used l-carnitine (150 to 250 mg/cat/day) and taurine (250 to 500 mg/cat/day) as dietary supplements. The physiologic role of carnitine in lipid oxidation is to transport long-chain fatty acids across the inner mitochondrial membranes. In severely affected cats, carnitine deficiency has not been demonstrated by determination of blood, liver tissue, and urine carnitine moieties.[8,9] It is possible that supplementation with l-carnitine ensures an optimal level of this substance in the cellular areas where demands for carnitine are greatest. Our clinical impression is that l-carnitine supplementation hastens the recovery of affected cats. Unfortunately, controlled studies have not been completed on this topic.

Taurine supplements are administered to reduce severely depleted blood taurine concentrations in affected cats.[9] The profoundly increased serum bile acids in affected cats are largely conjugated with taurine. This may provide some protection against bile salt–induced cholestatic injury.[9] Although serum arginine concentrations are also reduced in affected cats, provision of a well-balanced diet should replete any deficits. If a human enteral diet is used as a basic diet for cats with hepatic lipidosis, supplementation of arginine (1000 mg arginine/day) may be essential. Diets containing medium-chain triglycerides should be avoided because they appear to promote hepatic lipidosis in cats.[10] Because zinc deficiency develops in humans with severe liver disease[11] and because zinc deficiency leads to abnormalities in taste (dysgeusia), it is recommended that the diets of affected cats are supplemented with 7 to 8 mg of zinc per day.[12] Antibiotics capable of modifying enteric flora have been used by some clinicians on a prophylactic basis. Because many cats with severe lipidosis are weak and lethargic and often demonstrate neck ventroflexion, it is important that these patients are given water-soluble vitamin supplements, including thiamine. These cats also should be checked for hypokalemia. Thiamine supplements should be given at an initial dose of 100 mg intramuscularly or orally followed by 50 mg orally twice a day.

Currently, 60% of cats with severe hepatic lipidosis that receive aggressive supportive care recover.[1] Cats with idiopathic disease seem to have a better survival rate than cats with secondary lipidosis. Any cat undergoing caloric restriction for weight loss or any obese cat that suddenly becomes anorectic or develops recurrent vomiting should be evaluated for the presence of hepatic lipidosis. Monitoring the serum biochemical profile for characteristic changes in the serum enzymes of these cats and maintaining a high index of suspicion for syndrome development allow for early therapeutic intervention and better recovery.

REFERENCES

1. Center SA, Crawford MA, Guida L, et al: A retrospective study of cats (n=77) with severe hepatic lipidosis (1975–1990). *J Amer Coll Vet Intern Med*, in press.
2. Center SA: Hepatic lipidosis in the cat. *Proc 4th Annu Vet Med Forum ACVIM* 2:13-71–13-76, 1986.
3. Center SA, Dillingham S, Baldwin BH, et al: Serum gamma glutamyl transferase and alkaline phosphatase in cats with hepatobiliary disease. *JAVMA* 188:507–510, 1986.
4. Yaeger AE, Mohammed HO: The accuracy of ultrasonography in the detection of severe hepatic lipidosis in cats. *Am J Vet Res* 53:597–599, 1992.
5. Jones EA, Skolnick P, Gammal SH, et al: The γ-aminobutyric acid A (GABA A) receptor complex and hepatic encephalopathy: Some recent advances. *Ann Intern Med* 110:532–546, 1989.
6. Mathews KA, Ginnington AG: Percutaneous incisionless placement of a gastrostomy tube utilizing a gastroscope: Preliminary observations. *JAAHA* 22:601–610, 1986.
7. Bright RM, Burrows CF: Percutaneous endoscopic tube gastrostomy in dogs. *Am J Vet Res* 49:629–633, 1988.
8. Jacobs G, Cornelius L, Keene B, et al: Comparison of plasma, liver, and skeletal muscle carnitine concentrations in cats with idiopathic hepatic lipidosis and in healthy cats. *Am J Vet Res* 51:1349–1351, 1990.
9. Center SA, Thompson M, Wood PA, et al: Hepatic ultrastructural and metabolic derangements in cats with severe hepatic lipidosis. *Proc 9th Annu Vet Med Forum ACVIM* 193–196, 1991.
10. MacDonald ML, Anderson BC, Rogers QR, et al: Essential fatty acid requirements of cats: Pathology of essential fatty acid deficiency. *Am J Vet Res* 45:1310–1317, 1984.
11. Bode JC, Hanisch P, Henning H, et al: Hepatic zinc content in patients with various stages of alcoholic liver disease and in patients with chronic active and chronic persistent hepatitis. *Hepatology* 8:1605–1609, 1988.
12. Bauer JE: Feline lipid metabolism and hepatic lipidosis. *12th Annu Kal Kan Symposium* 75–78, 1989.

The Liver
Part I. Biochemical Tests for the Evaluation of the Hepatobiliary System*

Dennis J. Meyer, DVM
Department of Medical Sciences
University of Florida
Gainesville, Florida

Interpretation of the biochemical parameters of liver disease has taken on new meaning with an increased understanding of newly recognized disturbances of the hepatobiliary system. The study of liver disease in the dog and cat is in its infancy and is fraught with extrapolations from studies in humans. As the disease processes involving the hepatobiliary system of the dog and cat are unraveled, the diagnostic tests for liver disease will become more meaningful in the clinical evaluation of canine and feline patients.

Many liver enzymes and tests of hepatic function have been studied in search of a biochemical means of recognizing liver disease. This article focuses on the few tests that have proved to be valuable over time. These tests are categorized into three groups: serum activity of liver enzymes, tests that evaluate liver function (functional capacity), and supplementary diagnostic procedures. Included in the last group are the liver biopsy, selected angiography of the celiac axis, and splenoportography. These are not true liver tests, but they are important in the complete evaluation and sometimes for diagnosis of liver diseases.

The first two groups of tests are frequently referred to collectively as *liver function tests*. The term, although entrenched in the literature, is inappropriate since determination of the serum activity of liver enzymes is not a function test. Only the tests in the second group evaluate a metabolic (functional) capacity of the liver. Tests from all three groups are often necessary for complete evaluation of liver function and disease.

Anatomy

An understanding of certain anatomical features of the liver is a prerequisite for a discussion of liver tests and for an understanding of liver biopsy reports.

The liver is composed of four anatomical systems: hepatocytes, the biliary network, the vascular system, and Kupffer cells. Kupffer cells are a component of the monocyte phagocytic system (reticuloendothelial

---

*This article was published as Florida Agricultural Experiment Station journal series number 3956.

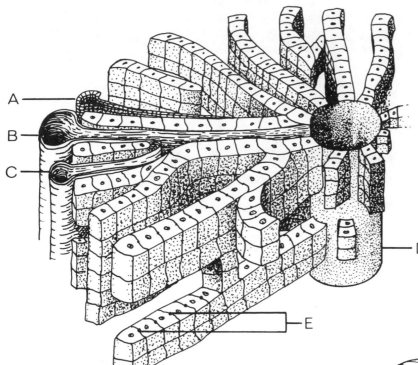

A —
B —
C —
D —
E —

Figure 1—The hepatic lobule. Several portal tracts (*A*, *B*, and *C*) located at the periphery empty blood into the central vein (*D*). *A* = bile duct, *B* = branch of the portal vein, *C* = branch of the hepatic artery, *E* = bile canaliculi.

system) and are involved in clearing living microorganisms and toxins of gut origin from the blood. They may also be involved in the mediation of chronic active liver disease.[1,2]

The Lobule

The basic anatomical unit of the liver is the lobule. It is composed of a central efferent vein surrounded by hepatocytes and portal tracts at the periphery of the lobule (Figure 1). The extensive vascular and sinusoidal network indicates the dependency of the hepatocytes on an adequate perfusion of blood to maintain functional integrity.

The liver is richly laced with an intrahepatic biliary network which progressively increases in ductal size and ultimately unifies to form the extrahepatic bile duct. The bile flow pattern is opposite that of the blood, i.e., bile flows away from the central vein toward the portal tract. This pattern explains why a severe lesion around the central vein (centrilobular) may not be associated with jaundice, while a relatively mild lesion around the portal tract (periportal) may cause sufficient obstruction of bile flow for icterus to develop.[3,4] Focal mechanical obstruction of small bile ducts, e.g., tumor metastasis, usually does not result in obstruction of bile flow since the intrahepatic canaliculi do not run between hepatocytes in a straight line but form an extensive and complicated three-dimensional network.

Portal Vascular System

Blood flows from most organs of the digestive system and the spleen through the portal vascular system to the liver (Figure 2). This vascular arrangement enables the

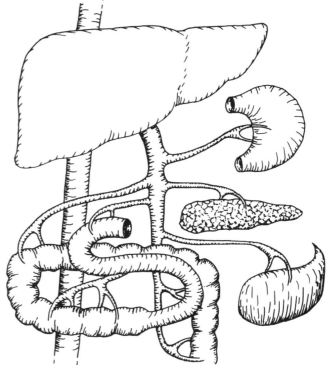

Figure 2—The portal vascular system receives blood from all parts of the gastrointestinal tract, pancreas, and spleen.

liver to act as a metabolic filter for detoxifying ingested substances. This is one reason for the frequent occurrence of nonspecific liver disease when the hepatobiliary system is directly damaged by a toxic agent.

Congenital anomalies of the portal vascular system[5] and acquired portal systemic shunts, which develop secondarily to hepatic cirrhosis, occur frequently in the dog. In both disorders, portal blood does not flow through the liver, and products of intestinal absorption bypass hepatic metabolism and exert toxic effects on the

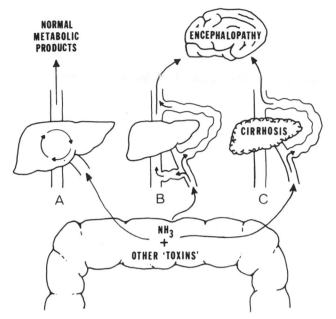

Figure 3—Portal systemic shunts. *A* = normal portal vascular system. Congenital (*B*) and acquired (*C*) shunts of the portal vascular system deprive the liver of an adequate total blood flow. Shunts carry potentially toxic products from intestinal digestion *around* the liver and into the general circulation, which may alter neuronal function in the central nervous system.

central nervous system by altering neuronal function (Figure 3). Signs that mimic primary central nervous system disturbances are frequently observed. This is the syndrome of hepatic encephalopathy.

The Hepatocyte

The hepatocyte contains many different kinds of specialized ultrastructural features (organelles), which reflects the numerous metabolic functions of the organ. No one hepatocyte is typical of the rest, but several general statements can be made about their structure and enzyme content.

The hepatocyte has two surfaces bordered by sinusoids. A portion of each of the interhepatocyte surfaces called the *canaliculus* is further modified to secrete bile (Figure 4). The cytoplasm also contains organelles which synthesize albumin and prothrombin (Figure 4). These two biochemical parameters can be used as indicators of liver function.

A large number of enzymes are located in the organelles and in the cytoplasm of the hepatocyte. Knowledge of the enzyme location in the cell and within the hepatic lobule aids in recognition of a particular disease process. However, the concept of the liver as a *bag of enzymes* has led to oversimplified explanations of the release of hepatic enzymes into the circulation in liver disease.

Figure 4—The hepatocyte. *A* = cell membrane, *B* = smooth endoplasmic reticulum, *C* = mitochondria, *D* = bile canaliculus, *E* = rough endoplasmic reticulum, *F* = Kupffer cell, *G* = bacteria.

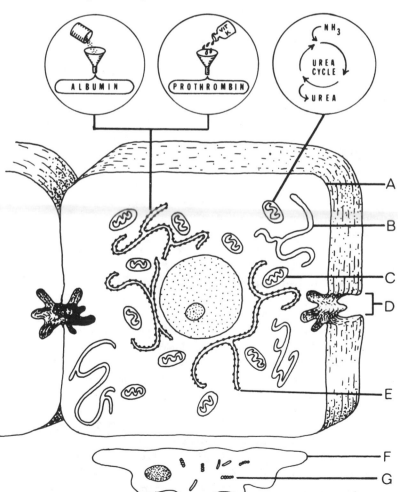

Factors such as hepatic concentration, intracellular distribution, permeability changes of the cell membrane, and plasma half-life times contribute to the serum enzyme activity measured for each species.

Tests for Serum Enzyme Activity

Many tests have been developed to indicate liver disease, but lack of specificity or sensitivity, technical difficulties in measurement, or inherent limitations of the enzymes themselves have limited the number of clinically useful tests to a handful.

Enzymes Indicative of Liver Cell Damage

The integrity of the hepatocyte membrane depends on adequate energy production by the mitochondria. Intracellular enzymes leak from the cell if membrane permeability is increased or the cell undergoes necrosis. The extent to which the serum enzyme activity increases depends on the severity and the number of cells damaged.

The aminotransferases are the major group of enzymes that reflect hepatocyte damage. Serum alanine aminotransferase (SALT; SGPT) is found solely in the cytoplasm, and serum aspartate aminotransferase (SAST; SGOT) is located in the cytoplasm and within the mitochondria. Serum activity of both enzymes is high in severe hepatocellular disease (Figure 5); however, there is little correlation between changes in serum transaminase activity and the extent of histopathologic changes.[4,6] If the hepatocellular damage is severe enough to cause jaundice, the peak SALT activity occurs at about the same time as the onset of jaundice. This may be observed, for example, following the administration of sodium caparsolate for the treatment of heartworms.

Determination of SALT activity is the preferred test in dogs and cats, because the enzyme is present in high concentration only in the hepatocytes, whereas AST is abundantly distributed in other tissues, particularly skeletal muscle. In addition, it has been observed that SALT activity may be increased in some canine liver diseases, while the SAST activity remains normal. The difference probably reflects the fact that an insult to the hepatocyte damages not only the cell membrane but also the mitochondria, resulting in the release of AST (Figure 5). In contrast, the SAST activity in cats is increased more consistently in certain liver diseases than is the SALT activity, but, as noted earlier, it is less liver specific.[7] This finding has not been reflected in cats with liver disease in the author's laboratory.

The plasma half-life for ALT, i.e., the time for the increased plasma activity of the enzyme to be halved, is approximately two and one-half hours.[8] Peak serum activity of the enzyme occurs within one to two days following a severe toxic insult such as oral ingestion of carbon tetrachloride and remains elevated for two to three weeks.[4,9,10] The persistence of increased serum enzyme activity beyond the calculated half-life probably reflects continued enzyme leakage occurring secondary to some nonspecific inflammatory reaction during the

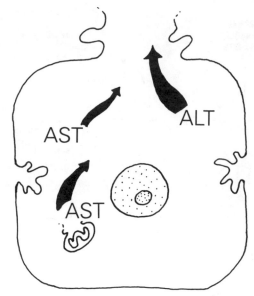

Figure 5—The hepatocyte. Disruption of the cell membrane releases ALT and some AST into the blood. Disruption of the mitochondria releases additional AST.

cellular reparative process (Figure 6). Altered cellular metabolism induced by hypoxia and metabolic inhibitors has been shown to result in enzyme leakage, which appears to stimulate enzyme synthesis until integrity of the cell membrane is restored.[11,12] Altered cell metabolism may partly explain the increased SALT activity associated with certain noninflammatory liver diseases such as congenital portal vascular anomalies,[13] the idiopathic feline hepatic lipidosis syndrome,[14] and steroid hepatopathy.[15,16]

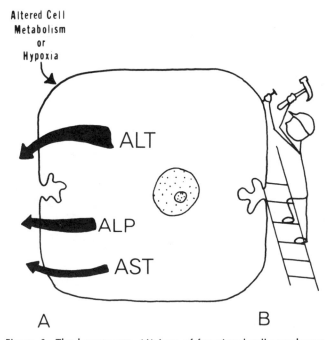

Figure 6—The hepatocyte. (A) Loss of functional cell membrane integrity (may appear normal microscopically), and (B) cellular repair (regeneration) may allow enzymes to *leak* into the peripheral circulation.

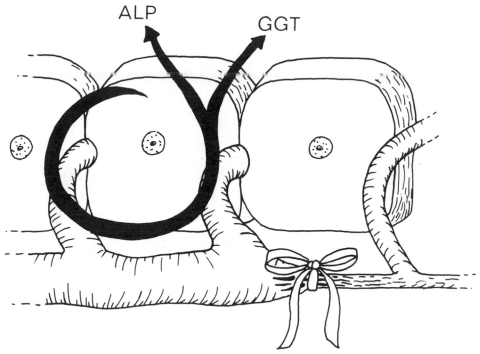

ALP   GGT

Figure 7—Impaired bile flow initiates an increase in the hepatic synthesis of ALP and GGT.

Enzymes Indicative of Impaired Bile Flow

Impairment of biliary flow causes bile stasis (cholestasis) in the ductal network above the obstruction and initiates a number of pathophysiological events. One intriguing process is stimulation of increased protein synthesis in the hepatobiliary tissue, which results in an increase in serum alkaline phosphatase (ALP).[17,18] The retention of bile also causes an increase in serum gamma-glutamyltransferase activity (GGT)[19] (Figure 7). The detergent action of the retained bile acids on the hepatocellular membrane is also involved in the elevation of both enzymes in the plasma. Very little, if any, of the increased serum ALP activity results from "retention" of the enzyme in the bile as had once been believed.

Isoenzymes of ALP are located in multiple tissues (e.g., bone, intestine, liver, certain neoplasms) and may contribute to the serum ALP activity determined by standard methods. Separation of the serum ALP into its isoenzymes has been reported to be diagnostically useful in dogs.[20,21]

Impairment of bile flow in the smaller biliary tributaries (intrahepatic cholestasis) often causes a slight increase in serum ALP activity without the development of jaundice. Jaundice associated with a markedly increased serum ALP activity suggests obstruction or inflammation of the larger bile ducts, especially the common bile duct (extrahepatic cholestasis). If jaundice develops subsequent to hepatocellular insufficiency resulting from inadequate numbers of hepatocytes (e.g., in cirrhosis or extensive necrosis), the serum ALP is usually only mildly elevated.[4,22]

There are several important species differences between the dog and cat regarding the interpretation of serum ALP activity. The serum ALP activity shows a less dramatic increase in cats than it does in dogs. Feline ALP has a much shorter plasma half-life, and less feline ALP is produced secondary to biliary obstruction than canine ALP.[23,24] Only slight to moderate increases of serum ALP activity may be associated with severe feline liver disease.[16]

The measurement of serum GGT activity in human patients with liver disease has been extensively studied;[25,26] this measurement can be readily determined in most commercial laboratories. Early studies in the dog[9,27,28] and cat[10] suggest that an increase in serum GGT activity is closely associated with an increase in serum ALP activity. Although some species differences were reported in these studies, clinical interpretation of serum GGT activity appears similar to that of serum ALP activity. Further clinical studies are necessary to determine the value of this liver test.

Effect of Some Commonly Used Drugs on Serum Liver Enzymes (Figure 8)

In the dog, glucocorticoids frequently cause increases in serum ALP and GGT activities.[16,27] A marked increase in serum ALP activity and a slight to moderate increase in SALT activity associated with hepatomegaly characterize the syndrome of steroid hepatopathy in the dog.[15] SALT and ALP activities usually return to normal within three to five weeks after discontinuation of the drug, but activity has been observed to persist for up to eight weeks following a single injection of a long-acting glucocorticoid.[28]

Another group of commonly used drugs that may increase the serum activity of the liver enzymes are the anticonvulsant drugs (primidone and diphenylhydantoin).[29] Sporadic but marked increases of both SALT

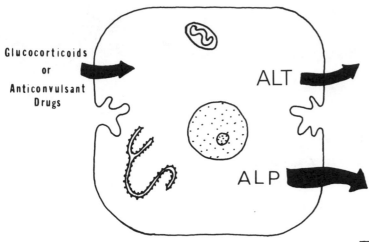

Figure 8—Glucocorticoids (exogenous or endogenous) and anticonvulsant drugs may cause an increase in serum ALP and ALT (SALT) activities.

and ALP activities may occur without clinical or histological evidence of liver disease. A few dogs develop drug-associated chronic active hepatitis.[30,31]

Tests of Liver Function Indicative of Liver Insufficiency

Tests that evaluate liver function depend on an adequate number of hepatocytes and blood flow. The two major causes of liver insufficiency in the dog are cirrhosis (reduced number of hepatocytes plus an acquired shunting of blood *around* the liver) and congenital portal vascular anomalies (Figure 3). Both of these common clinical conditions may be difficult to diagnose since serum enzyme activity may be normal or only slightly increased.

Sulfobromophthalein (BSP) Excretion[32]

BSP is a dye which the liver handles similarly to how it handles bilirubin (Figure 9). The BSP excretion test is a sensitive test for the evaluation of liver function in the dog. It is invalid in the jaundiced patient because the dye competes with bilirubin for hepatic uptake (see Step 1 in Figure 9). BSP excretion is also affected by low serum albumin, which causes an erroneously low value. The test is useful for evaluation of the dog with signs of central nervous system dysfunction secondary to suspected liver insufficiency.

Ammonia Tolerance Test (ATT)[32,35] and Serum Urea Nitrogen (SUN; BUN) Test

Ammonia is normally produced in the intestinal tract by bacterial degradation of protein and carried by the portal blood to the liver. There it is utilized for amino acid synthesis by the urea cycle with urea generated as one of the by-products (Figure 10). A normal liver can easily metabolize the increased ammonia resulting from a protein meal or the oral administration of an ammonium salt (the ammonia tolerance test) (Figure 10). The ammonia tolerance test is a particularly sensitive indicator of abnormal portal blood flow[33,34] and is especially useful for the evaluation of dogs suspected of having a congenital portal vascular anomaly.[35]

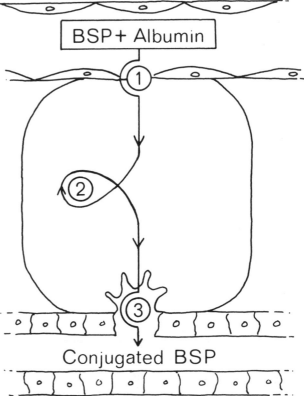

Figure 9—The excretion of BSP depends on (*1*) the serum albumin level and the blood flow to the liver for uptake by the hepatocyte, (*2*) an adequate number of functioning hepatocytes for the conjugation of BSP, and (*3*) a patent biliary system.

A deficiency of one of the enzymes in the urea cycle resulting in hyperammonemia has been reported in two dogs.[36] Other liver tests, SALT, ALP, and the BSP excretion test were normal in these dogs.[36]

The main limitation of the ammonia tolerance test is handling the samples. The heparinized samples should be kept on ice and the ammonia content should be determined within one hour after blood collection. The medical hospital or commercial laboratory used should be contacted with regard to the submission of the samples.

The formation of urea is related to the hepatic metabolism of ammonia. When ammonia metabolism is altered, a low serum urea nitrogen may be measured.

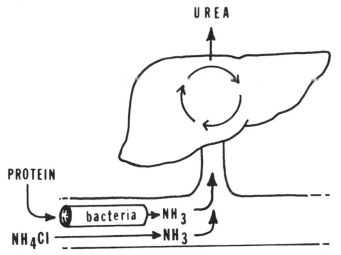

Figure 10—Ammonia is formed in the intestinal tract, absorbed, carried to the liver by the portal vascular system, and metabolized, forming urea.

A low SUN (<10 mg/dl) may be associated with prolonged anorexia or may result from liver insufficiency.[13] The SUN may be an unreliable index of renal function in patients with liver insufficiency; creatinine levels can be used instead of the SUN.

Albumin

The liver is the sole site of synthesis of albumin (Figure 4).[37] A low serum albumin concentration (<2.3 g/dl) may occur in dogs with liver insufficiency and may suggest congenital portal vascular anomalies in young dogs[13] and hepatic cirrhosis in older dogs. The canine liver has a tremendous reserve capacity for albumin synthesis, and a low serum albumin concentration is not usually noted until liver insufficiency is severe. Protein-losing diseases involving the kidney or intestinal tract should always be considered in the differential diagnosis when evaluating this biochemical parameter.

Prothrombin Time

Prothrombin is one of several vitamin K–dependent coagulation factors synthesized by the liver (Figure 4).[37] A prolonged prothrombin time occurs in the presence of a decreased hepatic cell mass (extensive necrosis or hepatic cirrhosis) or when there is insufficient bile (extrahepatic cholestasis) for the intestinal absorption of the fat-soluble vitamin K. Prothrombin time should be determined before a liver biopsy or exploratory laparotomy is performed in cases of suspected hepatobiliary disorders.

Bilirubin

Determination of total serum bilirubin concentration is a time-honored test of liver function. The total serum bilirubin measurement is comprised of unconjugated and conjugated bilirubin. Unconjugated bilirubin is formed from hemoglobin, metabolically altered, and excreted as conjugated bilirubin by the liver (Figure 11).

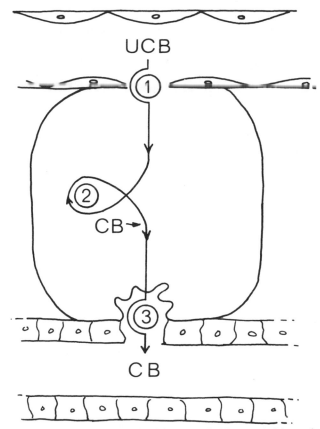

Figure 11—*Unconjugated* bilirubin (*UCB*) is (*1*) removed from the peripheral blood by the hepatocyte and (*2*) converted to *conjugated* bilirubin (*CB*), and (*3*) the *conjugated* bilirubin is excreted by the canaliculus into the biliary system.

Accumulation of bilirubin in the plasma and tissues is termed *jaundice* or *icterus*. The yellow discoloration of the tissues is clinically apparent when the total serum bilirubin concentration is greater than 2 to 3 mg/dl. Jaundice may develop from prehepatic causes (increased destruction of erythrocytes [unconjugated bilirubinemia predominates] or disease involving the hepatobiliary system). Conjugated bilirubinemia predominates when bile flow is impaired in the extrahepatic biliary system. When icterus is associated with a primary liver disorder, e.g., cirrhosis or severe hepatocellular degeneration, the predominant fraction comprising the hyperbilirubinemia is less predictable.

Most often the determination of the serum unconjugated and conjugated bilirubin concentration is not essential in evaluating the jaundiced patient. Other test parameters are often sufficient to direct further diagnostic efforts, such as a hemogram and serum haptoglobin for hemolytic disorders and the serum liver enzymes for hepatobiliary disorders.

Conjugated bilirubin is water soluble, and a small fraction is not bound to albumin,[38] which may allow the yellow pigment to appear in the urine. The dog has a low renal threshold for conjugated bilirubin, and a small amount may occasionally be detected in concentrated urine from a dog without liver disease.[39] Bilirubinuria resulting from a hepatobiliary disease precedes clinical detection of icterus in the dog and cat and is a useful screening test. Bilirubinuria in the cat strongly suggests a severe hepatic disturbance.[39] The yellow color of normal urine is due largely to the pigment urochrome. Therefore a chemical test is required to determine the presence of bilirubin in the urine. The tablet method[a] is a more sensitive and reliable test for detection of bilirubinuria than is the reagent strip method.[b,39] Since bilirubin is rapidly degraded when exposed to bright light, erroneously low results may be obtained if serum and urine samples are not properly handled.[40]

Urobilinogen is one product of bilirubin degradation by bacteria in the intestinal lumen. A small amount of the urobilinogen is absorbed by the intestine and excreted in the urine, and it can be measured by the reagent strip method. The test has been advocated as a useful indicator of extrahepatic bile duct patency in assessment of the jaundiced patient. A number of factors may alter the enterohepatic circulation of urobilinogen, e.g., diarrhea, constipation, and oral antibiotics, and can cause an unreliable test result. Urobilinogen is rapidly oxidized to urobilin when urine is exposed to air,[40] adding to the potential for misinterpretation of the test in the differential diagnosis of icterus.[41]

Serum Bile Acids

Bile acids are a component of bile which are synthesized in the liver, excreted into the intestine, efficiently reabsorbed into the portal blood, and *recycled* by the liver (enterohepatic circulation). Either portosystemic shunts or pathology of the hepatobiliary system prior to the development of hyperbilirubinemia can result in an increased fasting serum total bile acid concentration (FSBA).[42,43] The determination of the FSBA can contribute to the decision to obtain histologic confirmation of this last group of hepatic diseases. There is a high probability that histologic findings will define a lesion when the FSBA of a dog or cat is greater than 20 µmol/L.[42,44] Although the reported "normal" value for the FSBA in dogs or cats is (approximately) less than 5 µmol/L,[42–46] I and others have observed healthy dogs with FSBA values from 15 to 20 µmol/L.[6] When the FSBA concentration is between 5 and 20 µmol/L, I suggest one of the following: (1) evaluate the patient for extrahepatic diseases; (2) repeat the FSBA in two to four weeks; or (3) if the combined clinicopathologic findings support chronic hepatitis/cirrhosis or a congenital portal vascular anomaly,[47] pursue confirmation of the diagnosis.

In the medical literature, there is controversy concerning the diagnostic value of determining a postprandial serum total bile acid concentration (PPSBA).[48–51] In dogs, the PPSBA is reported to increase the sensitivity for the detection of cirrhosis and congenital portal vascular anomalies, especially when this concentration is greater than 25 µmol/L.[44] When using these guidelines,

it is prudent to recognize that healthy dogs are reported with PPSBA values of approximately 30 µmol/L.[45]

Supplementary Procedures

Liver tests can often detect and indicate a general type of liver disease. In some cases the information provided is adequate for patient management. In others, supplementary procedures such as liver biopsy or angiography are necessary to confirm a diagnosis or to suggest a prognosis.

Liver Biopsy

The liver biopsy provides a microscopic look at the type of pathological change present in the liver. The practical concerns regarding the liver biopsy are deciding when it is necessary, and the availability of a veterinary pathologist who is familiar with the evaluation of liver biopsy samples.

A liver biopsy is indicated for the evaluation of persistent, unexplained elevations of serum liver enzyme activity; the icteric patient suspected of hepatic disease; and hepatomegaly. A percutaneous liver biopsy with local anesthesia avoids general anesthesia and is convenient but should only be performed by the experienced clinician. The possibility of missing focal hepatic disturbances and the failure to obtain an adequate sample from a fibrotic liver limit the usefulness of the percutaneous technique.

Laparoscopy is useful for gross evaluation of the liver and improves the diagnostic yield of the needle biopsy. The expense of the equipment limits its widespread use. A laparotomy with general anesthesia is generally recommended for obtaining a liver biopsy because it allows for a visual and digital examination of the hepatobiliary system before the biopsy specimen is obtained.

There are two contraindications for liver biopsy: (1) if the prothrombin time is prolonged or the platelet count is less than $50,000/\mu l$ and (2) if extrahepatic obstruction of bile flow is suspected.

Radiology

Radiographic evaluation of the liver is frequently unrewarding. A small liver silhouette may supplement the biochemical information and be compatible with a diagnosis of cirrhosis or a congenital vascular anomaly, but interpretations are fraught with subjective error.

Special contrast radiographic procedures are necessary for the confirmation of congenital portal vascular anomalies. Cranial mesenteric angiography and splenoportography are procedures usually restricted to specialists.

Conclusion

The liver possesses diverse functions which have been utilized for evaluation of hepatic integrity and function. A few selected tests are used to identify disturbances of the hepatobiliary system and to suggest the type of liver disease. Further studies to establish the nature of the

---

[a]Ictotest®, Ames Co., Elkhart, IN 46515.
[b]Multistix®, Ames Co., Elkhart, IN 46515.

pathological changes in the liver and clarification of the types of liver disease will add new meaning to the use of the liver tests. The need is not for new liver tests but for more knowledgeable application of the tests currently available.

Acknowledgments

The author acknowledges the help of Pam Miller in preparing the drawings and Drs. Anne Chiapella and Colin Burrows for reviewing the manuscript.

REFERENCES

1. Rogoff TM, Lipsky PE: Role of the Kupffer cells in local and systemic immune responses. *Gastroenterology* 80:854-860, 1981.
2. Tanner A, Keyhoni A, Reiner R, et al: Proteolytic enzymes released by liver macrophages may promote hepatic injury in a rat model of hepatic damage. *Gastroenterology* 80:647-654, 1981.
3. Gopinath C, Ford EJH: Localization of liver injury and extent of bilirubinaemia in experimental liver lesions. *Vet Pathol* 9:99-108, 1972.
4. Van Vleet JF, Alberts JO: Evaluation of liver function tests and liver biopsy in experimental carbon tetrachloride intoxication and extrahepatic bile duct obstruction in the dog. *Am J Vet Res* 29:2119-2131, 1968.
5. Suter PF: Portal vein anomalies in the dog: Their angiographic diagnosis. *J Am Vet Radiol Soc* 16:84-97, 1975.
6. Visser MP, Krill MTA, Muijtjens AMM, et al: Distribution of enzymes in dog heart and liver; Significance for assessment of tissue damage from data on plasma enzyme activities. *Clin Chem* 27:1845-1850, 1981.
7. Hornbuckle WE, Allan GS: Feline liver disease, in Kirk RW (ed): *Current Veterinary Therapy VII*. Philadelphia, WB Saunders Co, 1980, pp 891-895.
8. Zinkle JG, Bush RM, Cornelius CE, Freedland RA: Comparative studies on plasma and tissue sorbital glutamic, lactic, hydroxybutyric dehydrogenase and transaminase activities in the dog. *Res Vet Sci* 12:211-214, 1971.
9. Noonan NE, Meyer DJ: Use of arginase and gamma glutamyltransferase as specific indicators of hepatocellular or hepatobiliary disease in the dog. *Am J Vet Res* 40:942-947, 1978.
10. Meyer DJ: Plasma gamma-glutamyltransferase in cats with toxic and obstructive hepatic disease. Submitted for publication.
11. Zierler KL: Increased muscle permeability to aldolase produced by depolarization and by metabolic inhibitors. *Am J Physiol* 193:534-538, 1958.
12. Ozawa K, Yamaolca Y, Nonby H, Honjo I: Insulin as the primary factor governing changes in mitochondrial metabolism leading to liver regeneration and atrophy. *Am J Surg* 127:669-675, 1974.
13. Griffiths GL, Lumsden JH, Valli VEO: Hematologic and biochemical changes in dogs with portosystemic shunts. *JAAHA* 17:705-710, 1981.
14. Burrows CF, Chiapella AM, Jezyk P: Idiopathic feline hepatic lipidosis: A syndrome. Submitted for publication.
15. Rogers WA, Ruebner BH: A retrospective study of probable glucocorticoid-induced hepatopathy in dogs. *JAVMA* 170:603-606, 1977.
16. Badylak SF, Van Vleet JF: Sequential morphologic and clinicopathologic alterations in dogs with experimentally induced glucocorticoid hepatopathy. *Am J Vet Res* 42:1310-1318, 1981.
17. Kaplan MM: Induction of rat liver alkaline phosphatase by bile duct ligation. *Yale J Biol Med* 52:69-75, 1979.
18. Toda G, Ikeda Y, Kako M, et al: Mechanism of elevation of serum alkaline phosphatase activity in biliary obstruction and experimental study. *Clin Chim Acta* 107:85-96, 1980.
19. Huseby N, Vik T: The activity of gamma-glutamyltransferase after bile duct ligation in guinea pig. *Clin Chim Acta* 88:385-392, 1978.
20. Hoffmann WE: The diagnostic value of canine serum alkaline phosphatase and alkaline phosphatase isoenzymes. *JAAHA* 13:237-241, 1977.
21. Rogers WA: Source of serum alkaline phosphatase in clinically normal and diseased dogs: A clinical study. *JAVMA* 168:934-937, 1976.
22. Meyer DJ, Inverson WO, Terrell TG: Obstructive jaundice associated with chronic active hepatitis in a dog. *JAVMA* 176:41-44, 1980.
23. Everett RM, Duncan JR, Prasse KW: Alkaline phosphatase, leucine aminopeptidase and alanine aminotransferase activities with obstructive and toxic hepatic disease in cats. *Am J Vet Res* 38:936-966, 1977.
24. Hoffmann WE, Renegar WE, Dorner JL: Serum half-life of intravenously injected intestinal and hepatic alkaline phosphatase isoenzymes in the cat. *Am J Vet Res* 38:1637-1639, 1977.
25. Goldberg DM, Martin JV: Role of gamma glutamyl transpeptidase activity in the diagnosis of hepatobiliary disease. Recent advances. *Digestion* 12:232-246, 1975.
26. Schmidt E: Strategy and evaluation of enzyme determinations in serum in disease of the liver and the biliary system, in Demers LM, Shaw LM (eds): *Evaluation of Liver Function: A Multifaceted Approach to Clinical Diagnosis*. Baltimore, Urban and Schwarzenberg, 1978, pp 79-101.
27. Shull RM, Hornbuckle W: Diagnostic use of serum gamma-glutamyltransferase in canine liver disease. *Am J Vet Res* 40:1321-1324, 1979.
28. Meyer DJ, Beauchamp RR: Prolonged liver test abnormalities and adrenocortical suppression in a dog following a single intramuscular glucocorticoid dose. In press.
29. Meyer DJ, Noonan NE: Liver tests in dog receiving anticonvulsant drugs (diphenylhydantoin and primidone). *JAAHA* 17:261-264, 1981.
30. Nash AS, Thompson H: Phenytoin toxicity: A fatal case in a dog with hepatitis and jaundice. *Vet Rec* 100:280-281, 1977.
31. Meyer DJ, Congdon L: Primidone-associated chronic active hepatitis in two dogs. Submitted for publication.
32. Duncan JR, Prasse KW: *Veterinary Laboratory Medicine: Clinical Pathology*. Ames, IA, The Iowa State University Press, 1977, pp 87-88.
33. Conn HO: Ammonia tolerance in assessing the patency of portacaval anastomosis. *Arch Intern Med* 131:221-226, 1973.
34. Adamsons RJ, Arifs S, Gabich A, et al: Arterialization of the liver in combination with a portacaval shunt in the dog. *Surg Gynecol Obstet* 140:594-600, 1975.
35. Meyer DJ, Strombeck DR, Stone EA, et al: Ammonia tolerance test in clinically normal dogs and in dogs with portosystemic shunts. *JAVMA* 173:377-379, 1978.
36. Strombeck DR, Meyer DJ, Freedland RA: Hyperammonemia due to a urea cycle enzyme deficiency in two dogs. *JAVMA* 166:1109-1111, 1976.
37. Asofsky R: Plasma protein synthesis by liver, in Becker FF (ed): *The Liver: Normal and Abnormal Functions*. New York, Marcel Decker Inc, 1974, pp 87-102.
38. Fevery J, Blanckaert N, Heirwegh KPM, DeGroote J: Bilirubin conjugates: Formation and detection, in Popper H, Schaffner F (eds): *Progress in Liver Diseases*, vol 5. New York, Grune & Stratton, 1976, pp 183-214.
39. Osborne CA, Steven JB, Lee GE, et al: Clinical significance of bilirubinuria. *Compend Contin Educ Pract Vet* 2:897-903, 1980.
40. Bold AM, Wilding P: *Clinical Chemistry Companion*. Philadelphia, JB Lippincott Co, 1978, pp 17, 76.
41. Duncan JR, Prasse KW: *Veterinary Laboratory Medicine: Clinical Pathology*. Ames, IA, The Iowa State University Press, 1977, pp 106-107.
42. Center SA, Baldwin BH, Erb HN, Tennant BC: Bile acid concentration in the diagnosis of hepatobiliary disease in the cat. *JAVMA* 189:891–896, 1986.
43. Center SA, Baldwin BH, Erb HN, Tennant BC: Bile acid concentrations in the diagnosis of hepatobiliary disease in the dog. *JAVMA* 187:935–940, 1985.
44. Center SA, ManWarren T, Slater MR, Wilentz E: Evaluation of twelve-hour preprandial and two-hour postprandial serum bile acid concentrations for diagnosis of hepatobiliary disease in dogs. *JAVMA* 199:217–226, 1991.
45. Counsell LJ, Lumsden JH: Serum bile acids—Reference values in healthy dogs and comparison of two kit methods. *Vet Clin Pathol* 17:71–74, 1988.
46. Johnson CA, Nachreiner RF, Refusal KR: Evaluation of feline postprandial bile acids (abstract). *J Vet Int Med* 5:131, 1991.
47. Meyer DJ, Coles EH, Rich LJ: *Veterinary Laboratory Medicine—*

Interpretation and Diagnosis. Philadelphia, WB Saunders Co, 1992, pp 55–70.

48. Greenfield SM, Soloway RD, Carithers RL Jr, et al: Evaluation of postprandial serum bile acid response as a test of hepatic function. *Dig Dis Sci* 31:785–791, 1986.

49. Simko V, Michael S: Bile acid levels in diagnosing mild liver disease. *Arch Int Med* 146:695–697, 1986.

50. van Blankenstein M, Frenkel M, van den Berg JWO, et al: Endogenous bile acid tolerance test for liver function. *Dig Dis Sci* 28:137–144, 1983.

51. Mannes GA, Stellaard F, Paumgartner G: Increased serum bile acids in cirrhosis with normal transaminases. *Digestion* 25:217–221, 1982.

The Liver
Part II. Biochemical Diagnosis of
Hepatobiliary Disorders in the Dog[*]

Dennis J. Meyer, DVM
Colin F. Burrows, BVetMed, PhD, MRCVS

Department of Medical Sciences
University of Florida
Gainesville, Florida

The liver can respond to injury in a limited number of ways: hepatocellular degeneration, hepatic fibrosis, the formation of regenerative nodules, and bile duct hyperplasia. Portal hypertension, resulting in altered portal blood flow, and cholestasis may occur subsequent to liver injury, depending on the type, severity, and duration of the insult. Liver tests reflect these pathologic processes; however, despite the diversity of causes of liver disorders, the disorders may appear clinicopathologically and histologically similar.

In this article, tests that the authors believe are useful for the clinical diagnosis of liver disease are evaluated. The pattern of test results may reveal that there is disease or damage to the liver, may indicate the extent of the damage or disease, and may differentiate between different groups of liver disease. The basic groups of liver disorders for which test result patterns are discussed include acute hepatitis (hepatocellular degeneration), cirrhosis, chronic active hepatitis, biliary obstruction, tumors, portal systemic vascular anomalies, and glucocorticoid hepatopathy. Illustrative case reports are included.

Acute Hepatitis and Acute Hepatocellular Degeneration

Acute hepatitis and acute hepatocellular degeneration are characterized by focal or diffuse damage to hepatocytes. The causes of hepatocellular disruption are many and varied and are often not determined. Some of the recognized agents include chemical solvents such as carbon tetrachloride,[1] mycotoxins such as aflatoxin,[2] drugs (e.g., acetaminophen[a] in the cat[3] and mebendazole[b] in the dog[4]), and viruses. The clinical signs, biochemical data, and histological findings do not usually indicate a specific cause which would result in a diagnosis of *toxic* hepatitis.

The predominant biochemical abnormality is an increased serum alanine aminotransferase (SALT; SGPT), the magnitude of which is

[*]This article was published as Florida Agricultural Experiment Station journal series number 3956.
[a]Tylenol®, McNeil Consumer Products Co., Fort Washington, PA 19034.
[b]Telmintic™, Pitman-Moore, Washington Crossing, NJ 08560.

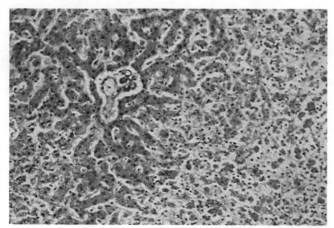

Figure 1—A canine liver specimen showing extensive acute hepatocellular degeneration. The dog had been icteric for one day. A blood sample did not clot, and the dog died six hours later. SALT = 8100 IU/L, serum ALP = 418 IU/L, total bilirubin = 3.3 mg/dl. No cause was determined.

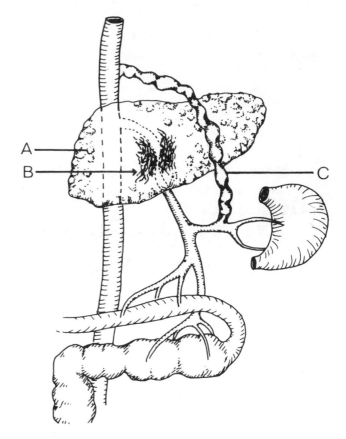

Figure 2—Hepatic cirrhosis. Structurally abnormal nodules, *A*, and fibrosis, *B*, may cause the development of an acquired portal systemic shunt, *C*.

dependent on the severity and extent of the hepatocellular damage. The serum alkaline phosphatase (ALP) and serum gamma-glutamyltransferase (GGT) are usually normal or only slightly elevated (Figure 1).

An increase in the serum bilirubin concentration—manifested as jaundice when greater than 2 mg/dl—may be noted (1) if the majority of hepatocellular damage occurs at the periphery of the lobule and the subsequent inflammatory process impairs the bile flow in the larger bile ducts, and (2) if severe, diffuse hepatocellular damage impairs bilirubin metabolism at one or more steps in the process of converting unconjugated bilirubin to conjugated bilirubin and excreting conjugated bilirubin into the biliary system (see Figure 11, Part I of this article). These types of intrahepatic cholestasis resolve if the liver is capable of repair (Case 1).

A liver function test such as the sulfobromophthalein sodium (BSP) excretion test is usually unnecessary for diagnosis, but the dye excretion is delayed if the hepatocellular damage is extensive.[1] Prothrombin deficiency can occur and may be the direct result of hepatocellular insufficiency or may be associated with disseminated intravascular coagulopathy. A prothrombin time should be determined if the patient has a tendency to bleed.

A liver biopsy is not essential in the diagnostic evaluation of the patient, but it is useful for assessing the severity and extent of the disease (Case 2). A liver biopsy is important if recurrent or persistent increases in SALT activity are documented (see chronic active hepatitis, below).

Hepatic Cirrhosis

Hepatic cirrhosis is the final, irreversible stage subsequent to many chronic liver diseases. Cirrhosis is a diffuse hepatic process characterized by fibrosis and an alteration in normal architecture by structurally abnormal nodules.[5] The causes of cirrhosis are varied and are seldom determined in individual cases.

Biochemical findings in association with the end-stage liver are often subtle. SALT and ALP activities may be normal or only slightly increased because of the reduced hepatic cell mass, the inaccessibility of the tissue enzyme to the systemic circulation, and minimal active inflammation.

The major biochemical abnormalities reflect the reduced functional capacity of the liver and the altered hepatic blood flow secondary to changes in architecture of the liver (Figure 2). A decreased serum urea nitrogen (SUN, or BUN) level and a decreased serum albumin concentration may be observed on the biochemical profile. An increased serum bilirubin concentration is another late indicator of liver insufficiency, and bilirubin can be detected in the urine before jaundice is evident (Case 3).

The BSP excretion test is the most reliable test for detecting hepatic insufficiency in the anicteric patient. A reduced number of hepatocytes, abnormal hepatic architecture, and an altered hepatic blood flow cause prolonged BSP excretion.

Jaundice may develop in the cirrhotic patient without prior clinical evidence of liver disease, and jaundice may require differentiation from extrahepatic impairment of bile flow. The increased total serum bilirubin concentration is often lower (usually <6 mg/dl) in the cirrhotic patient than it is in the patient with extrahepatic biliary obstruction. The absence of a marked

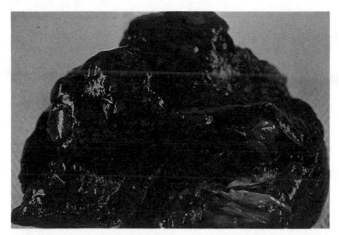

Figure 3—Macronodular cirrhosis in a dog. The nodules on the surface of the liver appear similar to the foci of metastatic disease (compare with Figure 5).

increase in serum ALP activity, a decreased SUN, and a decreased serum albumin concentration support a diagnosis of cirrhosis (Case 3).

Histologic confirmation of cirrhosis is important because, macroscopically, cirrhosis may resemble metastatic disease (Figure 3).

Chronic Active Hepatitis[c] (Chronic Hepatitis)

The term *chronic active hepatitis* is used to describe continuing inflammation of the liver. The cause is often unknown in individual cases. Chronic active hepatitis in the dog has been associated with leptospire infections;[13] primidone;[14,15] abnormal metabolism of copper in Bedlington terriers;[16] adenovirus infection;[17] and a syndrome in middle-aged, female Doberman pinschers[d] (Case 4). Doberman pinschers may be particularly susceptible to chronic hepatitis, as they were overrepresented in a recent review.[18]

The chronic inflammatory process varies among patients and with time. This variability is one reason why the syndrome is difficult to identify biochemically.

Chronic hepatitis should be suspected when recurrent, slight-to-moderate increases in SALT and serum ALP activities are observed. Histological examination of a liver biopsy is essential for confirmation of the diagnosis at this stage of the disease.

Continuation of the chronic inflammatory process for months to years disrupts normal liver architecture

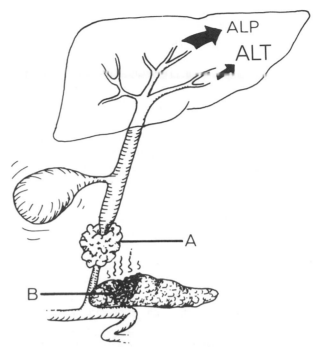

Figure 4—Extrahepatic impairment of bile flow. *A,* Neoplasia is often the cause of obstruction of the extrahepatic bile duct, resulting in a marked increase of serum ALP activity. *B,* Acute pancreatitis may biochemically mimic extrahepatic bile duct obstruction.

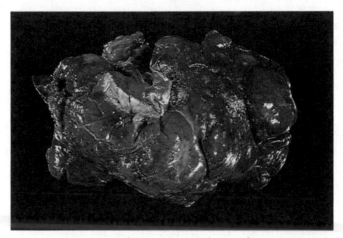

Figure 5—Hepatic neoplasia. Metastatic lesions from a pancreatic carcinoma can be seen on the surface of the liver (compare with Figure 3). Laboratory values prior to the liver biopsy were SALT = 265 IU/L, serum ALP = 88 IU/L, GGT = 7 Sigma units/L.

(Figure 3), and the earlier biochemical pattern of *low-grade* hepatocellular degeneration progresses to one of hepatic insufficiency. The disease may be difficult to detect biochemically at this stage because SALT and serum ALP activities may be normal or only slightly increased. However, decreased serum albumin and decreased SUN concentrations on the biochemical profile are suggestive of advanced liver disease. Earlier indicators of liver insufficiency are bilirubinuria and prolonged BSP excretion.

Extrahepatic Biliary Obstruction (Extrahepatic Impairment of Bile Flow)

Extrahepatic biliary obstruction refers to the

---

[c]The terminology regarding chronic active hepatitis poses some semantic confusion[6-8] and exemplifies the lack of understanding of this syndrome. A pathology report may summate the histological description of a liver biopsy sample as *hepatitis, chronic, active, with (or without) cirrhosis.* The descriptive terminology denotes histological findings (Cases 2 through 4), but it does not necessarily imply a specific clinical diagnosis, i.e., prednisolone-responsive, chronic active hepatitis, as reported in the dog.[9] Chronic active hepatitis is not a single disease but a progressive liver disease due to a variety of causes.[10] Chronic active hepatitis should be considered a syndrome in the dog until it is clarified clinically, biochemically, histologically, and immunologically. Prednisolone may be contraindicated in some forms of chronic active hepatitis in humans.[11,12]

[d]Since this article was written, an article has been published on this syndrome.[28]

impairment of bile flow in the biliary system between the liver and the duodenum. Tumors of the pancreas and the bile duct epithelia are the most common cause of extrahepatic disruption of bile flow (Figure 4, *A*).

Extrahepatic cholestasis causes a marked increase in the serum ALP and GGT activities. Bile acids in the retained bile cause hepatocellular injury,[19] resulting in a slight-to-moderate increase in SALT activity (Case 5).

The total serum bilirubin concentration is often markedly increased; the conjugated form predominates. However, measurement of unconjugated and conjugated bilirubin fractions is not essential in the differential diagnosis of an icteric patient with markedly increased serum ALP activity.

Urine tests for bilirubin are strongly positive. The absence of urobilinogen in the urine of an icteric patient is suggested as an indication of extrahepatic biliary obstruction. However, there is seldom complete obstruction of the flow of bile, and a positive test may result. Furthermore, false-negatives may occur when the enterohepatic circulation of urobilinogen is altered by variables such as oral antibiotics and diarrhea; thereby curtailing the clinical usefulness of the test.

Cholangitis may present a biochemical picture very similar to that of extrahepatic biliary obstruction. Cholangitis should be considered when an obstructive lesion involving the extrahepatic bile duct is not found at laparotomy. A liver biopsy provides histological confirmation.

Acute pancreatitis occasionally causes increases in SALT and ALP activities and in total serum bilirubin concentration. The biochemical test results may occasionally appear in a pattern similar to that of extrahepatic biliary obstruction or of chronic hepatitis with intrahepatic cholestasis. Acute onset of persistent vomiting preceding the development of jaundice is suggestive of acute pancreatitis. A marked increase in serum lipase and serum amylase activities may aid in the differential diagnosis. Suggested causes for the transient increases in test results associated with acute pancreatitis include inflammation of the peripancreatic tissue which compresses the bile duct and release of proteases into the portal blood which damage hepatobiliary tissue (Figure 4B).

Liver Tumors

Primary and metastatic tumors can occur in the liver. Metastatic tumors reportedly occur twice as frequently as primary tumors.[20] Tumors that do not cause extrahepatic biliary obstruction may cause increases in SALT and serum ALP activities and total serum bilirubin concentration which may appear in a pattern similar to that associated with chronic hepatitis. One or more of these tests are abnormal in approximately 50% of the dogs with metastatic tumors, but they are abnormal in 100% of the dogs with the less common but often massive primary hepatocellular carcinoma.[20,21]

Laparoscopy is an invaluable and efficient diagnostic procedure for evaluation of the liver for neoplastic disease. Laparoscopy equipment, though, is not routinely available to the practitioner, so laparotomy, which is the next best practical approach, can be performed. The gross appearance of neoplastic lesions may be similar to that of nodules associated with hepatic cirrhosis (Figure 5). Histologic evaluation can differentiate the two types of lesions.

Congenital Portal Systemic Vascular Anomalies

Congenital anomalies of the portal vascular system occur commonly in dogs. The cause of anomalous vascular development is unknown, but the miniature schnauzer, Doberman pinscher, and German shepherd appear to be overrepresented, in the authors' experience. Anomalous vascular development may involve one or more vessels of the hepatic portal circulation[22] (Figure 6).

Congenital anomalies are one disorder associated with the liver in which the signalment and history provide important clues to the diagnosis. Dogs are frequently young (<1 year), small for their age, less active than normal, and may be labeled *poor doers*. Neurological signs are common and include seizures, dementia, and personality changes.[23]

A misdiagnosis is easily made because few abnormalities are evident on the biochemical profile. The SALT,

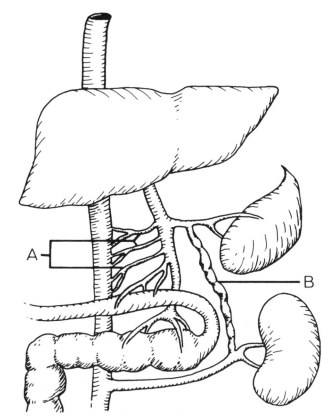

Figure 6—Congenital portal vascular shunts. Anomalous vascular development may involve any part of the portal system. *A*, Multiple mesenteric shunt vessels; *B*, splenorenal shunt vessels. Both were present in Case 6.

serum ALP, and serum GGT activities may be normal or only slightly increased.[23] The reasons for the serum enzyme increases in this noninflammatory liver condition are unknown, but an insufficient flow of blood through the liver probably causes a loss of hepatocellular membrane integrity and enzyme leakage. The decreased hepatic blood flow also deprives the hepatocytes of certain hormones in the portal blood, such as insulin, which are involved in the normal development and maintenance of the liver.[24]

The serum albumin and SUN concentrations are reportedly decreased in more than half of the cases.[23] The decreased concentrations occur because of hepatic atrophy and insufficient portal blood flow. These two parameters are valuable indicators of liver insufficiency on the biochemical profile.

The combination of a compatible history and one or more of the aforementioned biochemical abnormalities indicates the need for a function test such as the BSP excretion test or the ammonia tolerance test. Both of these tests depend on an adequate number of functioning hepatocytes and sufficient blood flow through the liver. The validity of the BSP excretion test can be affected by a decreased serum albumin concentration, resulting in an erroneously low value, i.e., the BSP excretion test results may appear normal. The ammonia tolerance test is considered to be a very sensitive indicator of portal systemic shunts and is not affected by decreased serum albumin concentration. The major practical limitation of the test is associated with sample handling. The laboratory should be consulted for specific instructions prior to performing the test.

Serum bile acid concentration, as measured in the authors' laboratory, has been markedly increased in dogs with portal systemic shunts. The measurement of serum bile acid concentration appears to be a valuable liver function test in the diagnosis of this disorder.

Visual confirmation of a portal vascular anomaly requires a cranial mesenteric angiogram or splenoportography.[22] An exploratory laparotomy seldom provides visual confirmation of the anomalous portal vascular development. Indentifying a suspected portal vascular anomaly is even more difficult at necropsy, due to vascular collapse (Case 6).

Glucocorticoid Hepatopathy

Glucocorticoids cause a morphological alteration in hepatocytes and an elevation in the clinicopathologic test results in the dog. Exogenous administration of glucocorticoids and naturally occurring hyperadrenocorticism can induce hepatopathy.[25,26] The reason for the predominantly noninflammatory hepatocellular lesion is unknown, but individual dog variation exists. Most dogs receiving glucocorticoids develop hepatocellular vacuolation; however, the severity of the condition varies, and the development of focal necrosis and hepatomegaly is less common.

Elevation of clinicopathologic test results occurs fre-

quently in dogs with elevated serum glucocorticoid concentrations. The extent of the increases shows individual variation and also varies with the type of glucocorticoid.

The serum ALP and GGT are the most consistently and markedly increased. The increased serum ALP activity is predominantly due to an isoenzyme of ALP which is produced by the liver following glucocorticoid administration.[25] The increase in serum ALP and GGT activities may be dramatic, similar to the increases associated with extrahepatic biliary obstruction and cholangitis. In contrast, the total serum bilirubin concentration remains normal in dogs with glucocorticoid hepatopathy. The serum ALP and GGT activities usually return to normal three to six weeks after glucocorticoid administration (Case 7).

SALT activity is less consistently increased, and the elevation is slight to moderate compared to serum ALP activity.

BSP excretion in dogs with glucocorticoid hepatopathy is also variable. In one study, experimentally induced glucocorticoid hepatopathy in a dog did not cause abnormal BSP excretion test results.[27] However, increased BSP retention has been reported in another study[26] and is more commonly associated with marked glucocorticoid-induced hepatomegaly in the authors' clinic.

A liver biopsy differentiates glucocorticoid-induced hepatopathy from other hepatic disorders. Electrophoresis of serum ALP when the activity level is elevated demonstrates that the steroid-induced isoenzyme predominates (Case 5).

Case Studies

The following cases were selected to supplement the preceding discussion. The histories, physical examinations, and laboratory data have been abstracted to accentuate the pertinent information. Normal serum biochemical values for the purposes of this discussion are listed in Table 1. Established normal serum biochemical values for veterinary practices may vary from these.

Case 1

A four-year-old, female miniature poodle was presented with acute hepatocellular degeneration or acute hepatitis, the cause of which was undetermined. History revealed that the dog had been observed vomiting once or twice three days ago, and it had been listless and anorectic. On physical examination the dog was found to have scleral icterus, and it was dehydrated. The laboratory data were

PCV	44%
SALT	1250 IU/L
Serum ALP	480 IU/L
Total bilirubin	6.2 mg/dl
SUN	47 mg/dl
Prothrombin time	32 seconds (control 12 seconds)

No liver biopsy was performed. Supportive care was given. Two weeks later, the dog appeared clinically normal. On follow-up, the laboratory data were

SALT	220 IU/L
Serum ALP	270 IU/L
Total bilirubin	0.5 mg/dl
SUN	14 mg/dl
Prothrombin time	13 seconds (control 12 seconds)

Case 2

A five-year-old, male, mixed-breed dog was presented with eosinophilic hepatitis associated with *Dirofilaria immitis*. Evaluation of the dog prior to initiating preventive heartworm treatment revealed the microfilaria of *Dirofilaria immitis*. There were no significant physical findings at the time of presentation. The laboratory data were

SALT	316 IU/L
Serum ALP	27 IU/L
Total bilirubin	0.1 mg/dl
Prothrombin time	9 seconds (control 12 seconds)

A percutaneous liver biopsy revealed hepatitis which was eosinophilic, chronic, active, focal, and moderate. The dog was treated with oral prednisolone and sodium carparsolate. The prednisolone was then gradually reduced. Following the completion of dithiazinine iodide, a second evaluation of the liver was performed. The laboratory data were

SALT	46 IU/L
Serum ALP	32 IU/L
Prothrombin time	8 seconds (control 12 seconds)

A percutaneous liver biopsy revealed a normal liver.

TABLE I

NORMAL SERUM BIOCHEMICAL VALUES FOR THE DOG*

Test	Dog
SALT (IU/L)	16–60
SAST (IU/L)	8–50
Serum ALP (IU/L)	14–80
SGGT (Sigma units/L)	<3
Total bilirubin (mg/dl)	0–0.6
BSP (% retention after 30 minutes)	<5
Albumin (g/dl)	2.4–3.4
SUN (mg/dl)	10–20
Ammonia tolerance test (µg/dl)	
0 minutes	<60
30 minutes	<130
Serum bile acids (µmoles/L)	
0 minutes	<40
2 hours postprandial	<60

*Established normal serum biochemical values for veterinary practices may vary from these.

Case 3

An eight-year-old male miniature poodle was presented with cirrhosis without icterus. A history revealed that the dog had had repeated episodes of lethargy and inappetence during the previous few months. It was occasionally observed to *wander, as if lost*. There were no significant findings on physical examination. The laboratory data were

SALT	72 IU/L
Serum ALP	232 IU/L
Serum GGT	3.2 Sigma units/L
Total bilirubin	0.6 mg/dl
Albumin	2.0 g/dl
SUN	8 mg/dl
BSP	11% retention after 30 minutes
Prothrombin time	10 seconds (control 11 seconds)
Urine bilirubin	+3 (sp. gr. 1.026)

In abdominal radiographs, the silhouette of the liver appeared small. The report from the pathologist regarding the percutaneous liver biopsy was hepatic cirrhosis, chronic, diffuse, moderate, with minimal inflammation.

Case 4

A six-year-old spayed female Doberman pinscher was presented with chronic active hepatitis and hepatic fibrosis. A history revealed that the dog had had recurrent episodes of lethargy and inappetence during the previous two months. On two occasions the local veterinarian had found the dog's SALT activity to be elevated. Icterus had been noted in the past three days, but the dog's appetite and activity appeared normal. On physical examination, the dog was found to have scleral icterus and slight weight loss. The laboratory data were

PCV	42%
SALT	432 IU/L
Serum ALP	145 IU/L
Serum GGT	3.5 Sigma units/L
Total bilirubin	19.5 mg/dl
Albumin	2.1 g/dl
SUN	15 mg/dl
Urine bilirubin	4+ (sp. gr. 1.021)
Prothrombin time	12 seconds (control 12 seconds)

The report from the pathologist regarding the percutaneous liver biopsy was hepatitis, chronic, active, multifocal, severe; cholestasis, intrahepatic, moderate, with portal fibrosis severe.

The copper content of the liver tissue was markedly increased (2200 µg/g dry weight liver).[e]

---

[e]This dog was one of three Doberman pinschers in which a markedly elevated liver copper content has been measured.

Case 5

An 11-year-old female standard poodle was presented with an extrahepatic biliary obstruction. A history revealed that the animal had been lethargic and had lost weight for five weeks. It had been icteric for the preceding two weeks. A physical examination confirmed the weight loss and revealed scleral icterus. An anterior mass was palpated. The laboratory data were

PCV	42%
SALT	236 IU/L
Serum ALP	3240 IU/L
Serum GGT	136 Sigma units/L
Total bilirubin	12.6 mg/dl
Prothrombin time	10.4 seconds (control 9.2 seconds)
Urine bilirubin	4+
Urine urobilinogen	normal

An exploratory laparotomy revealed a pancreatic tumor involving the bile duct.

Case 6

A two-year-old male German shepherd was presented with a congenital portal systemic vascular anomaly. A history revealed that the dog was inactive and a *poor doer*. It had occasionally walked into walls and had a seizure every three to four months. There were no significant findings on physical examination. The laboratory data were

SALT	180 IU/L
Serum ALP	134 IU/L
Albumin	1.9 g/dl
SUN	7 mg/dl
BSP	5.7% retention after 30 minutes
Ammonia tolerance test	0 minutes 88 μg/dl
	30 minutes 727 μg/dl
Serum bile acids	0 time 176.2 μmoles/L
	2 hours postprandial 376.9 μmoles/L

Angiography revealed a splenorenal shunt and multiple small mesenteric shunt vessels (Figure 6). The BSP value, although abnormal, is probably an erroneously low value due to hypoalbuminemia. The ammonia tolerance test value is clearly abnormal.

Case 7

An eight-year-old spayed female dachshund was presented with a steroid hepatopathy. An abdominal enlargement had been evident for one week, and the dog had been lethargic for the same period of time. Its appetite was normal, but its water intake had increased. The local veterinarian had palpated a markedly enlarged liver and had submitted serum for laboratory tests. Methylprednisolone acetate had been administered IM one week prior to the initial laboratory testing. The laboratory data were

	Initial	2 Weeks*	4 Weeks*
SALT (IU/L)	880	675	88
Serum ALP (IU/L)	2425	4072	162
Serum GGT (Sigma units/L)		43	2.7
Total bilirubin (mg/dl)	0.4	0.1	0.1
BSP (% retention after 30 minutes)	8		2
Serum bile acids (μmoles/L)		146	53

*Weeks following the administration of the glucocorticoid.

The pathologist's report on a percutaneous liver biopsy (taken after the initial laboratory data) was hydropic degeneration, hepatic, diffuse, and severe with hepatitis, acute, multifocal, and mild.

Acknowledgment

The authors acknowledge the many clinicians who provided the case material, especially Drs. Jack Samek, Ralph Beauchamp, and Cindy Seiler, Gainesville Animal Hospital, and Dr. LaVonn Congdon, Ft. Walton Beach, FL. They also thank Dr. Adolfo Garnica for his laboratory assistance.

REFERENCES

1. Van Vleet JF, Alberts JO: Evaluation of liver function tests and liver biopsy in experimental carbon tetrachloride intoxication and extrahepatic bile duct obstruction in the dog. *Am J Vet Res* 29:2119-2131, 1968.
2. Hayes AW, Williams WL: Acute toxicity of aflatoxin B_1 and rubratoxin in dogs. *J Environ Pathol Toxicol* 1:59-70, 1977.
3. St. Omer VV, McKnight ED, III: Acetylcysteine for treatment of acetaminophen toxicosis in cats. *JAVMA* 176:911-913, 1980.
4. Polzin DJ, Stowe CM, O'Leary TP, et al: Acute hepatic necrosis associated with the administration of mebendazole to dogs. *JAVMA* 179:1013-1016, 1981.
5. Scheuer PJ: *Liver Biopsy Interpretation*, ed 3. New York, Macmillan Publishing Co, 1980, pp 117-132.
6. Conn HO: Chronic hepatitis: Reducing an iatrogenic enigma to a workable puzzle. *Gastroenterology* 70:1182-1184, 1976.
7. MacKinnon M, Cooksley WGE, Reed WO, Hall P: Current concepts of chronic hepatitis. *Pathology* 13:227-288, 1981.
8. Ludwig J: Some names hang on like leeches. *Dig Dis Sci* 24:967-969, 1979.
9. Strombeck DR, Gribble D: Chronic active hepatitis in the dog. *JAVMA* 173:380-386, 1978.
10. Scheuer PJ: *Liver Biopsy Interpretation*, ed 3. New York, Macmillan Publishing Co, 1980, pp 102-116.
11. Lam KC, Lai CL, Ng RP, et al: Deleterious effect of prednisolone in HBsAg-positive chronic active hepatitis. *N Engl J Med* 304:380-386, 1981.
12. Redeker AG: Treatment of chronic active hepatitis: Good news and bad news. *N Engl J Med* 304:420-421, 1981.
13. Bishop L, Strandberg JD, Adams RJ, et al: Chronic active hepatitis in dogs associated with leptospires. *Am J Vet Res* 40:839-844, 1979.
14. Nash AS, Thompson H: Phenytoin toxicity: A fatal case in a dog with hepatitis and jaundice. *Vet Rec* 100:280-281, 1977.
15. Meyer DJ, Congdon L: Primidone-associated chronic active hepatitis in two dogs. Unpublished.
16. Twedt DC, Sternlieb I, Gilbertson SR: Clinical, morphologic and chemical studies on copper toxicosis of Bedlington terriers. *JAVMA* 175:169-275, 1979.
17. Gocke DJ, Morris TQ, Bradley SE: Chronic hepatitis in the dog: The role of immune factors. *JAVMA* 156:1700-1705, 1970.
18. Doige CE, Lester S: Chronic active hepatitis in dogs: A review of fourteen cases. *JAAHA* 17:725-730, 1981.

19. Iber FL: Cholestasis, in Foult WT (ed): *Diseases of the Liver*. New York, McGraw-Hill Book Co, 1968, pp 29-37.

20. Strombeck DR: Clinicopathologic features of primary metastatic neoplastic disease of the liver in dogs. *JAVMA* 173:267-269, 1978.

21. Patnaik AK, Hurvitz AI, Lieberman PH, Johnson GF: Canine hepatocellular carcinoma. *Vet Pathol* 18:427-438, 1981.

22. Suter PF: Portal vein anomalies in the dog: Their angiographic diagnosis. *J Am Vet Radiol Soc* 16:84-97, 1975.

23. Griffiths GL, Lumsden JH, Valli VEO: Hematologic and biochemical changes in dogs with portosystemic shunts. *JAAHA* 17:705-710, 1981.

24. Ozawa K, Yamaolca Y, Nonby H, Honjo I: Insulin as the primary factor governing changes in mitochondrial metabolism leading to liver regeneration and atrophy. *Am J Surg* 127:669-675, 1974.

25. Hoffman WE: The diagnostic value of canine serum alkaline phosphatase and alkaline phosphatase isoenzymes. *JAAHA* 13:237-241, 1977.

26. Rogers WA: Source of serum alkaline phosphatase in clinically normal and diseased dogs: A clinical study. *JAVMA* 168:934-937, 1976.

27. Badylak SF, Van Vleet JF: Sequential morphologic and clinicopathologic alterations in dogs with experimentally induced glucocorticoid hepatopathy. *Am J Vet Res* 42:1310-1318, 1981.

28. Johnson GF, Zawie DA, Gilbertson SR, Sternlieb I: Chronic active hepatitis in Doberman pinschers. *JAVMA* 180:1438-1442, 1982.

Feline Hepatic Lipidosis

KEY FACTS

- Idiopathic hepatic lipidosis, which frequently results in death, is often seen in cats.
- Most cats with idiopathic hepatic lipidosis are middle-aged, obese, and have been partially or completely anorectic for a prolonged period.
- Cytologic examination of hepatocytes obtained via fine-needle aspiration is often diagnostic of hepatic lipidosis.
- Nutritional support via a percutaneous gastrostomy tube markedly improves the prognosis for recovery.
- Recurrence of hepatic lipidosis is rare.

Global Veterinary Services
Houston, Texas
Brad S. Hubbard, DVM

Gulf Coast Veterinary Specialists
Houston, Texas
Jim C. Vulgamott, DVM

THE CAUSE of hepatic lipidosis, a common disease in cats,[1-5] is frequently not determined. Few retrospective studies of hepatic lipidosis cases have been done.[1,6] In addition, there is a lack of information describing the successful treatment of these critically ill patients. We believe that with appropriate and timely therapy, a significant percentage of cats with idiopathic hepatic lipidosis recover.

Between January 1986 and April 1989, we treated 130 cats with liver disease alone or in combination with other diseases. A review of the medical records of the 130 cats revealed that 70.0% had hepatic lipidosis, 11.5% had hepatic neoplasia, 10% had cholangiohepatitis complex, 1.5% had systemic mycosis, and the remaining 7.0% had other hepatopathies.

Hepatic lipidosis is defined as an acquired disorder of metabolism resulting in the hepatocellular accumulation of excessive quantities of triglycerides sufficient to be visualized by light microscopy.[3] In human medicine, the diagnosis of hepatic lipidosis is based on morphologic or biochemical evidence. Hepatic lipidosis is diagnosed by the presence of fat in 5% of hepatocytes (assuming an adequate liver biopsy has been done) or of more than 5 grams of lipid per 100 grams of fresh liver.[7] The various causes of hepatic lipidosis in humans and dogs include diabetes mellitus, toxins, hyperadrenocorticism, and anorexia.[3,7] In cats, however, the cause of hepatic lipidosis often cannot be determined. Forty-five cases of idiopathic hepatic lipidosis in cats are reviewed in this article.

PATHOPHYSIOLOGY

In healthy cats, a constant cycling of fatty acids occurs between adipose tissue, dietary lipid sources, and the liver. This exchange has multiple stages; a disruption in any one of the stages can result in excessive accumulation of triglyceride within hepatocytes. To understand the possible mechanisms of excessive triglyceride accumulation, normal fat metabolism and the role of the liver in energy production and storage must be appreciated.

In healthy animals, circulating fatty acids are carried in the blood stream bound to albumin. Fatty acids are taken up by the liver and oxidized for energy or incorporated into triglycerides. Triglycerides are bound to apoproteins, which form lipoprotein particles of the very low-density lipoprotein class (VLDL). Very low-density lipoprotein particles are secreted back into the circulation. If the rate of presentation of fatty acids to the liver exceeds the ability of the liver to oxidize or resecrete them, lipidosis occurs.[3] The liver is capable of extracting fatty acids from the blood stream at a rate that exceeds its capability to synthesize or excrete lipoproteins. In obese cats, hepatic lipidosis may result from increased mobilization of fatty acids from lipolysis of adipose stores, decreased hepatic fatty acid oxidation, or decreased ability to secrete lipoproteins into the circulation.

CLINICAL DESCRIPTION
History and Signalment

Cats with idiopathic hepatic lipidosis, although often obese, are commonly presented for anorexia. Depression and weight loss are also often seen.[3-5,8] In the cases reviewed, the duration of partial to complete anorexia ranged from several days to months. In 43% of the cats, a stressful event or events preceded the onset of clinical illness. Most often, the source of the stress was behavioral, that is, it was related to the move to a new house, the absence of the owner, or the addition of another pet to the household. In some cases, a physical source of stress could be identified, for example, a recent vaccination, dietary change, or exposure to organophosphates. Four of the cats had recently been treated with a flea dip containing organophosphates.

AFFECTED CATS were between 2 and 15 years of age (Figure 1). Ninety percent of the cats were between 2 and 8 years of age. The mean age of the cats was 4.6 years. There were 22 males and 23 females in the cases reviewed. All had been neutered. There was no breed predilection. At presentation, weights of the cats ranged from 3.5 to 13 pounds (1.6 to 5.9 kilograms) with a mean of 9.2 pounds (4.2 kilograms); weights of the cats before the onset of clinical illness ranged from 6 to 17 pounds (2.7 to 7.7 kilograms) with a mean of 11.9 pounds (5.4 kilograms).

Physical Findings

Depression was the most common physical examination finding. All but 6 of the 45 cats were clinically icteric. Most cats were obese. Muscle wasting was often severe, especially in the lumbar and proximal leg areas. In many cats, a large intraabdominal fat pad could be palpated and a large subcutaneous inguinal fat pad was present. When laparoscopy or a postmortem examination was performed, a large accumulation of intraabdominal fat was often seen. We believed that approximately 10% of the cats were of average weights before the onset of illness; the remainder were obese.

Based on the histories and clinical signs, it was assumed that some cats had hepatoencephalopathy. Although blood ammonia concentrations were not measured in any of the cases under review, it is known that blood ammonia concentrations may be elevated in anorectic cats (with or without hepatic lipidosis) because of an inability of the cat to synthesize the amino acid arginine.[9] Arginine functions in the conversion of ammonia to urea in the hepatic urea cycle.

Hepatomegaly was a rare finding in the cats. The liver, if palpable, was smooth and slightly softer than normal. None of the cats exhibited abdominal discomfort during

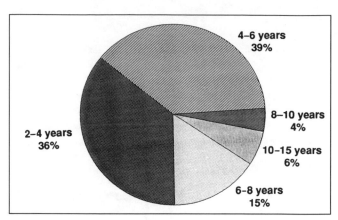

Figure 1—Age distribution of cats with idiopathic hepatic lipidosis.

palpation. All cats were afebrile. One of the cats had signs of peripheral vestibular dysfunction, which resolved with treatment for hepatic lipidosis.

Laboratory Findings

The most consistent findings were elevation in serum alkaline phosphatase activity and hyperbilirubinemia. These findings are in agreement with previous reports.[1,3,5,6] The mean serum alkaline phosphatase activity in the cases that we reviewed was 345 mg/dl (range = 13 to 2500 mg/dl). Serum concentrations of alanine transferase (mean = 185 mg/dl) were not as dramatically elevated as serum alkaline phosphatase, probably because lipidosis is more of an infiltrative than destructive process. The mean serum bilirubin concentration was 5.1 mg/dl (range = 0.2 to 14.2 mg/dl) (Figure 2).

EIGHT CATS had normal liver enzymes although cytologic or histopathologic examination of hepatocytes revealed significant liver disease. Four cats had blood glucose levels between 200 and 300 mg/dl. The results of urinalysis were consistently unremarkable with the exception that most cats had bilirubinuria and some had glucosuria. Ketonuria was not identified.

In addition, 13 cats had leukopenia, the significance of which is not known. Of the 27 cats tested, none were positive for feline leukemia virus (FeLV) infection. Cats were not tested for feline immunodeficiency virus (FIV) infection. Serum bile acid or blood ammonia concentrations were not determined. Although coagulation abnormalities may be observed in cats with hepatopathy,[1,9] none of the cats in our study had clinical evidence of coagulation disorders.

Ancillary Diagnostic Tests

In several cats, radiographs of the abdomen revealed minor alterations (e.g., mild hepatomegaly). Results of ultra-

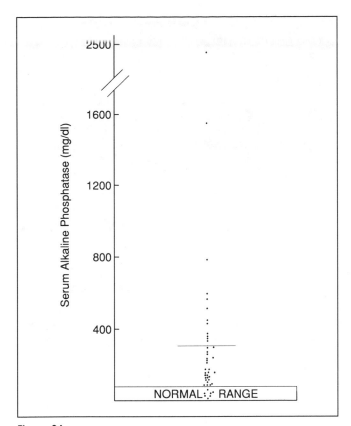

Figure 2A

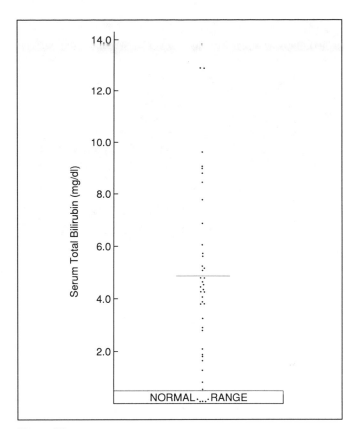

Figure 2C

Figure 2—Serum alkaline phosphatase activity (**A**) and alanine transferase (**B**) and total bilirubin (**C**) concentrations in 45 cats with idiopathic hepatic lipidosis. Mean values are indicated by horizontal lines.

sound examination of 13 cats were normal. Hepatic lipidosis may produce a diffuse increase in the echogenicity of liver tissue.[4]

Diagnostic Approach

The minimum data base for cats suspected of having hepatic lipidosis should include a complete history, thorough physical examination, complete blood count and biochemical profile, and a urinalysis. Cytologic examination of hepatocytes obtained via fine-needle aspiration should be performed. Ancillary diagnostic testing may include blood ammonia concentrations, thyroid hormone concentrations, FeLV and FIV testing, serum bile acid concentrations, serum electrophoresis, and coagulation studies. Radiography, ultrasonography, and laparoscopy can also provide additional useful information.

DIAGNOSIS

To make a definitive diagnosis of hepatic lipidosis, microscopic examination of hepatocytes is required. We believe that cytologic specimens obtained via percutaneous fine-needle aspiration of the liver are diagnostic in the majority of cases of idiopathic feline hepatic lipidosis (Figure

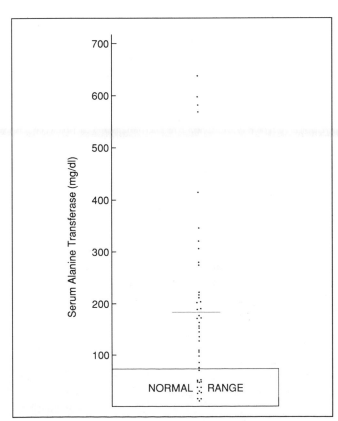

Figure 2B

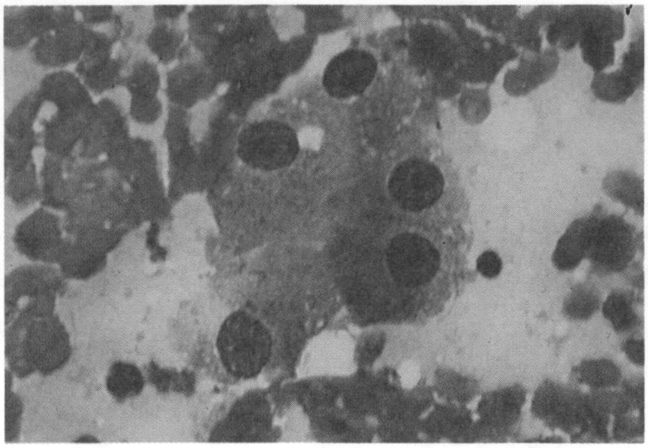

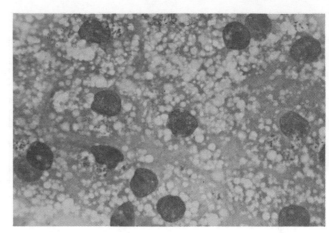

Figure 3A　　　　　　　　　　　　　　　　**Figure 3B**

Figure 3—Photomicrograph of normal (**A**) and abnormal (**B**) hepatocytes obtained via fine-needle aspiration. The abnormal hepatocytes are characteristic of severe hepatic lipidosis.

3). In 44% of the cases reviewed, a definitive diagnosis was established via laparoscopic liver biopsy. In the remaining 56%, the diagnosis was made based on examination of hepatocytes obtained via percutaneous fine-needle aspiration of the liver. In several instances, hepatocytes could not be obtained via fine-needle aspiration; thus, laparoscopic biopsy of the liver was performed.

BEFORE fine-needle aspiration of the liver, in most instances, sedation or tranquilization is not necessary and may be contraindicated because of the severe metabolic disturbances accompanying hepatic lipidosis. The cat is gently restrained in a sternal position and the liver is palpated. A 12-milliliter syringe with a 1-inch, 23-gauge needle is used for aspiration. The needle is directed toward the liver from a midlateral position caudal to the 13th rib. The needle is directed toward the diaphragm at a 45° angle from the left side of the cat. In some cases, the liver cannot be palpated and the fine-needle aspiration is performed in the approximate location of the liver. Routine aspiration is then performed. A small amount of blood-tinged tissue is often seen in the hub of the needle. The specimen is transferred to a standard microscope slide and a squash preparation is performed. The slide is then stained with a Romanovsky stain.

TREATMENT

Because the cause(s) cannot be identified, treatment of feline hepatic lipidosis is symptomatic. In our experience, treatment of hepatic lipidosis most often focuses on providing a high-protein, balanced diet and assuring adequate fluid and caloric intake. When vomiting could be controlled and adequate caloric and protein intake maintained, treatment was successful. Total caloric intake should be 80

to 100 kcal/kg/day. The adult cat's maintenance requirement for protein is 16% to 19% of its caloric requirement.

After the diagnosis of idiopathic hepatic lipidosis, the owner should be encouraged to allow placement of a feeding tube. A gastrostomy tube placed endoscopically has resulted in the most successful treatment with minimal stress to the cat. Of the 37 cats treated, 22 recovered. In 11 cats, treatment included placement of a pharyngostomy tube or intermittent orogastric feeding tube; only 2 of the 11 cats recovered. In 26 cats, treatment included placement of a gastrostomy tube; 20 of the 26 cats recovered. The technique for endoscopic placement of a gastrostomy tube has been illustrated elsewhere.[10] The procedure is technically easy and requires only 10 to 15 minutes of anesthetic time. Typically, the cat is not fed through the gastrostomy tube for 18 to 24 hours after placement, during which time a seal forms at the site of exit through the stomach and body wall. Two of the cats in the cases reviewed died after developing peritonitis secondary to leakage of ingesta into the abdominal cavity.

CATS WERE FED 30 to 60 milliliters of a blended gruel of 50% water and 50% Prescription Diet® feline p/d® (Hill's) three to six times daily. The food was warmed to body temperature before feeding. Vomiting, if it occurred, was controlled with metoclopramide at a dose of 2 to 3 milligrams subcutaneously 30 minutes before feeding.

Anorexia associated with idiopathic hepatic lipidosis usually persists for 2 to 20 weeks (mean = 7.4 weeks) after initiation of nutritional therapy. In the cases reviewed, when the cat's appetite returned, the quantity and frequency of tube feedings was gradually decreased. The feeding tube was left in place for 7 to 10 days after a normal appetite returned; the tube was then removed. A light plane of anesthesia using isoflurane gas was required. Gentle traction was maintained until the tube was extracted. Occasionally the mushroom tip of the gastrostomy tube broke off and remained in the stomach but no complications resulted.

ADDITIONAL MEASURES to be considered in the treatment of idiopathic feline hepatic lipidosis are presented in Ancillary Treatments. Lipotropic compounds, such as methionine and choline, should not be used in the treatment of any liver disease. The efficacy of these amino acids is under question. Methionine may precipitate or potentiate signs of hepatoencephalopathy by increasing the production of mercaptans, which inhibit normal brain activity.

DISCUSSION

Idiopathic hepatic lipidosis is a syndrome that results in severe liver dysfunction. It is characterized by prolonged anorexia, icterus, and weight loss. Currently, the specific cause(s) of hepatic lipidosis are unknown. The pathophysiology of hepatic lipidosis is an inadequate formation or release of hepatic lipoproteins by the hepatocytes, which results in an accumulation of triglycerides within hepatocytes. This sequence of events most commonly occurs in association with prolonged anorexia. Some authors have proposed that a deficiency of specific amino acids is a potential cause of hepatic lipidosis in cats.[5] A deficiency of either arginine or carnitine secondary to anorexia could conceivably result in hepatic lipidosis. Cats are unable to synthesize arginine and, when anorectic, rely on muscle catabolism for the production of arginine. Arginine is needed for urea cycle function. Arginine deficiency results in hyperammonemia and increased carbamoyl phosphate concentrations.[5] Carbamoyl phosphate is metabolized to orotic acid, which has been shown to interfere with lipoprotein synthesis.[2] Decreased lipoprotein synthesis can cause an accumulation of triglyceride within hepatocytes, i.e., hepatic lipidosis. L-carnitine is a quaternary amine with a major role in fatty acid metabolism. Lipid accumulation within liver, muscle, and nervous tissue is observed in human patients with L-carnitine deficiency.[7] Plasma, liver, and skeletal muscle L-carnitine levels were found to be normal in one study of 11 cats with idiopathic hepatic lipidosis.[1] Providing an adequate protein intake in cats with hepatic lipidosis should correct a deficiency of either of these amino acids in the anorectic patient.

Our review of cats with idiopathic hepatic lipidosis confirms that hepatic lipidosis is a syndrome affecting primarily middle-aged, obese cats that have been partially or completely anorectic for a prolonged period. Hepatic lipidosis is a noninflammatory hepatopathy with a high mortality. Physical examination findings usually include depression, icterus, and marked cachexia with preservation of inguinal

Ancillary Treatments

- **Minimize stress**
  The cat should be handled as infrequently as possible while hospitalized. Also, it should be kept in a quiet environment.

- **Alter blood ammonia concentration**
  Metronidazole at a dosage of 7.5 mg/kg three times daily or neomycin at a dosage of 20 mg/kg three times daily may be used to treat hepatoencephalopathy if it is present. Lactulose may be given orally at a dosage of 0.25 to 1 milliliters two or three times daily. Prescription Diet® Feline k/d® (Hill's) may also be used if signs of hepatoencephalopathy develop.

- **Stimulate appetite**
  Diazepam at a dose of 1 to 2 milligrams intravenously or oxazepam at a dosage of 3 to 5 milligrams orally, one to three times daily, can be used as appetite stimulants. The effects of diazepam are usually seen within minutes and persist for less than one hour after administration. Oxazepam is rarely effective in animals that do not respond to intravenous diazepam. Both diazepam and oxazepam are benzodiazepines and require hepatic biotransformation for inactivation and elimination from the body; therefore, they may be contraindicated in cats with severe hepatic lipidosis.[4]

- **Administer L-carnitine**
  L-carnitine at a dose of 50 to 100 mg/kg/day may facilitate hepatic lipid metabolism in cats with idiopathic hepatic lipidosis.

and intraabdominal fat stores. Most cats with hepatic lipidosis have hyperbilirubinemia and elevations in serum alkaline phosphatase.

Because epinephrine and glucocorticosteroids are released during prolonged anorexia, hyperglycemia may be present. Insulin therapy should be initiated only if careful monitoring of serial blood glucose levels can be assured. None of the cats that were treated successfully in the cases reviewed received insulin as part of their treatment. Leukopenia was observed in 27% of the cats. Leukopenia is a common finding in cows with hepatic lipidosis,[11] the significance of which is unknown. Radiographic or ultrasonographic abnormalities are not common with hepatic lipidosis.

The diagnosis of hepatic lipidosis relies on microscopic examination of hepatocytes. Fine-needle aspiration cytology should be attempted before other more invasive procedures. After the diagnosis of hepatic lipidosis is made, aggressive and long-term therapy must be instituted. In this review, the cats that were fed via a percutaneous gastrostomy tube had a better survival rate than cats fed via orogastric or pharyngostomy feeding tubes. Recurrence of hepatic lipidosis is rare.[1] There was recurrence of disease in only one of the surviving cats in our study.

About the Authors

When this article was submitted for publication, Dr. Hubbard was a resident in internal medicine at Gulf Coast Veterinary Specialists in Houston, Texas. Dr. Hubbard currently is the director of Global Veterinary Services in Houston, Texas. Dr. Vulgamott is affiliated with Gulf Coast Veterinary Specialists. Dr. Vulgamott is a Diplomate of the American College of Veterinary Internal Medicine.

REFERENCES

1. Jacobs G, Cornelius L, Allen S, Greene CL: Treatment of idiopathic hepatic lipidosis in cats: 11 cases (1986-1987). *JAVMA* 195:635-638, 1989.
2. Hardy PM: Diseases of the liver and their treatment, in Ettinger SJ (ed): *Textbook of Veterinary Internal Medicine.* Philadelphia, WB Saunders Co, 1989, pp 1479-1527.
3. Thornburg LP, Simpson S, Digilio K: Fatty liver syndrome in cats. *JAAHA* 18:397-400, 1982.
4. Center SA: Hepatic lipidosis in the cat. *Proc ACVIM*:71-79, 1986.
5. Center SA: Feline hepatic lipidosis is a common liver disorder. *Feline Health Top Vet* 4:1-6, 1989.
6. Cornelius LN, Rogers KS: Idiopathic hepatic lipidosis in cats. *Mod Vet Pract* 66:377-380, 1985.
7. Galambos JT: Alcoholic liver disease: Fatty liver, hepatitis, and cirrhosis, in Berk JE (ed): *Bockus Gastroenterology.* Philadelphia, WB Saunders Co, 1985, pp 2985-3048.
8. Cornelius L, Jacobs G: Feline hepatic lipidosis, in Kirk RW (ed): *Current Veterinary Therapy X.* Philadelphia, WB Saunders Co, 1989, pp 869-873.
9. Rogers KS, Cornelius L: Feline icterus. *Compend Contin Educ Pract Vet* 7:391-399, 1985.
10. Bright RM: Percutaneous endoscopic tube gastrostomy in dogs. *Am J Vet Res* 49:629-633, 1988.
11. Gerloff BJ, Herdt TN: Hepatic lipidosis from dietary restriction in nonlactating cows. *JAVMA* 185:223-224, 1984.

Hepatoencephalopathy *(continued from page 98)*

diazepine-like compounds in their plasma or CSF. The levels of benzodiazepine-like compounds found in the brains of humans and laboratory animals with HE are also lower than those that are usually associated with the neuropsychiatric effect caused by the administration of diazepam. Another problem with this hypothesis is that the origin of the endogenous benzodiazepine-like compounds has not been identified. Mammalian cells are not thought to synthesize 1,4 benzodiazepines de novo. It is possible that the compounds or their precursors are dietary in origin. Based on the above, endogenous benzodiazepines appear to play a central role in the development of HE; however, this theory does not answer all the questions regarding the pathogenesis of HE.

To summarize, HE is clinically manifested by diffuse CNS depression, the pathogenesis of which is multifactorial. Alterations in GABAergic neurotransmission are thought to play an important role in the development of CNS depression. Current research indicates that endogenous benzodiazepine-like compounds are involved in the pathogenesis of altered GABAergic neurotransmission.

John W. Tyler, DVM, ACVIM
Internal Medicine Specialty Service
St. Petersburg, Florida

BIBLIOGRAPHY

Basile AS: The contribution of endogenous benzodiazepine receptor ligands to the pathogenesis of hepatic encephalopathy. *Synapse* 7:141–150, 1991.
Basile AS, Hughes RD, Harrison PM, et al: Elevated brain concentrations of 1,4 benzodiazepines in fulminant hepatic failure. *New Engl J Med* 325(7):473–478, 1991.
Basile AS, Jones EA, Skolnick P: The pathogenesis and treatment of hepatic encephalopathy: Evidence for the involvement of benzodiazepine receptor ligands. *Pharmacol Rev* 43(1):27–71, 1991.
Bosman DK, Van Den Buijs CACG, De Haan JG, et al: The effects of benzodiazepine-receptor antagonist and partial inverse agonist on acute hepatic encephalopathy in the rat. *Gastroenterology* 101: 772–781, 1991.
Maddison JE: Hepatic encephalopathy, current concepts of the pathogenesis. *J Vet Intern Med* 6(6):341–353, 1992.
Maddison JE, Dodd PR, Johnston GAR, et al: Brain GABA receptor binding is normal in rats with thioacetamide-induced hepatic encephalopathy despite elevated plasma GABA-like activity. *Gastroenterology* 93:1062–1068, 1987.
Maddison JE, Dodd PR, Morrison M, et al: Plasma GABA, GABA-like activity and the brain GABA-benzodiazepine complex in rats with chronic hepatic encephalopathy. *Hepatology* 7:621–628, 1987.
Olasmaa M, Rothstein JD, Guidotti A, et al: Endogenous benzodiazepine receptor ligands in human and animal hepatic encephalopathy. *J Neurochem* 55(6):2015–2023, 1990.
Roy S, Pomier-Layrargues G, Butterworth RF, et al: Hepatic encephalopathy in cirrhotic and portacaual shunted dogs: Lack of changes in brain GABA uptake, brain GABA levels, brain glutamic acid decarboxylase activity and brain postsynaptic GABA receptors. *Hepatology* 4:845–849, 1988.

Icterus

KEY FACTS

- A thorough history and physical examination often suggest the underlying cause of icterus.
- Understanding the pathophysiology of bilirubin metabolism is essential in interpreting clinical pathology results.
- Diagnostic differentials for hyperbilirubinemia may be conveniently schematized into disorders of red blood cell destruction (hemolytic icterus), hepatocellular disease (hepatocellular icterus), and intrahepatic or extrahepatic obstructive disease (obstructive icterus).
- After a problem list has been made, the hematocrit and total protein can be assessed and hemolytic anemia as the cause of icterus can quickly be ruled in or ruled out.
- If hemolytic anemia is not the cause of icterus, disorders of hepatocellular or obstructive icterus may be differentiated through interpretation of clinical pathology results and radiographic and/or ultrasonographic findings.

University of Pennsylvania

Jamie G. Anderson, DVM, MS   Robert J. Washabau, VMD, PhD

ICTERUS (or jaundice) is a yellow discoloration of the serum and staining of soft tissue (e.g., sclera, mucous membranes, and skin). Icterus results from hyperbilirubinemia (total plasma bilirubin > 2 mg/dl), which occurs when the rate of production of bilirubin exceeds the rate of elimination. The intensity and distribution of tissue bile pigment staining depend on four important factors[1]: (1) the total serum bilirubin concentration; (2) the form of bilirubin (unconjugated or conjugated); (3) capillary perfusion and the ability to detect a yellow hue through normal pink mucous membranes; and (4) tissue composition (i.e., tissue high in fat is predisposed to deposition of lipid-soluble unconjugated bilirubin; tissue high in elastic fibers, such as sclera and skin, is predisposed to deposition of water-soluble conjugated bilirubin). Therefore, icterus would be expected to be most prominent at high serum bilirubin concentrations, in hemolytic anemia patients, and when the capacity of the liver to transport bilirubin is saturated.

BACKGROUND
Bilirubin Metabolism

An understanding of bilirubin metabolism is essential in interpreting clinical pathology results. A brief review of bilirubin biochemistry, transport, hepatocyte uptake, conjugation, biliary secretion, bile storage, duodenal delivery, bacterial deconjugation, reabsorption, enterohepatocyte recycling, and renal and fecal excretion follows. Bilirubin metabolism is summarized in Figure 1 and is discussed in detail elsewhere in the literature.[2]

Biochemistry. Bile pigments are derived from the metabolism of porphyrins (four pyrrole rings).[3] Heme, a complex of ferrous iron and protoporphyrin IX, is the most abundant porphyrin in animals. Sources of heme include hemoglobin, myoglobin, and other heme enzymes (cytochrome P-450, catalase, and peroxidase). Between 80% and 85% of serum bilirubin is produced from hemoglobin heme catabolism. The remaining 10% to 15% of serum bilirubin is produced from turnover of hepatic heme and hemoproteins, the most important of which is the cytochrome P-450 family.[4] Hemoglobin released from senescent erythrocytes (red blood cells) is phagocytosed by cells of the mononuclear phagocyte system in the liver, spleen, and bone marrow. Globin is enzymatically degraded to amino acids, iron is bound to transferrin and transported, and the heme is converted to biliverdin by heme oxygenase and subsequently to bilirubin by biliverdin reductase.

Transport. Bilirubin is released from the mononuclear phagocyte system tissue into the circulation, where it circulates bound to albumin.[5] This type of bilirubin is referred to as unconjugated, indirect-reacting, or lipid-soluble bilirubin. The bilirubin is relatively insoluble at physiologic pH and is deposited in soft tissue that is high in fat. Transport ends with the dissociation of albumin from bilirubin at the hepatic sinusoidal membrane.

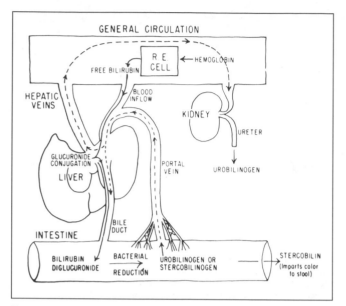

Figure 1—Diagram of normal bilirubin metabolism. (*R. E. cell* = reticuloendothelial cell or mononuclear phagocytic cell) (From Cornelius CE: Liver function, in Kaneko JJ, Cornelius CE (eds): *Clinical Biochemistry of Domestic Animals. Vol I*, ed 2. New York, Academic Press, 1970, pp 161-230. Reprinted with permission.)

Hepatocyte uptake. Hepatocyte uptake of bilirubin is a carrier-mediated process. The mechanism of carrier-mediated transport may exhibit saturation as it is shared by conjugated bilirubin and other organic anions, including bile acids, sulfobromophthalein sodium, and indocyanine green. Transfer of bilirubin across the hepatocyte membrane is bidirectional. Thirty percent of bilirubin initially removed by hepatocytes refluxes back into plasma.[6] Some conjugated bilirubin within this refluxed pool is freely filtered by the glomerulus.[2,6]

Conjugation. Conjugation renders bilirubin more water soluble, thereby facilitating the secretion of bilirubin in bile. Bilirubin is conjugated to glucuronic acid (and to a lesser extent, glucose) primarily via glucuronosyltransferase to form bilirubin monoglucoride and diglucuronide.[7,8] This form of bilirubin is referred to as conjugated, direct-reacting, or water-soluble bilirubin.

Biliary Secretion. Secretion of bilirubin across the canalicular membrane is the rate-limiting step in bilirubin metabolism. This active transport process occurs against a large concentration gradient.[9]

Posthepatic Bilirubin Metabolism. Bile is stored in the gallbladder until feeding initiates gallbladder emptying. Conjugated bilirubin in bile enters the duodenum via the biliary system and is not reabsorbed. Intestinal bacteria reduce most of the conjugated bilirubin to a group of colorless compounds known as urobilinogens. Urobilinogen is readily reabsorbed by the intestines. Most reabsorbed urobilinogen is resecreted in bile, but a small amount is excreted in the urine.[10] Some urobilinogen is not reabsorbed but is

instead passed in the feces either unchanged or further degraded into stercobilins, which impart color to the feces.

Pathophysiology of Bilirubin Disorders

Anatomically, the liver comprises hepatocytes, biliary epithelial cells, vascular system, and Kupffer's cells. The lobule (i.e., the basic anatomic unit of the liver) is composed of a central vein surrounded by hepatocytes, with portal vessels located at the periphery of the lobule. The intrahepatic biliary ductules enlarge in size and ultimately coalesce to form the extrahepatic bile ducts. Arterial and portal blood flows centripetally toward the central vein while bile flows centrifugally toward the portal triad. This anatomic distribution is the reason icterus does not readily develop with severe centrilobular lesions but is readily produced with mild periportal lesions that obstruct bile flow.[11,12] The vascular perfusion of the liver allows the liver to receive blood from the pancreas, spleen, and intestines and subserves its function in energy transport from the intestines. Kupffer's cells provide an immunologic surveillance of microorganisms and toxins of gastrointestinal origin. In addition, they may play a role in the pathogenesis of chronic active liver disease.[13,14]

THE PATHOGENIC mechanisms of hyperbilirubinemia may merely be disorders caused by red blood cell destruction (hemolytic icterus), hepatocellular disease (hepatocellular icterus), and intrahepatic or extrahepatic obstructive disease (obstructive icterus). Each of these is illustrated schematically in Figures 2 through 4, and the accompanying clinicopathologic changes are outlined in Figure 5.

HISTORY

A complete and detailed history is crucial to the diagnostic workup of the icteric patient. The owner should be questioned regarding the onset and chronicity of icterus. Signs related to hemolytic icterus may occur acutely and include weakness, anorexia, and pigmenturia in cases of intravascular hemolysis. Obstructive icterus is more likely to be chronic and progressive over several weeks with signs varying from vague inappetence and depression to severe vomiting and diarrhea.

Known exposure or the potential for exposure to toxins; medications; and such agents as methylene blue, lead, copper, benzocaine derivatives, propylthiouracil in cats as well as exposure to onions in cats and dogs may be implicated in hemolytic anemia. Exposure to agents associated with hepatobiliary disease (e.g., the anticonvulsants, inhalation anesthetics, and diethylcarbamazine) in dogs as well as exposure to acetaminophen in dogs and cats should be ruled out. The frequency and severity of vomiting and diarrhea should be characterized. The presence of vomiting and/or diarrhea is more suggestive of hepatocellular or obstructive icterus, although dogs and cats with acute hemolysis also

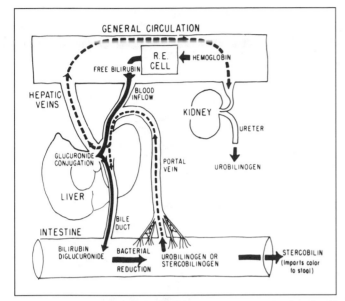

Figure 2—Hemolytic icterus. With accelerated red blood cell destruction, increases are noted in the quantities of unconjugated bilirubin in the serum (because the bilirubin does not undergo glomerular filtration), stercobilin in the feces (imparting a darker color to the feces), and urinary urobilinogen. (*R. E. cell* = reticuloendothelial cell or mononuclear phagocytic cell) (From Cornelius CE: Liver function, in Kaneko JJ, Cornelius CE (eds): *Clinical Biochemistry of Domestic Animals. Vol I*, ed 2. New York, Academic Press, 1970, pp 161-230. Reprinted with permission.)

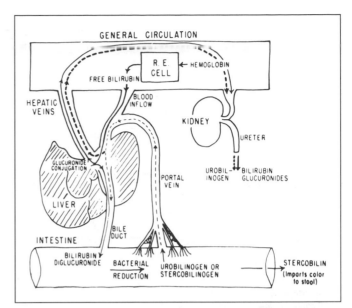

Figure 3—Hepatocellular icterus. With hepatocellular pathology, increased levels of conjugated bilirubin (direct-reacting) may be present in the serum; lesser amounts of unconjugated bilirubin (indirect-reacting) also may be elevated in the serum as a result of decreased uptake of the pigment. Conjugated bilirubin and urobilinogen are detected in the urine. Increased urinary urobilinogen may result from the inability of diseased hepatocytes to resecrete the urobilinogen compound in bile. (*R. E. cell* = reticuloendothelial cell or mononuclear phagocytic cell) (From Cornelius CE: Liver function, in Kaneko JJ, Cornelius CE (eds): *Clinical Biochemistry of Domestic Animals. Vol I*, ed 2. New York, Academic Press, 1970, pp 161-230. Reprinted with permission.)

are known to vomit occasionally. Owners should be asked if they have noted any evidence of gastrointestinal bleeding, such as hematemesis or hematochezia. Hematemesis or hematochezia could be evidence of a bleeding disorder associated with liver dysfunction. On the other hand, acholic feces may be observed with disorders associated with complete biliary outflow obstruction; however, this occurrence is uncommon in small animals. An attempt also should be made to document changes in body weight.

KNOWLEDGE of previous medical illness also may be pertinent to the diagnosis of underlying causes of icterus. Previous episodes of inflammatory bowel disease, acute pancreatitis, hematologic disorders, heart failure, or fatty liver could have some bearing on the current illness.

PHYSICAL EXAMINATION

The liver should be scrutinized carefully during the workup of an icteric patient. The size and shape of the liver and presence or absence of ascites should be assessed. Sites of bile pigment deposition also should be noted. Early sites of bile pigment deposition can be detected in the sclera; the nonpigmented thin skin of the inner pinnae; or, in cats, the soft palate.

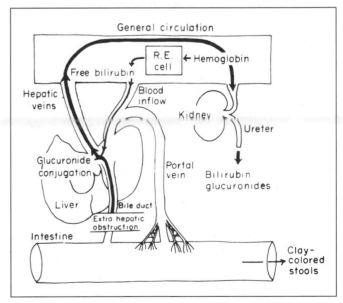

Figure 4—Obstructive icterus. Conjugated bilirubin is refluxed into the plasma. These bilirubin glucuronides subsequently undergo glomerular filtration. With complete biliary obstruction, urinary urobilinogen and fecal stercobilins are theoretically absent. (*R. E. cell* = reticuloendothelial cell or mononuclear phagocytic cell) (From Cornelius CE: Liver function, in Kaneko JJ, Cornelius CE (eds): *Clinical Biochemistry of Domestic Animals. Vol I*, ed 2. New York, Academic Press, 1970, pp 161-230. Reprinted with permission.)

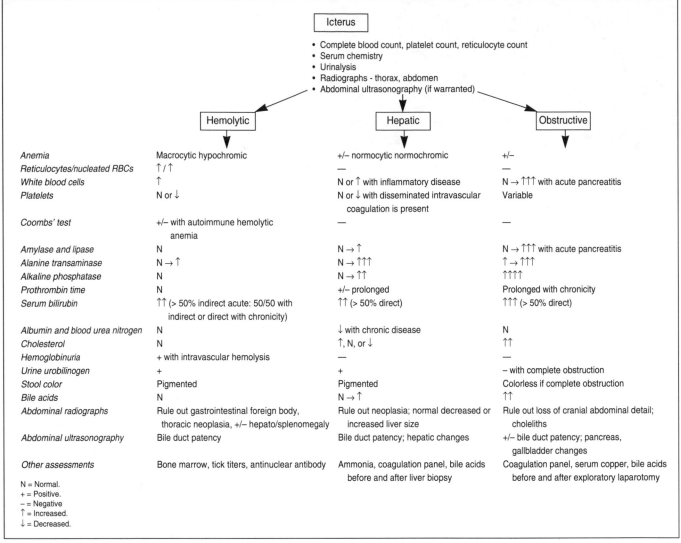

Figure 5—Diagnostic approach to the icteric small animal patient. A problem-solving approach is outlined for each pathogenic disorder (i.e., hemolytic icterus, hepatocellular icterus, and obstuctive icterus).

Any evidence of a hematologic disorder also should be noted during the examination. Clinical findings vary with the specific disease involved and its clinical course. General signs of anemia include lethargy, weakness, and pale mucous membranes. Fever is a fairly consistent clinical feature of hemolytic anemia. Splenomegaly and hepatomegaly could provide evidence of heightened reticuloendothelial activity in an animal affected with immune-mediated hemolytic activity; however, hepatomegaly also could be a sign of primary liver dysfunction.

If dictated by the history and physical examination, the status of the gastrointestinal tract, pancreas, and heart should be evaluated. The animal should be evaluated for hematemesis, hematochezia, cranial abdominal pain, abdominal enlargement, and heart murmurs and arrhythmias. Abdominal pain is usually a manifestation of an inflammatory disorder and is observed more frequently in animals with obstructive icterus than with hepatocellular icterus.

Other important clinical findings useful in differentiating the possible causes of icterus are signs of central nervous system dysfunction, such as intermittent depression, coma, head pressing, circling, ptyalism, and transient apparent blindness (amaurosis). These signs are sometimes seen with hepatic encephalopathy.

A thorough ophthalmoscopic examination is an important part of the physical examination, especially in cats. Ophthalmoscopy may identify ocular lesions with multisystemic disease processes (e.g., feline infectious peritonitis and lymphosarcoma) that cause icterus.

A list of diagnostic differentials can be made as soon as the detailed clinical history and physical examination are completed. The application of the well-known DAMNIT scheme to the pathophysiologic classification of icterus by

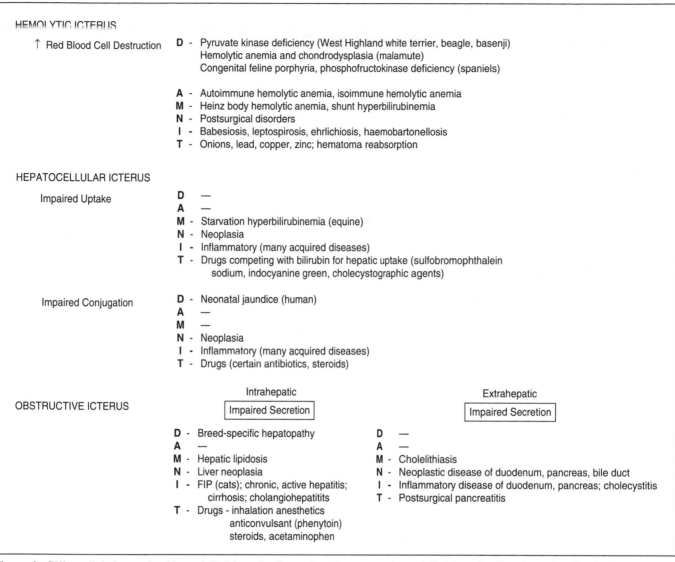

Figure 6—Differential diagnosis of hyperbilirubinemia. Examples of common hyperbilirubinemia disorders using the DAMNIT pathophysiologic classification scheme. (*D* = developmental, degenerative; *A* = autoimmune, allergic, anatomic; *M* = metabolic, mechanical; *N* = nutritional, neoplastic; *I* = inflammatory, infectious; *T* = toxic, traumatic)

suspected cause is outlined in this article. The DAMNIT scheme provides a methodical approach to diagnosis.

DIFFERENTIAL DIAGNOSIS

Icterus may be pathophysiologically classified according to the following suspected causes: (1) hemolytic icterus, (2) hepatocellular icterus, and (3) obstructive icterus. The DAMNIT scheme may then be used in the problem-oriented approach to medical diagnosis.

A reasonable list of differentials using the DAMNIT scheme is illustrated in Figure 6. In differentiating the underlying cause of hyperbilirubinemia, it must first be determined whether there is increased production of bilirubin as a result of excessive red blood cell destruction or whether there is impairment in hepatocellular transport of bilirubin in its uptake, conjugation, or secretion. If increased red blood cell destruction is suspected, hereditary enzymopathy, exposure to toxins, and postsurgical causes can probably be quickly ruled in or ruled out. A peripheral (e.g., ear) capillary venipuncture to evaluate blood may provide evidence of red blood cell parasitism. Immune-mediated hemolytic anemia is a common cause of increased red blood cell destruction resulting in hyperbilirubinemia.

Abnormal hepatocellular transport of bilirubin can be categorized based on the location of the impairment (Figure 6). Disorders of bilirubin uptake in small animals generally are limited to situations in which there is competition with bilirubin for the carrier-mediated transport system. Few differentials fall into the subcategory of impaired conjugation of bilirubin in small animals. After disorders of red blood cell destruction, impaired secretion of bilirubin is the most common cause of hyperbilirubinemia. Abnormalities in bilirubin secretion can be further subdivided into disorders of intrahepatic and extrahepatic cholestasis. In each category, infectious, inflammatory, and neoplastic disease processes must be considered. In generating differentials for intrahepatic cholestasis, particular attention should be paid to breed-specific hepatopathies and idiosyncratic drug reactions.

DIAGNOSTIC APPROACH

An algorithm detailing a rational diagnostic approach to the icteric small animal patient, based on suspected cause, is presented in Figure 5. The diagnostic approach begins with routine complete blood count, platelet count, reticulocyte count, serum chemistry screen, urinalysis, and radiographs of the chest and abdomen. As a result of hemolysis, macrocytic, hypochromic anemia with pronounced reticulocytosis, poikilocytosis, anisocytosis, large platelets, and regenerative leukocytosis may be seen in icteric animals. Spherocytosis and positive results from a Coombs' test frequently occur in immune-mediated hemolytic anemia.

Changes in erythrocytes also may be seen with hepatobiliary disease and may include target cells, spur cells, microcytes, and schistocytes. The white blood cell count may be normal or variably increased with inflammatory disease.

SERUM ENZYME activities consistent with changes in hepatocyte membrane permeability include alanine transaminase (ALT) and aspartate transaminase (AST). Serum enzyme activities consistent with impaired bile flow include alkaline phosphatase (ALP) and γ-glutamyl transpeptidase (GGT); however, activity of serum liver enzymes does not yield important information regarding functional liver mass. High serum enzyme activity is nonspecific and may reflect changes in hepatocellular membrane permeability, enzyme induction in the liver, or even changes in other organ systems.

Alanine Transaminase. Alanine transaminase is primarily a cystolic enzyme and is found in greatest concentration within hepatocytes. Elevation of alanine transaminase in the serum is a good screening test for hepatocellular pathology.[15] In general, the magnitude of the increase of the enzyme is proportional to the number of affected hepatocytes, although the increase is not a predictor of lesion reversibility.[16] Experimentally, serum alanine transaminase elevations persist for a number of days and then decline gradually after an acute hepatotoxic episode.[11] Alterations in cellular metabolism induced by hypoxia or metabolic inhibitors also cause enzyme leakage and may stimulate further enzyme synthesis until normal permeability properties of the hepatocyte membrane are restored.[17,18]

Aspartate Transaminase. Aspartate transaminase is located within the hepatocyte cytoplasm and mitochondria. Aspartate transaminase is not particularly liver specific—it is found in other tissues, including skin and skeletal muscle.[15,19]

Alkaline Phosphatase. Alkaline phosphatase is a cytoplasmic and microsomal membrane enzyme found in hepatocytes and biliary epithelial cells.[20-23] Elevation of this enzyme is a sensitive indicator of intrahepatic and especially extrahepatic cholestasis.[24] Isoenzymes of alkaline phosphatase also are produced by cells of the intestines, renal cortex, bone (osteoblasts), placenta, and leukocytes.[22,25] A steroid-inducible form of alkaline phosphatase also exists, evidenced by high alkaline phosphatase values in animals with steroid-induced hepatopathy.[26,27] The serum half-lives vary among isoenzymes.[28] Because of the short serum half-lives of the other isoenzymes, elevations in serum alkaline phosphatase nearly always originate from hepatocyte or biliary epithelium.

There are some important species differences in the interpretation of serum alkaline phosphatase.[29] The half-life of the enzyme in dogs is three days; in cats, the half-life is only six hours,[29,30] thereby making any elevation in alkaline phosphatase significant. In addition, less alkaline phosphatase is produced secondary to biliary obstruction in cats than in dogs,[30-32] and severe feline liver pathology may be present with only mild to moderate enzyme elevations.

In general, serum alkaline phosphatase activities are higher with periportal liver lesions than with centrilobular liver lesions. Cell swelling and pressure obstruction of small bile ductules in primary hepatocellular disease can result in sufficient intrahepatic cholestasis to elevate alkaline phosphatase.[37]

Gamma-Glutamyl Transpeptidase. Gamma-glutamyl transpeptidase is an enzyme found in highest concentrations in the kidneys, intestines, pancreas, and liver. Marked serum elevations are found only with liver disease.[33] Certain drugs, such as anticonvulsants, increase hepatic synthesis of this enzyme.[33] Increases in serum γ-glutamyl transpeptidase usually parallel alkaline phosphatase elevations in hepatocellular disease,[34-36] but measurement of γ-glutamyl transpeptidase is considered by some investigators to be less sensitive and, therefore, to offer no specific diagnostic advantage over measurement of alkaline phosphatase.

Serum Bilirubin. The total serum bilirubin represents the sum of the unconjugated and conjugated forms of bilirubin. General guidelines for correlating the relative amounts of the unconjugated and conjugated forms with specific sites of the lesion and suspected cause are as follows:

- Hemolytic icterus is suspected when more than 50% of the total serum bilirubin is unconjugated.
- Hepatocellular or obstructive icterus is suspected when more than 50% of the total serum bilirubin is conjugated.
- Patients with extreme conjugated hyperbilirubinemia are more likely to have complete extrahepatic obstruction.

Quantification of unconjugated and conjugated serum bilirubin concentrations is not, however, always essential in evaluating icteric animals, and other test parameters may be of greater value in the diagnostic workup. Indeed, many patients with liver disease may have normal total serum bilirubin concentrations.

A small amount of conjugated bilirubin may be detected in the concentrated urine of a dog without liver disease.[38] The renal threshold for conjugated bilirubin transport in cats is higher than in dogs, thereby suggesting that even small amounts of bilirubinuria indicate hepatic dysfunction in cats.[39]

Serum Proteins. The liver is the sole site of albumin synthesis.[2,40] The serum half-life of albumin is reported to be between 7 and 10 days. Reserve capacity for albumin synthesis is significant, and the degree of liver insufficiency must be severe for hypoalbuminemia to become apparent.

Aside from immunoglobulins, most globulins are synthesized by the liver. Increased globulin synthesis may occur as a result of systemic immune stimulation by gastrointestinal antigens normally removed from the portal blood during perfusion of the liver.[41] This has been shown experimentally in rats with portosystemic vascular shunts.[42]

THE CLOTTING FACTORS synthesized by the liver include factors I, II, V, VII, IX, and X. Clotting defects can become apparent in acute and chronic liver disease. The prothrombin time and partial thromboplastin time are useful diagnostic tests before hepatic biopsy or exploratory laparotomy are done as well as for cases in which hepatobiliary disease is suspected. Prolongation of prothrombin time and partial thromboplastin time may be evident with significant reduction in hepatic cell mass (e.g., cases of extensive necrosis or cirrhosis) and with insufficient biliary flow for intestinal absorption of vitamin K (e.g., extrahepatic cholestasis).[40] Bile duct obstruction can impair the bile-dependent intestinal absorption of fat-soluble vitamin K, which is essential for the synthesis of factors II, VII, IX, and X.[40]

Cholesterol. The liver is a major site of cholesterol metabolism. Normo-, hypo-, or hypercholesterolemia may be seen with liver disease. Hypercholesterolemia may occur with cholestasis caused by retention of cholesterol and increased production of cholesterol stimulated by retained lecithin present in bile.[41,43] In cats, it has been suggested that elevated serum cholesterol may be a better indicator of cholestatic disease than elevations of serum alkaline phosphatase.[44] Hypocholesterolemia may occur in severe liver disease as a result of decreased synthesis, decreased absorption from the gastrointestinal tract when fat digestion is impaired, and excessive conversion of cholesterol to bile acids (such as occurs with portacaval shunts).[41,45] With long-standing extrahepatic bile duct obstruction, the initial hypercholesterolemia may plateau and then decline as a function of decreased cholesterol intake, fat malabsorption, and hepatocellular dysfunction.

Blood Urea Nitrogen. Ammonia produced in the intestinal tract by bacterial degradation is absorbed and transported in portal blood to the liver. In the normal liver, ammonia reacts with carbon dioxide to form carbamoyl phosphate, which is subsequently converted to urea. Urea cycle activity becomes impaired during liver disease; for example, low blood urea nitrogen is a common clinicopathologic finding in animals with congenital portosystemic shunts.[46-48]

Glucose. The hypoglycemia observed with severe liver disease has a multifactorial pathogenesis. Depressed gluconeogenesis, however, is believed to be the most important biochemical defect.[37,41]

Bile Acids. Serum concentrations of bile acids depend on normal intestinal absorption of bile acids, adequate enterohepatic recirculation, functional liver mass, and biliary resecretion. Disturbance of any of these functions influences serum bile acid concentrations.[49-54] Some investigators believe that determination of preprandial and postprandial serum bile acid concentrations in combination with serum enzyme activities (alanine transaminase and alkaline phosphatase) and serum cholesterol is most helpful in differentiating hepatobiliary disorders.[54] For example, cholestatic jaundice of intrahepatic origin may be characterized by mild elevation in serum bile acids, moderate increases in alanine transaminase and alkaline phosphatase, and low cholesterol. With extrahepatic cholestasis, however, there would be marked elevations in serum bile acids (> 200 µMol/L),[54,55] elevated cholesterol, and higher alanine transaminase and alkaline phosphatase values. Interpretation of serum bile acid concentrations should be tempered by three important observations: (1) the general trends cited[54] may not be observed in an individual patient, (2) serum values may be low even when significant disease is present as a result of intestinal malabsorption of bile acids, and (3) serum values cannot differentiate individual disease entities because of the wide range in abnormal values.[50-52,54]

Urinary Urobilinogen. Determining urinary urobilinogen is a semiquantitative means of screening patients for obstructive jaundice.[2] The absence of urobilinogen in urine theoretically suggests that icterus has resulted from complete biliary obstruction; however, negative reporting of urine urobilinogen may occur under other circumstances. For example, (1) broad-spectrum antibiotic treatment suppresses intestinal bacterial flora responsible for reduction of conjugated bilirubin to urobilinogen, (2) rapid oxidation of urobilinogen occurs in urine left at room temperature and exposed to light, (3) acidic urine significantly increases reabsorption of urobilinogen in renal tubules, and (4) diurnal variations in glomerular filtration of urobilinogen occur.[2] Therefore, other evidence of biliary obstruction should be sought for patients with a negative urine urobilinogen test. In such patients, steatorrhea and/or acholic feces may be expected and abdominal ultrasonographic studies would also be very helpful in documenting biliary obstruction.

TABLE I
Relevant Laboratory Data of the Case Example

Parameter	Patient Values				Reference Range
	Day 1	Day 2	Day 3	Day 4	
Hematocrit (%)	52.6	44	—	34	34.5 ± 10.5
Red blood cell ($10^6/\mu l$)	9.7	9.14	—	—	7.5 ± 1.2
White blood cell ($/\mu l$)	7500	5600	—	—	12.5 ± 7.0
Albumin (g/dl)	3.2	3.2	—	—	2.7 – 3.6
Glucose (mg/dl)	71	105	—	—	65 – 135
Alanine transaminase (U/L)	770	750	—	—	13 – 57
Alkaline phosphatase (U/L)	312	250	—	—	2.2 – 38
Cholesterol (mg/dl)	251	198	—	—	75 – 150
Total bilirubin (mg/dl)	10.8	6.0	—	5.6	0.0 – 1.0
Amylase (U/L)	432	703	—	—	500 – 1050
Lipase (U/L)	—	431	—	—	298 – 1050
Prothrombin time (sec)	—	—	9.6	—	11.9 ± 0.6
Partial thromboplastin time (sec)	—	—	13.6	—	18.9 ± 1.4
Fibrin split products ($\mu g/ml$)	—	—	< 10	—	< 10
Bile acids (mMol/L)	—	—	—	189	< 5.0
Urine urobilinogen	—	1+	1+	—	Present
Urine bilirubin	—	3+	3+	—	—
Ammonia (mMol/L)	—	—	34	—	< 55

Serum Amylase, Lipase, and Trypsinogen. Acute pancreatitis is an important cause of extrahepatic biliary obstruction in cats and especially in dogs. Elevations in serum amylase, lipase, and trypsinogen may provide evidence of acute pancreatitis.[56-58] Elevations in serum activities of these enzymes are not, however, definitively diagnostic of the disorder. Diagnosis of acute pancreatitis requires careful integration of information derived from the history, physical examination, laboratory data (including pancreatic enzyme activities), and radiographic and/or ultrasonographic studies. Interpretation of activity of these serum enzymes should always be made in light of the other problems on the problem list.

Dye Retention. Several dye retention tests (e.g., sulfobromophthalein sodium and indocyanine green) have been described in assessment of liver function.[59,60] These tests are quite useful for assessment of nonicteric patients; however, because uptake and secretion of these dyes are competitive with bilirubin, no additional information would be obtained through these tests (i.e., an abnormal retention time would be expected in an icteric patient).[41]

CASE EXAMPLE

A seven-year-old, spayed female Domestic Shorthair cat was presented with a 10-day history of partial anorexia, four days of intermittent vomiting of a bile-colored fluid, and two days of visible icterus. The only other pertinent aspect of the history was mild weight loss because of an imposed dietary restriction. The cat resided indoors, and exposure to toxins was considered unlikely. Mild icterus was the only abnormality reported on physical examination by another veterinarian. Complete blood count, serum chemistry, and FeLV and FIV serologies were obtained (Table I).

At presentation, physical examination identified fever (103.2°F [40°C])); icteric sclerae, soft palate, mucous membranes, and pinnae (Figure 7); painful cranial abdomen; and hepatomegaly. The cat was alert, was slightly overweight (weighing 4.1 kg), had a fair hydration status, and had tachypnea (44 breaths/min). A minimum data base was obtained during admission, and the cat was treated with intravenous balanced electrolyte solutions at a rate of 25 ml/kg/hr.

The following problem list was made from information derived from the history, physical examination, and initial laboratory data:

1. Partial anorexia (10 days)
2. Vomiting (4 days)
3. Icterus (2 days)
4. Fever (resolved after intravenous fluid administration)
5. Mild obesity
6. Mild dehydration
7. Cranial abdominal pain
8. Tachypnea
9. Bilirubinuria
10. Elevated mean corpuscular volume
11. Elevated serum alanine transaminase
12. Elevated serum alkaline phosphatase

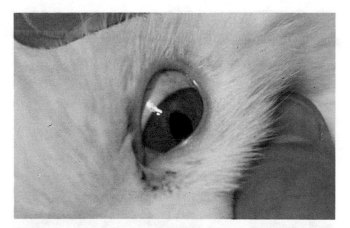

Figure 7A

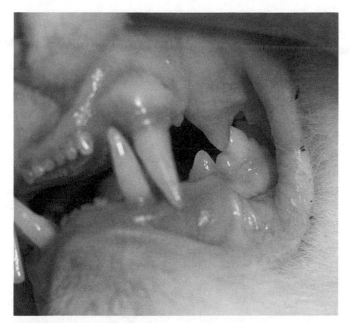

Figure 7B

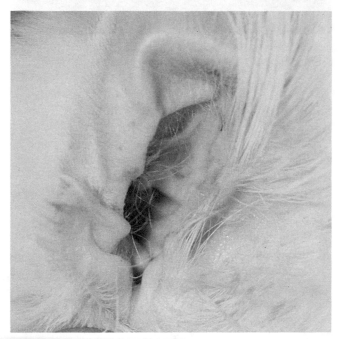

Figure 7C

Figure 7—(A) Sclera, **(B)** gingiva, **(C)** pinna, and **(D)** skin of the case example.

13. Hypercholesterolemia
14. Elevated serum total bilirubin
15. Positive FIV test.

Because there was no evidence supporting increased red blood cell destruction, hepatocellular or obstructive icterus was suspected. To further differentiate these two possibilities, the diagnostic plan included abdominal radiography, abdominal ultrasonography, coagulation panel, fasting plasma ammonia, and fasting serum bile acids. Serum thyroid hormones (T_3 and T_4), urinalysis, and culture also were submitted. The results of these diagnostic tests are summarized in Table I. Albumin, blood urea nitrogen, prothrombin time and partial thromboplastin time, and fasting plasma ammonia levels all were within the normal physiologic range;

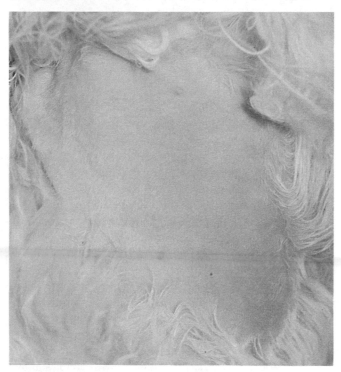

Figure 7D

however, fasting serum bile acids were extremely elevated—results suggestive of obstructive icterus. Urobilinogen was present in urine, suggesting that if biliary obstruction were present, it could not be complete. The bilious vomiting reported in the history also made complete biliary obstruction unlikely. Serum amylase and lipase activities also were within the normal physiologic range at the time of assessment. Mild hepatomegaly was the only abnormality reported on the abdominal radiographs; however, abdominal

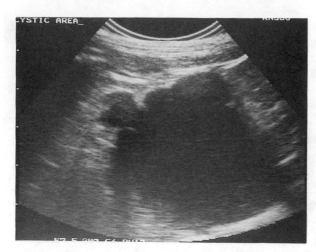

Figure 8—Abdominal ultrasonogram. A hypoechoic structure within the parenchyma of the pancreas was observed.

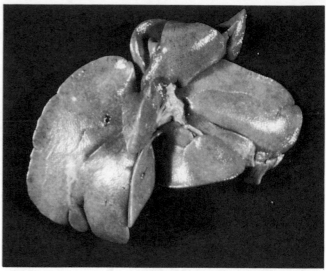

Figure 9—Postmortem liver of the case example. Note the large, rounded appearance.

ultrasonography revealed a 4-cm pancreatic cyst (Figure 8) and a distended gallbladder and common bile duct. The hepatic echogenicity was believed to be normal, and there was no peritoneal effusion or lymphadenopathy.

The expanded problem list now included:

16. Elevated fasting serum bile acids
17. Pancreatic cyst
18. Gallbladder distention
19. Common bile duct distention with possible obstruction.

Obstructive icterus was believed to be the cause of the animal's disorder because of normal hematocrit; normal albumin, blood urea nitrogen, prothrombin time and partial thromboplastin time, and ammonia; elevated serum cholesterol; highly elevated serum alkaline phosphatase and fasting serum bile acids; and abnormal pancreatic and common bile duct ultrasonographic findings.

The cat was treated with intravenous balanced electrolyte solutions with additional potassium supplementation as needed, vitamin K_1 (2.5 mg orally once daily), and ampicillin (10 mg/kg intravenously twice daily) before further investigation by means of exploratory laparotomy.

During surgery, the large pancreatic cyst was confirmed; the gallbladder was grossly distended with fluid, and bile could not be expressed through the common bile duct. The bile duct appeared to be occluded by a 1.0 x 0.5 x 0.5-cm firm nodule extending from the pancreatic cyst. A similar 1-cm nodule was identified in the omentum. Impression smears of the omental nodule examined during surgery revealed a monotonous population of pleomorphic carcinomatous cells. The liver parenchyma had a diffuse nutmeg appearance. Based on the extensive nature of the surgery required and the likelihood of regionally metastatic pancreatic adenocarcinoma complicated by hepatic lipidosis, the owners elected euthanasia. Pancreatic carcinoma with bil-

iary obstruction and severe hepatic lipidosis (Figure 9) were confirmed at necropsy.

The following problems from the problem list could be easily explained by the final diagnosis of pancreatic carcinoma with biliary obstruction and hepatic lipidosis: (1) anorexia, (2) vomiting, (3) icterus, (4) fever, (5) mild obesity, (6) mild dehydration, (7) cranial abdominal pain, (8) tachypnea, (9) bilirubinuria, (10) elevated mean corpuscular volume, (11) elevated alanine transaminase, (12) elevated alkaline phosphatase, (13) hypercholesterolemia, (14) elevated total bilirubin, and (15) elevated fasting serum bile acids. The positive result of the FIV test was believed to be a coincidental finding.

SUMMARY

The occurrence of icterus in small animal patients frequently represents a severe underlying disorder. A thorough history and physical examination often provide important clues to the underlying disorder. Understanding the pathophysiology of bilirubin metabolism in health and disease is important in developing a rational diagnostic approach to icterus. The DAMNIT scheme has been used here to generate a list of reasonable diagnostic differentials for icteric patients. The differentials can be conveniently schematized into disorders causing hemolytic, hepatocellular, or obstructive icterus.

About the Authors
Drs. Anderson and Washabau are affiliated with the Department of Clinical Studies, School of Veterinary Medicine, University of Pennsylvania, Philadelphia, Pennsylvania. Dr. Washabau is a Diplomate of the American College of Veterinary Internal Medicine.

REFERENCES

1. Pulley LT: Jaundice, in Ettinger SJ (ed): *Textbook of Veterinary Internal Medicine.* Philadelphia, WB Saunders Co, 1983, pp 110–115.
2. Cornelius CE: Liver function, in Kaneko JJ, Cornelius CE (eds): *Clinical Biochemistry of Domestic Animals. Vol I,* ed 2. New York, Academic Press, 1970, pp 161–230.
3. Plieninger H, El-Barkawi F, Ehl K, et al: Neue synthese und 14 C-markierung von bilirubin IX-alpha. *Justus Liebigs Ann Chem* 758:195, 1972.
4. Schmid R: Bilirubin metabolism. *Gastroenterology* 74:1307–1312, 1978.
5. Berlin N, Verk P: Quantitative aspects of bilirubin metabolism. *Blood* 57:983–999, 1981.
6. Chowdbury J, Wolkoff A, Arias I: Heme and bile pigment metabolism, in Arias I, Popper H, et al (eds): *The Liver Biology and Pathology.* New York, Raven Press, 1982, pp 309–332.
7. Fleischner GM, Arias IM: Structure and function of ligandin (Y-protein, GSH transferase B) and Z protein in the liver, in Popper H, Schaffner F (eds): *Progress in Liver Diseases. V.* New York, Grune & Stratton, 1976, pp 172–182.
8. Noir BA, Bilirubin conjugated in bile of man, rat and dog. *Biochemistry J* 1155:365, 1976.
9. Arias IM: Formation of bile pigment, in Code CF (ed): *Handbook of Physiology. Vol V,* sec 6. Washington, DC, American Physiology Society, 1968, pp 2347–2374.
10. Levy M, Lester R, Levinsky NG: Renal excretion of urobilinogen in the dog. *J Clin Invest* 47:2117, 1968.
11. Van Vleet JF, Alberts JO: Evaluation of liver function tests and liver biopsy in experimental carbon tetrachloride intoxication and extrahepatic bile duct obstruction in the dog. *Am J Vet Res* 29:2119–2131, 1968.
12. Gopinath C, Ford EH: Localization of liver injury and extent of bilirubinemia in experimental liver lesions. *Vet Pathol* 9:99–108, 1972.
13. Rogoff TM, Lipsky PE: Role of Kupffer cells in local and systemic immune responses. *Gastroenterology* 80:854–860, 1981.
14. Tanner A, Keyhoni A, Reiner R, et al: Proteolytic enzymes released by liver macrophages may promote hepatic injury in a rat model of hepatic damage. *Gastroenterology* 80:647–654, 1981.
15. Visser MP, Crill MA, Muiijtjens AM, et al: Distribution of enzymes in dog heart and liver; significance for assessment of tissue damage from data on plasma enzyme activities. *Clin Chem* 27:1845–1850, 1981.
16. Zinkl JG, Bush RM, Cornelius CE, et al: Comparative studies on plasma and tissue sorbitol, glutamic, lactic, and hydroxybutyric dehydrogenase and transaminase activities in the dog. *Res Vet Sci* 12:211–214, 1971.
17. Zierler KL: Increased muscle permeability to aldolase produced by depolarization and by metabolic inhibitors. *Am J Physiol* 193:534–538, 1958.
18. Ozawa K, Yamoica Y, Nonby H, et al: Insulin as the primary factor governing changes in mitochondrial metabolism leading to liver regeneration and atrophy. *Am J Surg* 127:669–675, 1974.
19. Meyer DJ: The liver. Part I. Biochemical tests for the evaluation of the hepatobiliary system. *Compend Contin Educ Pract Vet* 4(8):663–673, 1982.
20. Moore W, Feldman BF: The use of isoenzymes in small animal medicine. *JAAHA* 10:420–429, 1974.
21. Milne EM, Doxey DL: Alkaline phosphatase and its isoenzymes in tissues and sera of normal dogs. *Vet Res Commun* 10;229–236, 1983.
22. Hoffman WE: The diagnostic value of canine serum alkaline phosphatase isoenzymes. *JAAHA* 13:237–241, 1977.
23. Boyd JW: The mechanisms relating to increases in plasma enzymes and isoenzymes in diseases of animals. *Vet Clin Pathol* 12(2):9–24, 1983.
24. Brobst DF, Schall WD: Needle biopsy of the canine liver and correlation of laboratory data with histopathologic observations. *JAVMA* 161:382–388, 1972.
25. Rogers WA: Source of serum alkaline phosphatase in clinically normal and diseased dogs. A clinical study. *JAVMA* 168:934–939, 1976.
26. Badylak SF, Van Vleet JF: Sequential morphologic and clinicopathologic alterations in dogs with experimentally induced glucocorticoid hepatopathy. *Am J Vet Res* 42:1310–1318, 1981.
27. Hadley SP, Hoffmann WE, Kuhlenschmidt MS, et al: Effect of glucocorticoids on alkaline phosphatase, alanine aminotransferase, and gammaglutamyltransferase in cultured dog hepatocytes. *Enzyme* 43:89–98, 1990.
28. Hoffman WE, Dorner JL: Disappearance rates of intravenously injected canine alkaline phosphatase isoenzymes. *Am J Vet Res* 38:1553–1556, 1977.
29. Kramer JW, Sleight SD: The isoenzymes of serum alkaline phosphatase in cats. *Am J Vet Clin Path* 22:87–91, 1968.
30. Hoffman WE, Renegar WE, Dorner JL: Serum half-life of intravenously injected intestinal and hepatic alkaline phosphatase isoenzymes in the cat. *Vet Clin Pathol* 6:21–24, 1977.
31. Everett RM, Duncan JR, Prasse KW: Alkaline phosphatase, leucine aminopeptidase and ALT activities with obstructive and toxic hepatic disease in cats. *Am J Vet Res* 38:1637–1639, 1977.
32. Hoffman WE, Renegar WE, Dorner JL: Alkaline phosphatase and alkaline phosphatase isoenzymes in the cat. *Vet Clin Pathol* 6:21–24, 1977.
33. Ivanov E, Krustev L, Adjarov D, et al: Studies on the mechanism of the changes in serum and liver γ-glutamyl transpeptidase activity. *Enzyme* 21:8–20, 1976.
34. Noonan NE, Meyer DJ: Use of plasma arginase and gamma glutamyltranspeptidase as specific indicators of hepatocellular or hepatobiliary disease in the dog. *Am J Vet Res* 40:942–947, 1979.
35. Spano JS, August JR, Henderson RA, et al: Serum gamma-glutamyl transpeptidase in healthy cats and cats with induced hepatic disease. *Am J Vet Res* 44:2049–2053, 1983.
36. Center SA, Baldwin BH, Dillingham S, et al: Diagnostic value of serum gammaglutamyl transferase and alkaline phosphatase activities in hepatobiliary disease in the cat. *JAVMA* 188:507–510, 1986.
37. Shull RM, Hornbuckle W: Diagnostic use of serum gamma-glutamyltransferase in canine liver disease. *Am J Vet Res* 40:1321–1324, 1979.
38. Osborne CA, Steven JB, Lees GE, et al: Clinical significance of bilirubinuria. *Compend Contin Educ Pract Vet* 2(11):897–903, 1980.
39. Lees GE, Hardy RM, Stevens JB, et al: Clinical implications of feline bilirubinuria. *JAAHA* 20:765–771, 1984.
40. Asofsky R: Plasma protein synthesis by liver, in Becker FF (ed): *The Liver: Normal and Abnormal Functions.* New York, Market Decker, 1974, pp 87–102.
41. Hall RL: Laboratory evaluation of liver disease. *Vet Clin North Am [Small Anim Pract]* 15(1):3–19, 1985.
42. Keraan M, Meyers OL, Engelbracht GC, et al: Increased serum immunoglobulin levels following portocaval shunt in the normal rat. *Gut* 15:468–472, 1974.
43. Dowling RH: The enterohepatic circulation. *Gastroenterology* 62:122–140, 1972.
44. Center SA, Baldwin BH, King JM, et al: Hematologic and biochemical abnormalities associated with induced extrahepatic bile duct obstruction in the cat. *Am J Vet Res* 44:1822–1829, 1983.
45. Coyle JJ, Schwartz MZ, Marubbio AT, et al: The effect of portocaval shunt on plasma lipids and tissue cholesterol synthesis in the dog. *Surgery* 80:54–60, 1971.
46. Meyer DJ, Strombeck DR, Stone EA, et al: Ammonia tolerance tests in clinically normal dogs and in dogs with portosystemic shunts. *JAVMA* 173:377–379, 1978.
47. Vulgamott JC: Portosystemic shunts. *Vet Clin North Am [Small Anim Pract]* 15(1):229–242, 1985.
48. Griffiths GL, Lumsden JH, Valli VO: Hematologic and biochemical changes in dogs with portosystemic shunts. *JAAHA* 17:705–710, 1981.
49. DeNovo RC, Prasse KW: Comparison of serum biochemical and hepatic functional alterations in dogs treated with corticosteroids and hepatic duct ligation. *Am J Vet Res* 44:1703–1709, 1983.
50. Hauge JG, Adelkader SV: Serum bile acids as an indicator of liver disease in dogs. *Acta Vet Scand* 25:495–503, 1984.
51. Center SA, Baldwin BH, Erb HN, et al: Bile acid concentrations in the diagnosis of hepatobiliary disease in the dog. *JAVMA* 187:935–940, 1985.
52. Johnson SE, Rogers WA, Bonagura JA, et al: Determination of serum bile acids in fasting dogs with hepatobiliary disease. *Am J Vet Res* 46:2048–2053, 1985.
53. Meyer DJ: Liver function tests in dogs with portasystemic shunts:

Measurement of serum bile acid concentration. *JAVMA* 188:168–169, 1986.

54. Center SA, Van Warren T, Slater MR, et al: Evaluation of twelve-hour preprandial and two-hour postprandial serum bile acids concentrations for diagnosis of hepatobiliary disease in dogs. *JAVMA* 199(2):217–226, 1991.

55. Rutgers HC, Stradley RP, Johnson SE: Serum bile acid analysis in dogs with experimentally induced cholestatic jaundice. *Am J Vet Res* 49:317–320, 1988.

56. Strombeck DR, Farver T, Kaneko JJ: Serum amylase and lipase activities in the diagnosis of pancreatitis in dogs. *Am J Vet Res* 42:1966–1970, 1981.

57. Kitchell BE, Strombeck DR, Cullen D, et al: Clinical and pathologic changes in experimentally induced acute pancreatitis in cats. *Am J Vet Res* 47:1170–1173, 1986.

58. Simpson KW, Batt RM, McLean L, et al: Circulating concentrations of trypsin-like immunoreactivity and activities of lipase and amylase after pancreatic duct ligation in dogs. *Am J Vet Res* 50:629–632, 1989.

59. Himes JA, Cornelius CE: Hepatic excretion and storage of sulfobromophthalein sodium in an experimental hepatic necrosis in the dog. *Cornell Vet* 63:424–431, 1973.

60. Rakich PM, Prasse KW, Bjorling DE: Clearance of indocyanine green in dogs with partial hepatectomy, hepatic duct ligation, and passive hepatic congestion. *Am J Vet Res* 48:1353–1357, 1987.

New Tests *(continued from page 69)*

45. Abels J, Muckerheide MM, Van Kapel J, et al: A dual role for the dog pancreas in the absorption of vitamin B_{12}, in *Program, American Society of Hematology 17th Meeting*, Atlanta, 1974, p 95.

46. Horadagoda NU, Batt RM, Vaillant C, et al: Identification and characterization of a pancreatic intrinsic factor in the dog. *Am J Phys* 256:G517–G523, 1989.

47. Fyfe JC: Feline intrinsic factor (IF) is pancreatic in origin and mediates ileal cobalamin (CBL) absorption. *J Vet Int Med* 7:133, 1993.

48. Lindenbaum J: Malabsorption of vitamin B_{12} and folate. *Curr Concepts Nutr* 9:105–123, 1980.

49. Welkos SL, Toskes PP, Baer H, et al: Importance of anaerobic bacteria in the cobalamin malabsorption of the experimental blind loop syndrome. *Gastroenterology* 80:313–320, 1981.

50. Davenport DJ, Sherding RG: Clinicopathologic parameters of an experimental model of small intestinal bacterial overgrowth. *Proc 4th Annu Vet Med Forum ACVIM* 2:14–17, 1986.

51. Williams DA: Evaluation of radioassay methods for analysis of canine serum cobalamin and folate. *J Vet Int Med* 6:81, 1992.

52. Batt RM, McLean L, Rutgers HC, Hall EJ: Validation of a radioassay for the determination of serum folate and cobalamin concentrations in dogs. *J Small Anim Pract* 32:221–224, 1991.

53. Baker H, Schor SM, Murphy BD, et al: Blood vitamin and choline concentrations in healthy cats, dogs, and horses. *Am J Vet Res* 47:1468–1471, 1986.

54. Halsted CH, Beer WH, Chandler CJ, et al: Clinical studies of intestinal folate conjugase. *J Lab Clin Med* 107:228–232, 1986.

55. Bernstein LH, Gutstein S, Efron G, et al: Experimental production of elevated serum folate in dogs with intestinal blind loops: Relationship of serum levels to location of the blind loop. *Gastroenterology* 63:815–819, 1972.

56. Bernstein LH, Gutstein S, Efron G, et al: Experimental production of elevated serum folate in dogs with intestinal blind loops. 2. Nature of bacterially produced folate coenzymes in blind loop fluid. *Am J Clin Nutr* 28:925–929, 1975.

57. Bunch SE, Easley JR: Investigations of phenytoin-folate interactions in dogs. *Proc 4th Annu Vet Med Forum ACVIM* 2:14–18,1986.

58. Russel RM, Dhar GJ, Dutta SK, et al: Influence of intraluminal pH on folate absorption: Studies in control subjects and in patients with pancreatic insufficiency. *J Lab Clin Med* 93:428–436, 1979.

59. King CE, Toskes PP: Small intestine bacterial overgrowth. *Gastroenterology* 76:1035–1055, 1979.

60. Hoenig M: Intestinal malabsorption attributed to bacterial overgrowth in a dog. *JAVMA* 176:533–535, 1980.

61. Strombeck DR, Doe M, Jang S: Maldigestion and malabsorption in a dog with chronic gastritis. *JAVMA* 179:801–805, 1981.

62. Williams DA, Burrows CF: Short bowel syndrome—A case report in a dog and a discussion of the pathophysiology of bowel resection. *J Small Anim Pract* 22:263–275, 1981.

63. Simpson JW: Bacterial overgrowth causing malabsorption in a dog. *Vet Rec* 110:335–336, 1982.

64. Watson ADJ, Church DB, Middleton DJ, et al: Weight loss in cats which eat well. *J Small Anim Pract* 22:473–482, 1981.

65. Hoskins JD, Turk JR, Turk MA: Feline pancreatic insufficiency. *VM SAC* 77:1745–1748, 1982.

66. Tangner CH, Turrel JM, Hobson HP: Complications associated with proximal duodenal resection and cholecystoduodenostomy in two cats. *Vet Surg* 11:60–64, 1982.

67. Lewis LD, Boulay JP, Chow FHC: Fat excretion and assimilation by the cat. *Feline Pract* 9:46–49, 1979.

68. Sherding RG, Stradley RP, Rogers WA, et al: Bentiromide:xylose test in healthy cats. *Am J Vet Res* 43:2272–2273, 1982.

69. Hawkins EC, Meric SM, Washabau RJ, et al: Digestion of bentiromide and absorption of xylose in healthy cats and absorption of xylose in cats with infiltrative intestinal disease. *Am J Vet Res* 47:567–569, 1986.

70. Tams TR: Chronic feline inflammatory bowel disorders. Part I. Idiopathic inflammatory bowel disease. *Compend Contin Educ Pract Vet* 8:371–378, 1986.

71. Tams TR: Chronic feline inflammatory bowel disorders. Part II. Feline eosinophilic enteritis and lymphosarcoma. *Compend Contin Educ Pract Vet* 8:464–471, 1986.

72. Edwards DS, Russell RG: Probable vitamin K-deficient bleeding in two cats with malabsorption syndrome secondary to lymphocytic-plasmacytic enteritis. *J Vet Int Med* 1:97–101, 1987.

73. Hall EJ, Batt RM: Abnormal intestinal permeability in a wheat-sensitive enteropathy of Irish setter dogs. *Gastroenterology* 92:1422, 1987.

Surgical Management of Hepatic and Biliary Disease in Cats

KEY FACTS

- Definitive diagnosis of hepatic disease in cats often requires hepatic biopsy.
- Biopsy of the liver during exploratory laparotomy allows examination of the entire liver and biopsy of isolated lesions.
- Thickening of bile associated with inflammation and infection can result in biliary obstruction in cats.
- A primary objective of surgical treatment of biliary obstruction is to provide a patent conduit for the discharge of bile.

University of Wisconsin
Dale E. Bjorling, DVM, MS

DISEASES of the liver and biliary tract are common causes of illness in cats. Although clinically apparent icterus may suggest that the cause of illness is a hepatic or biliary disorder, hepatic and biliary disease may cause such nonspecific signs as malaise, anorexia, depression, lethargy, vomiting, diarrhea, or ascites. Hepatic or biliary disease may be accompanied by abdominal pain, abdominal enlargement (caused by hepatomegaly or ascites), thrombocytopenia, or abnormalities in the coagulation process.

PREOPERATIVE AND POSTOPERATIVE CONSIDERATIONS

The presence of hepatic or biliary disease is usually confirmed by laboratory analysis of blood samples. Most cats with liver disease are initially treated medically unless a mass lesion or biliary obstruction is identified. Placement of a feeding tube (nasogastric, pharyngostomy, or gastrostomy) to allow enteral hyperalimentation should be considered as part of the medical treatment of patients with hepatobiliary disease. Although many cats respond to medical therapy and improved alimentation, definitive diagnosis and treatment often require surgery.

Liver biopsy has been recommended as part of the routine evaluation of cats with bile acid concentrations that exceed 20 μmol/L.[1] Leakage of bile or biliary obstruction that does not respond to medical therapy should be managed surgically. Liver biopsy can be performed percutaneously; ultrasonographically guided biopsy has improved the safety and accuracy of this procedure. Isolated lesions may be overlooked, however, and continued hemorrhage or leakage of bile may occur. After ultrasonographically guided biopsy of the liver in a cat, I have performed surgery to treat continued leakage of bile from the hepatic parenchyma with no apparent damage to a large biliary duct.

Surgical intervention to establish the diagnosis and treat disease should be considered early in the course of therapy, before the patient's condition has deteriorated to the point that the risks of anesthesia and surgery make survival unlikely. Preanesthetic evaluation of cats with hepatobiliary disease should focus on hydration, coagulation function, anemia, hypoproteinemia, plane of nutrition, and general metabolic status. Cats with hepatobiliary disease are often dehydrated and in poor condition nutritionally.[2] Hepatic disease can contribute directly to hypoproteinemia and coagulopathy, or these may result from peritonitis or extension of primary disease. Leakage of sterile bile into the abdominal cavity for a brief period causes chemical peritonitis. Contamination of the abdominal cavity by bacteria (from damaged hepatic parenchyma, the biliary system, or direct migration across the bowel wall because of exposure to bile) leads to bacterial peritonitis, a much more serious consequence.[3,4]

Originally published in Volume 13, Number 9, September 1991

Cytologic and enzymatic evaluation of abdominal fluid before surgery may suggest leakage of bile or peritonitis. Samples of abdominal fluid obtained before or during surgery or tissue samples collected during surgery should be submitted for aerobic and anaerobic microbial culture and antibiotic sensitivity testing. Gram-positive and gram-negative organisms as well as anaerobic organisms are frequently cultured from hepatic abscesses or bile from cats with biliary obstruction or disruption. Broad-spectrum antibiotic therapy is thus necessary.

Oral or intravenous metronidazole (20 mg/kg twice daily) may be given to treat infection caused by anaerobic organisms. Other antibiotics (intravenous gentamicin [6 mg/kg] once daily or cefazolin [20 mg/kg] four times daily) should be given concurrently to control aerobic organisms. Cefazolin is a first-generation cephalosporin and does not have as broad a spectrum of efficacy against gram-negative organisms as gentamicin does. Alternatively, intravenous cefotetan (30 mg/kg three times daily) can be used. Cefotetan is a second-generation cephalosporin and, although more expensive, has better efficacy against gram-negative and anaerobic organisms than the first-generation cephalosporins do. Because of its mode of action, gentamicin given once daily is more effective and causes less renal toxicity than a similar total dose given at more frequent intervals.[5] If a positive bacterial culture has been obtained, antibiotic therapy should be continued after surgery for at least 10 days; extended treatment may be required for established infection.

AFTER SURGERY, cats should be carefully evaluated for recurrence of biliary obstruction or continued leakage of bile. Many cats with hepatobiliary disease are in a poor state of nutrition. The stress of surgery may further aggravate this state, and consideration should be given to placing a feeding tube before or after surgery to support enteral alimentation.[6]

ANATOMY

The anatomy of the feline liver is similar to that of the canine liver.[7] The lobes of the liver of a cat are generally narrower than those of a dog; this facilitates hepatic lobectomy. In cats, the right lateral and medial lobes are more difficult to remove than the other lobes because of their broad attachment to the rest of the liver and the caudal vena cava.

The anatomy of the biliary tract is more variable in cats than in dogs (Figure 1). From one to five lobar biliary ducts may join the common bile duct, and duplication of the gallbladder has been reported.[8] The major pancreatic duct usually joins the common bile duct before the point at which the common bile duct enters the duodenum; occasionally, the major pancreatic duct shares an opening with the common bile duct. Only 20% of cats have an accessory (or minor) pancreatic duct; when present, this duct enters the duodenum two centimeters distal to the major papilla.[8,9] Diseases of the biliary tract in cats thus are often accompanied by pancreatic disease.

THE LIVER receives three to five proper hepatic arteries from the common hepatic artery. At the hilus, the portal vein gives rise to two or three major branches before dividing into intrahepatic vessels. As in dogs, the hepatic veins in cats are short and often broad and enter the caudal vena cava at or near the diaphragm.[8]

HEPATIC BIOPSY AND PARTIAL HEPATECTOMY

Small samples of the liver may be obtained and biopsy may be performed on isolated lesions of the liver with various biopsy needles and dermal punches. Jamshidi needles can be used to collect small tissue samples, and Keyes or Baker cutaneous biopsy punches can be used to obtain larger (2- to 12-mm diameter) samples. The hepatic veins are most superficial on the caudal (or visceral) surface of the liver; this area should generally be avoided with biopsy needles and punches.

It has been suggested that defects created in the liver with biopsy punches can be filled with absorbable gelatin sponges.[10] I prefer to close the defects with 2-0 or 3-0 absorbable sutures placed deeply in a horizontal mattress or cruciate pattern. If necessary, continued hemorrhage or leakage of bile from needle biopsy sites can be controlled in a similar manner.

The periphery of the liver lobes is easy to biopsy during surgery with minimal risk of hemorrhage or leakage of bile[11] (Figure 2). The tip of the lobe may be encircled with an absorbable suture (3-0 or 4-0). As the suture is tightened, the parenchyma is crushed; vessels and bile canaliculi are occluded. The isolated liver tissue distal to the ligature is sharply excised. Although excessive damaged hepatic parenchyma should not remain, a small amount (3 to 5 mm) of parenchyma should be left distal to the ligature to ensure that the ligature is not cut as the tissue is removed or that the ligature does not slip.

Larger biopsy samples may be obtained from the tips of liver lobes by placing interlocking sutures or horizontal mattress sutures proximal to the line of excision. Isolated lesions located on the periphery of liver lobes (away from the tips) can be removed by placement of a row of interlocking or overlapping mattress sutures and subsequent excision (Figure 2). Vessels in the hepatic parenchyma that continue to bleed should be individually ligated.

Treatment of hepatic abscesses, trauma, or masses may require lobectomy. In cats, entire lobes of the liver can be removed by isolating and ligating the associated vessels and bile ducts. The left lateral and medial lobes, the quad-

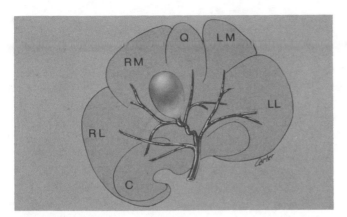

Figure 1—Biliary drainage of the liver. One to five lobar ducts may be present in cats (four are shown here). The duct from the right division of the liver usually joins the short cystic duct first; this is the beginning of the common bile duct. *C* = caudate lobe; *RL* = right lateral lobe; *RM* = right medial lobe; *Q* = quadrate lobe; *LM* = left medial lobe; and *LL* = left lateral lobe. (From Bjorling DE, Prasse KW, Holmes RA: Partial hepatectomy in dogs. *Compend Contin Educ Pract Vet* 7(3):258, 1985. Reprinted with permission.)

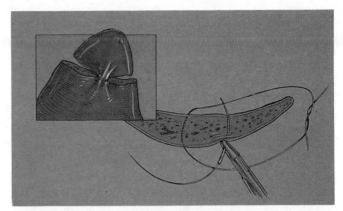

Figure 2A

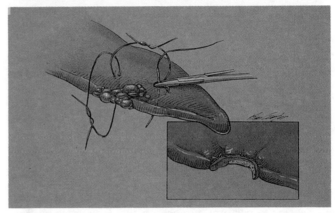

Figure 2B

Figure 2—Biopsy of the liver. (**A**) A biopsy may be obtained from the tip of a liver lobe by placing two interlocking sutures, which are tightened and tied to occlude vessels and bile ducts. (**B**) Biopsy can be performed on lesions on the periphery of the lobe by placing a row of mattress sutures to control hemorrhage and leakage of bile. (From Bjorling DE: Partial hepatectomy and hepatic biopsy, in Bojrab MJ (ed): *Current Techniques in Small Animal Surgery*, ed 3. Philadelphia, Lea & Febiger, 1990, pp 291–295. Reprinted with permission.)

rate lobe, and most of the caudate lobe can be removed by placing an encircling silk ligature (1-0 or 2-0) near the hilus, tightening the ligature, and excising the lobe.[7] Displacement of this ligature will result in profuse hemorrhage; particular care should be taken to avoid damage or displacement of the ligature.

Liver lobes can be removed by compressing the parenchyma near the hilus with the surgeon's fingers or an instrument to isolate vessels and bile ducts (the finger fracture technique). The vessels and bile ducts are individually ligated and divided. Vessels in the parenchyma that continue to bleed are ligated.

REMOVAL of most of the right medial or lateral lobe usually requires careful dissection of the hepatic parenchyma from its attachment to the caudal vena cava and the rest of the liver. Vessels and bile ducts are ligated as they are encountered. The hepatic veins tend to be short and broad; secure placement of encircling ligatures thus is difficult. The vessels should be grasped and oversewn or ligated with transfixation ligatures.[7] The liver has a remarkable capacity for regeneration; in dogs, as much as 70% to 80% of the liver has been successfully removed during a single operation.[12,13]

SURGERY OF THE BILIARY TRACT

Disorders of the biliary tract that require surgical correction include disruption, obstruction, or destruction of a portion of the tract by primary or adjacent disease. Disruption of the biliary tract in cats is most often the result of

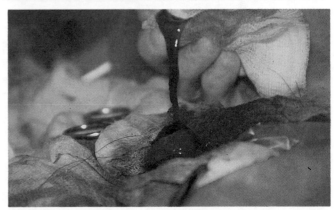

Figure 3—Inspissated bile being removed via cholecystotomy. The patient had biliary obstruction, and the bile had a mucinous character. In some cats with cholangiohepatitis, the bile can be even thicker and have a claylike consistency. (Courtesy of R. C. DeNovo, DVM, College of Veterinary Medicine, University of Tennessee)

trauma or prolonged obstruction. Cholangiohepatitis with inspissation of bile[2,14] (Figure 3), cholelithiasis,[15-17] infestation with liver flukes,[18,19] and compression by extraluminal masses[20,21] may cause obstruction of the biliary tract in cats. Primary neoplastic disorders of the tract are uncommon; diseases of the pancreas, duodenum, or liver that affect the tract are more common.

The primary goals of surgical treatment of biliary disease are to establish a diagnosis, to prevent continued leakage of bile into the abdomen, and to provide a patent conduit for discharge of bile into the gastrointestinal tract. Principles of surgery of the biliary tract have been described in the literature.[22] Bile samples can be collected for cytologic evaluation and aerobic or anaerobic culture by needle aspiration or via cholecystotomy. If bile is aspirated from the gallbladder, I prefer to pass the needle through a purse-string suture of 5-0 nonabsorbable material placed in the dome of the gallbladder. After a bile sample has been obtained, the suture is tightened and tied to prevent continued leakage of bile.

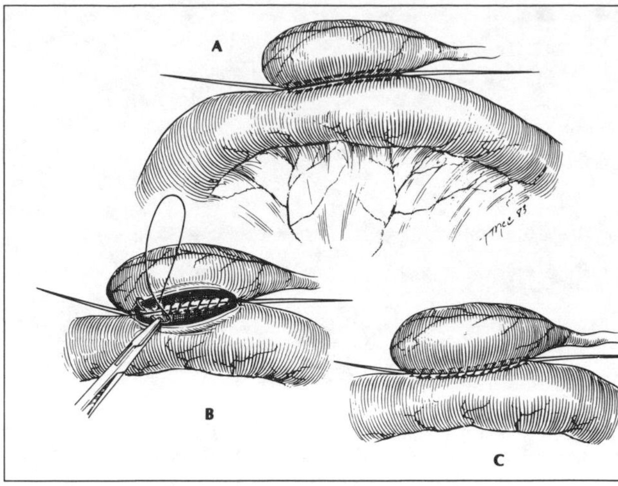

Figure 4—Cholecystenterostomy. (A) The gallbladder is sutured to the bowel, and parallel incisions are made. (B) The cut edge of the gallbladder is sutured to the corresponding edge of the bowel. (C) The stoma is encircled by the second suture line. (From Blass CE: Surgery of the extrahepatic biliary tract. *Compend Contin Educ Pract Vet* 5(10):806, 1983. Reprinted with permission.)

IN NORMAL CATS, the bile ducts are small. It is usually easier to perform surgery on the ducts after obstruction has caused distention. Magnification facilitates detection and surgical treatment of disorders of the biliary tract. If a lobar duct has been damaged, it is often more prudent to ligate the duct than to attempt to repair it. In dogs, auxiliary channels apparently conduct bile to the biliary tract after ligation of hepatic ducts; however, transient icterus may be observed after ligation of lobar ducts.[23-25] Ligation of all hepatic ducts should be avoided.

CHOLECYSTOTOMY, CHOLEDOCHOTOMY, AND LACERATIONS OF THE GALLBLADDER AND BILE DUCTS

The most common indications for making an incision into the gallbladder (cholecystotomy) or common bile duct (choledochotomy) are the presence of inspissated (thickened) bile, choleliths, or liver flukes. Before the gallbladder is incised, it should be dissected free of its attachment to the liver. Stay sutures (5-0) are placed on both sides of the proposed site of incision. The gallbladder should be isolated with laparotomy pads to minimize contamination of the abdomen.

After the gallbladder has been opened (Figure 3), samples of bile should be obtained for microbial culture and cytologic evaluation. The cystic duct, lobar ducts, and common bile duct should be cannulated (via a 3.5 or 5 French soft catheter) and flushed with sterile saline to en-

sure patency. Occasionally, it is necessary to open the duodenum to allow retrograde passage of a catheter into the common bile duct. The incision into the gallbladder is closed with a 4-0 or 5-0 absorbable suture in a simple continuous pattern, and the duodenum is closed routinely.

Incisions into the biliary ducts should be made in a longitudinal direction. After removal of sludged bile, choleliths, or flukes, a catheter is passed in both directions to ensure patency. The incision is closed with a 4-0 or 5-0 absorbable suture in a simple interrupted or continuous pattern. In small ducts, closure of the longitudinal incision in a transverse manner (by apposing the two ends of the incision) will increase the diameter of the duct at the point of closure.

To divert the flow of bile past the surgical site and maintain the biliary tract in a decompressed state, a short and soft 3.5 or 5 French catheter can be placed between the gallbladder and duodenum. Bowel motility will cause the catheter to be displaced in a few days, and it will be passed with the feces. Alternatively, a catheter can be passed across the wall of the gallbladder and the abdominal wall, allowing bile to be drained to the skin surface. A collection device should be attached to the catheter. These catheters are often difficult to manage in clinical patients; it has been suggested that the catheters are unnecessary in veterinary surgery.[21]

Lacerations of the gallbladder and bile ducts are debrided and closed as described. Alternatively, lobar ducts can be ligated on both sides of the defect. Severe damage to the gallbladder may necessitate cholecystectomy, and destruction of a portion of the common bile duct must be treated by choledochoenterostomy or cholecystenterostomy.

CHOLECYSTECTOMY

Removal of the gallbladder (cholecystectomy) in cats is not technically difficult and is associated with few complications. The most common indications are trauma, prolonged distention caused by biliary obstruction, and infection of the gallbladder associated with cholangiohepatitis. The gallbladder is dissected free of its attachment to the liver, and the cystic duct and cystic artery are ligated. Care should be taken to preserve the lobar ducts.

CHOLEDOCHOENTEROSTOMY AND CHOLECYSTENTEROSTOMY

Loss of function of the common bile duct as it approaches the duodenum is the primary indication for surgical creation of (1) a new opening into the duodenum for the remnant of the common bile duct (choledochoduodenostomy) or (2) a new opening into the duodenum or jejunum for the gallbladder (cholecystenterostomy). Both of these procedures are complicated by the need to preserve the major pancreatic duct. If it is patent, the distal common bile duct should be preserved with the major pancreatic duct. It may be necessary to ligate the major pancreatic duct; pancreatitis and pancreatic exocrine insufficiency should be anticipated.

CHOLEDOCHOENTEROSTOMY is easiest to perform and produces the fewest complications if the common bile duct is dilated. The distal end of the duct is isolated, and a 5- to 10-millimeter longitudinal incision is made in the end of the duct. The proximal duodenum is repositioned to allow anastomosis of the common bile duct to the duodenum without tension on the suture line.

A transverse incision is made into the lumen of the duodenum. The length of the incision should approximate half the circumference of the distal common bile duct, including the longitudinal incision. An anastomosis is created between the duodenum and common bile duct using a 3-0 or 4-0 synthetic absorbable or monofilament nonabsorbable suture in a simple interrupted pattern. To facilitate complete closure, suturing should begin at the point farthest from the surgeon. A single layer of sutures is usually adequate. Alternatively, a longitudinal incision can be made into the common bile duct and duodenum, and a choledochoduodenostomy can be performed without transecting the common bile duct.[26]

In cats, a cholecystenterostomy can be performed using the proximal duodenum or jejunum. It is desirable to place the opening of the gallbladder as close to the stomach as possible. The gallbladder is dissected free of its attach-

ments to the liver and is positioned near the selected section of bowel (Figure 4). The serosal surface of the gallbladder is sutured to the bowel near the mesentery with a 3-0 or 4-0 synthetic absorbable suture. The suture line should extend for three to four centimeters, and the needle should be left attached to the suture for later completion of the line.

PARALLEL incisions 2.5 to 3.0 centimeters long are made in the bowel and gallbladder within two to three millimeters of the original suture line. A stoma between the bowel and gallbladder is created by suturing the cut edge of the bowel to that of the gallbladder. I prefer to begin at the most oral extent of the incisions and to continue in an aboral direction, suturing the two edges closest to the original suture line first. The same suture material is used in a simple continuous pattern. After this suture line is complete, the original line is completed to encircle the sutures that create the stoma. The result is a two-layer closure.

Leakage of bile or intestinal contents is a potential complication of this surgical technique. This complication has been uncommon in my experience. Much more common complications are pancreatic exocrine insufficiency (caused by obstruction of the major pancreatic duct) and reflux of bowel contents or obstruction of the stoma; either of these complications may lead to cholangitis.[27] Pancreatic exocrine insufficiency is observed almost immediately after surgery; cholangiohepatitis may not develop for several days to weeks. Pancreatic exocrine insufficiency can be treated satisfactorily by adding pancreatic enzymes to the food of the patient.[27]

In dogs, it has been recommended that the stoma between the bowel and gallbladder be at least 2.5 centimeters long to minimize the potential for obstruction of bile flow or retention of bowel contents in the gallbladder.[28] To create a larger stoma between the bowel and gallbladder, it may help to remove an ellipse of tissue from the gallbladder rather than making a simple incision.[29] If a satisfactory opening remains, the cholangitis that is observed after cholecystenterostomy usually responds to antibiotic therapy.[27]

About the Author

Dr. Bjorling, who is a Diplomate of the American College of Veterinary Surgeons, is affiliated with the Department of Surgical Sciences, School of Veterinary Medicine, University of Wisconsin, Madison, Wisconsin.

REFERENCES

1. Center SA: Serum bile acid concentrations for hepatobiliary function testing in cats, in Kirk RW (ed): *Current Veterinary Therapy. X. Small Animal Practice*. Philadelphia, WB Saunders Co, 1989, pp 873-878.

2. Zawie DA, Shaker E: Diseases of the liver, in Scherding RG (ed): *The Cat: Diseases and Clinical Management*. New York, Churchill Livingstone, 1989, pp 1015-1036.
3. Cain JL, Lubat JA, Cohn I: Bile peritonitis in germ-free dogs. *Gastroenterology* 53:600-603, 1967.
4. Dineen P: The importance of the route of infection in experimental biliary tract obstruction. *Surg Gynecol Obstet* 119:1001-1008, 1964.
5. Nordstrom L, Ringberg H, Cronberg S, et al: Does administration of an aminoglycoside in a single daily dose affect its efficacy and toxicity? *J Antimicrob Chemother* 25:159-173, 1990.
6. Crowe DT: Enteral nutrition for critically ill or injured patients—Parts I, II, and III. *Compend Contin Educ Pract Vet* 8(9-11):603-612, 719-732, 826-836, 1986.
7. Bjorling DE: Partial hepatectomy in dogs. *Compend Contin Educ Pract Vet* 7(3):257-267, 1985.
8. Schummer A, Nickel R, Sack WO: *The Viscera of the Domestic Mammals*, ed 3. Berlin, Verlag Paul Parey, 1979, pp 134-136.
9. Crouch JE, Lackey MD: *Text-Atlas of Cat Anatomy*. Philadelphia, Lea & Febiger, 1969, pp 145-146.
10. Walshaw R: Liver and biliary system: Surgical diseases, in Slatter DH (ed): *Textbook of Small Animal Surgery*. Philadelphia, WB Saunders Co, 1985, pp 798-827.
11. Bjorling DE: Partial hepatectomy and hepatic biopsy, in Bojrab MJ (ed): *Current Techniques in Small Animal Surgery*, ed 3. Philadelphia, Lea & Febiger, 1990, pp 291-295.
12. Francavilla A, Porter KA, Benichou J, et al: Liver regeneration in dogs. *J Surg Res* 25:409-419, 1978.
13. Islami AH, Pack GT, Schwartz MK, et al: Regenerative hyperplasia following major hepatectomy: Chemical analysis of the regenerated liver and comparative nuclear counts. *Ann Surg* 140:85-89, 1959.
14. Kelly DF, Baggott DG, Gaskell CJ: Jaundice in a cat associated with inflammation of the biliary tract and pancreas. *J Small Anim Pract* 16:163-172, 1975.
15. Hirsch VM, Doige CE: Suppurative cholangitis in cats. *JAVMA* 182:1223-1226, 1983.
16. O'Brien TR, Mitchum GD: Cholelithiasis in a cat. *JAVMA* 156:1015-1017, 1970.
17. Wolf AM: Obstructive jaundice in a cat resulting from choledocholithiasis. *JAVMA* 185:85-87, 1984.
18. Jenkins CC, Lewis DD, Brock KA, et al: Extrahepatic biliary obstruction associated with *Platynosomum concinnum* in a cat. *Compend Contin Educ Pract Vet* 10(5):628-632, 1988.
19. Lewis DT, Malone JB, Taboada J, et al: Cholangiohepatitis and choledochectasia associated with *Amphimerus pseudofelineus* in a cat. *JAAHA* 27:156-162, 1991.
20. Barsanti JA, Higgins RJ, Spano JS, et al: Adenocarcinoma of the extrahepatic bile duct in a cat. *J Small Anim Pract* 17:599-604, 1976.
21. Martin RA, MacCoy DM, Harvey HJ: Surgical management of extrahepatic biliary tract disease: A report of eleven cases. *JAAHA* 22:301-307, 1986.
22. Blass CE: Surgery of the extrahepatic biliary tract. *Compend Contin Educ Pract Vet* 5(10):801-808, 1983.
23. Sleight DR, Thomford NR: Gross anatomy of the blood supply and biliary drainage of the canine liver. *Anat Rec* 166:153-160, 1970.
24. MacKenzie RJ, Furnival CM, O'Keane MA, et al: The effect of hepatic ischemia on liver function and the restoration of liver mass after 70 percent partial hepatectomy in the dog. *Br J Surg* 62:431-437, 1975.
25. Siegel B: Partial hepatectomy in the dog: A revised technique based on anatomic consideration. *Arch Surg* 87:788-791, 1963.
26. Bradley EL: A technique for choledochoduodenostomy. *Am Surg* 48:599-600, 1982.
27. Tangner CH, Turrel JM, Hobson HP: Complications associated with proximal duodenal resection and cholecystoduodenostomy in two cats. *Vet Surg* 11:60-64, 1982.
28. Tangner CH: Cholecystoduodenostomy in the dog. Comparison of two techniques. *Vet Surg* 13:126-134, 1984.
29. Rutledge RH: Sphincteroplasty and choledochoduodenostomy for benign biliary obstructions. *Ann Surg* 183:476-480, 1976.

The Pathophysiology of Acute Mechanical Small Bowel Obstruction

Gary C. Lantz, DVM
Assistant Professor of Surgery
School of Veterinary Medicine
Purdue University
West Lafayette, Indiana

Small bowel obstruction is a frequent occurrence in small animal practice. It is essential that the clinician have a working knowledge of the pathophysiologic events that can occur in the patient with bowel obstruction. This knowledge helps the diagnostician maintain an index of suspicion for obstruction and reinforces the important concepts of early diagnosis and rapid, systematic therapeutic intervention. This paper will briefly review the physiologic alterations that occur in the patient with an obstructed small bowel.

The diagnosis of small intestinal obstruction is based on history, physical examination, and radiography. Clinical signs may include lethargy, anorexia, vomiting, diarrhea, and abdominal distention. Clinical findings include abdominal pain, dehydration, and shock. The manifestations of small bowel obstruction depend upon such factors as the duration, location, and degree of obstruction and the amount of damage to the blood supply.

The two major classifications of bowel obstruction are *simple* and *strangulated*.[1] Simple obstruction is partial or complete luminal blockage which results in fluid and electrolyte loss. The mesenteric circulation is not involved. With strangulated obstruction there may or may not be luminal blockage, but there is some interruption of the mesenteric blood supply.

Simple Obstruction

The definition of simple obstruction must be qualified by stating that the intramural circulation may potentially be impaired by bowel distention occurring proximal to the obstruction or by direct pressure applied against the wall by an intraluminal mass, i.e., a foreign body (Figure 1). Compromise of wall integrity can result in the loss of lumen contents and peritonitis. The consequences of this complication will be discussed under the section on strangulation obstruction.

Distention starts in the portion of the intestine immediately proximal to the obstruction. Fluid and gas contribute to the distention (Figure 2). The fluid is comprised of the normal amounts of daily digestive secretions (Table I) and increased local bowel secretions. The composition and sources of the intraluminal gas are listed in Table II. The type of diet or residual materials within the intestinal lumen do not significantly alter the gas composition.[3]

Originally published in Volume 3, Number 10, October 1981

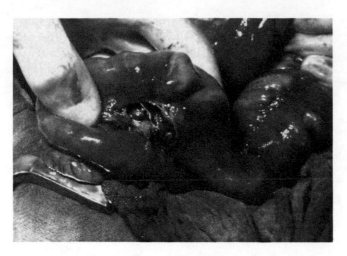

Figure 1—Pressure necrosis and perforation of the intestinal wall secondary to an intraluminal foreign body.

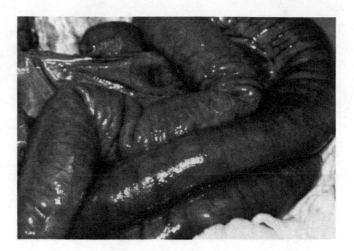

Figure 2—Gas- and fluid-distended small bowel proximal to a manually reduced distal jejunal intussusception.

The effects of distention are related to duration of the obstruction and intraluminal pressure. Normal small bowel intraluminal pressure ranges from 2 to 4 mm Hg.[4,5] Experimentally created simple small bowel obstruction demonstrated intraluminal pressures between 5 and 10 mm Hg[4-6] that were maintained for the 72-hour duration of the experiments. Intraluminal pressure proximal to the obstruction may gradually increase as a result of further accumulation of gas and fluid.[7,8] This increased pressure can cause venous congestion and additional fluid loss in the form of bowel wall edema and extravasation into the peritoneal cavity.[1,9] The intraluminal pressure is influenced by eructation, vomiting, and the passage of flatus and diarrhea. Distention can cause vascular compromise and anoxia in the involved intestinal segment. Rapid artificial distention causes lymphatic and capillary stasis at 30 mm Hg, totally occludes venous drainage at 50 mm Hg, and stops arterial flow at 90 mm Hg.[7,9] Studies have determined that small bowel obstruction involves a slow, moderate increase in intraluminal pressure.[4,6,10-13] No gross signs of wall devitalization were observed as a result of natural distention occurring after the development of experimental simple obstruction. Continued distention can interfere with the transfer and utilization of oxygen in the wall. This may be related to a distention-altered *autoregulatory* mechanism controlling oxygen extraction at the capillary level.[13] Therefore, the distended intestine is anoxic and vulnerable to devitalization. Sustained, intraluminal pressures during spontaneous simple obstruction could contribute to wall anoxia and devitalization and subsequent contamination of the peritoneal cavity with intraluminal contents. A literature search has failed to discover any documentation of intraluminal pressures during spontaneous obstruction in animals.

Systemic alterations during intestinal distention are primarily from fluid and electrolyte losses. Severe distention can limit normal diaphragmatic excursions and compromise respiration. Distention may also reduce venous return to the heart.[14]

Fluid and electrolyte loss from simple obstruction causes hypovolemia and acid-base imbalance.[15-22] The volume of fluid lost depends on the level, duration, and completeness of the obstruction. Loss occurs from vom-

TABLE I

DAILY VOLUME OF DIGESTIVE SECRETIONS THAT ENTER THE INTESTINE OF A 20-KG DOG*

Source	Volume (ml)
Saliva	300
Gastric	600
Bile	300
Pancreatic	600
Small intestine	300
TOTAL	2100

*From Strombeck D: *Small Animal Gastroenterology.* Davis, CA, Stonegate Publishing, 1979, p 174. Adapted with permission.

TABLE II

COMPOSITION AND SOURCE OF GAS IN SMALL BOWEL DISTENTION[2,3]

Composition
  Nitrogen—70%
  Carbon dioxide—6 to 9%
  Oxygen—10 to 12%
  Hydrogen—1 to 3%
  Methane—less than 1%
  Hydrogen sulfide—1 to 10%

Source
  Swallowed air—72%
  Formed in the body—28%
  Diffusion of gas from blood into bowel lumen—70%
  Intraluminal decomposition of food material—30%

iting, diarrhea, and sequestration of fluid within the intestinal lumen. Intestinal wall edema is due to vascular congestion from increased intraluminal pressures. Wall edema contributes a little to the fluid loss. Insensible water loss and inadequate water intake contribute to the dehydration.

The classic clinical course of upper (duodenum and proximal jejunum) small bowel obstruction is described as frequent vomiting that is initiated soon after the onset of obstruction.[18,23] Studies do not consistently support this finding in the dog.[19,20] Vomiting may occur infrequently and cease within 48 to 72 hours after the onset of obstruction. In general, the closer the obstruction is to the pylorus, the more severe is the vomiting. The major lethal factor of an upper small bowel obstruction is hypovolemia. With severe vomiting and no treatment, death occurs in three to four days.[18] The fatal nature of this hypovolemia and electrolyte loss is substantiated by the fact that infusion of physiologic saline or replacement of the vomitus into the intestine through an enterotomy below the obstruction prolongs life for three to four weeks.[18,23]

Low (distal jejunum and ileum) small bowel obstruction is infrequently associated with vomiting.[21] If vomiting does occur, its onset is approximately two to three days after the onset of obstruction and it is intermittent.[16] Distention may be gaseous in the initial 12 to 36 hours and it is later accompanied by the loss of varying quantities of fluid into the bowel lumen.[19,21,23] Dogs with experimentally produced simple low obstructions are more lethargic than those with high obstruction. They exhibit steady weight loss, they drink but do not eat, and they die of the effects of starvation rather than of fluid and electrolyte loss. They may survive for three or more weeks.[17,19,20,24]

The distended bowel gradually loses its ability to absorb (24 to 144 hours postobstruction),[21,25] and local intestinal secretion is increased (24 to 60 hours postobstruction).[16,21,26] Although these alterations are observed with distention, the complete mechanism is not fully understood.[6,16,21,26,27] Additional factors believed to contribute to increased secretion and decreased absorption include increased concentrations of intraluminal bacterial toxins,[27] bile acids, and fatty acids,[28] and products of tissue ischemia.[26] The intraluminal fluid volume increases as the obstruction becomes more prolonged.[19] The sequestered fluid moves proximally and, in low bowel obstruction, eventually reaches nondistended intestine with normal absorptive capabilities. This portion of fluid and electrolytes is absorbed. In high obstruction, if fluid reaches the proximal duodenum, vomiting and permanent fluid and electrolyte loss occur. Fluid and electrolyte loss is not as severe in low obstructions as it is in upper obstructions.

Fluid initially sequestered in the bowel lumen in low obstruction is isotonic and very similar to plasma in its composition.[16,21,29,30] There is a gradual increase in secretion of sodium, potassium, and albumin into the lumen.[19,21,25,29] This sequestration and increased secretion of fluid, electrolytes, and protein cause a net loss of these materials. Analysis of intraluminal fluid after a low obstruction of 72 hours duration reveals a mean sodium level of 140.3 mEq/liter, potassium level of 16.8 mEq/liter, and albumin level of 36.4 mg/ml.[19] Bicarbonate-rich secretions from the upper intestinal tract are entrapped at the level of the obstruction. The effects of bicarbonate loss, dehydration, and starvation contribute to the development of metabolic acidosis.

Fluid and electrolyte losses that occur with vomiting in high obstructions are dependent on the relationship between the obstruction and the pylorus. Vomiting that occurs secondary to a high duodenal obstruction results in a loss of primarily gastric secretions and an initial metabolic alkalosis. Continued fluid depletion through vomiting, insensible loss, lack of intake, and catabolism of body energy stores causes the later development of metabolic acidosis. Vomiting associated with obstruction at other levels of the proximal intestinal tract results in the loss of basic duodenal fluids and gastric contents. Acid-base values in these patients may range from normal to metabolic acidosis in the initial phase; however, metabolic acidosis will be found later resulting from continued fluid loss and starvation.

Initially, violent peristalsis occurs proximal to the obstruction in an attempt to move the blockage.[9,23] Hyperperistalsis is replaced by rhythmic or nonrhythmic pressure increases of low magnitude in the distended segment. This motor activity can be maintained throughout the course of noncomplicated simple obstruction, but it may be masked by passive backflow of luminal contents.[4,31] Peristaltic activity in the remainder of the intestinal tract may not be affected.[32] Hyperperistalsis in conjunction with a linear foreign body occurs proximal and distal to the obstruction and contributes to laceration of the bowel wall.

The pathophysiology of simple obstruction is summarized in Figure 3.

Strangulation Obstruction

The most serious complication of intestinal obstruction is compromise of the blood supply to the involved bowel segment. This interference can incorporate the mesenteric vessels and result in devitalization of the entire involved intestinal segment or it may be confined to a discrete localized area of bowel wall as with foreign body pressure necrosis. Examples of strangulated obstruction include intussusception, traumatic avulsion of a segment of mesentery, mesenteric arterial thrombosis, intestinal volvulus, and strangulated hernia. Strangulation obstruction can result in a rapidly fatal outcome if it is not promptly relieved. Death is caused by hypovolemia and the events that occur following devitalization of intestinal wall. The clinical course depends on the degree of vascular compromise, the volume of blood and plasma loss, and the absorption of bacteria and toxins.

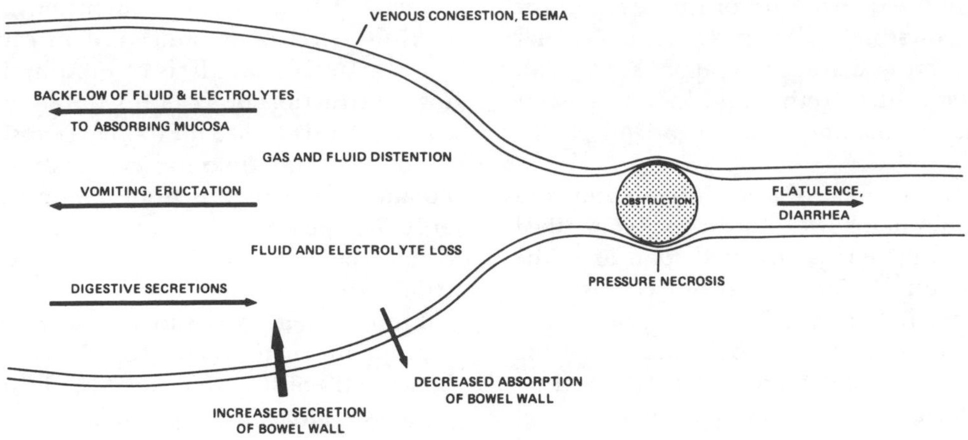

Figure 3—The pathophysiology of simple bowel obstruction.

Partially or totally obstructed venous drainage (i.e., in strangulated hernias and intussusceptions) is the most frequently encountered vascular impairment causing strangulation obstruction in small animals. In the presence of venous obstruction, an intact arterial supply allows the sequestration of blood within the intestinal wall and the subsequent development of wall edema. Bowel distention with gas and fluid occurs proximal to the obstruction, as in simple obstruction. Anoxia and wall necrosis result from the stagnation of blood flow (Figure 4). Blood loss into the bowel lumen and peritoneal cavity[1,9,18,23,33] and the transmural passage of intraluminal bacteria and toxins [34-36] ensue.

The accompanying blood loss and hypovolemia may contribute significantly to the patient's death.[1,18,23,33] Blood loss has been reported to be as high as 61% of total blood volume when large areas of intestine are strangulated.[1] Fluid loss into the bowel proximal to the obstruction and extravasation into the peritoneal cavity also contribute to hypovolemia.[33]

The gross pathologic changes that occur in the bowel after experimental venous ligation are proportional to the duration of the venous obstruction.[36] Immediate observations of the involved bowel segment in one study included marked increase in peristaltic activity and a shortening of the bowel segment.[36] Cyanosis was evident and petechial hemorrhages were developing in the adjacent mesentery and serosa within five minutes. Motility ceased, and the wall was visibly thickened and dark red to blue black in color. Wall edema and hemorrhage and mucosal epithelial sloughing were noted between one and three hours. At four hours the loop had almost regained its normal length, it was turgid, and whole blood was accumulating within the bowel lumen. The wall was greatly thickened from the sequestered mural blood (Figure 5). At 8 to 12 hours the bowel segment was black, maximally distended, and elongated 25 to 50% of its original length. Gross disintegration of the tissues was evident at 20 hours. Histologic examination of the tissues at this time showed masses of bacteria and red cells in all layers of the bowel wall.

Intestinal obstruction alters the concentration and distribution of intestinal bacteria.[37] Normal peristalsis is necessary for the maintenance of normal bacterial concentrations and position in the intestine.[28] Abnormal peristalsis throughout the intestinal tract is found in strangulation obstruction. A large proliferation of resident bacteria in the involved bowel segment takes place. Organisms that are normally confined to the terminal intestinal tract can be found in various levels of the small bowel. The major intestinal flora in dogs comprises clostridia, coliforms, and streptococci.[38] These organisms and bacilli markedly increase in numbers in the area of strangulation[37-39] and are predominant in blood cultures.[36,39] The stagnated luminal contents and devitalized intestinal wall are excellent growth media.[40] Small intestinal bacterial concentrations that normally range from 10^2 to 10^4/g of residual secretion may range from 10^8 to 10^{11}/g of residual secretion.[38] Maximal intraluminal bacterial concentration can be achieved within six hours of the onset of strangulation.[38]

The major toxin-producing organisms are *Escherichia coli* and clostridia. The virulence of *E. coli* is greatly enhanced in the presence of hemoglobin.[11] The mechanisms behind this enhancement are believed to be that hemoglobin acts as a bacterial nutrient, interfering with phagocytosis and/or inhibiting the peritoneal absorption of organisms and subsequent transfer to the reticuloendothelial system for destruction. There is also evidence that hemoglobin may increase the virulence of other gram-negative organisms.[12] A minimum concentration of 4 mg% of hemoglobin is needed to increase virulence.[13] Blood may be continually discharged into the peritoneal cavity and bowel lumen from the congested devitalized wall. The blood and bacteria easily mix. Clostridial exotoxins may contribute to hemoglobin release via hemolysis.

Clostridia are producers of potent exotoxins and proliferate in the presence of devitalized tissue. The most lethal strain is *Clostridium perfringens*. It is rapidly fatal in the presence of dead tissue and is a massive gas producer.[44] Clostridial organisms can be injected

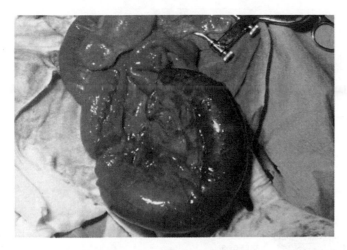

Figure 4—Necrotic intussusception. Approximately 75 ml of a dark pink peritoneal fluid was retrieved from the peritoneal cavity.

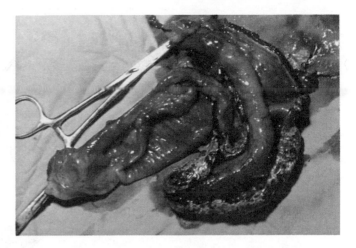

Figure 5—The intussuscipiens (receiving sheath) of the intussusception in Figure 4 has been opened. The thickened, blood-engorged wall is shown. Intraluminal blood can be seen.

intraperitoneally in sublethal concentrations; however, when injections are combined with a sterile, devitalized portion of intestine, death is rapid.[40] Death of animals treated for strangulation obstruction has been attributed to preformed and absorbed clostridial toxins produced in dead tissues.[39,40]

Anoxia of the intestinal wall allows a breakdown of the mucosal barrier that normally prevents absorption of bacteria and toxins.[6,45] Products of bacterial metabolism, primarily the clostridia, probably aid in the devitalization of the bowel wall.[11,23,46,47] Bacteria and toxins quickly diffuse transmurally into the peritoneal cavity. These organisms and toxins are rapidly absorbed through the peritoneum and enter the systemic circulation. Absorption does not occur from venous or lymphatic drainage of the involved bowel segment.[1,47,48] Studies have shown that within five minutes of ligation of the anterior mesenteric artery, bacterial toxins are found in the systemic circulation.[48] It is much longer before toxins are demonstrated in the portal circulation. This illustrates that the intestinal wall barrier is compromised by anoxia and allows transmural migration and transperitoneal absorption of luminal contents. The result in the untreated animal is an endotoxinlike shock syndrome and death.[2,35,49,50,57] An additional source of toxins is thought to be the necrotic bowel wall.[23,40]

The fluid that fills the lumen of the strangulated segment during early obstruction (two to four hours) is small in quantity, odorless, and red black in color. Fluid volume increases as the damage to the bowel wall becomes more severe, allowing greater loss of plasma and whole blood. At 12 hours, the fluid is black, has a foul odor, and is at maximum volume.[35] High concentrations of intraluminal bacteria are present.

Free peritoneal fluid (strangulation fluid) begins to accumulate in the initial two to four hours after obstruction.[35] This fluid, a transudate from serosal vessels that results from venous congestion or obstruction, is pink, clear, and odorless. The fluid is initially abundant but decreases in amount as the devitalization process progresses, possibly due to thrombosis of the serosal vessels and continued peritoneal absorption. Peritoneal fluid is sterile for 4 to 20 hours after strangulation.[35] There is an abrupt change in the appearance of the fluid corresponding to rapid clinical deterioration. The fluid becomes black and has a very foul odor and a high concentration of bacteria and toxins. The alteration is due to the filtration of lumen contents through devitalized bowel wall. Death follows in one to four hours. Strangulation fluid is lethal. When it is injected intraperitoneally into clinically normal dogs, death occurs rapidly.[51] The toxic component of strangulation fluid is removed by filtration[43,52] or centrifugation.[47] Fluid prepared by one of these two methods is not lethal. One investigator refutes these findings and has demonstrated that preformed clostridia toxins present in filtered fluid render the fluid highly toxic.[53]

Strangulated low intestinal obstruction experimentally created in 30-cm lengths of small bowel in the dog caused death in 7 to 24 hours.[35] Strangulation of 60-cm segments caused death in 16 to 35 hours.[18] These animals appeared in relatively good condition until one to four hours before death. At that time, severe, continuous vomiting of dark, foul-smelling fluid commenced. The respiratory and pulse rates increased and the blood pressure fell. These parameters showed a dramatic fall prior to death. Rectal temperature ranged from 103° to 107.6°F. Experimentally, death can be averted by collecting all the peritoneal fluid in a plastic bag wrapped around the strangulated segment.[43] Death is delayed by the administration of systemic antibiotics which suppress bacterial growth and thereby prolong the integrity of the bowel wall.[23,39] The toxic factor(s) form in the lumen of the bowel and can only migrate out when the bowel wall integrity has been destroyed by vascular compromise and products of bacterial growth.[23] The cause of death is probably a combination of hypovolemia, living bacteria and their toxins, and products of tissue necrosis.[11,39,43,50-55]

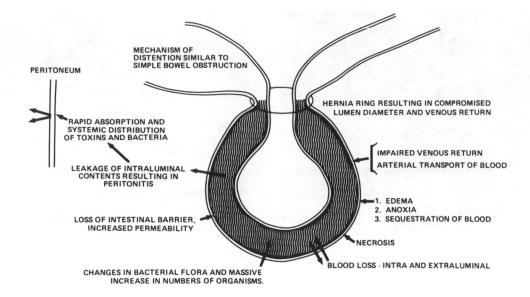

MECHANISM OF
DISTENTION SIMILAR TO
SIMPLE BOWEL OBSTRUCTION

PERITONEUM

HERNIA RING RESULTING IN COMPROMISED
LUMEN DIAMETER AND VENOUS RETURN

RAPID ABSORPTION AND
SYSTEMIC DISTRIBUTION
OF TOXINS AND BACTERIA

IMPAIRED VENOUS RETURN
ARTERIAL TRANSPORT OF BLOOD

LEAKAGE OF INTRALUMINAL
CONTENTS RESULTING IN
PERITONITIS

1. EDEMA
2. ANOXIA
3. SEQUESTRATION OF BLOOD

LOSS OF INTESTINAL BARRIER,
INCREASED PERMEABILITY

NECROSIS

BLOOD LOSS - INTRA AND EXTRALUMINAL

CHANGES IN BACTERIAL FLORA AND MASSIVE
INCREASE IN NUMBERS OF ORGANISMS.

Figure 6—The pathophysiology of strangulated obstruction.

The pathophysiology of strangulation obstruction is summarized in Figure 6.

Clinical Applicability

Specific diagnostic and therapeutic discussions are available,[28,58-60] so they will not be reviewed here in detail. Some important general considerations regarding diagnosis and treatment will be mentioned.

Throughout the discussion of obstruction pathophysiology, events were roughly coordinated with time. The time frames are relatively short and should indicate to the clinician that the obstruction should be relieved as soon as possible. Common errors in the management of small bowel obstruction are listed in Table III.

Initial patient management consists of a complete history and physical examination. Blood and urine studies are helpful in making a differential diagnosis. Survey abdominal radiographs or possibly contrast radiography of the gastrointestinal system are needed to confirm the diagnosis. Differentiation between a mechanical ileus related to an intestinal obstruction and a nonmechanical ileus from other causes is essential in order to prevent needless surgery. The patient should be carefully monitored to detect clinical findings suggesting intestinal strangulation (Table IV). Laboratory data suggestive of strangulation include leukocytosis with left shift (early course) or leukopenia (later course), low hematocrit, and pink to dark red peritoneal fluid with peritoneal lavage.

The majority of patients presented with an obstruction are clinically dehydrated. Replacement therapy is instituted immediately and continued during the diagnostic period. In general, a solution equivalent to lactated Ringer's is used. Normal saline is the fluid of choice in the early course of obstruction with vomiting. A minimum of 80% of the calculated fluid deficits is replaced prior to surgical intervention. Perioperative fluid administration will help assure adequate tissue perfusion. The rate of initial administration may be as high as 90 mg/kg/hour; however, central venous pressure should be monitored to prevent volume overload. The

TABLE III

COMMON ERRORS AND PROBLEMS IN THE
MANAGEMENT OF SMALL BOWEL OBSTRUCTION[57]

1. Delay in diagnosing bowel obstruction

2. Difficulty in differentiating simple from strangulated obstruction

3. Improper preoperative fluid and electrolyte administration

4. Inappropriate timing of surgical intervention

5. Poorly performed surgery

6. Failure to provide adequate postoperative supportive care

TABLE IV

CLINICAL FINDINGS SUGGESTING
INTESTINAL STRANGULATION[57,58]

1. Abdominal tenderness and/or localized pain

2. Fever

3. Subnormal temperature

4. Palpable abdominal mass or irreducible hernia

5. Rectal blood

6. Tachycardia

7. Slow capillary refill, pale mucous membranes

8. Increased respiratory rate

9. Shock

volume of urine production and the hematocrit can be used as rough guides for monitoring hydration. Whole blood transfusions may be needed for patients with a strangulated obstruction. In the majority of cases, administering fluids to restore hydration and electrolyte balances and relief of the obstruction correct acid-base abnormalities. Metabolic acidosis is the most commonly encountered alteration.

Some intestinal foreign bodies may pass through the intestine. Patients with this condition require continual monitoring, baseline laboratory data (minimally, a CBC, BUN, and urinalysis), periodic radiography to determine if the object is moving through the intestine, fluid administration to maintain hydration, and consideration of antibiotics as described below. The decision to pursue this conservative therapy is based upon initial physical examination findings of a near normal patient. Failure to radiographically demonstrate movement of the object within the intestine over an eight-hour period or nonexcretion within 36 hours indicates that surgical removal is necessary. Surgery is also indicated at any time during the observation period if abnormal findings such as abdominal pain, fever, vomiting, and lethargy appear.

Surgical correction is required for most small bowel obstructions. Preoperative parenteral antibiotics (i.e., kanamycin, gentamicin, ampicillin, chloramphenicol) are administered and continued after correction of the obstruction. Antibiotics are justified for three reasons. First, an enterotomy or bowel resection is often required and this carries the risk of peritoneal contamination. Second, in the presence of strangulation, intraluminal bacteria are proliferating and the bowel wall viability is compromised. Bacterial leakage is a threat. The third reason is that foreign bodies may abrade the mucosa or cause pressure necrosis, allowing systemic absorption of bacteria. Aspiration pneumonia, secondary to vomiting, can occur and this necessitates careful attention to respiratory status. Proper surgical technique and exploration of the entire abdominal cavity is essential.

Postoperative fluid and nutritional support and close observation are necessary as with any surgical patient. Oral food and water are started the first postoperative day. The food should be soft and given in small, frequent quantities during the day. Intestinal motility is usually returned to near normal by the first or second postoperative day. If ileus persists, the possibility of peritonitis or recurrent intestinal obstruction (i.e., intussusception or volvulus) should be investigated by radiography, peritoneal lavage, laboratory data, and observation of patient lethargy. Low serum potassium can also contribute to decreased bowel motility.

In conclusion, acute mechanical small bowel obstruction is a disease that may have fatal results shortly after onset. The clinician must maintain an index of suspicion for bowel obstruction, make a rapid diagnosis, and quickly apply appropriate therapy in accordance with the pathophysiology of the condition.

REFERENCES

1. Noer R: Intestinal obstruction, in Cole WH, Zollinger RM (eds): *Textbook of Surgery*, ed 9. New York, Appleton-Century-Crofts, 1970, pp 810-812.
2. Danhop IE: Mechanism of intestinal gas formation with reference to carbon dioxide. *South Med J* 56:768-776, 1968.
3. Hibbard J: Gaseous distention associated with mechanical obstruction of the intestine. *Arch Surg* 33:146-167, 1936.
4. Ohman U: Studies of small intestinal obstruction I. Intraluminal pressure in experimental low small bowel obstruction in the cat. *Acta Chir Scand* 141:413-416, 1975.
5. Owings JC, et al: Intraintestinal pressure in obstruction. *Arch Surg* 17:507, 1928.
6. Mickovitch V, et al: Morphology and function of the dog ileum after mechanical occlusion. *Clin Sci Molec Med* 50:123-130, 1976.
7. Ruf W, et al: Intestinal blood flow at various intraluminal pressure in the piglet with closed abdomen. *Ann Surg* 191:157-163, 1980.
8. Sperling L, et al: Intra-enteric pressure in experimental and clinical obstruction. *Proc Soc Exp Biol Med* 32:1504-1509, 1936.
9. Nadrowski L: Pathophysiology and current treatment of intestinal obstruction. *Rev Surg* 31:381-407, 1974.
10. Ohman U: Studies on small intestinal obstruction II. Blood flow, vascular resistance, capillary filtration and oxygen consumption in denervated small bowel with obstruction. *Acta Chir Scand* 141:417-423, 1975.
11. Shirota A, et al: Experimental studies on acute strangulated intestinal obstruction in germ free animals. *Int Surg* 53:223-229, 1970.
12. Ohman U: Studies on small intestinal obstruction VI. Blood circulation in moderately distended small bowel with obstruction. *Acta Chir Scand* 141:771-779, 1975.
13. Ohman U: Blood flow and oxygen consumption in the feline small intestine: Responses to artificial distention and intestinal obstruction. *Acta Chir Scand* 142:329-333, 1976.
14. Wangensteen D: *Intestinal Obstruction*, ed 2. Springfield, IL, Charles C Thomas, 1942.
15. Billig D, et al: Hemodynamic abnormalities secondary to extracellular fluid depletion in intestinal obstruction. *Surg Gynecol Obstet* 128:1274-1282, 1969.
16. Drucker W, et al: Physiology and pathophysiology of intestinal fluids. *Curr Probl Surg* :34-36, 1964.
17. Enquist I, et al: Changes in body fluid spaces in dogs with intestinal obstruction. *Surg Gynecol Obstet* 127:17-22, 1968.
18. Surgical physiology of intestinal obstruction, in Markowitz J, et al (eds): *Experimental Surgery*, ed 5. Baltimore, Williams & Wilkins Co, 1964.
19. Mishra N, et al: The effects of distention and obstruction on the accumulation of fluid in the lumen of small bowel of dogs. *Ann Surg* 180:791-795, 1974.
20. Nepomuceno O, et al: Extracellular volume changes in experimental high small bowel obstruction. *Am J Surg* 117:643-646, 1969.
21. Shields R: The absorption and secretion of fluid and electrolytes by the obstructed bowel. *Br J Surg* 52:774-779, 1965.
22. Welbourn R: Management of water and electrolyte in acute intestinal obstruction. *West Afr Med J* 17:199-202, 1968.
23. Miller L: The pathophysiology and management of intestinal obstruction. *Surg Clin North Am* 42:1285-1309, 1962.
24. Ming S, et al: Evolution of lesions of intestinal ischemia. *Arch Pathol Lab Med* 101:40-43, 1977.
25. Surg T, et al: Intravenous fluid infusion in small bowel obstruction. *Am J Surg* 121:91-95, 1971.
26. Mickovitch V, et al: The consequences of ischemia after mechanical obstruction of the dog ileum. *Res Exp Med (Berl)* 168:45-55, 1976.
27. Field M: Intestinal secretion. *Gastroenterology* 66:1063-1084, 1974.
28. Strombeck D: *Small Animal Gastroenterology*. Davis, CA, Stonegate Publishing, 1979, pp 291-300.
29. Matsubara K: Experimental studies of intestinal obstruction in dogs: Its clinical and hematological findings on ileum obstruction. *Jpn J Vet Res* 22:102, 1974.
30. Thurman J, et al: Physiologic changes affecting anesthetic management in gastrointestinal obstruction. *Vet Clin North Am* 3:65-78, 1973.
31. Nylander G, et al: Gastric emptying and propulsive intestinal motility in experimental intestinal obstruction. *Acta Chir Scand* 134:135-145, 1968.

32. Dixon J, et al: Intestinal motility following luminal and vascular occlusion of the small intestine. *Gastroenterology* 58:673-678, 1970.
33. Scott H: Intestinal obstruction; Experimental evidence on the loss of blood in strangulation obstruction. *Arch Surg* 36:816-837, 1938.
34. Cuevas P, et al: Role of intraintestinal endotoxin in death from peritonitis. *Surg Gynecol Obstet* 134:953-957, 1972.
35. Nemir P, et al: The cause of death in strangulation obstruction: An experimental study. *Ann Surg* 130:857-873, 1949.
36. Yale C: Experimental strangulated intestinal obstruction. *Surgery* 66:338-344, 1969.
37. Yale C, et al: The importance of six common bacteria in intestinal strangulation. *Arch Surg* 104:438-442, 1972.
38. Cohn I, et al: Imbalance of the normal microbial flora, influence of strangulation obstruction upon the bacterial ecology of the small intestine. *Am J Dig Dis* 10:873-882, 1965.
39. Bornside G, et al: Intestinal bacteriology of closed loop, strangulated obstruction in dogs. *Gastroenterology* 41:245-250, 1961.
40. Cohn I, et al: The role of *Clostridium welchii* in strangulation obstruction. *Ann Surg* 134:999-1006, 1951.
41. Youmans R, et al: The potentiation of bacterial contamination by hemoperitoneum. *J Surg Res* 4:567-568, 1964.
42. Bornside G, et al: Hemoglobin as a bacterial virulence enhancing factor in fluids produced in strangulation intestinal obstruction. *Am Surg* 34:63-67, 1968.
43. Yull A, et al: The peritoneal fluid in strangulation obstruction. The role of the red blood cell and *E. coli* bacteria in producing toxicity. *J Surg Res* 4:223-232, 1962.
44. Yale C, et al: The importance of clostridia in experimental intestinal strangulation. *Gastroenterology* 71:793-796, 1976.
45. Johnson D, et al: Experimental studies of fluid pathophysiology in small intestinal obstruction in the rat IV. Effects of intraluminal hyperosmolality and simultaneous intravenous infusions in mucosal micromorphology. *Scand J Gastroenterol* 13:373-384, 1978.
46. Tanturi C, et al: Lecithinase and hyoluronidase in experimental intestinal obstruction. *Surg Gynecol Obstet* 90:171-174, 1950.
47. Turner M, et al: A study of the lethal mechanisms in experimental closed loop strangulated obstruction of the small intestine. *Am J Surg* 102:560-568, 1961.
48. Cuevas P, et al: Route of absorption of endotoxin from the intestine in nonseptic shock. *J Reticuloendothel Soc* 11:535-538, 1972.
49. Barnett W: Shock in strangulation obstruction: Mechanisms and management. *Ann Surg* 157:747-758, 1963.
50. Weipers W, et al: A comparison of the toxic effects of intestinal obstruction fluid with those of certain endotoxins. *J Pathol* 110:295-304, 1972.
51. Nagy L, et al: A study of bacteria and lethal factors in fluids from experimental intestinal obstruction in dogs. *J Pathol Bacteriol* 95:199-210, 1968.
52. Saltz N, et al: The bacterial factor in the lethality of experimental strangulation obstruction. *Surg Gynecol Obstet* 121:319-325, 1965.
53. Bornside G, et al: Enhanced bacterial virulence in fluids produced in strangulation intestinal obstruction. *Soc Exp Biol Med* 121:551-555, 1966.
54. Amundsen E, et al: The toxicity of fluid from experimentally strangulated intestinal loops in the rat. *J Surg Res* 4:306-313, 1964.
55. Trippestad A, et al: The role of hemoglobin for the lethal effect of intestinal strangulation fluid. *J Surg Res* 10:465-470, 1970.
56. Laws H: Management of small bowel obstruction. *Am Surg* 44:313-317, 1978.
57. Leffall L, et al: Clinical aids in strangulation intestinal obstruction. *Am J Surg* 120:756-759, 1970.
58. Larsen LH, Bellenger CR: Stomach and small intestine, in Archibald J (ed): *Canine Surgery*. Santa Barbara, American Veterinary Publications Inc, 1974, pp 576-602.
59. Hornbuckle WE, Klein LJ: Obstruction of the small intestine, in Kirk RW (ed): *Current Veterinary Therapy VI*. Philadelphia, WB Saunders Co, 1977, pp 952-958.
60. O'Brien T: Small intestine, in *Radiographic Diagnosis of Abdominal Disorders in the Dog and Cat: Radiographic Interpretation, Clinical Signs, Pathophysiology*. Philadelphia, WB Saunders Co, 1978, pp 279-351.

The Omentum—The Forgotten Organ: Physiology and Potential Surgical Applications in Dogs and Cats

KEY FACTS

- The omentum has applications in surgery because it can fill dead space, function despite the presence of infection, adhere to other organs, and induce vascularization.
- Omental pedicle grafts allow mobilization of the omentum to distant recipient sites.
- Omental grafts improve the results of gastrointestinal, vascular, and reconstructive surgery.

Purdue University
Giselle Hosgood, BVSc, MS

OMENTAL GRAFTS are often used in gastrointestinal, vascular, and reconstructive surgery in humans and are becoming increasingly important in veterinary surgical procedures. As new techniques for reconstructive and vascular surgery in veterinary patients are developed, surgical applications of the omentum will become increasingly important.

ANATOMY

The greater and lesser omenta[1] (which originate from the dorsal and ventral mesogastria, respectively) make up the organ called the omentum. The lesser omentum is the mesogastric portion extending between the lesser curvature of the stomach and the initial part of the duodenum. The greater omentum is made up of a large bursal portion and smaller splenic and veil portions. Each portion is composed of a double peritoneal sheet that is transparent except for streaks of fat around the traversing blood vessels.

The bursal portion of the greater omentum is of most clinical and surgical significance and is therefore referred to as the omentum. The bursal portion attaches cranioventrally to the greater curvature of the stomach and extends caudally as far as the urinary bladder.

The omentum reflects on itself as it returns to the dorsal region of the stomach, thus covering the intestines with a double layer—the visceral and parietal leaves. The potential cavity between the two leaves is the omental bursa or the lesser peritoneal cavity. The opening of the bursa is the epiploic foramen. In humans and dogs, the size of the omentum is directly related to body weight.[2,3]

Histology

The omentum is a mesothelial membrane with microvilli and glycocalices, which provide a slippery surface that allows passive movement of the omentum through the peritoneal cavity.[4] The omenta of mice, rabbits, dogs, and humans display small (0.5 to 3.0 mm in diameter) aggregates of lymphoid tissue; these aggregates are known as milk spots.[5,6] The milk spots may be as small as two cells thick but increase in size and number in response to inflammatory stimuli.[7] The omental mesothelium is discontinuous over the milk spots and thus enables cells and particulate matter to gain access to the peritoneal cavity.[8]

Blood Supply

In dogs and cats, the major arterial supply of the bursal

portion of the greater omentum is via the epiploic branches of the right and left gastroepiploic arteries. A large epiploic branch emerges from the right gastroepiploic artery and runs caudally in the parietal leaf of the omentum near its right border. A second vessel originating in a similar position runs in the visceral leaf near its right border. Comparable vessels of the left side originate from the splenic artery[1] (Figure 1). In addition to the anastomoses between the epiploic vessels, there is a rich collateral circulation provided by small vessels and capillaries.[5]

The venous drainage mimics the arterial vessels. The right and left gastroepiploic veins drain directly into the portal system via the gastroduodenal and splenic veins, respectively.[1]

Lymphatic Drainage

Lymphatic drainage of the canine omentum originates from the blind bulbous capillaries in the milk spots; these capillaries empty into narrow, one-way collecting channels that run alongside the arteries and veins and anastomose with lymphatics of the serosa of the stomach and spleen.[6] These lymphatics then drain to the subpyloric and splenic lymph nodes, which drain into the celiac nodes, which drain into the thoracic duct.

A secondary lymphatic drainage route is via the wall of the omental bursa to the lacunae (specialized lymphatics) of the visceral surface of the diaphragm. This route is the major efferent lymphatic route of the peritoneal cavity.[9]

Innervation

Omental innervation is restricted to autonomic innervation of the blood vessels.[5]

FUNCTION
Fat Storage

Varying amounts of fat are located around the omental vessels. The omentum is one of the main fat repositories in obese animals.[1]

Immune Function

The normal omental stroma contains mesothelial and histiocytic cells, whereas the milk spots contain cells of lymphoid and myeloid origin—mainly monocytes and macrophages. Other cells found in the omentum are T and B lymphocytes and mast cells.[5] The T and B lymphocytes are a significant source of antibody formation after intraperitoneal immunization.[10] Mast cells are present throughout the peritoneum but are concentrated in the omental milk spots and omental perivascular tissue.[11] Inflammation induces degranulation; because of the perivascular location of the mast cells, endothelial and mesothelial permeability is increased.[12]

The cells of the milk spots have free access to the peritoneal cavity and are apparently the focus of peritoneal phagocytic activity.[13] Stimulated human and murine omental macrophages produce interferon and colony-stimulating factors.[5] Macrophages also play a role in fibroblast func-

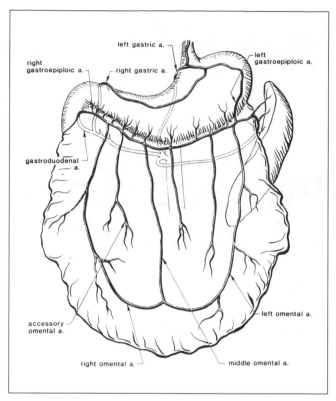

Figure 1—Anatomy and blood supply of the greater omentum.

tion and proliferation; these processes are important in infection control and wound healing in the peritoneal cavity.[5]

Angiogenesis

The omentum is a source of revascularization after injury in the peritoneal cavity[14]; it induces, promotes, and effects angiogenesis.[5] Cells normally active in angiogenesis include activated peritoneal macrophages,[15] mast cells,[16] and lymphocytes,[17] which are all present in the omentum. A lipid angiogenic factor that was isolated from cats induces angiogenesis in rat corneas.[18] The dense superficial capillary network of the omentum is also a site of capillary bud formation after stimulation.[5]

Adhesion

Normal peritoneal mesothelial cells have high fibrinolytic activity.[19] Damage to the mesothelial membrane inhibits this activity and potentiates adhesion formation.[19,20] The omentum is particularly prone to adhesion formation because it can move freely throughout the peritoneal cavity.[5] Adhesion is essential for revascularization[21] and may also provide protection by localizing a contaminant and the subsequent inflammatory response.[19]

SURGICAL APPLICATIONS

Surgical applications of greater omental grafts use the fat-storage, immunogenic, angiogenic, and adhesive properties of the omentum to fill dead space, allow graft function despite the presence of infection, induce vascularization, and adhere to and support other organs during

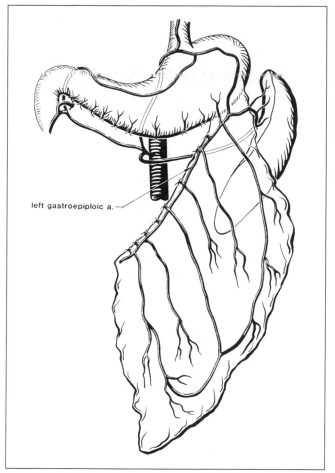

Figure 2A

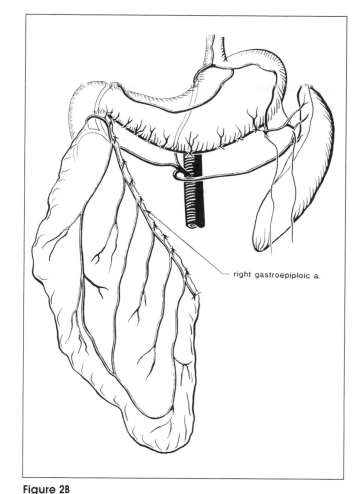

Figure 2B

Figure 2—A greater omental pedicle graft can be based on the left (**A**) or right (**B**) gastroepiploic artery.

healing. These properties have applications in reconstructive surgery, for support of gastrointestinal and vascular anastomoses, and for support of damaged tissue and organs.

Most of the techniques have progressed from experimental efforts to clinically useful procedures in humans; however, techniques in veterinary surgery have not been fully developed.

Creation of the Omental Graft

For surgery within the abdomen, the proximity of the lesion to the free edge of the greater omentum may exclude the need for omental mobilization.[5] The free edge of the omentum is simply placed at the recipient site.[22,23] When lengthening of the omentum is required, an omental pedicle graft based on the right or left gastroepiploic artery is created[5,24,25] (Figure 1). The epiploic branches to the greater curvature of the stomach are ligated, and then the left or right gastroepiploic artery is ligated at its origin[5,25] (Figure 2). Further elongation of the pedicle can be achieved in humans by division within the omentum (Figure 3). Division results in a graft that is longer but is also narrower and more prone to necrosis.[5]

FREE OMENTAL GRAFTING with microvascular transfer is an alternative to further omental division in humans.[2] Because techniques for vascular anastomosis are becoming more common in veterinary surgery, this technique may become useful. After the omental graft is harvested and the recipient site prepared, the omental graft is transferred and the gastroepiploic artery is anastomosed to a major host artery.[5]

Exteriorization of the Omental Pedicle Graft

Exteriorization of the omental pedicle graft for abdominal, thoracic, and head and neck procedures requires a separate abdominal incision placed as close as possible to the recipient site. The incision is made large enough to avoid obstructing vascular flow, and care is taken to avoid torsion of the omental pedicle.

If the recipient site is far from the exit point in the abdominal wall, the omentum is passed through a subcutaneous tunnel.[5,26] In thoracic procedures, the omentum can be passed into the thoracic cavity through a substernal tunnel at the margin of the diaphragm or through lateral diaphragmatic incisions. The omental pedicle is then passed through an appropriate intercostal space.[27]

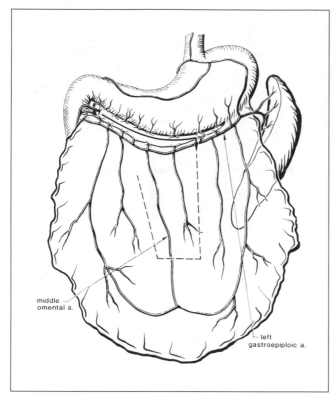

middle
omental a.

left
gastroepiploic a.

Figure 3—In humans, the omental pedicle can be lengthened further by division within the greater omentum. This technique may or may not be applicable in small animals.

Reconstruction
Body Wall Defects

Omental pedicle grafts have been used to cover full-thickness abdominal or thoracic wall defects in humans and have been used experimentally and clinically in dogs.[26-29] The omental graft is placed over polypropylene mesh (Marlex®—Ethicon) and sutured in place.[27,30] The omentum is then covered by skin grafts (advancement skin flaps, free full-thickness or split-thickness skin grafts, or pedicle skin grafts).[26,27,30]

Immediate or delayed (2 to 14 days) skin grafting has been used in humans.[5] For delayed grafting, the exposed omentum is covered by a thin, transparent polyethylene membrane (Opsite®—Smith and Nephew Medical) to prevent drying and allow granulation. Mesh grafting is then preferred because it allows greater coverage with a given amount of skin and permits exudate (which may be profuse from the omentum) to escape.[5]

In dogs with experimentally created diaphragmatic defects that were closed with a left or right gastroepiploic omental pedicle sutured to the periphery of the defect, negative intrathoracic pressure was achieved in 24 hours.[25] The omentum became thicker and firmer and at 60 days showed strong fibrous adhesions and foci of fibrous metaplasia in the normal adipose tissue.[25]

Protection of Vasculature

Exposed vessels and vascular anastomoses have a greater propensity for spontaneous rupture.[31] Pedicle omental grafts have been used to cover vessels, particularly to prevent rupture of vessels in surgical reconstructions of the human head and neck.[31]

Where lengthening techniques are inadequate, free grafts with microvascular anastomoses have been used.[5] As microvascular surgical techniques for veterinary patients are developed, omental protection may become a useful adjunct in many procedures.

Other Reconstructive Procedures

In humans, omental grafting has value in support of reconstructions of the axillae, groin, limbs, and face and for chronic limb ulcers in patients with peripheral arterial disease. Free revascularized omental grafts are most often used. Where skin coverage is not possible, the omental surface is covered with moist, nonadherent dressings until a granulation bed can support skin grafts.[5] Similar procedures may become applicable in small animal surgery as reconstructive techniques are developed.

Abdominal Surgery
Reinforcement of Gastrointestinal Anastomoses

Omental wrapping is the most valuable adjunct procedure for protection of gastrointestinal anastomoses[31] and is used routinely in dogs and cats.[23,30] The rationale for use of the omentum to reinforce anastomoses is based on the following considerations:

- The omentum adds a supplementary layer that provides a seal after adherence to the outer layer of the anastomosis.[5]
- New blood vessels arising from the omental vessels may provide additional blood supply to the anastomosis.[5]
- Phagocytic and other immune functions of the omentum may result in local containment of anastomotic leakage.[5]
- Adhesions contribute to the strength of anastomoses.[32]

THE FREE EDGE OF the omentum is wrapped around the anastomoses and may[22] or may not[23] require loose suturing to the intestinal serosa. To reduce the risk of stricture formation, the omentum should not be wrapped tightly or wrapped 360° around the anastomosis.[33,34] Pedicle omental grafts may be used if additional length of the omental segment is required. Free omental grafts have no role in anastomosis protection because fat necrosis is inevitable and the resultant inflammation may weaken anastomoses.[33]

Extraperitoneal Anastomoses

In humans, extraperitoneal anastomoses of the esophagus, rectum, or colon are associated with an increased occurrence of anastomotic breakdown because of the lack of serosa or parietal peritoneum that is capable of rapid regeneration.[5,31] Omentum has been used successfully to reinforce esophageal anastomoses in human patients[35,36] and in experiments in dogs.[37,38]

Colorectal anastomosis beyond the peritoneal reflections is also associated with high morbidity in humans.[5] Omental pedicles have shown clinical value in reinforcing these anastomoses.[39-41] Although the morbidity associated with extraperitoneal anastomoses in dogs and cats is not documented, the use of omental grafts to support such anastomoses may be beneficial.

Placement of Gastrostomy or Enterostomy Tubes

Enteral tube placement is common in small animal surgery. The omentum can provide a seal and prevent leakage from the entry sites of gastroenterostomy tubes. The omentum is interposed between the body wall and the gastric or enteric serosa.[23,42] The omentum may also help prevent leakage from the stoma after the tubes are removed.

Tube Gastropexy

In gastrostomy-tube gastropexy, the interposition of omentum between the gastric serosa and the body wall may promote adhesion formation.[23] Gastropexy is most commonly performed after correction of gastric dilatation-volvulus in dogs.

Hemostasis

The omentum acts as a natural hemostatic agent[5] and is used in humans to control hemorrhage from parenchymal lacerations of the liver[43,44] and spleen.[45-47] The omentum can also be used to control hemorrhage in veterinary surgery.

The omentum is beneficial in filling dead space in hepatic lacerations. It also aids in the control of oozing hemorrhage when applied to a raw organ surface that is not amenable to suture closure. The omentum is also a rich source of macrophages.[43]

FOR CASES OF SPLENIC INJURY, the omentum can reinforce a suture line[45,46] or the entire fragmented spleen can be wrapped in the omentum and held in place with encircling sutures.[47] The omentum can also be used to cover the cut surface of the kidney after partial nephrectomy.[48]

Revascularization

The ability of the omentum to form a seal and also to stimulate revascularization is useful in the application of the omentum to the surface of organs (e.g., the stomach, bowel, or urinary bladder) that have questionable viability and that cannot be resected.[31] The omentum has also been used to seal small gastric and duodenal perforations in humans; but jejunal defects are associated with a high incidence of leakage, and serosal patching with an adjacent bowel loop is apparently more successful for repair of these perforations.[5] Omental coverage of nonresectable tissue of questionable viability may be beneficial in veterinary surgery.

Bladder Reconstruction

Omentum is suitable as a substitute for the bladder wall. In experimental partial cystectomies in dogs, a pedicle omental graft has been used to cover the defect.[49] The graft rapidly adhered to the defect and was covered with luminal epithelium by 15 days after surgery.[49] Although the margins of the defect no longer have muscular support, collapse and contraction of the omental graft can be prevented by anchoring the margins to other tissue.[5,48]

Thoracic Cavity Surgery

In human thoracic surgery, omental grafts can be used to support repairs of esophageal perforation, to provide blood supply to the mediastinal area when infection is present, to cover bronchial and arterial stumps after pneumonectomy, to support repairs of bronchopleural fistulas, and to obliterate dead space and provide vascular support after cervical exenteration.[5] In veterinary surgery, similar applications of omental grafts may be possible.

COMPLICATIONS

Although partial necrosis of the omentum occurs infrequently, it is the most common complication of omental grafting in humans and might occur in veterinary surgical patients. This complication is most often the result of excessive tension on the vascular pedicle. Partial necrosis may also result from compression or strangulation at the site of emergence and has been associated with the use of a long, narrow subcutaneous tunnel.[50] The omentum, however, is resilient. After the necrotic tissue is excised, the defect will fill with healthy granulation tissue.[5] Other complications reported to occur in humans include incisional hernia, gastric stasis, intestinal obstruction, hemorrhage, colonic ischemia, gastric devascularization, tumor recurrence, and wound infection.[5]

CONCLUSION

The omentum has important potential applications in veterinary surgery. Such simple procedures as support of gastrointestinal anastomosis are already used. Other simple techniques for gastrointestinal and abdominal organs are also available for use in veterinary surgery. Omental grafting has a significant role in reconstructive surgery in humans; and as this discipline in veterinary surgery expands, the extent of the omentum's applicability should become well recognized.

About the Author
When this article was submitted for publication, Dr. Hosgood was affiliated with the Department of Veterinary Clinical Sciences of the School of Veterinary Medicine, Purdue University, West Lafayette, Indiana. She is currently with the Department of Veterinary Clinical Sciences of the School of Veterinary Medicine, Louisiana State University, Baton Rouge, Louisiana.

REFERENCES

1. Evans HE, Christensen GC: *Miller's Anatomy of the Dog*, ed 2. Philadelphia, WB Saunders Co, 1979, pp 467–471.
2. Martin PE, Prevotel M, Poey V, Rivera DC: Dimensiones del velo omental del perro y su relacion con el peso y la longitud corporal. *Zentralbl Veterinarmed [C] Anat Histol Embryol* 114:215–220, 1985.
3. Das SK: The size of the greater omentum and methods of lengthening it for transplantation. *Br J Plast Surg* 29:170–174, 1976.
4. Andrews PM, Porter KR: The ultrastructural morphology and possible function of mesothelial microvilli. *Anat Rec* 177:409–426, 1973.
5. Williams R, White H: The greater omentum: Its applicability to cancer surgery and cancer therapy. *Curr Probl Surg* 23:789–865, 1986.
6. Nylander G, Tjernberg B: The lymphatics of the greater omentum: An experimental study in the dog. *Lymphology* 1:3–7, 1969.
7. Borisov AV: Lymphatic capillaries and blood vessels of milky spots in the human greater omentum. *Fed Proc* 23:150–154, 1964.
8. Hodel C: Ultrastructural studies in the absorption of protein markers by the greater omentum. *Eur Surg Res* 2:435–449, 1970.
9. Higgins GM, Bain CG: The absorption and transference of particulate material by the greater omentum. *Surg Gynecol Obstet* 50:851–860, 1930.
10. Walker FC, Rogers AW: The greater omentum as a site of antibody production. *Br J Exp Pathol* 42:222–231, 1961.
11. Yong LC, Waltkins S, Wilhelm DL: The mast cell: Distribution and maturation in the peritoneal cavity of the adult rat. *Pathology* 7:307–318, 1975.
12. Simionescu M, Simionescu N: Organization of cell junctions in the peritoneal mesothelium. *J Cell Biol* 74:98–110, 1977.
13. Beelen RHJ, Fluitsma DM, Hoefsmit ECM: The cellular composition of omentum milky spots and the ultrastructure of milky spot macrophages and reticulum cells. *J Reticuloendotheliol Soc* 28:585–599, 1980.
14. Ellis H: The causes and prevention of intestinal adhesions. *Br J Surg* 69:241–243, 1982.
15. Polverini PJ, Cotran RS, Gimbrone MA, et al: Activated macrophages induce vascular proliferation. *Nature* 269:804–806, 1977.
16. Azizkhan RG, Azizkhan JC, Zetter GR, et al: Mast cell heparin stimulates migration of capillary endothelial cells in vitro. *J Exp Med* 152:931–944, 1980.
17. Sidky YA, Auerbach R: Lymphocyte-induced angiogenesis: Quantitative and sensitive assay of the graft vs. host reaction. *J Exp Med* 141:1084–1100, 1975.
18. Goldsmith HS, Griffith AL, Kupferman A, Catsimpoolas N: Lipid angiogenic factor from omentum. *JAMA* 252:2034–2036, 1984.
19. Ryan GB, Grobety J, Majno G: Mesothelial injury and recovery. *Am J Pathol* 171:93–112, 1973.
20. Hau T, Haaga JR, Aeder MI: Pathophysiology, diagnosis and treatment of abdominal abscesses. *Curr Probl Surg* 21:1–83, 1984.
21. Myllarniemi H, Karpinen V: Vascular pattern of peritoneal adhesions. *Br J Surg* 55:605–608, 1968.
22. Krahwinkel DJ, Richardson DC: Surgery of the small intestine, in Bojrab MJ (ed): *Current Techniques in Small Animal Surgery*, ed 2. Philadelphia, Lea & Febiger, 1983, pp 162–174.
23. van Sluijs FJ, Happe RP: The stomach: Surgical diseases, in Slatter DK (ed): *Textbook of Small Animal Surgery*. Philadelphia, WB Saunders Co, 1985, pp 684–717.
24. Alday ES, Goldsmith HS: Surgical technique for omental lengthening based on arterial anatomy. *Surg Gynecol Obstet* 135:103–107, 1972.
25. Bright RM, Thacker HL: The formation of an omental pedicle flap and its experimental use in the repair of a diaphragmatic rent in the dog. *JAAHA* 18:283–289, 1982.
26. Bright RM, Birchard SJ, Long GG: Repair of thoracic wall defects in the dog with an omental pedicle flap. *JAAHA* 18:277–282, 1982.
27. Mathiesen DJ, Grillo HC, Vlahakes GJ, Daggert WM: The omentum in the management of complicated cardiothoracic problems. *J Thorac Cardiovasc Surg* 95:677–684, 1988.
28. Jurkiewicz MJ, Arnold PG: The omentum: An account of its use in the reconstruction of the chest wall. *Ann Surg* 185:548–554, 1977.
29. Dupont C, Menard Y: Transposition of the greater omentum for reconstruction of the chest wall. *Plast Reconstr Surg* 49:263–267, 1972.
30. Bright RM: Reconstruction of thoracic wall defects using Marlex mesh. *JAAHA* 17:415–420, 1982.
31. Samson R, Pasternak BM: Current status of surgery of the omentum. *Surg Gynecol Obstet* 149:437–442, 1979.
32. Vance JF, Williams HTG: Mechanical support of healing small intestinal anastomoses in the rat. *Can J Surg* 15:101–107, 1972.
33. Carter DC, Jenkins DHR, Whitfield HN: Omental reinforcement of intestinal anastomoses. An experimental study in the rabbit. *Br J Surg* 59:129–133, 1972.
34. McLachlin AD, Denton DW: Omental protection of intestinal anastomoses. *Am J Surg* 125:134–140, 1973.
35. Fekete F, Breil P, Rouse H, et al: EEA stapler and omental graft in esophagogastrectomy. *Ann Surg* 193:825–830, 1981.
36. Hugh TB, Lusby RJ, Coleman MJ: Antral patch esophagoplasty (a new procedure for acid-peptic esophageal stricture). *Am J Surg* 137:221–225, 1979.
37. Goldsmith HS, Kiely AA, Randall HT: Protection of intrathoracic esophageal anastomosis by omentum. *Surgery* 63:464–466, 1968.
38. Moore TC, Goldstein J: The use of intact omentum for closure of full-thickness esophageal defects. *Surgery* 193:825–830, 1981.
39. Greenberg BM, Low D, Rosato EF: The use of omental grafts in operations performed upon the colon and rectum. *Surg Gynecol Obstet* 161:487–489, 1985.
40. Goldsmith HS: Protection of low rectal anastomosis with intact omentum. *Surg Gynecol Obstet* 144:584–586, 1977.
41. Lantner B, Robert AM: Use of omental pedicle graft to protect lower anterior colonic anastomosis. *Dis Colon Rectum* 22:448–451, 1979.
42. Crane SW: Placement and maintenance of a temporary feeding tube gastrostomy in the dog and cat. *Compend Contin Educ Pract Vet* II(10):770–776, 1980.
43. Pachter HL, Spencer FC: Recent concepts in the treatment of hepatic trauma. *Ann Surg* 190:423–425, 1979.
44. Stone NH, Lamb JM: Use of pedicled omentum as an autogenous pack for control of hemorrhage in major injuries of the liver. *Surg Gynecol Obstet* 141:92–96, 1975.
45. Burrington JD: Surgical repair of a ruptured spleen in children. *Arch Surg* 112:417–418, 1977.
46. Sherman NJ, Asch MJ: Conservative surgery for splenic injuries. *Pediatrics* 61:247–252, 1978.
47. Buntain WL, Lynn HB: Splenorrhaphy: Changing concepts for the traumatized spleen. *Surgery* 86:748–760, 1979.
48. Turner-Warwick R: The use of the omental pedicle graft in urinary tract reconstruction. *J Urol* 116:341–347, 1976.
49. Goldstein MB, Dearden LC: Histology of omentoplasty of the urinary bladder in the rabbit. *Invest Urol* 3:460–469, 1966.
50. Petit JY, Lacour MD, Margulis A, et al: Indications and results of omental pedicle grafts in oncology. *Cancer* 44:2343–2348, 1979.

UPDATE

A recent study has confirmed that the omental pedicle in dogs can be lengthened without vascular compromise and will attain sufficient length to reach any region of the body.[1] The omental pedicle is established by first releasing the dorsal leaf from its pancreatic attachments and extending it caudally. An inverted L-shaped incision is then made just caudal to the gastrosplenic ligament. This allows the left side of the omentum to be rotated caudally to achieve full extension.[1] This technique may facilitate the use of the omentum for reconstructive procedures distant to the abdomen.

REFERENCE

1. Ross WE, Pardo AD: Evaluation of an omental pedicle extension technique in the dog. *Vet Surg* 22:37–43, 1993.

Intussusception in Dogs and Cats

University of Florida
Daniel D. Lewis, DVM
Gary W. Ellison, DVM, MS

Louisiana State University
Matt G. Oakes, DVM

KEY FACTS

❏ Although intussusceptions are reported as sequelae to a number of disease conditions, the vast majority are idiopathic.

❏ Clinical signs depend on the anatomic level, completeness, and duration of obstruction.

❏ Preoperative considerations should include patient hydration, electrolyte imbalances, acid-base status, and possible sepsis.

❏ Surgical management involves reduction and/or resection and anastomosis, followed by prophylactic enteropexy or enteroplication.

The word *intussusception* is derived from the Latin words *intus* (within) and *suscipere* (to receive). Intussusception is defined as a prolapse or invagination of one portion of the gastrointestinal tract into the lumen of an adjoining segment.[1] The invaginated segment, consisting of an entering tube and a returning tube, is termed the *intussusceptum*, while the receiving sheath is called the *intussuscipiens*. Thus, a simple intussusception is composed of three layers of bowel wall from its outer surface to its inner lumen. The junction of the entering and the returning segments is called the *apex* of the intussusception, whereas the junction of the returning segment and the intussuscipiens is termed the *neck*.[2] Intussusceptions usually occur in the direction of normal peristalsis, with the proximal intussusceptum invaginating into the distal intussuscipiens. Aboral invaginations are designated as *direct* or *forward* intussusceptions. An *indirect* or *retrograde* intussusception is an invagination of a distal segment of the gastrointestinal tract into a proximal segment.[3] Compound or double intussusceptions occasionally occur in which the entire intussusception undergoes a second invagination at the same site and there are five layers of bowel wall rather than three as in a simple intussusception.[4-7] Multiple intussusceptions at more than one location in the gastrointestinal tract also have been reported.[6-9] Multiple intussusceptions may occur as agonal events and can be recognized as such as they are easily reduced and lack appreciable inflammation.[7]

CLASSIFICATION AND LOCATION

Intussusceptions are classified according to their location in the alimentary tract. The first term in this nomenclature refers to the segment of the gastrointestinal tract forming the apex. The latter term in the compound classification refers to the recipient segment. Gastroesophageal, pylorogastric, enteroenteric, enterocolic, and colocolic intussusceptions have been reported in small animals. "Cecal inversion," in which the inverted cecum forms the apex of a cecocolic intussusception, can occur in small animals.[6,8,10-13]

Most intussusceptions in small animals are enterocolic.[6,8,10-12] Two retrospective studies have been published concerning gastrointestinal intussusception in small animals. Wilson and Burt reviewed 50 intussusceptions in 45 animals (40 dogs, 5 cats)[12] and Weaver reviewed an additional 26 intussusceptions (all dogs).[14] In Wilson and Burt's study, enterocolic intussusception was the predominant type (35 enterocolic, 14 enteroenteric, and 1 pylorogastric intussusceptions were reported). All ileo-colic lesions were primary, whereas several of the enteroenteric intussusceptions were considered agonal changes or secondary to a primary enterocolic intussusception.[12] In Weaver's study, only half (13) of the intussusceptions were enterocolic, but 3 of the 13 enteroenteric intussusceptions were short intussusceptions involving the mid or terminal ileum.[14]

INCIDENCE AND PREDISPOSING CAUSES

Puppies and kittens have a much higher incidence of intussusception than adult animals. Thirty-seven of the 45 animals in Wilson and Burt's study were less than one year of age.[12] Nineteen of 26 dogs in Weaver's study were less than six months of age.[14] In a recent review of gastroesophageal intussusception, 80% of the dogs were less than three months of age.[15] There is no apparent sex predisposition in dogs or cats.[12] Siamese cats and German shepherd dogs are more frequently affected than other breeds.[12] German shepherd dogs appear to be at risk for developing gastroesophageal intussusception.[15]

Intussusception has been reported as a sequela to a number of conditions, including intestinal parasitism, linear foreign bodies,[6,12,16] viral-induced enteritis caused by canine distemper[3,6,9,11,12,17] or parvovirus,[17] and prior abdominal surgery.[18,19] Mural lesions associated with intussusceptions in dogs and cats include polypoid masses, congenital enterocysts, intestinal granulomas, and intestinal neoplasia.[3,12,17,20,21] There is an association between esophageal diseases, such as megaesophagus, and gastroesophageal intussusception.[15] The majority of intussusceptions seen in young animals are idiopathic.[3,6,9,11,12,17]

PATHOPHYSIOLOGY

The events involved in the development of intussusceptions remain speculative. Reymond proposed that intussusceptions begin as either an inhomogeneity in a bowel segment or a mechanical linkage of nonadjacent bowel segments.[22,23] The local inhomogeneity may represent a bowel segment that is either flaccid or indurated (e.g., infiltrative bowel disease, a segment of spastic bowel, or a surgical or cicatricial lesion) or a region in which the gastrointestinal tract undergoes a sudden anatomic change in diameter (e.g., the ileocolic or gastroesophageal junction). Mechanical linkage of nonadjacent segments of bowel can be intraluminal (e.g., pedunculated polyps, linear foreign bodies, or parasites) or extramural (e.g., fibrous adhesions or bands). Either of these situations can result in a kink or a fold in the bowel wall that can serve as a precursor for intussusception development. Invagination commences as a result of peristaltic contraction,[22,23] and the progression can be rapid, involving several centimeters of intestinal tract within hours.[11] The initial invaginating segment remains the apex of the intussusception throughout its development. The distance the intussusceptum can invaginate is limited by mesenteric tension; beyond this point, further invagination requires rupture of the mesentery.[7]

Invagination and intussusception result in luminal obstruction, which may be partial or complete. Obstruction usually results in distention of the bowel segment proximal to the intussusception. The degree of distention is dependent on the duration and completeness of obstruction and is caused by gas and fluid accumulation within the bowel lumen. The gas that accumulates proximal to the obstruction is derived from aerophagia, gaseous diffusion from the intestinal microcirculation, and gas produced by digestive fermentation.[9] Gaseous distention causes increased intraluminal pressure.[24] Intestinal secretory and absorptive function is retained in the face of mild increases in intraluminal pressure. Continued increases in intraluminal pressure eventually exceed venous and lymphatic hydrostatic pressure, resulting in intestinal edema. Mucosal absorptive capacity is then lost, resulting in sequestration of fluid within the bowel lumen.[25]

The intussusceptum is particularly prone to vascular compromise. The venous and lymphatic drainage, because of their low hydrostatic pressure, are susceptible to early compromise. Compromised venous and lymphatic return in the presence of an intact arterial circulation results in intramural hemorrhage and edema. Large volumes of blood can be lost into the bowel lumen.[24,26] Exudation of fibrin from serosal surfaces contributes to the development of adhesions which eventually render the intussusception irreducible. If intramural pressure exceeds arterial pressure or if thrombosis occurs within the strangulated segment, full-thickness necrosis may result. Perforation is rare because the ensheathing intussuscipiens generally remains viable.[6] It has been reported that "self-cures" may take place if the neck of the intussusception is sealed off with fibrinous adhesions and the nonviable intussusceptum is sloughed, reestablishing the patency of the intestinal lumen.[6,7,17]

CLINICAL EXAMINATION

Clinical signs accompanying intussusceptions depend on the anatomic level, completeness, and duration of the obstruction. Regurgitation, persistent violent vomiting followed by unproductive retching, dyspnea, hematemesis, and abdominal discomfort are the initial clinical signs associated with gastroesophageal intussusception.[15,27,28] Auscultation of the thorax may reveal dull lung fields.[28] Dogs with gas-

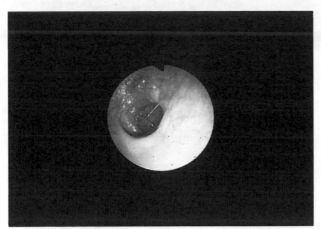

Figure 1—Endoscopic visualization of a cecal inversion. The "umbiliform" structure present on the wall of the ascending colon is the ileocolic sphincter. (Courtesy of Dr. C. F. Burrows, University of Florida)

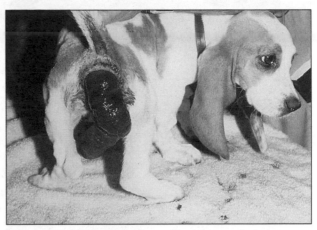

Figure 2—Twelve-week-old puppy with a prolapsed enterocolic intussusception.

troesophageal intussusceptions deteriorate rapidly and the outcome is almost universally (95.5%) fatal. Less than 20% of affected dogs are diagnosed antemortem.[15]

The cardinal signs of intestinal intussusception are recurrent or sporadic vomiting, bloody mucoid diarrhea, and a palpable cylindrical or "sausage-shaped" abdominal mass.[11] The mass is usually palpated in the cranial abdomen because most intussusceptions involve the ileocolic region. Occasionally intussusceptions escape palpation because of a remote craniodorsal position. Abdominal pain is not a consistent finding.[12]

High intestinal intussusception results in more severe, acute symptoms than low obstruction.[24] Frequent vomiting is common with upper (pyloric, duodenal, and proximal jejunal) gastrointestinal obstruction. Without treatment, death may occur within 72 to 96 hours as the result of lethal hypovolemia, electrolyte disturbances, and acid-base imbalances.[29] Vomiting is not consistently associated with low obstruction. When present, vomiting is less acute and more intermittent than with upper intestinal obstruction.[27] Dogs with experimentally induced low intestinal obstruction may survive three weeks or longer and die of starvation rather than dehydration or electrolyte imbalances.[30–32] A chronic history of sporadic vomiting, anorexia, and hematotenesmus is typically associated with enterocolic or colocolic intussusception.[17] Animals with cecal inversion present with a history of chronic intermittent hematochezia and soft stools. Clinical signs generally persist despite prior medical therapy.[13,33] Colonoscopy using a flexible fiberoptic endoscope has been a useful procedure in diagnosing cecocolic intussusception (Figure 1).[13]

Occasionally in animals with enterocolic[14] or colo-

colic[3] intussusception, the intussuscepted bowel may protrude through the anus (Figure 2) and must be differentiated from a rectal prolapse.[11] This is accomplished by passing a blunt probe between the protruding segment and the anal sphincter. If the probe can be passed cranial to the pubis without reaching a fornix, then the protruding bowel is the apex of an intussusception rather than a rectal prolapse.[11]

RADIOGRAPHIC EXAMINATION

Definitive radiographic diagnosis of an intussusception on plain radiographs may be difficult.[3] Gastroesophageal intussusception should be suspected when there is esophageal dilatation and a soft tissue density within the thoracic esophagus adjacent to the diaphragm (Figure 3A). The gas-filled gastric fundus may be absent or reduced in size (Figure 3B). A positive-contrast esophagram may delineate the apex of the intussusceptum. In addition, the lungs should be carefully evaluated for evidence of aspiration pneumonia.[28]

In many cases of intestinal intussusception, gas and fluid accumulate proximal to the intussusception, producing signs of obstructive bowel disease. The degree of bowel distention reflects the completeness and duration of obstruction. When the obstruction is complete, the intestinal tract distal to the intussusception may be devoid of fecal material. The intussusception may be apparent as a well-defined mass in the cranioventral or central abdomen. The apex of the intussusception might be outlined if sufficient gas accumulates in the distal intestinal segment (Figure 4). In animals with an enterocolic intussusception, the gas shadows of the cecum and ascending colon often are absent.

Contrast studies can be used to differentiate an intussusception from other forms of obstructive bowel disease. Upper gastrointestinal studies usually are not

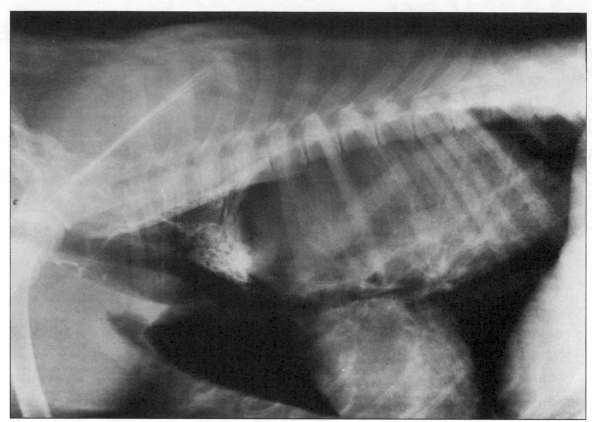

Figure 3A

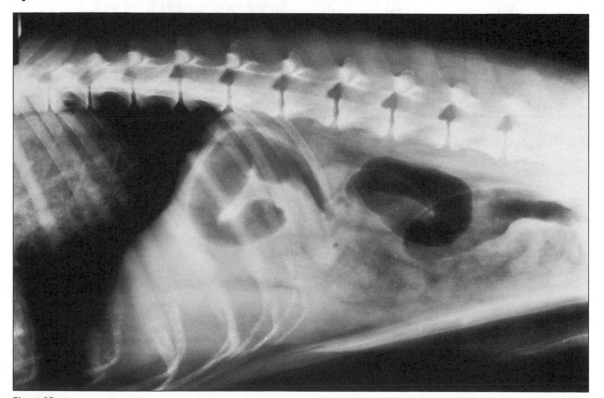

Figure 3B

Figure 3—(A) Lateral thoracic radiograph of a dog with a gastroesophageal intussusception. Note the dilated esophagus (with food material present in the cranial thoracic esophagus) and the large, soft tissue-dense mass present in the distal esophagus. **(B)** Lateral abdominal radiograph of the same dog. Note the absence of a gas-filled gastric fundus. (Courtesy of Dr. D. A. Hager, University of Florida)

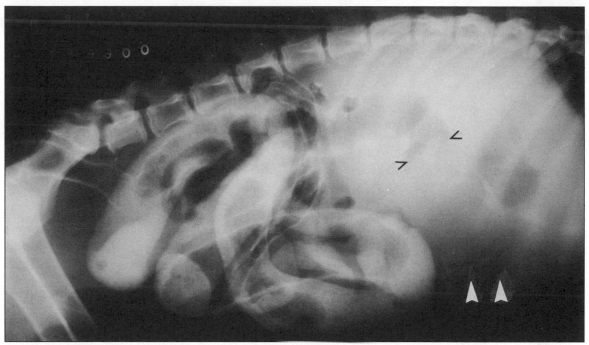

Figure 4—Lateral abdominal radiograph of a dog with ileocolic intussusception. Intestinal obstruction is apparent. There is ileus of the small intestine and the colon is devoid of feces. The apex of the intussusception is readily apparent (*black arrows*). A "coil spring" pattern is produced by gas trapped between the plicated wall of the intussusceptum and the intussuscipiens (*white arrows*).

rewarding if the obstruction is complete. In the presence of ileus, contrast material may not reach the level of obstruction because of the lack of peristaltic contraction. If the obstruction is incomplete and the lumen of the intussusceptum is patent, a ribbon of contrast material may be visible within the intussusceptum aboral to a dilated bowel segment. Contrast material also may accumulate in the lumen between the intussusceptum and the intussuscipiens (Figure 5). The lesion may not become evident until as late as 24 hours after administration of the contrast material.

Enterocolic and colocolic intussusceptions are more successfully identified by barium enema or pneumocolon than upper gastrointestinal studies. The intussusception may be visualized as the contrast interface outlines the apex of the intussusceptum (Figure 6). The appearance of this interface has been described at times as resembling the numeral 3. Gas or contrast material may dissect between the returning sheath of the intussusceptum and the intussuscipiens, creating a "coil spring" appearance (Figure 4).[3]

Barium enema is a technique used to reduce enterocolic intussusception in human infants.[34–36] Most enterocolic intussusceptions in dogs and cats are chronic and, therefore, the presence of inflammation, edema, and fibrous adhesions would likely preclude hydrostatic reduction.[12]

PREOPERATIVE MANAGEMENT

Preoperative considerations should include patient hydration, electrolyte imbalances, acid-base status, and possible sepsis. The preanesthetic evaluation should include a complete blood count, serum electrolyte values, and an acid-base determination (if available). A search for predisposing factors should be initiated.

Vomiting associated with gastroesophageal, pylorogastric, and high duodenal intussusceptions can be profuse and fluid loss may consist primarily of gastric secretions high in H^+, Cl^- and K^+. When vomitus consists primarily of gastric fluids, metabolic alkalosis may exist initially but continued vomiting, anorexia, and ongoing insensible losses cause metabolic acidosis to develop. Dehydration can be severe. Vomiting associated with obstruction distal to the proximal duodenum results in metabolic acidosis secondary to the loss of alkaline duodenal fluids. Dehydration and electrolyte derangements usually are not as severe with low intestinal obstruction.[24] because vomiting is typically intermittent. Intravenous fluid therapy with correction of volume and electrolyte depletion should be initiated prior to anesthesia. A balanced electrolyte solution, such as lactated Ringer's, will adequately correct the situation in mildly affected animals. Potassium should be supplemented as necessary. In animals with severe hypochloremia or hyponatremia,

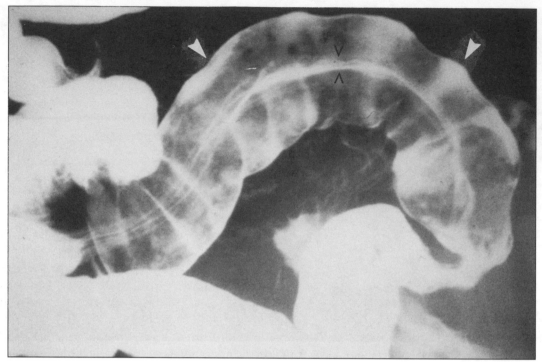

Figure 5—Close-up of a lateral abdominal radiograph of a dog with an ileocolic intussusception following oral barium administration showing the patent lumen of the intussusceptum (*black arrows*) and the contrast interface between the intussusceptum and intussuscipiens (*white arrows*).

0.9% NaCl is administered. If substantial acidosis exists (pH <7.2 and base deficit > –10 mEq/L), conservative sodium bicarbonate therapy is indicated.[37] Acid-base determinations in clinical cases of vomiting have revealed metabolic acidosis to occur only slightly more frequently than metabolic alkalosis. Thus, indiscriminate sodium bicarbonate therapy for these cases is not advised.[38]

Antimicrobial therapy should be instituted before surgical intervention. Most intussusceptions require resection and anastomosis, and entrance into the alimentary tract lumen constitutes a clean-contaminated surgical wound; therefore, antimicrobial prophylaxis is justified.[39] Alterations in the normal gastrointestinal bacterial flora occur with impairment of local circulation. If circulatory impairment progresses to necrosis, the devitalized tissue provides an excellent medium for bacterial growth. Coliform and clostridial organisms increase in number.[40] The mucosal barrier (which normally functions to prevent the absorption of bacteria and toxins) is disrupted, allowing transmural migration into the peritoneal cavity to occur. Rapid absorption through the peritoneum into the systemic circulation can result in septicemia and possible endotoxic shock.[24] Parenteral bactericidal antibiotic therapy is advocated. Gentamicin sulfate (Gentocin® Solution—Schering), 2 to 4 mg/kg IV or IM every six hours, alone or in combi-

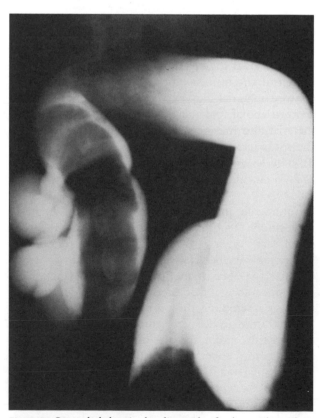

Figure 6—Lateral abdominal radiograph of a dog with an ileocolic intussusception after administration of a barium enema. (Courtesy of Dr. N. Ackerman, University of Florida)

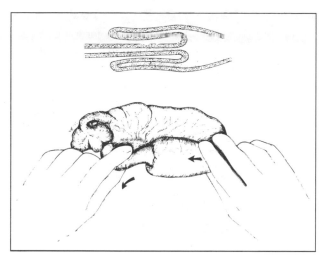

Figure 7—Manual reduction of an intestinal intussusception. The intussusceptum is gently milked from the intussuscipiens with minimal traction placed on the proximal segment. (Reprinted, with permission, from Krahwinkel DJ, Richardson DC: Intestines, in Bojrab MJ (ed): *Current Techniques in Small Animal Surgery*, ed 2. Philadelphia, Lea & Febiger, 1983, pp 162–173)

nation with sodium cephalothin (Keflin®—Eli Lilly), 15 mg/kg IV every six hours, or penicillin G potassium (E.R. Squibb & Sons), 20,000 units/kg IV every six hours is recommended, especially in those animals exhibiting signs of sepsis or endotoxic shock.[41,42]

SURGERY

Surgical correction with successful long-term survival of a gastroesophageal intussusception has yet to be reported in the veterinary literature. In one clinical report, a gastroesophageal intussusception in a dog was reduced via a midline laparotomy by applying traction to the pylorus. A circumcostal gastropexy was performed to prevent recurrence. The dog died of aspiration pneumonia five days after surgery. At necropsy, the gastropexy was intact and the stomach was viable and in a normal position.[15] It has been suggested that fundoplication be performed in addition to gastropexy because incompetence of the esophageal hiatus is incriminated in the development of gastroesophageal intussusception.[15]

The surgical management of intestinal intussusception involves either reduction of the intussusception or intestinal resection and anastomosis, or both, followed by enteropexy or enteroplication to prevent recurrence.[17] The abdomen is approached via a standard midline laparotomy. The laparotomy incision should be of sufficient length to allow examination of the entire abdomen. The abdomen is packed with moist laparotomy pads to prevent contamination. The involved bowel loop is exteriorized and the in-

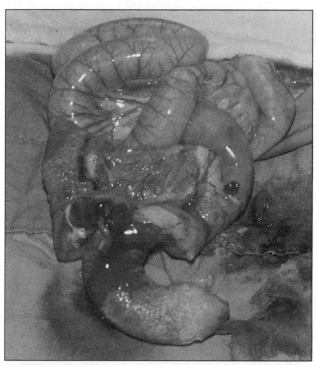

Figure 8A

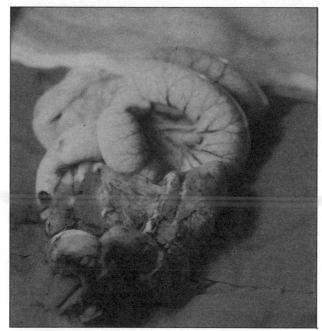

Figure 8B

Figure 8—(**A**) Intussusception after reduction. The reduced intussusceptum is in the near field. (**B**) Intussusception following reduction after administration of sodium fluorescein under illumination of an ultraviolet light source. Note the lack of fluorescence in the reduced intussusceptum.

tussusception is further isolated and packed off from the peritoneal cavity.[11]

In acute cases, manual reduction may be accomplished by gently milking the apex of the intussusceptum from within the ensheathing intussuscipiens. Minimal traction is placed on the proximal segment while the invaginated segment is pushed from the apex of the intussusception (Figure 7). Excessive traction may result in tearing of compromised intestine.[8,17] After reduction, bowel viability must be ascertained.

Various parameters and techniques have been proposed to determine intestinal viability. Color, perfusion, and muscular peristalsis of the involved segment should be evaluated after the intussusception has been reduced (Figure 8A). Viable bowel will respond to a mechanical stimulus. Pinching the bowel should result in peristaltic contractions. If bowel integrity is still in question, intravenous vital dyes can be used to assess viability. Sodium fluorescein (Alcon Laboratories), 20 mg/kg, may be administered via any peripheral vein. Two minutes after injection, the intestines should be illuminated with a 3600 Å-wavelength ultraviolet light. Normal healthy bowel will exhibit a uniform bright green fluorescence. The segment in question may show a mottled pattern with decreased fluorescence while other areas of bowel exhibit no fluorescence (Figure 8B). If these areas of nonfluorescence exceed 3 mm, or if only tissues adjacent to the mesenteric border fluoresce, or there are areas of total nonfluorescence, then the segment is not viable and should be resected.[43,44] The segment to be resected should include a minimum of 1½ cm of healthy bowel on either side of the devitalized tissue.[17]

In chronic intussusceptions in which mature adhesions preclude manual reduction, resection and anastomosis are performed.[3,17,43,45] Typhlectomy should be performed in dogs with cecocolic intussusceptions.[6,13,33] Resection and anastomosis of intussusceptions have been purported to lessen the incidence of recurrence when compared with simple manual reduction alone.[6,46]

Recurrent intussusception is common following surgical correction,[3,8–12,14,17,46–48] thus a prophylactic surgical procedure should be performed to prevent recurrence.[17,46–48] Various enteroplication or enteropexy techniques have been described.[46–53]

In 1937 Noble introduced a procedure to create planned adhesions in an attempt to decrease the incidence of recurrent intestinal obstruction in humans.[49] The Noble plication involves folding the intestine and its mesentery into neatly stacked rows. A continuous catgut suture is begun near the root of the mesentery and continued to the mesenteric border of the intestine to appose adjacent mesenteric folds. The same suture is continued along the serosal surfaces of adjacent bowel loops midway between the mesenteric

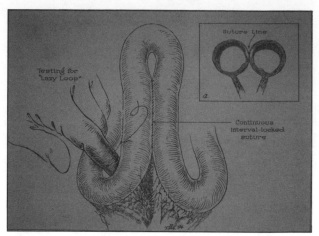

Figure 9—The Noble plication technique. A continuous suture is begun near the root of the mesentery to appose adjacent mesenteric folds and continued midway between the mesenteric and antimesenteric border. The "lazy loop" helps prevent intestinal obstruction. (Reprinted, with permission, from Smith GK: The Noble plication procedure. *Arch Surg* 70(6):801–807, 1955)

and antimesenteric border. All sutures should penetrate the submucosa without entering the lumen of the bowel. The suture is terminated approximately 2 cm before the apex of the fold (Figure 9) to prevent the formation of an abrupt change in direction of the intestine that might precipitate subsequent obstruction.[46,49–51]

The Childs-Phillips plication uses transmesenteric plication alone to limit intestinal mobility.[52] The intestine is neatly folded upon itself into rows and a series of three or four nonabsorbable sutures is placed through the mesentery approximately 4 cm from the mesenteric border of the intestine. The sutures are first secured by taking a generous through and through bite in the mesentery near the ileocolic junction. Passage of the suture is facilitated by using a large, gently curved, tapered needle (Figure 10A). The mesenteric vessels must be avoided. All sutures are passed successively through the mesentery of each row before proceeding to the adjacent row (Figure 10B). The sutures are either transfixed to the final mesenteric fold or are tied on each other, holding the intestines in loosely arranged rows (Figure 10C). Strangulation of the mesenteric vessels can occur if the sutures are tied too tightly.[46,47,49–52]

Ragins et al compared the Noble and the Childs-Phillips procedures clinically in humans and experimentally in dogs. Clinically, they found the Noble procedure had several disadvantages. The operating time was longer. Many patients experienced prolonged ileus and partial obstruction postopera-

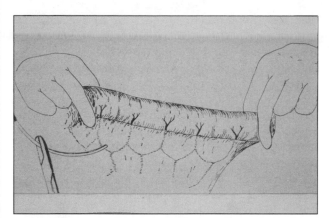

Figure 10A

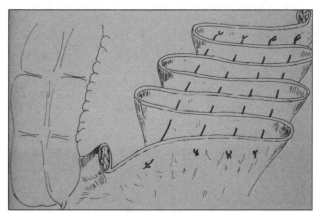

Figure 10B

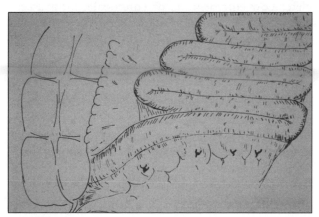

Figure 10C

Figure 10—The Childs-Phillips plication. (**A**) A large, gently curved needle is used to pass the suture through the mesentery. Care is taken to avoid the mesenteric vessels. (**B**) Rows of intestine are serially sutured and folded into gently stacked loops. (**C**) The sutures are tied upon themselves. Care is taken not to strangulate the mesenteric circulation. (Reprinted, with permission, from Ferguson AT, Reihmer VA, Gasper MR: Transmesenteric plication for small intestinal obstruction. *Am J Surg* 114(2):201–288, 1967)

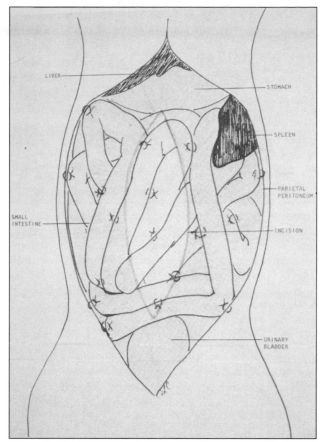

Figure 11—The creation of random serosal to serosal adhesions every 8 to 12 cm using simple interrupted sutures. (Reprinted, with permission, from Wolfe DA: Recurrent intestinal intussusception in the dog. *JAVMA* 171(6): 553–556, 1977)

tively. Some patients experienced postprandial cramping and abdominal pain. Fistula formation was a common sequela. Significant alterations of intestinal motility, assessed by controlled transit time studies and cinefluoroscopy, were not observed with either technique in dogs two months after surgery.[53]

Enteropexy, performed by creation of random serosal-to-serosal adhesions by suturing adjacent intestines together or to the abdominal peritoneum (Figure 11) has been reported in two dogs. The adhesions were created using simple interrupted silk sutures every 8 to 12 cm. The entire length of the small bowel from the duodenocolic ligament to the ileocolic junction should be sutured to decrease the potential for strangulation of bowel between adhered intestines.[46]

The enteroplication technique preferred by the authors places the intestines side to side, forming a series of gentle loops. The intestines are sutured together midway between the mesenteric and anti-

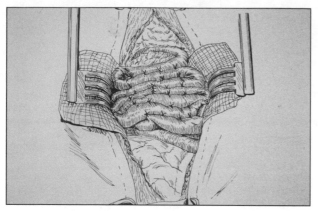

Figure 12—The creation of planned serosal adhesions by folding the bowel into gentle loops. Simple interrupted sutures are placed midway between the mesenteric and antimesenteric borders. (Reprinted, with permission, from Engen MH: Bowel plication for preventing recurrent intussusception, in Bojrab MJ (ed): *Current Techniques in Small Animal Surgery,* ed 2. Philadelphia, Lea & Febiger, 1983, p 183)

mesenteric borders with absorbable suture in a simple interrupted or continuous pattern (Figure 12). Sutures should penetrate the submucosal layer but not the lumen of the bowel.[47,48] The entire length of the jejunum and ileum should be plicated.[48]

A recent retrospective study examined postsurgical recurrences of intussusception in dogs with enteroplication compared with dogs that were not plicated at surgery. Intussusception recurred in 27% of the dogs that did not have enteroplication, but did not recur in any dog following enteroplication. Enteroplication caused no apparent adverse effects and significantly decreased the probability of recurrent intussusception.[48]

POSTOPERATIVE MANAGEMENT

After surgery, animals should be allowed water per os within the first 12 to 24 hours. An early return to oral feeding is advised to stimulate normal gastrointestinal motility and avoid ileus.[45] Food should be offered within 24 to 48 hours in the form of a "gruel." Multiple, small meals should be continued for three to four days. Intravenous fluid therapy should be continued as necessary to maintain hydration and electrolyte balance. If a predisposing cause for intussusception has been established (e.g., endoparasites) appropriate therapy should be instituted.[17]

The use of anticholinergic drugs is controversial. Proponents advocate their use to counteract the hyperspasmodic state, thus decreasing the incidence of

recurrence of intussusception.[17] In an experimental study, kidney transplants were performed in 54 dogs. Intussusceptions developed postoperatively in 8 dogs. Subsequently, 16 dogs had transplants after being premedicated with anticholinergics and no intussusceptions occurred. Prevention of intussusception was attributed to the use of anticholinergics.[19] Anticholinergics, however, decrease intestinal motility and can precipitate ileus, and some investigators feel that their use should probably be avoided.[17,54,55]

Recurrence of intussusception often occurs within three days after the initial surgery, but it can occur as late as 20 days postoperatively. Resumption of vomiting, diarrhea, or the presence of a palpable abdominal mass should alert the clinician of possible recurrence of intussusception. In one study in which no form of prophylactic enteropexy was performed, 20% of the dogs underwent a second operation for recurrence. One dog experienced three episodes of recurrence.[14] Recurrent intussusceptions typically occur proximal to the anatomic location of the original intussusception[17] and can be retrograde.[3]

CONCLUSIONS

The prognosis associated with intussusception is dependent on the anatomic location, duration, and completeness of obstruction and the predisposing cause. Gastroesophageal intussusception carries a grave prognosis. Animals with pylorogastric or high enteroenteric intussusception deteriorate rapidly without therapy, particularly if obstruction is complete. Low enteroenteric or enterocolic intussusception may have a more protracted clinical course. Underlying systemic diseases, such as canine distemper or parvovirus enteritis, increase morbidity and mortality.[17] Fluid and electrolyte therapy will minimize mortality associated with intussusception. Only 35% of the afflicted animals recovered in Wilson and Burt's study, but many of the animals that did not recover died or were euthanatized without surgical intervention because of financial or humane reasons.[12] The 65% recovery rate in Weaver's study was attributed to aggressive fluid therapy and sound surgical technique.[14]

About the Authors

Drs. Lewis and Ellison are affiliated with the Department of Small Animal Medical Sciences, College of Veterinary Medicine, University of Florida, Gainesville, Florida. Dr. Oakes is affiliated with the Department of Veterinary Clinical Sciences, School of Veterinary Medicine, Louisiana State University, Baton Rouge, Louisiana. Drs. Lewis and Ellison are Diplomates of the American College of Veterinary Surgeons.

REFERENCES

1. *Dorland's Illustrated Medical Dictionary*, ed 26. Philadelphia, WB Saunders Co, 1981, pp 676–677.
2. Shanks SC, Kerley P: *A Textbook of X-Ray Diagnosis*, ed 4, vol IV. Philadelphia, WB Saunders Co, 1970, pp 425–430.
3. O'Brien TR: *Radiographic Diagnosis of Abdominal Disorders in the Dog and Cat: Radiographic Interpretation: Clinical Signs: Pathophysiology*. Davis, CA, Cell Park Vet Co, 1978, pp 311–320.
4. Bellenger CR, Middleton DJ, Ilkiw JE, et al: Double intussusception followed by reintussusception in a kitten. *Vet Rec* 110:323–324, 1982.
5. Wolfe DA: Compound intussusception. *VM SAC* 73(4):455–459, 1978.
6. Larsen LH, Bellenger CR: Stomach and small intestine, in Archibald J (ed): *Canine Surgery*, ed 2. Santa Barbara, CA, American Veterinary Publications, 1974, pp 583–585.
7. Jubb KVF, Kennedy PC: *Pathology of Domestic Animals*, ed 2. San Francisco, Academic Press, 1970, p 95.
8. Krahwinkel DJ, Richardson DC: Intestines, in Bojrab MJ (ed): *Current Techniques in Small Animal Surgery*, ed 2. Philadelphia, Lea & Febiger, 1983, pp 162–173.
9. Tangner CH: A review of canine intestinal intussusception. *Southwest Vet* 34(3):203–207, 1982.
10. Strombeck DR: *Small Animal Gastroenterology*. Davis, CA, Stonegate Publishing, 1979, p 295.
11. Butler NC: Surgery of the small intestine. *Vet Clin North Am [Small Anim Pract]* 2(1):160–161, 1972.
12. Wilson GP, Burt JK: Intussusception in the dog and cat: A review of 45 cases. *JAVMA* 164(5):515–518, 1974.
13. Miller WN, Jathcock JT, Dillon AR: Cecal inversion in eight dogs. *JAAHA* 20(6):1009–1013, 1984.
14. Weaver AD: Canine intestinal intussusception. *Vet Rec* 100(24):524–527, 1977.
15. Leib MS, Bass CE: Gastroesophageal intussusception in the dog: A review of the literature and a case report. *JAAHA* 20(5):783–790, 1984.
16. Reed JH, Catcott EJ: Intestinal diseases, in Catcott EJ (ed): *Feline Medicine and Surgery*, ed 2. Santa Barbara, CA, American Veterinary Publications, 1975, pp 163–164.
17. Ellison GW: Nontraumatic surgical emergencies of the abdomen, in Bright R (ed): *Contemporary Issues in Small Animal Practice*, vol 2. New York, Churchill Livingstone, 1986, pp 127–173.
18. Kipins RM: A case of postoperative intussusception in a dog. *JAAHA* 13(2):197–199, 1977.
19. Olsen PR, Boserup F, Mikkelsen AM, et al: Intussusception following renal transplant in dogs. *Nord Vet Med* 29(1):36–40, 1977.
20. Runyon CL, Merkley DF, Hagemose WA: Intussusception associated with a paracolonic enterocyst in a dog. *JAVMA* 185(4):443, 1984.
21. Prier JE, Prier SC: Intestinal granuloma in a cat with intussusception and prolapse. *Calf Vet* 5:17, 1980.
22. Reymond RD: A mechanism of the kink formation which precedes intussusception. *Invest Radiol* 6(1):61–64, 1971.
23. Reymond RD: The mechanism of intussusception: A theoretical analysis of the phenomenon. *Br J Radiol* 45(1):1–7, 1972.
24. Lantz GC: The pathophysiology of acute mechanical small bowel obstruction. *Compend Contin Educ Pract Vet* 3(10):910–916, 1981.
25. Chambers JN: Diseases of the intestines, in Bojrab MJ (ed): *Pathophysiology in Small Animal Surgery*. Philadelphia, Lea & Febiger, 1981, pp 112–117.
26. Noer R: Intestinal obstruction, in Cole WH, Zollinger RM (eds): *Textbook of Surgery*, ed 9. New York, Appleton-Century-Crofts, 1970, pp 810–812.
27. Watrous B: Esophageal disease, in Ettinger SJ (ed): *Textbook of Veterinary Internal Medicine*, ed 2. Philadelphia, WB Saunders Co, 1983, pp 1220–1223.
28. Suter PF, Lord PF: *Thoracic Radiography*. Wettswill, Switzerland, Peter F. Suter, 1984, pp 331–334.
29. Markowitz J, Archibald J, Downie HC: *Experimental Surgery*, ed 5. Baltimore, The Williams & Wilkins Co, 1964, pp 185–192.
30. Shields R: The absorption and secretion of fluid and electrolytes by the obstructed bowel. *Br J Surg* 52(10):744–779, 1965.
31. Enquist IF, Baumann FG, Rehder E: Changes in body fluid spaces in dogs with intestinal obstruction. *Surg Gynecol Obstet* 122(1):17–22, 1968.
32. Mishra NK, Appert HE, Howard JM, et al: The effects of distention and obstruction on the accumulation of fluid in the lumen of small bowel of dogs. *Ann Surg* 180(6):791–795, 1974.
33. Leighton RL: Cecal inversion in dogs. *VM SAC* 78(4):521–524, 1983.
34. Raidlovo PJ, Smith H: Intussusception: Analysis of 98 cases. *Br J Surg* 68(9):645–648, 1981.
35. Gierup J, Jorulf H, Livaditis A: Management of intussusception in infants and children: A survey based on 288 consecutive cases. *Pediatrics* 50(4):535–546, 1972.
36. Franken CA, Smith LW, Chernish SM, et al: The use of glucagon in hydrostatic reduction of intussusception: A double blind study of 30 patients. *Radiology* 146(3):687–689, 1983.
37. Haskins SC: Fluid and electrolyte therapy. *Compend Contin Educ Pract Vet* 6(3):244–260, 1984.
38. Cornelius LM, Rawlings CA: Arterial blood gas and acid-base values in dogs with various diseases and signs of disease. *JAVMA* 178(9):992–995, 1981.
39. Riviere JE, Kaufman GM, Bright RM: Prophylactic use of systemic antimicrobial drugs in surgery. *Compend Contin Educ Pract Vet* 3(4):345–354, 1981.
40. Yale CE, Balish E: The importance of six common bacteria in intestinal strangulation. *Arch Surg* 104(4):438–442, 1972.
41. McAnulty JF: Septic shock in the dog: A review. *JAAHA* 19(6):827–836, 1983.
42. Hardie EM, Rawlings CA: Septic shock. Part II. Prevention, recognition and treatment. *Compend Contin Educ Pract Vet* 5(6):483–492, 1983.
43. Ellison GW, Volcinen MC, Park RD: End to end intestinal anastomosis in the dog: A comparative fluorescein dye, angiographic and histopathologic evaluation. *JAAHA* 18(5):729–736, 1982.
44. Wheaton LB, Strandberg JD, Hamilton SR, et al: A comparison of three techniques for intraoperative prediction of small intestinal injury. *JAAHA* 19(6):897, 1983.
45. Richardson DC: Intestinal injury: A review. *Compend Contin Educ Pract Vet* 3(3):259–270, 1981.
46. Wolfe DA: Recurrent intestinal intussusception in the dog. *JAVMA* 171(6):553–556, 1977.
47. Engen MH: Bowel plication for preventing recurrent intussusception, in Bojrab MJ (ed): *Current Techniques in Small Animal Surgery*, ed 2. Philadelphia, Lea & Febiger, 1983, p 183.
48. Oakes MG, Lewis DD, Hosgood G, Beale BS: Enteroplication for the prevention of recurrent intussusceptions in dogs. *JAVMA* (accepted for publication), 1993.
49. Noble TB: Plication of small intestine as prophylaxis against adhesions. *Am J Surg* 35(1):41–44, 1937.

(continues on page 190)

The Use and Misuse of Abdominal Drains in Small Animal Surgery

Gayle S. Donner, DVM
Gary W. Ellison, DVM, MS
Department of Surgical Sciences
College of Veterinary Medicine
University of Florida
Gainesville, Florida

The need to drain the peritoneal cavity following abdominal surgery has long been a subject of controversy. In 1905 Yates stated that, "There is probably no detail in modern surgical pathology that deserves more thorough comprehension, but which is less definitely understood by the average teacher, practitioner and student than the nature of the reaction of the peritoneum to drainage."[1] This statement is equally true today.

Intraperitoneal drains are commonly and often empirically inserted for one of the following reasons: (1) to drain localized fluid collections, such as abscesses; (2) to drain the general peritoneal cavity in the treatment of diffuse peritonitis; or (3) prophylactically, to drain fluids that may appear in the peritoneal cavity subsequent to operation. The purpose of this article is to present a rational approach to drainage of the abdominal cavity based on a review of the literature and on current surgical practice.

History of Drainage

The concept of drainage is as old as surgery itself. The earliest recorded use of drains is attributed to Hippocrates (ca 460–377 BC), who used hollow tubes to treat empyema. In the second century AD, Celsus and Galen used conical tubes of brass and lead to drain ascites, which is the first recorded use of an intraperitoneal drain. This form of therapeutic tapping continued to be practiced for the next 1500 years. Heister introduced the principle of capillary drainage in 1719, using a gauze wick inside a metal tube. Penrose, for whom the most popular and widely used latex drain is named, modified this concept in 1890 by using gauze inside a thin rubber tube.

Truly successful drainage of the abdominal cavity remained elusive because the drains often became plugged and thus ineffective. In fact, these early drains frequently led to increased complications and mortality from dehiscence, herniation, or infection—paradoxically, the very complications that the drains were intended to prevent.[2] The modern evolution of abdominal drains has resulted from attempts to overcome the problems of low efficiency and high morbidity, with varying degrees of success.

Principles of Drainage

Pleural drainage is usually successful because it is based on a thorough understanding of the physics of the pleural cavity. Abdominal drainage is less reliable, as comparatively little is known about the forces that make the drain work. From a mechanical view, the abdomen is like a fluid-filled container with two flexible walls. There are two separate pressure zones: within the lumen of the gastrointestinal tract, which has a positive atmospheric pressure; and within the peritoneal cavity, which has an extraluminal subatmospheric pressure between -5 and -8 cm H_2O (the pressure is more negative in the cranial abdomen near the diaphragm).[2] In essence, the peritoneal cavity resembles a plastic intravenous-fluid–filled vacuum bottle. The mechanism of emptying the fluid contents of the peritoneal cavity is the same as that required for draining fluid from the infusion bottle. To initiate outflow of fluid, an air vent must first be established to break the vacuum and create a positive atmospheric pressure within the cavity.[3]

A positive-pressure pneumoperitoneum results after laparotomy, and the air is reabsorbed after several days. This postoperative pneumoperitoneum is responsible for the onset of peritoneal drainage.[3,4] It can be maintained and prolonged with appropriate drain modifications.

Types of Drains

Abdominal drainage is classified into two broad categories, passive drainage and active drainage (Figure 1). Passive drains function by overflow and are assisted by gravity. They cannot counteract the negative atmospheric pressure in the abdomen and therefore do not actively drain an area but rather provide a tract of least resistance along which excess fluid accumulation can flow. This may be satisfactory initially if a large enough fluid volume is present to create positive pressure in the abdominal or abscess cavity. Passive drains placed uphill are deprived of the effect of gravity.

The best example of a passive drainage system is that using a Penrose drain. The drain is composed of rubber latex that is very soft and pliable and thus does not have a tendency to erode into adjacent viscera or vasculature. As an abdominal drain, its acceptance is based more on safety than efficacy. As early as 1905, Yates demonstrated that passive drains are sealed from the rest of the abdominal cavity in dogs as early as six hours after placement. In addition, the serous drainage noted is, for the most part, not from the general peritoneal cavity itself but secondary to the local irritation of the peritoneum in contact with the drain.[5] Experiments by Yates proved that passive drainage of the general peritoneal cavity is impossible.[6] His work has withstood the test of time, as more recently it has been demonstrated that when Penrose drains are placed within the abdominal cavity of healthy dogs, the omentum completely plugs the site of the entry hole into the peritoneal cavity and incompletely surrounds the drain by 24 hours. At 48 hours, the Penrose drain is completely surrounded by fibrin and omentum and becomes effectively isolated from the peritoneal cavity. Purulent discharge is seen around a drain that is retained for four days or longer.[7]

Recently there has been a trend toward replacing rubber latex with silicone as a drain material, as silicone is more

inert and does not incite a fibrin reaction in the peritoneal cavity.[8] Passive silicone drains placed in the contaminated abdomen of dogs remain patent for at least seven days postoperatively.[9]

Active or suction drainage is classified into two types, either simple closed drainage or sump drainage, depending on whether air is admitted into the wound. Suction at the end of drainage tubes first became popular in the 1960s to increase the efficiency of drainage when large quantities of fluid collection were suspected. These drains depend on an external source of suction to create negative pressure within the wound.

A closed suction system consists of a tube with single or multiple side holes, attached to a source of negative pressure that is not open to the atmosphere. This negative pressure may be applied by a prevacuumed (Redi-Vac®—Orthopedic Equipment Company) or a spring-loaded (Hemo-Vac®—Zimmer Manufacturing Company) compressible plastic receptacle (Figure 2). One major drawback of using closed suction in the abdomen is the reduced pliability of the drain. If the drain is sufficiently rigid to maintain patency under general suction, then it has a tendency to erode through adjacent soft tissue as well.[10,11] If the drain is soft, it will collapse under suction and become ineffective. Another disadvantage of the closed suction

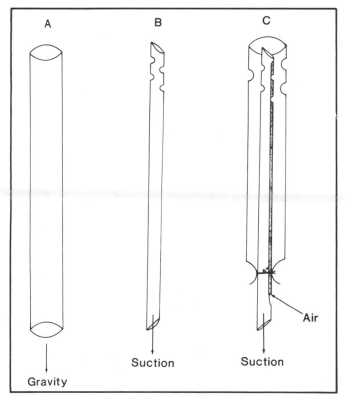

Figure 1—Types of abdominal drains: *A*, passive drain, *B*, active drain—closed suction, *C*, active drain— triple-lumen sump drain. The three lumens shown in *C* function in the following manner: to actively suction abdominal fluid out of the wound, to allow room air into the wound to break the negative vacuum pressure in the peritoneum, and to surround the rest of the drain as a cushion to protect surrounding viscera.

system for abdominal surgery is that the application of continuous suction to the drain improves its efficiency for only a short period of time, as it results in suction of viscera, omentum, or wound wall toward the holes of the drainage catheter, thereby occluding it.[10]

Closed-suction drains were originally used very successfully in orthopedic and plastic surgery for deep wounds and subcutaneous drainage of skin flaps. They were quickly adopted for abdominal surgery use, only to be abandoned in favor of sump drainage shortly thereafter. The popularity of the closed suction system has persisted in other areas of soft tissue surgery and orthopedic surgery, as they have consistently resulted in less wound infection and hematoma and seroma formation when compared with passive drainage systems.[12]

Sump drainage has greatly increased the efficiency of abdominal drainage because it conforms to the principles of physics that govern optimal fluid drainage of the peritoneal cavity. It is a modification of the closed system tube whereby a second lumen is added that serves as an external air vent to break the intraperitoneal vacuum. This double-lumen tube, known as a sump tube, permits the access and circulation of air to the area of drainage. This prevents occlusion of the tube fenestrations by collapsed tissue and thereby improves the rate of drainage and patency of the system. Sump drainage is two to four times as efficient as closed suction or passive Penrose drainage of the abdomen.[12-14]

The major disadvantage of the sump system is its poor adaptability to many veterinary hospital situations. The small portable units that work adequately in closed suction systems cannot cope with the volumes of air produced by the air-vent system and so they are not applicable to the

sump drain.[15] Either built-in hospital wall suction units or large motor-driven portable suction machines are necessary (Figure 3). Another disadvantage of sump drains is the need to allow large quantities of room air to enter the peritoneal cavity via the air inlet. Large air flows have been shown to increase the risk of intraperitoneal infection.[16] The risk of airborne infection can be reduced by using bacterial filters in the air inlets.[17] As with closed suction tubes, the rigidity of sump tubes at first remained a problem. This problem has been partially overcome by surrounding the double-lumen sump with a fenestrated third lumen composed of soft rubber that acts as a cushion to minimize the risk of erosion of adjacent viscera or blood vessels. Triple-lumen sump drains are available commercially in a variety of designs (Figure 4),[10,18] or can be made very simply and inexpensively using a Foley catheter, a small-sized rubber urethral catheter, and a Penrose drain (Figures 5 and 6).[11,19,20]

The veterinarian confronted with the task of draining an abdomen is faced with a dilemma. Passive Penrose drains,

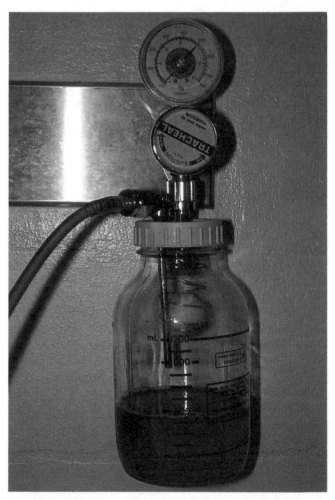

Figure 3—A hospital wall suction unit, necessary for sump suction drainage. The suction source for closed drains (as shown in Figure 2) is unable to apply adequate suction to sump drains. The large volumes of room air that enter via the sump drain's air vent lumen and then exit out the suction lumen would rapidly fill up the closed suction system's receptacle, effectively eliminating this source of negative pressure suction.

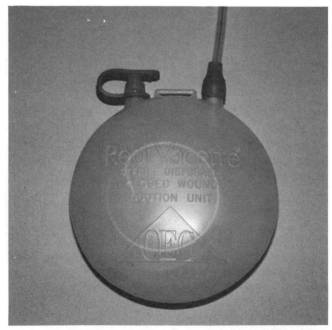

Figure 2—The closed-suction drain's compressible plastic receptacle functions both as the source of a moderate amount of suction and as the receptacle for the drained fluid.

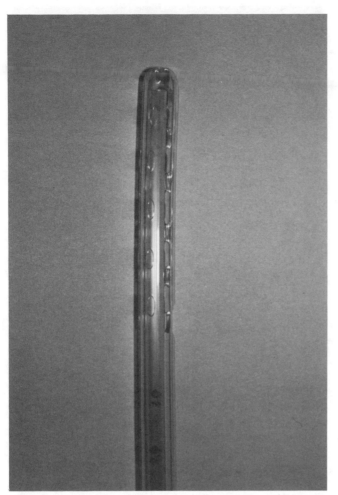

Figure 4—The tip of a commercially available triple-lumen sump drain (Argyle Saratoga® Sump Drain—Sherwood Medical) is much more rigid than a passive Penrose drain.

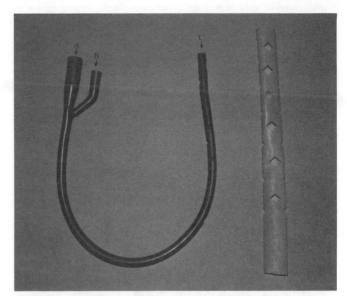

Figure 5A

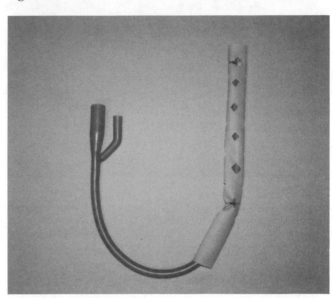

Figure 5B

Figure 5—(**A**) Example of an easily made triple-lumen sump drain. A Foley catheter (*left*) has been modified into a double-lumen sump drain within a fenestrated Penrose drain (*right*), which functions as the surrounding cushioning third lumen. Suction is applied to the Foley catheter at *A*. Room air enters the wound at *B*. The balloon tip of the Foley catheter has been cut off, and fenestrations added at *C*. A gauze sponge may be placed optionally around the Foley catheter, within the Penrose drain, for additional cushioning. (**B**) The Foley catheter is inserted within the Penrose drain.

the drainage system that is the safest and easiest to manage, are also the least efficient. Sump suction drains, the system that is the most effective, are also the most complex in terms of equipment, constant patient and drain management, and expense. In essence, the ideal abdominal drainage system readily adaptable for everyday veterinary use has not yet been developed.

Drain Complications

With the advent of sump suction, abdominal drainage has been greatly improved; but, while fairly efficient drainage is now possible, the next major factor to be considered is the possible harmful effect that drains may have on the patient. The danger of drain-tip erosion into adjacent soft tissue has already been discussed. This problem has been reported clinically in humans[5,21] and confirmed experimentally in pigs and rabbits.[14,22] Drain-tip erosion is not entirely confined to rigid suction drains, however, as Penrose drains can on rare occasion cause similar damage.[23] Another rare but possible complication is the occurrence of omental or intestinal herniation and incarceration through the drain exit hole.[24,25] A retained drain is also another pos-

sible problem—either one that has slipped entirely within the abdominal cavity or one that has been accidentally sutured to a deep fascia layer during closure (Figure 7). Both of these complications probably occur more frequently than has been reported in the literature.[26] The avoidance of a second surgical procedure to retrieve the drain by using various types of endoscopic equipment for retrieval through the original drain tract has recently been reported.[26–28]

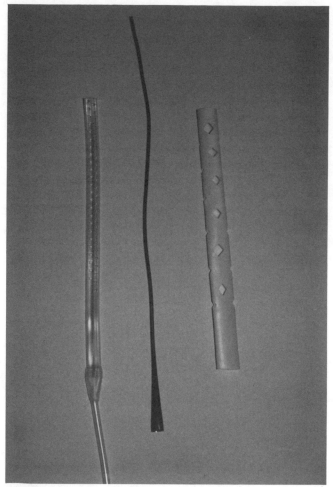

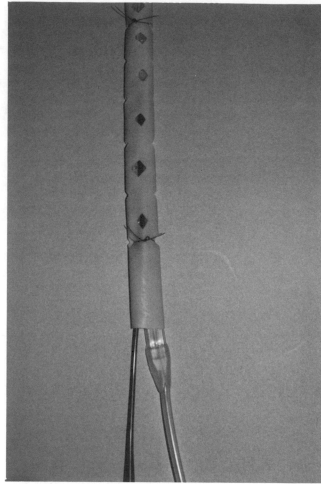

Figure 6A

Figure 6B

Figure 6—(**A**) Another method of constructing a triple-lumen sump drain. The drain is fashioned in a similar manner as described in Figure 5, except a soft red rubber urethral catheter (*middle*) and a closed suction Silastic drain catheter (*left*) replace the Foley catheter. The urethral catheter acts as an air vent, and suction is applied to the end of the closed suction catheter. (**B**) The urethral catheter and the Silastic drain catheter are inserted within the Penrose drain.

Perhaps the most common drain-associated complication is that of ascending infection. Nora[29] demonstrated that pathogenic bacteria ascend a Penrose drain into the abdomen of dogs. After seven days, 90% of the experimental dogs had positive intraabdominal cultures of the same bacteria type as that placed on the exterior tip of the drain.[29] This finding has been confirmed in rabbits as well.[30] Agrama[7] noted that infection always occurred around Penrose drains left in situ for four or more days in dogs. Cultures of the drain tract yielded a mixed flora, including β-hemolytic *Streptococcus,* enterococcus, *Escherichia coli*, and *Staphylococcus.*[7]

The use of a closed-suction drainage system does not guard totally against ascending infection, as it is necessary to disconnect the drain catheter in order to create or reestablish the vacuum in the fluid receptacle; hence it is not always a closed drainage system. It is theoretically possible, therefore, for bacteria to gain entry when the system is open to the atmosphere as the plastic bottle is being compressed.[31] Experimentally, it is possible for bacteria to migrate up static serum in standard polyethylene suction tub-

ing within 24 hours.[32] Sump suction airborne contamination can be decreased with the use of a bacterial filter.[33]

Prophylactic Drainage

Surgical drainage is used for either prophylactic or therapeutic purposes. The therapeutic use of drains for the removal of intraperitoneal collections of fluid, such as pus, blood, urine, or bile, is well established. The prophylactic use of drains, placed in anticipation of an intraperitoneal fluid collection, remains controversial. It has become increasingly more evident that drains are not always a reliable indicator of intraperitoneal events; a lack of drainage does not always indicate that bile, blood, urine, or intestinal content leakage has not occurred.[15,24] This fact, coupled with the increased incidence of complications associated with prophylactic drainage, has resulted in a tendency toward the discontinuation of drain placement in the absence of obvious fluid collections at the time of surgery.

Four commonly performed human surgical procedures in which it is routine to place prophylactic drains are splenectomy, appendectomy, cholecystectomy, and colonic

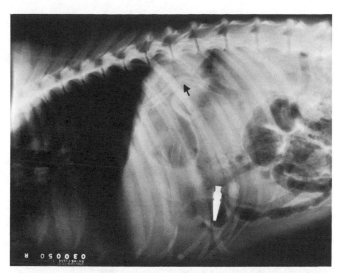

Figure 7—This canine patient dislodged and swallowed a Penrose drain that had been placed during prostatic abscess surgery (*black arrow*). The drain can be seen in the stomach in this radiograph. It must be differentiated from a drain that has slipped back into the abdominal cavity, which would need to be retrieved.

anastomosis. Recently, the surgical literature has suggested that the routine use of prophylactic drainage should be reconsidered.

Splenectomy

In contrast to animals, the spleen is retroperitoneal in humans, and a large retroperitoneal dead space remains following its removal. Drain placement is aimed at preventing fluid accumulation in this space. Another reason advanced for the use of drains in this procedure is to provide an exit for pancreatic juice if the tail of the pancreas is injured in the course of the splenectomy. Even when care has been taken to avoid this damage, an increased concentration of amylase has been found in the drainage fluid, leading to a strong tendency toward the use of drains. It has been found, however, that the use of drains has resulted in either no comparative improvement in patient outcome[34] or a much higher incidence of subphrenic abscesses and drain tract infections compared with patients in whom drains have not been used.[35,36] These findings have been confirmed experimentally in animals as well. Penrose drains placed following splenectomy in dogs and rabbits caused up to a 90% infection rate compared with no infections in the undrained group.[29,30]

Appendectomy

Wound infection is the most common complication and intraabdominal abscesses or generalized septicemia is the most common cause of mortality following operation for a perforated appendix. The use of drains has not decreased either of these complications to any appreciable degree.[37-39]

Cholecystectomy

Traditionally, drains have been used after routine cholecystectomy because the major cause of mortality after this operation is leakage of bile into the peritoneal cavity. The intended use of the drain is to allow early detection of this leakage and thus prevent bile peritonitis should leakage occur. Multiple retrospective studies, however, have documented that the omission of drains has resulted in a significant reduction in postoperative morbidity.[40-44] Furthermore, if bile leakage or sepsis should occur, it often does not exit the drain site, or it exits from the surgical incision.[43,45] Many surgeons refute these results; and the use of drains following routine cholecystectomy still remains a common, although controversial, practice.

Colonic Anastomosis

The rationale of those who favor drains is that leakage that occurs subsequent to colonic repair or anastomosis can be detected earlier, thus allowing diversion of the fecal stream from the rest of the peritoneal cavity. Drains have been especially favored where the anastomotic integrity has been compromised. The evidence is overwhelming that drains actually hinder colonic healing. Numerous studies on dogs have documented that Penrose drains placed on and up to 2 cm from the incision line have a disastrous effect on the anastomosis. The drain appears to prevent sealing of a possible anastomotic leak by interposing between the suture line and adjacent omentum. As a result, the drain often causes rather than prevents colonic leakage.[46-50] Unlike the Penrose drain, Silastic drains have a minimal effect on colonic healing.[47,50]

If it is acceptable to extrapolate results from human medicine and canine experiments and apply them to veterinary patient management, then it appears that the use of prophylactic surgical drainage of the abdomen is usually *unwarranted* and may be *detrimental*. As comparatively little is mentioned in the veterinary literature about the prophylactic use of drains, it may be reasonable to conclude that their lack of use is generally well accepted by veterinary surgeons.

Therapeutic Drainage

Drainage of the abdomen for therapeutic purposes is a more commonly performed and accepted surgical practice. It is most frequently employed in veterinary medicine for the treatment of intraabdominal, particularly prostatic, abscesses. More recently, it has been found to be beneficial as an adjunctive treatment for severe pancreatitis and diffuse septic peritonitis in the modified form of postoperative peritoneal lavage.[51] Multiple ingress and egress Silastic drains, sump drains, or peritoneal dialysis catheters are used for this procedure.[52-54]

In the past, resistance to the use of peritoneal lavage stemmed from the belief that irrigation would disseminate localized infection throughout the abdominal cavity, thereby making it more difficult for the body's defense mechanisms to eliminate the infection. In actuality, bacteria spread from the site of contamination, even without the presence of lavage, as a result of the existence of an intraperitoneal circulation.[55]

Furthermore, it has been demonstrated in dogs that irrigating the peritoneal cavity after local intraperitoneal inoculation of bacteria does not increase the mortality rate.[56] It is beyond the scope of this article to present an in-depth discussion of the indications, contraindications, controversial applications, and techniques of therapeutic peritoneal lavage. In general, the procedure is gaining more acceptance as a means of diluting and removing pathogenic bacteria, destructive enzymes, and debris from the abdomen.

While marsupialization is one accepted method of treatment for large prostatic abscesses, drainage via tubes or catheters is necessary when the abscess is too small to suture directly to the ventral abdominal wall. The properties that make the Penrose drain unsuitable for general peritoneal drainage make it well suited for drainage of localized, walled-off abscesses, such as those that occur in the prostate. The latex tube drain acts as a foreign body in the peritoneal cavity, and the fibrous reaction that occurs around the drain tract results in an externalization from the peritoneal cavity and local drainage of the abscess cavity contents in contact with the drain to the exterior. The placement of Penrose drains through the prostatic abscess to the exterior of the abdomen is one successful drainage method.[57,58] Direct drainage through a Foley catheter secured to the abscess cavity with a purse-string suture is another option.[59] After the drain is removed the extraperitoneal exit persists for two to three days to allow for continued drainage. The use of a drain for the treatment of noninfected prostatic cysts runs the risk of causing an ascending infection and peritoneal cavity inflammation by the cystic fluid. Marsupialization, when possible, is the preferred method of treatment.

New Concepts in Abdominal Drainage

Several new approaches to therapeutic abdominal drainage in human surgery have been developed recently and may have application to selected cases in veterinary surgery. Intraabdominal abscesses are now being diagnosed, localized, and drained via guidance from computerized tomography and/or ultrasonography. The abscess cavity is flushed through the drain; and the drain is removed when drainage ceases and the abscess cavity is obliterated, usually in 30 to 60 days. This new procedure has obviated the need for exploratory laparotomy in many patients.[60-64]

In patients with severe life-threatening necrotizing intraabdominal sepsis, postoperative closed peritoneal lavage has been replaced by open peritoneal drainage. In such cases, the abdominal cavity is not closed following surgical exploration. Rather, the abdominal incision is covered with gauze sponges and not sutured to allow optimum exposure for thorough, frequent peritoneal debridement and lavage and complete drainage of purulent debris. The incision is either left open to heal by second intention or closed at a later date, as dictated by patient progress. This radical procedure is starting to be considered as an option in veterinary medicine,[65] as the results so far in human medicine have demonstrated a significant decrease in mortality in patients with an otherwise very guarded prognosis. The inherent postoperative management and complications have

been imposing with this procedure and include evisceration, tremendous colloid and crystalloid fluid loss, incisional herniation, iatrogenic bacterial contamination, and fistula formation of exposed bowel.[66-70]

Drain Selection and Placement

Once the decision to use an abdominal drain has been made, it is imperative that the appropriate drain be selected for the proposed task. If localized drainage of a discrete abscess is desired, then a Penrose drain should suffice. If a large quantity of fluid or diffuse abdominal drainage over an extended period of time is expected, then a sump drain should be used. A Penrose drain should not be expected to drain the entire peritoneal cavity satisfactorily (Figure 8).

The drain should exit via a stab incision separate from the surgical incision line. Placing the drain in the incision results in a much higher incidence of wound infection.[71] A drain tract through the suture line is also a potential source of weakness and increases the chance of visceral herniation through the incision.[5,24] Care should be taken to avoid the epigastric vessels by placing the stab incision lateral to the border of the rectus muscle. Traction should be applied to bring the abdominal wall layers into normal alignment before making the stab incision to avoid a "scissors" effect of the drain tract when the main wound is closed. The drain should be placed along the shortest and most direct route from the drainage site to the outside. No drain kinking should occur when the viscera are replaced and the surgical wound closed. If a passive drainage system is used, then the drain should exit the most dependent site of the abdomen.

The drain should be fixed securely to the skin with a nonabsorbable suture of adequate strength and should incorporate a radiopaque marker to detect a suspected inadvertent loss of the drain into the abdomen. Penrose drains routinely contain a radiopaque marker. The drain exit site should be kept clean. A bandage around the abdomen may help to decrease contamination from the external environ-

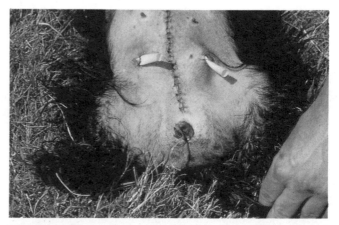

Figure 8—The use of an abdominal drain in this female Scottish terrier was inappropriate on two accounts. First, a Penrose drain was used to drain the peritoneal cavity of diffuse peritonitis; and, second, the drain was placed adjacent to a colonic anastomosis incision.

ment and help prevent the animal from gaining access to the drain.

In general, the drain should be removed as soon as possible, usually within 24 hours after significant drainage ceases. It must be remembered that the drain itself elicits a foreign body response and even in the absence of disease a small amount of serous discharge occurs. Conversely, a lack of drainage does not always indicate that excess abdominal fluid is not present.

If a drain is inadvertently removed prematurely, the clinical situation must be carefully evaluated to decide if drain replacement is necessary.[72] As the anatomic surface of the peritoneal membrane approximates that of the total body surface area[55] and the healthy canine peritoneal cavity is capable of absorbing fluid at a rate of 3% to 8% of the body weight per hour,[1] not every patient needs its abdominal drain replaced to remove the excess fluid accumulation that may still be present.

Summary

The rationale for using an abdominal drain deserves close scrutiny. Drains are foreign bodies and may serve as two-way streets for bacteria. This must be considered when weighing the benefits of drainage for a given clinical situation. As with the use of antibiotics, the presence of a drain should not be substituted for proper surgical management. When appropriately used, however, the abdominal drain is a valuable addition to the surgical armamentarium of the veterinarian.

REFERENCES

1. Yates JL: An experimental study of the local effects of peritoneal drainage. *Surg Gynecol Obstet* 1:473–492, 1905.
2. Moss JP: Historical and current perspectives on surgical drainage. *Surg Gynecol Obstet* 152:517–527, 1981.
3. Gold E: The physics of the abdominal cavity and the problem of peritoneal drainage. *Am J Surg* 91:415–417, 1956.
4. Gedda S, Van Der Linden W: What makes the peritoneal drain work? Pressure in the subhepatic space after biliary surgery. *Acta Chir Scand* 149:703–706, 1983.
5. Hermann G: Intraperitoneal drainage. *Surg Clin North Am* 49:1279–1288, 1969.
6. Golovsky D: Observations on wound drainage with a review of the literature. *Med J Aust* 1:289–291, 1976.
7. Agrama HM, Blackwood JM, Brown CS, et al: Functional longevity of intraperitoneal drains, an experimental study. *Am J Surg* 132:418–421, 1976.
8. Baker JL, Eisenberg HV: A new silicone drain. *Plast Reconstr Surg* 61:297, 1978.
9. Santos OA, Hastings FW, Mohamad KM: Effectiveness of silicone as an abdominal drain. *Arch Surg* 84:643–645, 1962.
10. Formeister JF, Elias EG: Safe intraabdominal and efficient wound drainage. *Surg Gynecol Obstet* 142:415–416, 1976.
11. Vercouterer AL, Humphrey R: Improved method for intraabdominal drainage. *Surg Gynecol Obstet* 158:587–588, 1984.
12. Golden GT, Roberts TL III, Rodeheaver G, et al: A new filtered sump tube for wound drainage. *Am J Surg* 129:716–717, 1975.
13. Hanna EA: Efficiency of peritoneal drainage. *Surg Gynecol Obstet* 131:983–985, 1970.
14. Robbs JV, MacIntyre IM: The efficacy of intraperitoneal drains—An experimental study. *S Afr J Surg* 17(4):191–197, 1979.
15. Duthie HL: Current concepts in drainage of the abdomen. *N Engl J Med* 287:1081, 1972.
16. Baker BH, Brochardt KA: Sump drains and airborne bacteria as a cause of wound infections. *J Surg Res* 17:407–410, 1974.
17. Spengler MD, Rodeheaver GT, Edlich RF: Performance of filtered sump wound drainage tubes. *Surg Gynecol Obstet* 154:333–336, 1982.
18. Abramson DJ: A combined soft tissue and suction drain. *Surg Gynecol Obstet* 125:365–366, 1967.
19. Ranson JH: Safer intraperitoneal sump drainage. *Surg Gynecol Obstet* 137:841–842, 1973.
20. Tribble DE: An improved sump drain-irrigation device of simple construction. *Arch Surg* 105:511–513, 1972.
21. Scott JW: Suction drainage complication. *Br J Surg* 68:825, 1981.
22. Johansson L, Nystrom PO, Lennquist S: Drainage of the abdominal cavity after abdominal missile trauma—A comparison of intestinal damage of three evacuation systems. *Acta Chir Scand* 508(Suppl):371–372, 1982.
23. Hubbard JG: Bladder perforation secondary to surgical drains. *J Urol* 121:521–522, 1979.
24. O'Connor TW, Hugh TB: Abdominal drainage—A clinical review. *Aust NZ J Surg* 49:253–260, 1979.
25. Teasdale C, Kenyon GS, Jones SM: External strangulated small-bowel hernia after intraperitoneal drainage. *Lancet* 1:459, 1982.
26. Soper LE, Nacheff NM, Rydell WB: An endoscopic technique for removal of suture bound surgical drains. *Surg Gynecol Obstet* 141:925–926, 1975.
27. Cos LR, Davis RS: Release of sutured Penrose drain by optical urethrotome. *J Urol* 21:528, 1983.
28. Kalies DW, Small MP: Panendoscopic removal of sutured retained Penrose drain. *South Med J* 68:1155–1156, 1975.
29. Nora PF, Vanecko RM, Bransfield JJ: Prophylactic abdominal drains. *Arch Surg* 105:173–176, 1972.
30. Cerise EJ, Pierce WA, Diamond OL: Abdominal drains—their role as a source of infection following splenectomy. *Ann Surg* 171:764–769, 1970.
31. Milson I, Gustafsson A: An evaluation of a post-operative vacuum drainage system. *Curr Med Res* 6:160–164, 1979.
32. Casey BH: Bacterial spread in polyethylene tubing—a possible source of surgical wound contamination. *Med J Aust* 2:718, 1971.
33. Worth MH, Anderson HW: The effectiveness of bacterial filtration in vented wound drains. *J Surg Res* 27:405–407, 1979.
34. Pachter HL, Hofstetter SR, Spencer FC: Splenorrhaphy versus splenectomy and postsplenectomy drainage: Experience in 105 patients. *Ann Surg* 194:262–269, 1981.
35. Cohn LH: Local infections after splenectomy. *Arch Surg* 90:230–232, 1965.
36. Doud FS, Fishcer DC, Hafner CD: Complications following splenectomy with specific emphasis on drainage. *Arch Surg* 92:32–36, 1966.
37. Farrar DJ, Maybury NK, Sanson JR: The use of closed wound suction drainage after appendectomy. *Br J Clin Pract* 27:63–65, 1973.
38. Grenall MJ, Evans M, Pollock AV: Should you drain a perforated appendix? *Br J Surg* 65:880–882, 1978.
39. Haller JA, Shaker IJ, Donahoo MD, et al: Peritoneal drainage versus nondrainage for generalized peritonitis from ruptured appendicitis in children. *Ann Surg* 177:595–600, 1973.
40. Chilton CP, Mann CV: Drainage after cholecystectomy. *Ann R Coll Surg Engl* 62:60–65, 1980.
41. Goldberg IM, Goldberg IP, Liechty RD, et al: Cholecystectomy with and without surgical drainage. *Am J Surg* 130:29–32, 1975.
42. Kassum DA, Gagic NM, Menson GT: Cholecystectomy with and without drainage. *Can J Surg* 22:358–360, 1979.
43. Kambouris EA, Carpenter WS, Allaben AD: Cholecystectomy without drainage. *Surg Gynecol Obstet* 137:613–617, 1973.
44. Ross FP, Quinlan RM: Eight hundred cholecystectomies—A plea for many fewer drains. *Arch Surg* 110:721–724, 1975.
45. Stone HH, Hooper A, Millikan WJ: Abdominal drainage following appendectomy and cholecystectomy. *Ann Surg* 187:606–612, 1978.
46. Berliner SD, Burson LC, Lear PE: Use and abuse of intraperitoneal drains in colon surgery. *Arch Surg* 89:686–690, 1964.
47. Crowson WN, Wilson CS: An experimental study of the effects of drains on colon anastomosis. *Am Surg* 39:597–601, 1973.
48. Lennox MS: Prophylactic drainage of colonic anastomosis. *Br J Surg* 71:10–11, 1984.
49. Manz CW, Tendresse C, Sako Y: The detrimental effects of drains on colonic anastomosis, an experimental study. *Dis Colon Rectum* 13:17–35, 1970.

50. Smith SR, Connolly JC, Gilmore OJ: The effect of surgical drainage materials on colonic healing. *Br J Surg* 69:153–155, 1982.
51. Parks J, Gahring D, Greene R: Peritoneal lavage for peritonitis and pancreatitis in twenty-two dogs. *JAAHA* 9:442–446, 1973.
52. Jennings WC, Wood CD, Guernsey JM: Continuous postoperative lavage in the treatment of peritoneal sepsis. *Dis Colon Rectum* 25:641–643, 1982.
53. Ranson JH, Spencer FC: The role of peritoneal lavage in severe acute pancreatitis. *Ann Surg* 187:565–575, 1978.
54. Rosato EF, Oram-Smith JC, Mullis WF: Peritoneal lavage treatment in experimental peritonitis. *Ann Surg* 175:384–387, 1972.
55. Hau T, Ahrenholz DH, Simmons RL: Secondary bacterial peritonitis—The biologic basis of treatment. *Curr Prob Surg* 16(10):1–65, 1979.
56. Havnovian AP, Saddawi N: An experimental study of the consequences of intraperitoneal irrigation. *Surg Gynecol Obstet* 134:575–578, 1972.
57. Christie TR: Prostate gland and testes, in Bojrab MJ (ed): *Current Techniques in Small Animal Surgery*, ed 2. Philadelphia, Lea & Febiger, 1983, pp 360–369.
58. Zolton GM, Greiner TP: Prostatic abscesses—A surgical approach. *JAAHA* 14:698–702, 1978.
59. Aultman SH, Betts CW: An unusual case of a prostatic cyst: Utilization of a suprapubic catheter. *JAAHA* 14:638–644, 1978.
60. Glass CA, Cohn I: Drainage of intraabdominal abscesses—A comparison of surgical and computerized tomography guided catheter drainage. *Am J Surg* 147:315–317, 1984.
61. Halasz NA, Van Sonnenberg E: Drainage of intraabdominal abscesses, tactics and choices. *Am J Surg* 146:112–115, 1983.
62. Martin EC, Fankuchen E, Neff RA: Percutaneous drainage of abscesses—A report of 100 patients. *Clin Radiol* 35:9-11, 1984.
63. Pruett TL, Rotstein OD, Cross J: Percutaneous aspiration and drainage for suspected abdominal infection. *Surgery* 96:731–737, 1984.
64. Van Sonnenberg E, Mueller PR, Ferrucci JF: Percutaneous drainage of 250 abdominal abscesses and fluid collections. *Radiology* 151:337–341, 1984.
65. Orsher RJ, Rosen F: Open peritoneal drainage in experimental peritonitis in dogs. *Vet Surg* 13(4):222–226, 1984.
66. Anderson ED, Mandelbaum DM, Ellison EC, et al: Open packing of the peritoneal cavity in generalized bacterial peritonitis. *Am J Surg* 145:131–135, 1983.
67. Bohnen JM, Meakins JL: Treatment of intra-abdominal sepsis. *Can J Surg* 27:222-225, 1984.
68. Broome A, Hansson L, Lundgren F, et al: Open treatment of abdominal septic catastrophies. *World J Surg* 7:792–796, 1983.
69. Duff JH, Moffat J: Abdominal sepsis managed by leaving the abdomen open. *Surgery* 90:774-778, 1981.
70. Maetani S, Takayoshi T: Open peritoneal drainage as effective treatment of advanced peritonitis. *Surgery* 90:804–809, 1981.
71. Cruse PJ, Foord R: A five-year prospective study of 23,649 surgical wounds. *Arch Surg* 107:206–210, 1973.
72. Levy M: Intraperitoneal drainage. *Am J Surg* 147:309–314, 1984.

Intussusception in Dogs and Cats *(continued from page 181)*

50. Seabrook DB, Wilson N: Prevention and treatment of intestinal obstruction by the use of the Noble procedure. *Am J Surg* 88(1):186–189, 1954.
51. Smith GK: The Noble plication procedure. *Arch Surg* 70(6):801–807, 1955.
52. Ferguson AT, Reihmer VA, Gaspar MR: Transmesenteric plication for small intestinal obstruction. *Am J Surg* 114(2):203–288, 1967.
53. Ragins N, Freeman L, Coomaraswamy R, et al: Clinical and experimental comparison of the Noble and the Childs-Phillips plications of the small bowel. *Am J Surg* 111(4):555–558, 1966.
54. Strombeck DR: *Small Animal Gastroenterology*. Davis, CA, Stonegate Publishing, 1979, pp 188–190.
55. Willard MD: Newer concepts in treatment of secretory diarrheas. *JAVMA* 186(1):86–88, 1985.

Partial Hepatectomy in Dogs

D. E. Bjorling, DVM, MS
Department of Small Animal Medicine

K. W. Prasse, DVM, PhD
Department of Pathology

R. A. Holmes, DVM
Department of Parasitology

College of Veterinary Medicine
University of Georgia
Athens, Georgia

The removal of one or more lobes of the liver may be necessary in the treatment of hepatic trauma, abscesses, or neoplasia, or for research purposes. Several techniques, including parenchymal crushing,[1,2] anatomic dissection,[3-5] and mass ligation,[6] have been described for the excision of entire liver lobes. The canine liver is divided into distinct lobes, which makes removal of individual lobes possible. Certain details of the anatomy of the liver require careful attention to avoid surgically related complications. Anticipation of metabolic derangements following partial hepatectomy facilitates their detection and prompt treatment. Removal of large portions (70% to 80%) of the liver is tolerated, and the capacity of the canine liver for regeneration is well documented.[6,7]

This article outlines the surgical anatomy of the liver and discusses surgical considerations and preoperative and postoperative evaluation of dogs requiring partial hepatectomy.

Anatomy

The canine liver is composed of six lobes grouped into three major divisions: The left lateral and medial lobes form the left division; the quadrate and right medial lobes are considered the central division; and the right division consists of the right lateral and caudate lobes (Figure 1). The left division contributes about 40% of the liver mass, and the right and central divisions comprise approximately 30% each.[6] The papillary process of the caudate lobe extends from left to right dorsal to the portal vein and receives its blood supply from the vessels supplying the left division.[8] Deep fissures separate the lobes of the liver, but the parenchyma of the lobes becomes continuous near the hilus. The lobes of the left and central divisions maintain their distinct nature to a greater degree than do the lobes of the right division. As the caudal vena cava passes the liver, it is enveloped by the caudate and right lateral lobes.[9] These lobes do not have a discrete attachment to the rest of the liver, but rather are joined to it over a broad area near the caudal vena cava.

The liver is attached to the diaphragm by the right and left triangular ligaments. The right is relatively small, and the left provides the main attachment of the liver to the diaphragm.[8] The hepatorenal ligament extends from the right kidney to the caudate lobe. The lesser omentum is formed by the hepatogastric and hepatoduodenal ligaments, which extend to the hilus of the liver from the lesser curvature of the stomach, the pylorus, and the duodenum.[10]

Originally published in Volume 7, Number 3, March 1985

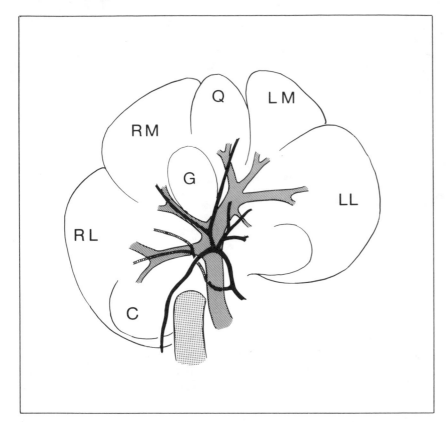

Figure 1—The three divisions of the liver are the left (left lateral and medial lobes), central (quadrate and right medial lobes), and right (right lateral and caudate lobes). The most frequently observed pattern of the common and proper hepatic arteries is shown. The arteries are black, the portal vein and its branches are gray, and the caudal vena cava is stippled. C = caudate lobe, RL = right lateral lobe, RM = right medial lobe, G = gall bladder, Q = quadrate lobe, LM = left medial lobe, and LL = left lateral lobe.

The hepatic artery arises from the celiac artery and enters the free margin of the hepatoduodenal ligament at the antimesenteric border of the duodenum.[8,10] The common hepatic artery has one to five branches (most commonly three), which usually supply first the right, then the left, and finally the middle divisions of the liver (Figure 1).[8,11] After giving off the proper hepatic arteries, the common hepatic artery continues as the gastroduodenal artery.[9]

The portal vein is very consistent in its course. Near the hilus it divides into a right branch that goes to the right division of the liver and a larger left branch that continues to the central and left divisions (Figure 1).[8,11]

The caudal vena cava receives six to eight major hepatic veins.[4,8] To determine the distribution of hepatic veins, the authors dissected the hepatic venous outflow tracts of 15 dogs. Although many minor variations were found, the distribution of the larger veins was fairly constant and similar to that previously outlined.[12] The most commonly encountered configuration will be described.

The entry points of the hepatic veins into the vena cava form a partial spiral around the vena cava (Figure 2 [insert]). The left division of the liver is drained by a single vein that receives individual veins from the left lateral and medial lobes (Figure 2). A vein that leaves the quadrate lobe and left border of the right medial lobe usually enters the caudal vena cava slightly caudal and medial to the vein from the left division (Figure 3). The remainder of the right medial lobe is drained through a single vein. The quadrate lobe can have a separate vein, while there are one or two veins in the right medial lobe. The right lateral and caudate lobes are each drained primarily through a single vein (Figure 4). These two veins enter the right lateral aspect of the caudal vena cava in close proximity to one another, and occasionally they arise together from a single broad trunk on the right lateral surface of the caudal vena cava. The most caudal hepatic vein is small and passes from the caudate lobe to the right lateral or dorsal aspect of the caudal vena cava. Other small hepatic veins vary in their number and location. The hepatic veins of the right division are almost entirely surrounded by hepatic parenchyma.

The gall bladder lies in a depression between the quadrate and right medial lobes. The cystic duct is extremely short and is joined close to the gall bladder by two ducts from the central division to become the common bile duct (Figure 5).[8,11] Halfway between the gall bladder and the duodenum, the common bile duct receives one duct from the left division and one duct from the right division. When less than four major hepatic ducts are present, the pattern of biliary drainage is variable. Sleight and Thomford[8] described an "auxiliary retroportal system" in the dog that connects the intrahepatic ducts. This may provide a route of drainage for bile when the primary ducts are blocked. The common bile duct passes within the hepatogastric ligament to the duodenum.

Preoperative Evaluation

If time and the animal's condition permit, preopera-

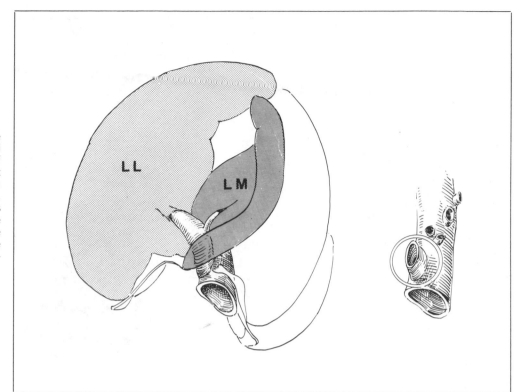

Figure 2—Venous drainage of the left division of the liver as viewed from the diaphragmatic surface of the liver. The vein from the left medial (*LM*) is slightly smaller than that from the left lateral (*LL*) lobe. The distribution of hepatic veins around the ventral surface of the hepatic vena cava is seen on the right. The primary vein from the left division (*circled*) is most cranial.

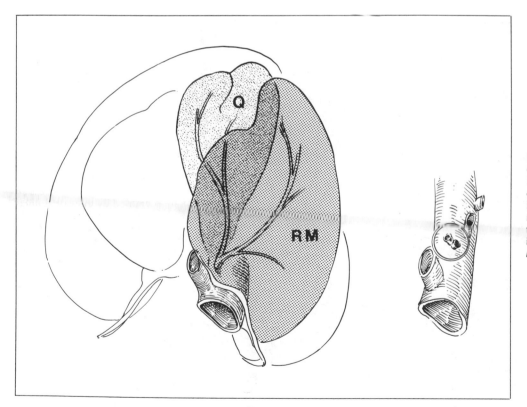

Figure 3—Venous drainage of the central division of the liver. The illustration on the left shows a common trunk draining both lobes. The quadrate (*Q*) and right medial (*RM*) lobes can have veins that enter the caudal vena cava independently (*circled in right illustration*).

tive evaluation should be as thorough as possible. Liver disease may be associated with hypoproteinemia (primarily hypoalbuminemia), fasting hypoglycemia, derangements of clotting factors, or ascites.[13]

The general condition of the patient and the relative normalcy of the remaining hepatic tissue have a more profound effect on survival than the amount of liver removed.[14] Dogs with experimentally produced liver cirrhosis can tolerate removal of no more than 40% of the liver.[15] After two weeks of total biliary obstruction, no dogs survived either 40% or 70% hepatectomy without biliary decompression, whereas 40% and 70% hepatec-

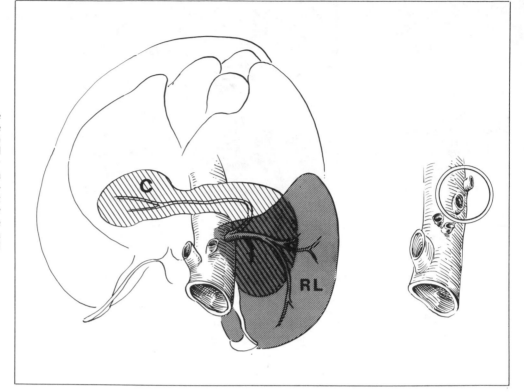

Figure 4—Venous drainage of the right division of the liver. The caudate (C) and right lateral (*RL*) lobes are primarily drained through two large veins that enter the right side of the caudal vena cava at a common trunk (*left illustration*) or independently (*right illustration, circled*). The papillary portion of the caudate lobe (*labeled* C) is often served by a single vein that enters the caudal vena cava dorsally.

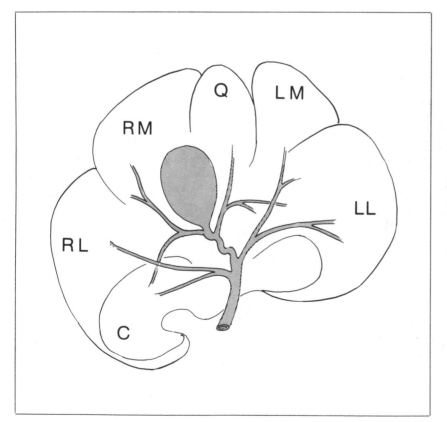

Figure 5—Biliary drainage of the liver. There is an overlapping of areas drained by individual ducts near the hilus. The central division most commonly has two ducts that join the cystic duct to form the common bile duct. The left and right divisions of the liver have individual ducts that join the common bile duct in its mid region.

tomy cases had corresponding survival rates of 71% and 33% when accompanied by biliary decompression.[16] When serum albumin was less than 2 g/dl, no dogs survived 70% hepatectomy, and only two of five dogs survived 40% hepatectomy despite biliary decompression.[16]

Sulfobromophthalein (BSP—Hynson, Westcott & Dunning) is an organic dye that is extracted from the blood and metabolized by the liver. When this dye is given intravenously, its disappearance from the plasma can be used to estimate functional mass of the liver.[17] Secretion of the dye into bile appears to be the rate-limiting step in the extraction of BSP from plasma.[13,18] At the commonly used dose (5 mg/kg), if hepatic blood flow is normal, clearance of BSP from the blood is prolonged after the common bile duct is ligated or two thirds of the liver mass is removed.[18] When functional liver mass is diminished, however, the remaining hepatic tissue is more efficient at BSP excretion; BSP removal was seen to continue at 60% of normal levels despite the removal of two thirds of the liver.[18]

Indocyanine green (ICG) is another dye used to determine the functional liver mass. A dose of 10 mg ICG/kg body weight given intravenously is believed to saturate nearly all the available hepatic receptors.[16,19] The rate of ICG clearance reflects the number of receptors available. The authors evaluated the effects of acute reduction of hepatic mass in anesthetized dogs on clearance of ICG given at a dosage recommended by the manufacturer for clinical testing (Cardo-Green®—Hynson, Westcott & Dunning; 0.5 mg/kg).[20] Forty percent hepatectomy resulted in a 29% decrease in the rate of plasma clearance of ICG; 60% hepatectomy led to a 75% decrease in ICG clearance from that of normal anesthetized dogs. Ligation of the hepatic artery or disruption of portal blood flow to the liver results in increased blood flow in the remaining hepatic vasculature.[21,22] Mean ICG clearance was not affected after ligation of the hepatic artery or diversion of portal blood flow.[20]

Plasma ammonia levels have also been used to evaluate hepatic function. High fasting plasma ammonia concentration or abnormal increases observed with an ammonia tolerance test indicate decreased functional hepatic mass or portosystemic shunting.[13,23] Plasma ammonia was significantly increased in anesthetized dogs that had 60% hepatectomies or portocaval shunts.[20] There was no difference in ammonia tolerance values when controls were compared with dogs with 40% hepatectomy or hepatic artery ligation.[20]

It has been stated that one-stage prothrombin time and activated partial thromboplastin time are seldom increased in dogs with hepatic disease.[13] However, one study of 32 dogs with naturally occurring hepatic disease found abnormal values for these coagulation tests in 66% (21) of the animals if plasma was diluted with buffered saline solution prior to testing.[24] A subsequent study of 28 dogs with naturally occurring hepatic disease demonstrated abnormal plasma concentrations of coagulation factors in 93% (26) and prolonged prothrombin times and activated partial thromboplastin times in 50% (14) and 70% (20), respectively.[25] Low fibrinogen levels are most commonly due to increased utilization of fibrinogen. Plasma concentrations of fibrinogen remain normal until hepatic function is almost lost.[13] An increased tendency toward hemorrhage

has not been observed in dogs with liver disease despite abnormal results of coagulation testing.[24,25] Intraoperative hemorrhage while performing liver resection in humans is not usually due to alteration in the clotting mechanism.[14]

Surgical Considerations

The use of pentobarbital anesthesia in experimental dogs in the authors' laboratory resulted in prolonged recovery after 40% and 60% hepatectomies. Recovery from anesthesia was rapid when a combination of thiopental sodium (11 mg/kg) and lidocaine (8.8 mg/kg) was used for induction[26] and anesthesia was maintained with halothane and oxygen. With the use of lidocaine, the dosage of barbiturate can be reduced.

Removal of an isolated portion of a liver lobe is not difficult and can be achieved by parenchymal crushing techniques.[1,2] Excising one or more entire lobes is more difficult. The most common complication of hepatic lobectomy is hemorrhage.[14,27] Quattlebaum and Quattlebaum have outlined the major technical points of removing large portions of the liver, as follows[3]:

1. Adequate exposure
2. Incision of the peritoneal attachment of the liver to improve its mobilization
3. Dissection of the porta hepatis and ligation of the vessels associated with the tissue being removed
4. Separation of the hepatic parenchyma with a blunt rather than sharp instrument
5. Control of hemorrhage from small vessels.

Adequate exposure is essential to any surgery, but it is particularly important when operating on the liver. A ventral midline incision can be extended cranially, splitting the sternum if necessary. In most dogs, incising the cartilaginous portion of the xiphoid provides adequate exposure of the liver. If further visualization is needed, a transverse paracostal incision or a diaphragmatic incision can be made after the abdomen is opened. Incisions in the diaphragm to improve exposure of the liver should be directed toward the postcaval foramen.

The liver can be retracted caudally and its attachment to the diaphragm divided. The liver can then be maintained in a caudal and ventral position by placing laparotomy pads dorsal to it and between the diaphragm and liver.

The branches of the portal vein, hepatic artery, and biliary tree associated with the portion of liver being removed should be identified, ligated, and severed. The distribution of the portal vein is usually easy to follow, but careful attention should be paid to selectively ligating only those branches of the hepatic artery and bile duct that lead to the affected tissue. Inadvertent ligation of a portion of the arterial blood supply to hepatic parenchyma remaining in the dog may be of little consequence.[28] Ligation of hepatic ducts draining part of the remaining liver has led to jaundice that apparently was not alleviated by compensatory flow through the auxiliary channels previously mentioned.[5,29] Care should be taken to avoid obstruction of the biliary tract because this promotes the development of suppurative cholangitis.[30]

In small dogs, either of the left liver lobes can be removed following placement of a single encircling ligature in an area that has been bluntly crushed with an instrument or fingers.[6] This technique should not be used when removing the lobes of the central or right divisions of the liver. The hepatic veins of these two divisions (especially the right) are short and broad, and when cut they will retract from within a single ligature, resulting in profuse hemorrhage. It is far safer to reflect the hepatic parenchyma from the caudal vena cava, identify the appropriate hepatic veins, and ligate or oversew them. Dissection of the hepatic parenchyma from the caudal vena cava should be cautiously performed using a blunt forceps (right angle or Mixter). Parenchyma remaining near the hilus of the liver can be gently crushed with an instrument or digital pressure to isolate the vascular supply and biliary drainage. The vascular supply and biliary duct(s) of the lobe(s) to be removed should be ligated with nonabsorbable suture (usually silk). Hepatic veins that are too short or broad to safely accept a ligature are grasped with a vascular forceps and oversewn.

Abdominal exploration following trauma may be complicated by ongoing hepatic hemorrhage. Temporary inflow occlusion can be achieved by passing a finger around the free edge of the lesser omentum into the epiploic foramen and compressing the hepatic artery, portal vein, and common bile duct between the thumb and forefinger (Pringle maneuver).[28,31] Occlusion of the hepatic artery and portal vein can be safely continued for 15 minutes.[32] Prolonged periods of ischemia must be accompanied by diversion of the portal blood to the systemic circulation to prevent congestion of the vasculature of the bowel and resultant shock.[33] Total ischemia of the liver remnant and diversion of the portal flow for up to one hour following 70% hepatectomy have not adversely affected liver function or capability to regenerate.[29,34]

Ligation of the common hepatic artery[35] or selective ligation of hepatic lobar arteries[28,36] has been recommended to control intrahepatic hemorrhage. It has been stated that ligation of the common hepatic artery in the dog can lead to rapid proliferation of endogenous clostridial organisms[28] or fatal gangrenous necrosis of the liver[37]; however, if the collateral arterial supply of the liver is left undisturbed and prophylactic antibiotics are given, the mortality is extremely low after experimental ligation of the hepatic artery in dogs.[38,39] Antibiotic administration does not prevent hepatic necrosis resulting from ligation of the hepatic artery.[39] While ligation of the portal vein results in increased hepatic arterial flow,[21,22] portal blood flow may[21] or may not[22] increase after ligation of the hepatic artery. Loss of hepatic arterial blood supply is compensated for by hypertrophy of collateral arteries.[35,39] Glucagon decreases mesenteric vascular resistance, thereby increasing portal flow and oxygen delivery to the liver via the portal system.[40] Glucagon may be of value in the prevention of ischemic damage to the liver after ligation of the hepatic artery.[31,35]

Postoperative Clinicopathologic Evaluation

Regeneration of the liver commences within 24 hours of partial hepatectomy in the dog and peaks at three days.[6] Although the remaining hepatocytes show increased mitotic activity,[6,7] regeneration actually takes the form of compensatory hypertrophy and hyperplasia of remaining hepatocytes.[6] Histologically, the hepatocytes are enlarged and show lipid infiltration and depletion of glycogen stores.[6] Restoration of liver mass progresses rapidly, and in the dog, hepatic weight approaches or exceeds prehepatectomy weight by the sixth week after 70% hepatectomy.[19,29,34]

Hypoglycemia has been described as a common occurrence within 48 hours of partial hepatectomy in humans[14,27] and in dogs.[41,42] Other sources do not indicate that profound hypoglycemia inevitably follows removal of a major portion of the liver.[29,34,43,44] Itatsu et al[41] found a 50% decrease in plasma glucose three hours after removal of 70% of the liver in dogs, but plasma glucose rose to 75% of preoperative values by six hours after surgery. The fall in plasma glucose was eliminated by the intravenous infusion of 10% glucose at a rate of 1 g glucose/kg/hour during surgery.[41] Plasma glucose levels following partial hepatectomy appear to depend on the amount of liver removed and the time of sampling. The lowest plasma glucose levels are found in the early postoperative period after the removal of large (70% or more) portions of the liver.[14,41,43,44] It has been recommended that postoperative glucose supplementation be empirically based on the amount of liver removed.[14]

Glucagon levels in portal blood increase within hours after partial hepatectomy.[6,41,42] This is commonly interpreted as an attempt to compensate for low plasma glucose levels,[6,41] but glucagon and insulin may stimulate hepatocellular regeneration.[42] Starzl et al[45] stated that insulin was the primary hormone preventing liver atrophy and stimulating hepatic regeneration, and they speculated that multiple hormonal factors might be involved. The increase in glucagon in the portal circulation after hepatectomy is eliminated by intravenous administration of 10% glucose, indicating that the initial glucagon increase is a response to decreased plasma glucose.[41]

Plasma protein concentrations in peripheral blood decrease after partial hepatectomy primarily because of low levels of albumin.[14,29,35,43,44] In humans, low serum albumin after partial hepatectomy has been associated with anasarca and ascites.[14,27,46] Ascites also has been attributed to increased portal pressure after hepatic resection.[14]

Bilirubin is only mildly increased after removal of as much as 90% of the liver, and it usually returns to normal within one week.[14,29,34,44] Persistent high levels of serum bilirubin indicate obstruction of hepatic ducts or the common bile duct or ongoing hepatic inflammation.[14]

Serum alkaline phosphatase (SAP) and serum alanine aminotransferase (SALT) are greatly increased within 24 to 72 hours of removal of 70% or more of the liver in dogs.[29,34] Mild increases of SAP and SALT can persist as long as six weeks after partial hepatectomy in the dog.[29,34] High levels of SALT after the first postoperative week may indicate continued hepatic necrosis.[44]

The rates of clearance of BSP and ICG from plasma after hepatic resection correspond with regeneration of the liver.[13,17,21,31,34] The plasma clearance of both BSP and ICG is prolonged following 70% hepatectomy in the dog. Plasma clearance of a high-dose bolus (10 to 15 mg/kg) of ICG gives a good indication of the amount of functional hepatic mass present during regeneration of the liver; clearance of lower doses of ICG is affected by altered blood flow as well as by functional mass.[19]

Hemorrhagic diathesis reportedly is common after hepatic resection in humans.[44,47] While this appears to be an inevitable consequence of total hepatectomy in the dog,[4] removal of large portions of the liver does not usually lead to abnormal postoperative clotting patterns.[6,19,29,34,47] Clotting factors V and VII are reduced after 70% hepatectomy in the dog, but platelet counts and fibrinogen levels remain in the normal range.[47-49] If the liver remnant (30%) is deprived of blood flow for 60 minutes or longer, fibrinogen levels drop and a further decrease is observed in factor V postoperatively.[47] This results in prolonged prothrombin times and abnormal kaolin-cephalin clotting times but does not cause a clinically apparent increased bleeding tendency.[47] It should be stressed that intraabdominal hemorrhage during surgery and after partial hepatectomy is most commonly due to failure of ligatures.

Postoperative Management

As previously mentioned, hypoglycemia commonly occurs after partial hepatectomy.[41,42] Intravenous administration of isotonic dextrose in water at a rate reported to prevent hypoglycemia (1 g glucose/kg/hour; 20 ml 5% dextrose/kg/hour) would result in a rate of fluid administration double that usually recommended during routine anesthesia and surgery.[41,50] Isotonic dextrose given at the standard rate (10 ml/kg/hour) lessens the severity of hypoglycemia observed after partial hepatectomy, and the rate of administration during surgery can be increased to compensate for blood loss. Postoperatively, intravenous fluids should be given at maintenance levels (40 to 60 ml/kg/day) for at least the first 24 hours. The choice of fluids postoperatively depends on blood glucose and serum electrolyte values.

Albumin supplementation has not been necessary after partial hepatectomy in normal healthy dogs.[19,29,34] Even when serum albumin levels are low postoperatively, they usually return to normal within two to three weeks after hepatic resection.[29,34,43] After partial hepatectomy, serum albumin concentrations are best maintained within the normal range by supplemental enteral alimentation or by early resumption of a normal diet.[14,46]

Antibiotic therapy initiated during surgery should be continued for two to three days postoperatively. If an abscess has been removed or suppurative cholangitis is present, prolonged antimicrobial therapy may be required. The choice of antibiotic is ideally based on aerobic and anaerobic culturing and sensitivity testing. While bile from normal dogs is usually sterile, bile peritonitis is associated with gram-positive aerobic and anaerobic organisms.[51] Penicillin alone[39] or in combination with dihydrostreptomycin[38] has been used to prevent fatal sepsis after ligation of the hepatic artery in dogs. The portal venous blood flow appears to be an important route of migration of bacteria to the liver,[30] and infections of the liver and biliary tract in humans commonly involve gram-negative organisms.[52] Penicillin alone may not have an adequate spectrum of activity to prevent infections of the liver and biliary tract. Aminoglycosides are very useful in the treatment of peritonitis but are excreted into bile in small amounts.[53] Cephalosporins have a satisfactory antibacterial spectrum and are excreted into bile in high concentrations.[54] Chloramphenicol reaches high levels in liver tissue,[55] has a broad spectrum of antimicrobial activity, and is effective against anaerobic organisms commonly isolated from dogs.[56]

Other postoperative treatment should be administered as indicated by the animal's clinical appearance and laboratory test results. Persistent high levels of SAP or bilirubin may suggest biliary obstruction. Elevated SALT concentrations, leukocytosis, and fever are associated with ongoing hepatic necrosis, possibly due to abscess formation. Definitive treatment of biliary obstruction or hepatic abscessation after partial hepatectomy requires surgical exploration of the liver and associated structures.

REFERENCES

1. Dingwall JS, deBier J, Archibald J: A new technique for liver resection in the dog. *J Small Anim Pract* 7:429-433, 1970.
2. Lin T-Y: A simplified technique for hepatic resection: The crush method. *Ann Surg* 180:285-290, 1974.
3. Quattlebaum JK, Quattlebaum JK Jr: Technique of hepatic lobectomy. *Ann Surg* 149:648-650, 1959.
4. Starzl TE, Bernhard VM, Benvenuto R, et al: A new method for one-stage hepatectomy for dogs. *Surgery* 46:880-886, 1959.
5. Siegel B: Partial hepatectomy in the dog: A revised technique based on anatomic consideration. *Arch Surg* 87:788-791, 1963.
6. Francavilla A, Porter KA, Benichou J, et al: Liver regeneration in dogs: Morphologic and chemical changes. *J Surg Res* 25:409-419, 1978.
7. Islami AH, Pack GT, Schwartz MK, et al: Regenerative hyperplasia following major hepatectomy: Chemical analysis of the regenerated liver and comparative nuclear counts. *Ann Surg* 140:85-89, 1959.
8. Sleight DR, Thomford NR: Gross anatomy of the blood supply and biliary drainage of the canine liver. *Anat Rec* 166:153-160, 1970.
9. Evans HE, Christensen GC: *Miller's Anatomy of the Dog*, ed 2. Philadelphia, WB Saunders Co, 1979, pp 492-501.
10. Nickel R, Schummer A, Seiferle E, et al: *The Viscera of the Domestic Mammals*. New York, Springer-Verlag, 1973, pp 134-156.
11. Cerrany C, Barinka K: Topography of vessels in the porta hepatis of a dog for experimental purposes. *Acta Vet Bruno* 40:259-272, 1971.
12. Schmidt S, Suter PF: Angiography of the hepatic and portal venous system in the dog and cat: An investigative method. *Vet Rad* 21:57-77, 1980.
13. Strombeck DR: *Small Animal Gastroenterology*. Davis, CA, Stonegate Publishing, 1979, pp 489-503.
14. Stone HH, Long WI, Smith RB, et al: Physiologic considerations in major hepatic resections. *Am J Surg* 117:78-84, 1969.
15. Kohno A, Mizumoto R, Honjo I: Changes after major resection of experimental cirrhotic liver. *Am J Surg* 134:248-252, 1977.
16. Mizumoto R, Kawarada Y, Yamawaki T, et al: Resectability and functional reserve of the liver with obstructive jaundice in dogs. *Am J Surg* 137:768-772, 1979.
17. Brody DH, Leichter L: Clearance tests of liver function. *Med Clin North Am* 63:621-630, 1979.
18. Klaassen CD: Comparison of the effects of two-thirds hepatectomy and bile duct ligation on hepatic excretory function. *J Pharmacol Exp Ther* 191:25-31, 1974.
19. Rikkers LF, Moody FG: Estimation of functional reserve of normal and regenerating dog livers. *Surgery* 75:421-429, 1974.
20. Prasse KW, Bjorling DE, Holmes RA, et al: Indocyanine green clearance and ammonia tolerance in partially hepatectomized and hepatic devascularized, anesthetized dogs. *Am J Vet Res* 44:2320-2323, 1983.
21. Kock NC, Hahnloser P, Roding B, et al: Interaction between portal venous and hepatic arterial blood flow: An experimental study in the dog. *Surgery* 72:414-419, 1972.
22. Richardson PDI, Withrington PG: Liver blood flow I. Intrinsic nervous control of liver blood flow. *Gastroenterology* 81:159-173, 1981.
23. Schall WD: Laboratory diagnosis of hepatic disease. *Vet Clin North Am* 6:679-686, 1976.
24. Badylak SF, Van Vleet JF: Alterations of prothrombin time and activated partial thromboplastin time in dogs with hepatic disease. *Am J Vet Res* 42:2053-2056, 1981.
25. Badylak SF, Dodds J, Van Vleet JF: Plasma coagulation factor abnormalities in dogs with naturally occurring hepatic disease. *Am J Vet Res* 44:2336-2340, 1983.
26. Rawlings CA, Kolata RJ: Cardiopulmonary effects of thiopental/ lidocaine combination during anesthetic induction in the dog. *Am J Vet Res* 44:144-149, 1983.
27. McDermott WV, Greenberger NJ, Isselbacher KJ, et al: Major hepatic resection: Diagnostic techniques and metabolic problems. *Surgery* 54:56-64, 1963.
28. Crane SW: Evaluation and management of abdominal trauma in the dog and cat. *Vet Clin North Am* 10:655-690, 1980.
29. MacKenzie RJ, Furnival CM, O'Keane MA, et al: The effect of hepatic ischaemia on liver function and the restoration of liver mass after 70 percent partial hepatectomy in the dog. *Br J Surg* 62:431-437, 1975.
30. Dineen P: The importance of the route of infection in experimental biliary tract obstruction. *Surg Gynecol Obstet* 119:1001-1008, 1964.
31. Madding GF, Lim RC, Kennedy PA: Hepatic and vena caval injuries. *Surg Clin North Am* 57:275-289, 1977.
32. Dunham CM, Militello P: Surgical management of liver trauma. *Am Surg* 48:435-440, 1982.
33. Rafucci FL, Wangensteen OH: Tolerance of dogs to occlusion of entire afferent vascular inflow to the liver. *Surg Forum* 1:191-193, 1951.
34. MacKenzie RJ, Furnival CM, Wood CB, et al: The effects of prolonged hepatic ischaemia before 70 percent partial hepatectomy in the dog. *Br J Surg* 64:66-69, 1977.
35. Lewis FR, Lim RC, Blaisdell FW: Hepatic artery ligation: Adjunct in the management of massive hemorrhage from the liver. *J Trauma* 14:743-754, 1974.
36. Mays ET: Lobar dearterialization for exsanguinating wounds of the liver. *J Trauma* 12:397-407, 1972.
37. Rubin GJ, Jones BD: The liver, in Bojrab MJ (ed): *Pathophysiology in Small Animal Surgery*. Philadelphia, Lea & Febiger, 1981, pp 129-141.
38. Popper HL, Jefferson NC, Necheles H: Interruption of all arterial blood supply to the liver not compatible with life. *Am J Surg* 84:429-431, 1952.
39. Kamen J: Morphology of functional relations between the arteria hepatica and the vena portae. *Zentralbl Veterinarmed [A]* 16:323-329, 1969.
40. Kock NG, Roding B, Hahnloser P, et al: The effect of glucagon on hepatic blood flow. *Arch Surg* 100:147-153, 1970.
41. Itatsu T, Kishimoto T, Shintani T, et al: The release and metabolism of pancreatic hormones after major hepatectomy in the dog. *Endocrinol Jpn* 26:319-324, 1979.
42. Caruana JA, Gage AA: Increased uptake of insulin and glucagon by the liver as a signal for regeneration. *Surg Gynecol Obstet* 150:390-394, 1980.
43. Aronsen KF, Ericsson B, Phil B: Metabolic changes following major hepatic resection. *Ann Surg* 169:102-110, 1969.
44. Vajrabukka T, Bloom AL, Sussman M, et al: Postoperative problems and management after hepatic resection for blunt injury to the liver. *Br J Surg* 62:189-200, 1975.
45. Starzl TE, Porter KA, Kashiwagi N, et al: Portal hepatotrophic factors, diabetes mellitus and acute liver atrophy, hypertrophy and regeneration. *Surg Gynecol Obstet* 141:843-850, 1975.
46. Starzl TE, Putnam CW, Groth CG, et al: Alopecia, ascites, and incomplete regeneration after 85 to 90 percent liver resection. *Am J Surg* 129:507-590, 1975.
47. Furnival CM, MacKenzie RJ, Blumgart LH: The mechanism of impaired coagulation after partial hepatectomy in the dog. *Surg Gynecol Obstet* 143:81-86, 1976.
48. Nilehn JE, Aronsen KF, Ericsson B: Changes in blood clotting factors after massive liver resection and total hepatectomy in dogs. *Acta Chir Scand* 133:183-188, 1967.
49. Hafstrom L, Lede R, Stehlin JS, et al: Influence of hydrocortisone on blood clotting and fibrinolysis after a standard resection of the liver in dogs. *Surg Gynecol Obstet* 139:860-866, 1974.
50. Muir WW, DiBartola SW: Fluid therapy, in Kirk RW (ed): *Current Veterinary Therapy VIII*. Philadelphia, WB Saunders Co, 1983, pp 28-40.
51. Cain JL, Lubat JA, Cohn I: Bile peritonitis in germ-free dogs. *Gastroenterology* 53:600-603, 1967.
52. Dye M, MacDonald A, Smith G: The bacterial flora of the biliary tract and in man. *Br J Surg* 65:285-287, 1978.
53. Stone HH, Kolb LD, et al: Use of aminoglycosides in surgical infections. *Ann Surg* 183:650-653, 1976.
54. Ratazan KR, Baker HB, Lauredo I: Excretion of cefamandole, cefazolin, and cephalothin into T-tube bile. *Antimicrob Agents Chemother* 13:985-991, 1978.
55. Sisodia CS: Pharmacotherapeutics of chloramphenicol in veterinary medicine. *JAVMA* 176:1069-1073, 1980.
56. Berg JN, Fales WH, Scanlan CM: Occurrence of anaerobic bacteria in diseases of the dog and cat. *Am J Vet Res* 40:876-880, 1979.

UPDATE

Partial hepatectomy is still performed infrequently for clinical disorders in dogs.[1-5] Nonetheless, recent reports have described a variety of techniques that may improve the results of this procedure. In particular, stapling devices or ultrasonic dissection/suction devices may decrease the time it takes to perform a partial hepatectomy and reduce the possibility of subsequent surgical complications. These alternatives require specialized equipment, however.

Thoracoabdominal stapling devices have been used to perform partial hepatectomy with good results.[2,6-8] Although postoperative inflammation of the hepatic bed may be lessened when staples are used instead of traditional suture techniques, the subsequent complications and amount of blood loss will be similar with either technique. The primary advantage of stapling devices appears to be reduced operating time.

Ultrasonic dissection/suction devices have been used to remove parenchyma along the proposed line of resection, which exposes or "skeletonizes" vessels that can then be occluded with sutures or vascular clips.[9-12] Ultrasonic energy is used to disrupt the parenchyma, which is simultaneously aspirated from the irrigated operative field.

Partial hepatectomy can be performed with the Nd:YAG laser. Because this technique results in significant tissue necrosis, care must be taken to avoid inadvertent damage to large vessels before ligation.[13,14]

Studies comparing various techniques of partial hepatectomy have observed that only ultrasonic dissection and suction devices will cause less blood loss and tissue necrosis than other methods.[14,15] These observations, in conjunction with the cost of the equipment, suggest that many veterinarians will continue to perform partial hepatectomy using traditional techniques of tissue dissection and suture application.

Hemorrhage has long been recognized as a significant complication during and after partial hepatectomy. To facilitate partial hepatectomy in dogs, temporary vascular occlusion can be done by applying tourniquets or forceps to the hepatic artery, portal vein, and caudal vena cava (caudal and cranial to the liver).[5] Temporary vascular occlusion also can be achieved by selective placement of balloon-tipped catheters.[16,17]

It has been suggested that the hepatic artery can be permanently ligated in dogs to decrease hemorrhage during treatment of neoplastic or traumatic disorders of the liver with few untoward effects.[18] Selective angiographic embolization of branches of the hepatic artery has been reported to decrease blood loss during hepatic resection in humans.[19] Neither technique has widespread use in veterinary practice, however.

Hemorrhage seeping from exposed parenchyma can obscure the operative field and result in significant blood loss. To control parenchymal hemorrhage without causing permanent parenchymal damage, the hepatic parenchyma can be compressed using one of several methods.[20-22] With each of these methods, a broad band is applied across the parenchyma proximal to the line of resection. This arrests hemorrhage without crushing the parenchyma. This technique also may control hepatic hemorrhage caused by traumatic injuries to the parenchyma. In humans, uncontrollable hemorrhage caused by hepatic parenchymal injuries has been treated by packing the abdomen with laparotomy pads, closing the wound, and returning the patient to the operating room at a later date for removal of the pads and treatment of the injuries. The efficacy of this procedure has been questioned, and it has been reported that packing the abdomen to control hepatic hemorrhage does not decrease mortality and may cause sepsis.[23] Applying a band across the hepatic parenchyma to control hemorrhage temporarily or for prolonged periods may be a viable alternative.

REFERENCES

1. Bailey MQ, Willard MD, McLoughlin MA, et al: Ultrasonographic findings associated with congenital hepatic arteriovenous fistula in three dogs. *JAVMA* 192:1099–1101, 1988.
2. Lewis DD, Ellison GW, Bellah JR: Partial hepatectomy using stapling instruments. *JAAHA* 23:597–602, 1987.
3. Kosovsky JE, Manfra-Marretta S, Matthiesen DT, et al: Results of partial hepatectomy in 18 dogs with hepatocellular cancinoma. *JAAHA* 25:203–206, 1988.
4. Kuntze A, Kuntze O: Partial hepatectomy in a dog. *Monat Veterinar* 44:253–254, 1989.
5. Whiting PG, Breznock EM, Moore P, et al: Partial hepatectomy with temporary hepatic vascular occlusion in dogs with hepatic arteriovenous fistulas. *Vet Surg* 15:171–180, 1986.
6. Lewis DD, Bellenger CR, Lewis DT, et al: Hepatic lobectomy in the dog: A comparison of stapling and ligation techniques. *Vet Surg* 19:221–225, 1990.
7. Zilling T, Walther BS, Holmin T: Left-sided hepatectomy with a linear stapling device: An experimental study on pigs. *HPB Surg* 6:51–55, 1992.
8. Zilling T, Walther BS, Holmin T: Segmental liver resection with linear stapling device: An experimental study on pigs. *In Vivo* 4:273–275, 1990.
9. Hodgson WJ, Morgan J, Byrne D, et al: Hepatic resections for primary and metastatic tumors using the ultrasonic surgical dissector. *Am J Surg* 163:246–250, 1992.
10. Kochin EJ, Gregory CR: Surgical attenuation of intrahepatic portosystemic shunts using the cavitron ultrasonic surgical aspirator. *Vet Surg* 20:340, 1991.
11. Little JM, Hollands MJ: Impact of the CUSA and operative ultrasound on hepatic resection. *HPB Surg* 3:271–277, 1991.
12. Millat B, Hay JM, Descottes B, et al: Prospective evaluation of ultrasonic surgical dissectors in hepatic resection: A cooperative multicenter study. *HPB Surg* 5:135–144, 1992.
13. Joffe SM, Brackett KA, Sankar, et al: Resection of the liver with the Nd:YAG laser. *Surg Gynecol Obstet* 163:437–442, 1986.
14. Tranberg KG, Rigotti P, Brackett KA, et al: Liver resection: A comparison using the Nd:YAG laser, an ultrasonic surgical aspirator, or blunt dissection. *Am J Surg* 151:368–373, 1986.
15. Ottow RT, Barbieri SA, Sugarbaker PH, et al: Liver transection: A controlled study of four different techniques in pigs. *Surgery* 97:596–601, 1985.
16. Okuda K, Makayama T, Taniwaki S, et al: A new technique of hepatectomy using an occlusion balloon catheter for the hepatic vein. *Am J Surg* 163:431–434, 1992.
17. Shimamura Y, Gunven P, Takenaka Y, et al: Selective portal branch occlusion by balloon catheter during liver resection. *Surgery* 100:938–941, 1986.
18. Gunn C, Gourley IM, Koblik PD: Hepatic dearterialization in the dog. *Am J Vet Res* 47:170–175, 1986.
19. Robinette DR, Gardner CC Jr, Thomas HA: Selective hepatic arterial embolization as an adjunct to hepatic resection. *South Med J* 80:1302–1304, 1987.

(continues on page 281)

Radiology of Acute Abdominal Disorders in the Dog and Cat (Part 1)

Lawrence J. Kleine, DVM, MS
Associate Professor and Head, Radiology
Tufts University
School of Veterinary Medicine
North Grafton, Massachusetts

Acute abdominal disorders are among the most difficult problems to diagnose in small animal practice. Even though the clinical signs are of short duration, the underlying lesion may be either acute or chronic. Since many of these disorders must be treated promptly to prevent rapid deterioration of the patient's condition, a practical approach is urged. It is suggested that an attempt be made to classify the disorder as *inflammatory, hemorrhagic, obstructive,* or *traumatic.* This initial approach may permit management decisions which will reduce morbidity without excluding other diagnoses. An exact diagnosis can often be made only during an exploratory laparotomy or after biopsy or necropsy.

The inevitable question that must be answered is, should surgery be performed? Survey radiography and specific radiographic procedures often provide crucial data which not only categorize the disorder but determine if surgery is needed. Utilization of special techniques in the diagnosis of acute abdominal disorders is limited by the animal's inability to tolerate stress. These individuals must be handled gently because of their painful and often precarious metabolic state. Yet radiographic examinations must be thorough if morbidity and mortality are to be reduced to a minimum.

Clinical Aspects and Physical Examination—First priority in caring for the dog or cat with an acute abdominal disorder is to determine the necessity for support of both the respiratory and circulatory systems. Such intervention is accomplished by administration of oxygen, colloid or crystalloid fluids, and by maintaining body temperature. After emergency care a more thorough physical examination should be carried out to estimate the need for other tests. The importance of repeating the physical examination cannot be overemphasized in reevaluating the dog or cat's condition.

Careful inspection of the animal's conformation gives an indication of the nature and presence of any abnormality. A recumbent posture may indicate weakness, spinal injury, or pain, and if there is a unilateral painful condition, the affected side is generally kept uppermost. Kyphosis may indicate back or kidney pain. Rapid shallow breathing often accompanies abdominal pain regardless of the organ involved, making a short x-ray exposure time essential. Wounds, bruising, or pain should lead to further examination for internal injuries that are not immediately apparent.

Originally published in Volume 1, Number 7, July 1979

Thorough but careful palpation of the external surface of the body and abdomen is essential for adequate diagnosis. However, routine abdominal palpation may be difficult or even impossible in the injured animal because of pain. Therefore, changing the position, such as laying the animal on its back so that it cannot tense its abdominal muscles, or the use of analgesics may aid in this critical part of the examination.[3]

Body temperature and pulse are criteria used in determining the seriousness and location of an injury. A rapid pulse rate, rising rectal temperature, and concomitant radiographic and clinical signs of obstruction are highly suggestive of small bowel infarction. Simple laboratory tests such as packed cell volume and white blood cell count are useful in determining the likely source, and sometimes the seriousness of the condition. Blood gas evaluations are needed, not only for diagnosis, but as aids in deciding the type of fluid to be administered. When peritoneal effusion is suspected, paracentesis with laboratory examination of any fluid thus obtained may be diagnostic.

General Radiographic Technique—The primary considerations in selecting x-ray exposure factors are the thickness and composition of the tissue being examined. A general technique chart will usually suffice for abdominal radiography. However, if the x-ray generator can produce a short exposure time at high milliamperage it may be desirable to produce a second chart utilizing low kilovoltage technique with a high milliampere-second setting in order to enhance patient contrast. A high milliampere-second setting is necessary to compensate for the decreased radiographic density that would otherwise result from lowering the kilovoltage. If the exposure is longer than 1/10th of a second there will be an inherent lack of sharpness due to motion of viscera during the exposure.

The primary x-ray beam should be collimated only to the area of interest. This reduces the secondary radiation exposure to personnel who restrain the animal and also increases detail on the x-ray film by reducing scatter. The most important factor in reducing scatter, and thereby increasing detail, is the use of a grid. Grids should be used when the area being radiographed is thicker than 10 cm. The grid will absorb scattered radiation that would otherwise fall on the x-ray film thereby reducing contrast and image sharpness. Either a stationary or moving (Bucky) grid can be used. The higher the grid ratio[a] the greater the amount of scatter that will be reduced. When a grid is used, the radiation necessary to produce the image must be increased to compensate for primary beam absorption.

With low output equipment compromise is necessary so that increased radiation exposure does not require a length of exposure time that increases the possibility of motion. For lower power equipment a 5 to 1 stationary table-top grid may be the best compromise, whereas with maximum power equipment a 10 to 1 high speed movable grid may be more desirable.

Both ventrodorsal and lateral projections are necessary for evaluation of the abdomen. One view or the other will not usually give a satisfactory evaluation. Gas within the gastrointestinal tract or the abdominal cavity will rise and fluid will fall; therefore, in the left lateral radiograph one would expect air to rise into the pylorus and fluid to fall into the fundus of the stomach. The reverse is true in the right lateral projection. Bearing these facts in mind, one may choose whether the right or left lateral view is more desirable under a particular set of circumstances. In some cases, both projections are needed.

The ventrodorsal view is generally preferred over the dorsoventral view because in the former the animal may be stretched somewhat thus reducing the amount of tissue to be penetrated by the x-ray beam. It is also usually easier to position the animal correctly in the ventrodorsal view because the landmarks for positioning are more readily seen. Oblique views project an image of the structures that lie at the margin of the abdomen but would be otherwise partially obliterated by overlying viscera in the standard ventrodorsal and lateral projections.

Special views such as recumbent lateral or horizontal beam radiographs are useful in determining whether a particular opacity is fluid or solid. Horizontal beam radiography is also used to demonstrate air-fluid levels in the intestine or free gas in the abdominal cavity.

Radiographic Examination of the Gastrointestinal Tract Utilizing Contrast Medium—There are several reasons why barium is the most commonly used contrast medium in the gastrointestinal tract. Not only is barium unexcelled as a coating agent of mucosal surfaces, it is readily obtainable and inexpensive. As long as it remains in the gastrointestinal tract, it is nontoxic and its transit time through the gastrointestinal tract is predictable.[8] On the other hand, the organic iodides intended for gastrointestinal use are hypertonic and have a tendency to draw fluid into the gastrointestinal tract.[11] In the case of a debilitated patient this feature is highly undesirable and may lead to increased morbidity. In addition, the transit time of organic iodides through the gastrointestinal tract is less predictable than that of barium, they are more expensive, have a bitter taste, and generally do not provide satisfactory mucosal coating.

However, since these agents are much less irritating to peritoneal and pleural surfaces than barium, it would seem that organic iodides have a place in contrast studies of the gastrointestinal tract where perforation is suspected. A caveat to consider is that these contrast agents are generally

---

[a]This is the ratio between the height and distance between the lead strips that form the grid.

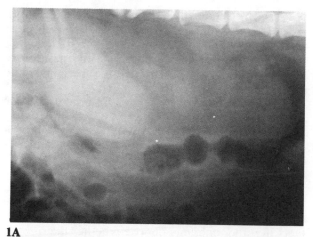

1A

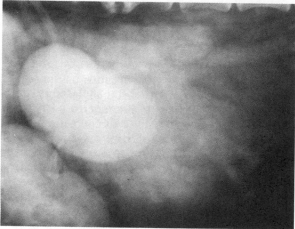

1B

Fig 1–This 13-year-old Beagle had an abdominal mass and pitting rear leg edema. Since only one kidney was seen in the survey radiograph **A** an excretory urogram was performed **B**. Both kidneys were outlined and the mass contains contrast medium. A few hours later the dog suddenly became weak, pale, and died. The mass was a post caval aneurysm.

diluted by fluid that accumulates proximal to the site of obstruction or perforation, and therefore the site of perforation may not be seen radiographically. Moreover, one must recognize that these agents are rapidly absorbed from the peritoneal surface, so that if perforation is present it may not be visualized because of rapid reabsorption of the contrast medium across the peritoneal membrane.

It is *not* true that contrast visualization of the kidneys, ureters, and urinary bladder during organic iodide upper gastrointestinal examination (UGI) indicates gastrointestinal tract perforation. Occasionally the organic iodide is absorbed by the mucosa of the small intestine and excreted by the kidneys.[10] For these reasons organic iodides have a restricted role in gastrointestinal radiography of the dog and cat.

Spilling of barium into the peritoneal cavity as the result of perforation may not be as serious as once thought if lavage of peritoneal surfaces is carried out at exploratory laparotomy immediately upon recognition of such a perforation.[13] Because

of the hazards of barium granulomas in the peritoneum and the possibility of not visualizing the perforation when organic iodides are used, it may be desirable to perform exploratory laparotomy based on clinical and survey radiographic findings rather than performing any type of contrast examination when perforation is suspected.

Pure USP barium sulfate is generally an unsatisfactory product for use in an UGI. Commercial barium preparations which are micropulverized and have added suspending agents are much more desirable. Their transit time through the gastrointestinal tract is more predictable and there is much less tendency for these agents to precipitate during the examination.

Barium products may be mixed by the user or may be purchased already mixed. Since the latter are uniform in consistency, they are usually the best and most convenient choice for UGI in the dog and cat. If barium is mixed manually, the manufacturer's instructions should be carefully followed. Vigorous agitation in a blender will produce the most uniform suspension. The contrast medium should be weighed and mixed with the appropriate volume of water.

Before administering any oral contrast agent for the UGI the stomach and small intestine should be free of food and the colon should not contain feces. Without proper preparation, transit of barium through the gastrointestinal tract will be impeded. Furthermore, dense ingesta may overlap and obliterate lesions so that radiographic examination is not only not useful, but possibly misleading.

However, since many patients suffering from acute abdominal conditions cannot receive enemas or laxatives because of the nature of their illness, it may be necessary to perform contrast examination without bowel preparation. Under these circumstances the radiographic study may be limited in its accuracy and if the examination is inconclusive it should be repeated later if the animal's condition will permit.

In general, it is preferable to give a large amount of barium (11 to 15 ml per kg of body weight) for the UGI. Contrast medium is administered by stomach tube to encourage passage through the gastrointestinal tract as a bolus. This permits better evaluation of the gastrointentinal tract than when barium is present in all parts of the GI tract simultaneously. A more accurate judgement of transit time is obtained if the contrast medium is deposited in the stomach quickly.

If the stomach is the primary area of interest, the UGI technique can be modified by administering a small amount of contrast medium (4 to 7 ml per kg of body weight). The animal is then rotated and radiographed in the dorsoventral, ventrodorsal, right, and left lateral projections. Ventrodorsal-oblique views may also be useful if a lesion near the cardia is suspected. After these radiographs are made, the UGI may be continued by administering another 9 to 11 ml per kg of body weight of con-

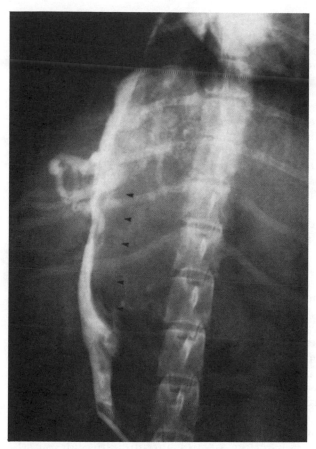

Fig 2—A 7-year-old spayed female Dachshund was examined for ascites and rear leg edema and weakness. The post-vena-cava gram indicates a large filling defect (*arrows*) due to invasion of the vena cava by an adrenal pheochromocytoma. Acute weakness was due to bleeding from the neoplasm.

trast medium by stomach tube and repeating the radiographic procedure. This technique permits evaluation of the stomach in several planes in both the distended and undistended states. Further examination of the stomach can be accomplished by instilling room air or carbon dioxide through the stomach tube or by mixing barium suspension with an effervescent agent.[b]

During the UGI examination, radiographs in both the ventrodorsal and lateral projections are generally made at each of the following times: immediately, 30 minutes, 60 minutes, 3 hours, 6 hours, and 24 hours. However, in each case the examination is tailored to the animal's needs and consideration is given to the expected pathologic change. If the passage of contrast medium is exceptionally rapid, radiographs should be taken more frequently early in the course of the examination. If transit time is slow some of the early films may be eliminated. Both ventrodorsal and lateral radiographs are essential for complete examination of the gastrointestinal tract. Some examiners choose to increase their millampere-seconds by 25% or kilovoltage by 10% to provide penetration of the barium column, permitting better evaluation of the intestinal wall during the UGI.

If the colon is the primary area of interest the best radiographic examination is a barium enema rather than the UGI. The consistency of contrast medium is not uniform when it finally reaches the colon in the UGI, so that its coating characteristics are altered, and there is a longer wait to visualize the colon when barium is given orally rather than by enema.

The barium enema procedure is generally performed under anesthesia and should not be preceded by punch biopsy of the colon or vigorous colonoscopy because the colon can be weakened, increasing the danger of perforation with subsequent spilling of barium into the peritoneum. There is no uniform opinion as to the length of time that should elapse before a barium enema can be given after these procedures, however, a delay of 7 days is preferred.

The most satisfactory barium enema technique is to use a commercially available plastic bag which contains dry barium and has plastic tubing with an attached inflatable cuff.[c] After suspending the barium in water, the tubing is inserted in the rectum so that the cuff lies just beyond the pelvic brim. The cuff is inflated to maintain the position of the tubing and to prevent leakage of barium from the patient during the examination. For small dogs or kittens a bulb syringe inserted into the rectum may serve the same purpose as an inflatable cuff, but air administration is difficult to control when the examination is performed in this manner. The barium is instilled by gravity flow, until the colon and rectum are outlined by contrast. This generally requires 22 to 33 ml of contrast medium per kg of body weight. When the colon has been filled, radiographs are made in the right and left lateral projections and the ventrodorsal and dorsoventral projections.

Barium is drained from the colon by placing the administration bag lower than the level of the dog. Gentle abdominal palpation helps to empty the colon and rectum. Usually 15 to 20 minutes is required to drain most of the contrast medium. After removing the barium, all projections are repeated. Finally the colon is insufflated with carbon dioxide or room air and the four projections are repeated again. This final procedure provides double contrast and distends the colon, providing superior mucosal detail.

Radiographic Examination of the Urogenital Tract Using Contrast Medium—Contrast radiographic examination of the urinary tract is essential in diagnosing many cases of acute abdominal disease. The male canine urethra is most clearly seen when 5 to 10 ml of a sterile aqueous iodine solution, with an iodine concentration of approximately 200 mg per ml, is administered by uri-

[b]E-Z Gas, E-Z-EM Company, Inc., Westbury, NY 11590

[c]Barium enema, E-Z-EM Company, Inc., Westbury, NY 11590

nary catheter into the distal urethra while occluding the urethral orifice. X-ray exposure is made at the conclusion of this procedure. The entire urethra and neck of the urinary bladder are outlined to show filling defects or mucosal irregularities.

The urinary bladder is drained and an attempt is made to flush out blood clots or debris with sterile saline. The bladder is then distended with either gas or organic iodine contrast medium until back pressure is exerted on the syringe by the medium, or until the volume of contrast medium administered equals the estimated capacity of the urinary bladder. The potential hazard of fatal air embolism resulting from air insufflation of the urinary bladder, particularly in patients with hematuria, must be considered. Less risk is associated with carbon dioxide insufflation of the bladder. Radiographs are made in the ventrodorsal and lateral projections. Ventrodorsal oblique views are needed if a bladder neck lesion is suspected.

Excretory urography is done to evaluate the kidneys and ureters. For this procedure, aqueous organic iodine contrast medium, at a dose of 250 to 900 mg of iodine per kg body weight, is injected rapidly intravenously. The lower dosage is suggested in giant breeds of dogs and when the pyelographic phase of the urogram is the area of primary interest. The upper dose range is utilized when working with small dogs and cats, when hypotension or uremia are present, or when the nephrographic phase of the urogram is of greatest importance.

The contrast medium can be administered through an indwelling venous catheter rather than a needle to facilitate visualization of the vascular phase of the urogram in the immediate radiographs. Ordinarily, compression techniques are not used because of the diminished visibility which results when there is overlapping of small bowel silhouettes on the kidneys, and because tranquilization is usually necessary for effective compression.

In the conventional intravenous urogram both ventrodorsal and lateral radiographs are obtained at the following times after injection of the contrast medium: immediately, 10 minutes, 30 minutes and 60 minutes. If a lesion is suspected in the trigone area, ventrodorsal oblique radiographs which include the pelvic canal should be taken in addition to the standard lateral and ventrodorsal views. The nephrographic phase is best seen in the immediate radiographs while the pyelographic phase is best seen at 10 and 30 minutes. The one hour radiograph is used to evaluate the renal silhouettes for the presence of a pyelographic phase and prolonged distortion of pelvic diverticula.

In cases of a prolonged nephrogram or pyelogram, additional radiographs are generally taken at 2 and 4 hours. A crude measure of renal function is given by the quantity and density of contrast medium in the kidneys and urinary bladder. The ureters are seldom visualized completely in a single exposure regardless of its timing because the contrast medium is carried away from the kidney in peristaltic waves.

Cholecystography—Where ultrasound is available, it has largely replaced cholecystography in gallbladder evaluation. The oral cholecystogram is generally used to evaluate dogs and cats for cholecystitis. For performing oral cholecystography, 200 mg of iopanic acid tablets[d] per kg of body weight are given per os, and radiographs are then made 10 to 14 hours later. If the gallbladder is not visualized, radiographs are repeated in 24 hours. There are many causes of nonvisualization of the gallbladder, but most can be readily eliminated on a clinical basis. Among these causes are: drug not administered, drug vomited after administration, proximal duodenal obstruction, malabsorption syndrome, insufficient liver excretion of drug, obstruction of cystic duct, absence of gallbladder, and cholecystitis.

When the gallbladder is not visualized by the oral technique, an intravenous cholecystogram using meglumine iodipapide[e] may then be performed. The contrast medium is administered intravenously at a dose rate of 0.5 ml per kg of body weight over a period of ten minutes. Radiographs are made 30, 60 and 180 minutes after injection. This procedure outlines the intrahepatic bile ducts, and may permit the examiner to determine whether or not intrahepatic bile duct obstruction is present.

Angiography–Angiography is used extensively in man to evaluate abdominal trauma.[9] However, this technique has not found wide acceptance in small animal practice because of the need for special equipment and expertise not generally available to the private practitioner. In renal infarction or rupture of the renal pedicle angiography is the preferred method of diagnosis. There are other vascular lesions that may require angiography for ante mortem diagnosis (Figs 1 and 2).

When aortic embolism is suspected the most accurate radiographic approach to the problem is to catheterize the aorta through a carotid artery approach. However, a simpler and usually satisfactory technique is to use a venous catheter inserted by means of the cephalic or jugular vein, making a rapid injection of approximately 2 ml of contrast medium per kg of body weight. Radiographs are made between 7 and 20 seconds following the administration of the medium, which will not be as dense as with the aortic approach, but usually will outline any major obstruction of the abdominal aorta.

ACKNOWLEDGMENT
The author gratefully acknowledges the help of Paula Ruel, BSN, RN, in the preparation of the manuscript.

[d]Telepaque, Winthrop Laboratories, New York, NY 10016
[e]Cholegraffin, Squibb & Sons, Princeton, NJ 08540

REFERENCES

1. Dixon JA, et al: Intestinal motility following vascular occlusion of small intestine. *Gastroenterology* 58: 673-678, 1970

2. Donahue JK, Hunter C and Balch HH: Significance of fluid levels in x-ray films of the abdomen. *New Eng J Med* 259: 13-15, 1958.

3. Hornbuckle WE, Kleine LJ: Obstruction of the small intestine, in *Current Veterinary Therapy VI*, Kirk R(ed): Philadelphia, WB Saunders Co, 1977, pp 952-958.

4. Kleine LJ, Hornbuckle WE: Acute pancreatitis: radiographic findings in 182 dogs. *J Am Vet Rad Soc* 19: 102-106, 1978.

5. Kleine LJ: Radiographic Diagnosis of urinary tract trauma in the dog and cat. *Sm An Vet Med Update Series* 7:2-6, 1978.

6. Kleine LJ: Radiography in the diagnosis of intestinal obstruction in dogs and cats. *Compen Contin Educ for Sm An Pract*, 1: 44-51, 1979.

7. Laufman H; Intestinal strangulation. *Surg Gynec and Obst* 135: 271-272, 1972

8. Miller RE, Skucas J: *Radiographic Contrast Agents*. Baltimore, University Park Press, 1977.

9. Osborn D, et al: Role of Angiography in abdominal nonrenal trauma. *Rad Clin N Amer* 11: 579-592, 1978.

10. Poole CA, Rowe MI: Clinical evidence of intestinal absorption of gastrograffin. *Radiology* 118: 151-153, 1976.

11. Rowe MI, et al: Gastrograffin induced hypertonicity: the pathogenesis of neonatal hazard. *Am J Surg* 125: 185-188, 1973.

12. Wolfe DA, Meyer WC: Obstructing intestinal abscess in a dog. *JAVMA* 166: 518-519, 1975.

13. Zhuetlin N, Lasser EC, Rigler LG: Clinical studies on effect of barium in the peritoneal cavity following rupture of the colon. *Surg* 32: 967-979, 1952.

Radiology of Acute Abdominal Disorders in the Dog and Cat (Part II)

Lawrence J. Kleine, DVM, MS
Associate Professor and Head, Radiology
Tufts University
School of Veterinary Medicine
North Grafton, Massachusetts

In acute abdominal disorders survey film findings are exceptionally important because contrast examinations may be impossible to perform due to the animal's poor condition or the need for a rapid diagnosis. When the radiographic findings are correlated with physical and laboratory tests a decision whether a contrast examination should be performed can be made. Survey radiographs also indicate whether the initial radiographic technique was correct and whether factors are present that will preclude a contrast examination or will prevent adequate visualization of the various abdominal structures during the contrast examination. These factors include the presence of feces or excessive gas in the intestine and the presence of gas in the intraperitoneal space.

Each examiner should develop a method of evaluating radiographs to determine whether they are of adequate technical quality and also to evaluate the films so that no abnormality will be overlooked. Clinical judgement is used to assign proper significance to any abnormalities that are found.

When examining the radiograph one should first visualize those structures external to the abdomen, including the bony portion of the spinal column, the ribs and the ilia. Next, the abdominal wall should be evaluated for any break in its integrity, changes in opacity (Fig 1) or the presence of a foreign body. The diaphragmatic silhouette should be examined and the general abdominal configuration evaluated. A search should be made for evidence of free gas or fluid within the peritoneal cavity. Free gas tends to accumulate in the subdiaphragmatic area between the liver and the diaphragm in both the ventrodorsal and lateral projections. Horizontal beam radiography in a recumbent lateral or standing position may be useful in further delineating small amounts of gas. Another manifestation of free intraperitoneal gas is the formation of small bubbles due to gas becoming trapped within the mesentery. These bubbles will tend to occupy a central position in the abdomen, may have the same stippled appearance as hemorrhage of the omentum and be difficult for the inexperienced observer to discern.

Next, the appearance of the retroperitoneum and kidneys should be evaluated for masses or uneven opacity which generally indicates extravasation of fluid. The uneven appearance does not reveal the

Originally published in Volume 1, Number 8, August 1979

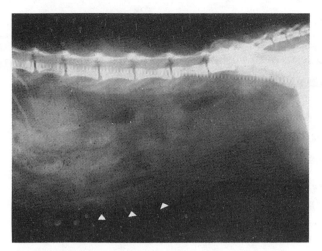

Fig 1—A one-and-a-half-year old cat experienced pain when its abdomen was touched. In abdominal radiographs an irregular opacity was present in the ventral subcutaneous soft tissues (*arrows*). The microscopic diagnosis was pansteatitis.

nature of the fluid but merely its presence. It may be hemorrhage, an exudate or a transudate. After the evaluation of the skeletal structures of the abdomen, the abdominal wall, the abdominal cavity and retroperitoneum, each abdominal viscus in turn should be examined. The entire gastrointestinal tract including the stomach, small intestine and colon should be evaluated. In addition, special attention should be paid to the liver, spleen and pancreas.

Stomach

The normal gastric silhouette lies parallel to the arch of the rib in the lateral radiograph, except in deep-chested dogs, where it is nearly perpendicular to the sternum. Hepatomegaly displaces the pyloric antrum in a dorsocaudomedial direction causing the fundic-pyloric axis to lie more parallel to the spine than usual. When gastric thickening or edema of mucosal folds is suggested, no specific conclusions can be drawn with respect to the cause. This finding is often associated with vomiting, regardless of whether the vomiting is due to pyloric or intestinal obstruction, irritation of the gastrointestinal tract, or secondary to metabolic upset such as uremia. In chronic uremia, gastric mineralization may occur.

Direct trauma to the stomach is seldom easily evaluated radiographically. Granular material within the stomach is sometimes the result of gastric hemorrhage which may be secondary to trauma, inflammatory disease or a neoplasm. In gastric perforation free air is usually released into the abdominal cavity. Volvulus of the stomach results because of rotation of the stomach around the mesenteric axis. The pylorus comes to lie in a more dorsal and cranial position than normal on the left of the midline. When this occurs neither air nor fluid can easily leave the stomach and further distension leads to toxemia and strangulation. There is reduced venous blood flow to the

heart due to compression of the caudal vena cava. Gastric volvulus can be recognized by the displacement of the pylorus and by a dense line along the cranial aspect of the gastric silhouette, resulting from the folding of the pylorus upon the body of the stomach.

Diaphragmatic hernia is a very common acute abdominal injury. It is most often recognized radiographically by the presence of abdominal viscera within the thoracic cavity or by the absence of viscera which would normally be present in the abdomen. These displaced viscera usually partially obliterate the cardiac silhouette. Transudation of fluid into the pleural or intraperitoneal space occurs if there is incarceration of a viscus within the thoracic cavity. A gastric diaphragmatic hernia must be recognized as a surgical emergency because it can be rapidly fatal, leading to strangulation, toxemia, interference with lung expansion, and reduced cardiac filling.

Vomiting is the most frequent clinical sign associated with a gastric foreign body, pyloric obstruction, or mucosal irritation.

Intussusception of the stomach into the esophagus is a rare condition that can be rapidly fatal if not recognized early.

Any time shock or difficult breathing is present, the gastric silhouette may be greatly distended with air.

While neoplasms are not generally considered the cause of acute abdominal disease, if they cause obstruction, massive blood loss, or perforation, clinical signs will be acute.

The stomach may be indirectly involved in either pancreatic or hepatic masses or pancreatitis.[4] In these situations gastric displacement is a prominent finding. With a pancreatic mass or pancreatitis the pylorus may be displaced to the left. Other findings that may be associated with pancreatitis include spreading of the angle between the descending duodenum and the greater curvature of the stomach and lack of definition in the cranial abdominal quadrant due to inflammatory response of the tissues in that region[4] (Fig 2).

Small Intestine

Injury to the small intestine due to blunt trauma is not common because of its ability to be displaced. With a large perforation of the intestine free gas is found in the intraperitoneal space, whereas when small tears occur the free gas may be confined to small bubbles trapped in the mesentery and omentum.

Weeks or months following trauma, an abdominal mass may develop due to adhesions between the lacerated portion of intestine, mesentery, and omentum. Obstruction can occur because of narrowing of the lumen due to fibrosis. Bruising of the intestine may not produce any immediate radiographic abnormality except for a slight loss of contrast due to hemorrhage. An organizing intramural hematoma is capable of producing small bowel obstruction after a period of several hours.

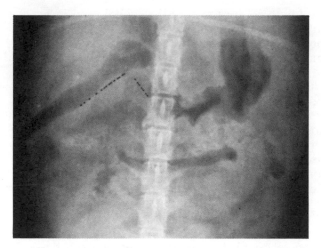

Fig 2—This 6-year-old male miniature poodle had an acute episode of hematemesis. The duodenum and stomach were both displaced caudally by the enlarged liver. In addition, the duodenal-gastric angle was widened (*dotted line*). The microscopic diagnosis was acute, necrotizing pancreatitis.

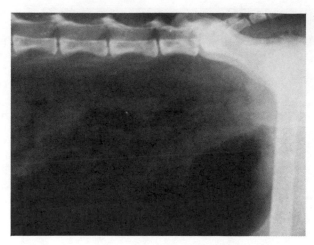

Fig 4—This 3-year-old cat presented with stranguria and ventral-caudal abdominal swelling after an automobile accident. The small intestine was displaced into a ventral hernia. A pneumocystogram demonstrated herniation of the urinary bladder also. There was rupture of the prepubic tendon.

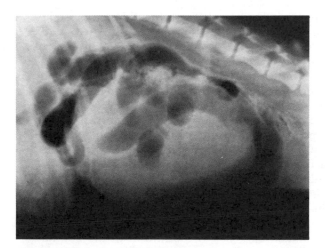

Fig 3—In this lateral abdominal radiograph of a four-year-old male miniature poodle, a large oval midabdominal mass is apparent. There is also gaseous distension of the small intestine. These findings, in the presence of clinical signs of intestinal obstruction, are highly suggestive of small bowel infarction. Surgical examination revealed an 18 cm segment of infarcted jejunum.

If massive infarction of the intestine occurs one expects to find both gas and fluid distending the small intestine due to paralysis and diminished absorption of material from the infarcted segment (Fig 3).[1] Small areas of infarction may not produce any radiographic findings initially but fibrosis can cause obstruction in the subsequent days and weeks.

Small Bowel Herniation

Small bowel herniation through an opening in the diaphragm is one of the most common results of blunt abdominal trauma. Paracostal, abdominal and inguinal herniae containing small intestine are less common but the importance of finding such lesions cannot be overemphasized (Fig 6). Incarceration with or without volvulus in the hernia may result in obstruction and vascular compromise with subsequent toxemia.

Foreign Bodies and Intussusceptions

Foreign bodies and intussusceptions are also considered under the broad definition of trauma. Foreign bodies are the most common cause of intestinal obstruction in the dog and cat, and the size and nature of ingested objects defy the imagination. The most common complication of foreign body ingestion is obstruction of the intestinal lumen. The radiographic signs are those of distension with delayed transit of material through the gastrointestinal tract (Fig 5). When a linear foreign body such as a string is ingested, the small intestine becomes hyperactive and becomes *bunched* as peristalsis causes the bowel to move along the string (Fig 6). Perforation may occur soon after such hyperperistalsis is initiated.

In early intussusception, obstruction may not be complete but vascular compromise can produce infarction and necrosis. Usually a tubular structure of fluid opacity is visualized in mid abdomen, with gas accumulation proximal to the point of obstruction. A barium enema should be diagnostic in cases of cecocolic or ileocolic intussusception (Fig 7). In intussusceptions confined to the small intestine, an UGI may be necessary to reach a definitive diagnosis.

Tumors

Tumors of the small intestine cause acute or chronic clinical signs by obstruction or blood loss from an ulcerated surface. Intestinal adenocarcinoma and lymphoma are the most common

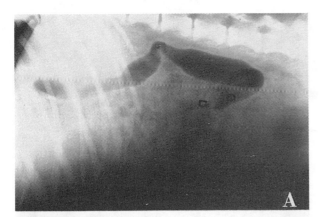

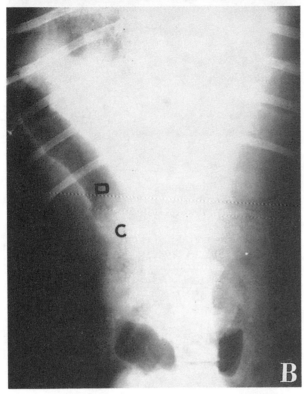

Fig 5 A and B—This 11-year-old terrier dog had an acute onset of vomiting. The gas distended duodenum (*D*) and the obstructing foreign body (*C*, corn cob) are clearly seen.

gastrointestinal neoplasms seen in this practice.

Adynamic (Paralytic) Ileus

Adynamic (paralytic) ileus occurs from peritonitis, shock, intestinal obstruction and administration of anticholinergic drugs. In paralytic ileus it may be difficult to determine whether dilated loops of intestine that contain gas are small bowel or colon. As a general rule, small bowel occupies a more central position in the abdomen while the laterally located loops are more likely to be colon.

Simple and Strangulated Obstruction

Intestinal obstruction regardless of its cause may be either simple or strangulated. In simple obstruction there is closure of a loop at a single site, whereas in strangulation there is closure of a loop at two sites resulting in interference with intestinal blood supply. When the ischemic area becomes

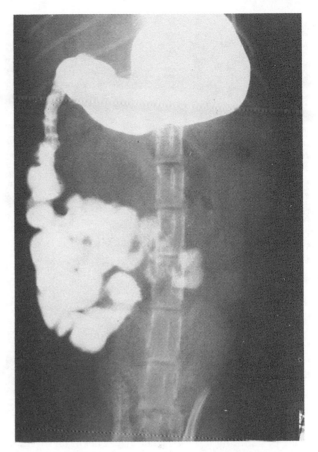

Fig 6—Acute abdominal pain and vomiting were prominent signs in a 9-month-old female cat. A 30-minute radiograph in the UGI shows convolutional plication of the proximal small intestine, highly suggestive of a linear foreign body. An 8-inch string was removed surgically.

infarcted, perforation rapidly follows.[1,7] Horizontal beam radiography may demonstrate intralumenal air-fluid levels at different heights in the same loop and can be an invaluable technique in the diagnosis of strangulation obstruction (Fig 8).[2]

Inflammatory Disease

Inflammatory disease of the small intestine is common in dogs and cats but does not always produce radiographic signs. The expected signs include thickening of intestinal walls and evidence of hyperperistalsis during contrast examination (Figs 9 and 10). Abscesses of the small intestine may protrude into the lumen and become large enough to cause obstruction.[12] Often there is resolution before obstruction develops, but fibrosis and occasionally stenosis are possible sequelae to this condition. Adhesions secondary to surgical procedures, previous inflammatory diseases, or external trauma will occasionally produce obstruction of the small intestine. Dogs can develop obstruction due to adhesions as long as three months after a traumatic incident.

Pancreatitis is capable of producing secondary changes in the intestinal tract and this assists in making the diagnosis. The duodenum may be somewhat thickened and distended and displaced to the right. An uneven granular opacity may be

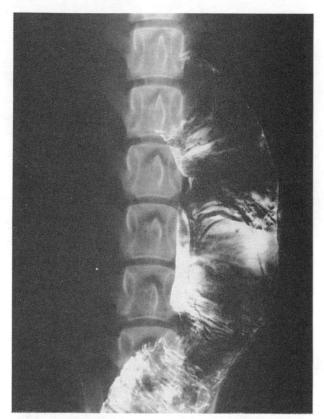

Fig 7—This 4-month-old Golden Retriever had several bouts of vomiting and diarrhea. An abdominal mass was palpated and a barium enema was performed. The multiple circumferential filling defects in the colon were caused by invagination of the small intestine into the lumen of the colon. A large percentage of the small intestine was involved in the intussusception.

present in the left cranial quadrant of the abdomen due to inflammatory disease within the peripancreatic tissues.[4]

Cecum and Colon

Blunt abdominal trauma seldom produces any radiographic changes in the cecum or colon. Penetrating foreign bodies may perforate either of these structures and produce pneumoperitoneum with associated bacterial contamination of the peritoneal cavity. Foreign bodies causing clinical signs in the cecum and colon are much less common than those in the stomach or small intestine.

Volvulus and Intussusception

Volvulus of the cecum associated with neoplasm initiates dramatic distension. Cecocolic intussusception may be a chronic disease with vague signs such as vomiting, intermittent abdominal pain and diarrhea. Cecocolic intussusception is therefore a difficult condition to diagnose clinically, but is easily recognized with a barium enema by noting a coiled filling defect in the ascending and transverse colon. Occasionally the diagnosis can be strongly suspected based on survey film findings of a soft tissue mass (invaginated cecum) in a gas filled ascending or tranverse colon (Fig 11).

Inflammatory Lesions and Tumors

Inflammatory lesions of the cecum are most

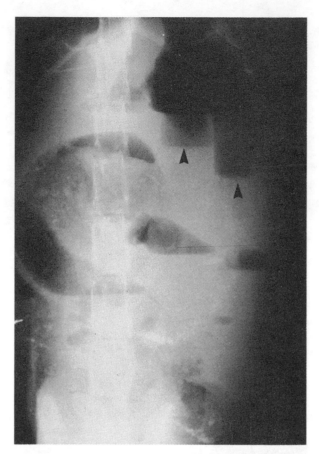

Fig 8—A 13-year-old cat had clinical signs of acute small bowel obstruction. A horizontal beam dorsoventral radiograph demonstrated multiple intralumenal air-fluid levels (*arrows*) in a loop of intestine in the left cranial abdomen. There was strangulating obstruction of the midjejunum.

often due to parasitic infestation or extension of enterocolitis.

Histiocytic colitis is expected to produce ulceration and thickening of the colon and this may be detected by barium enema. Tumors in the cecum

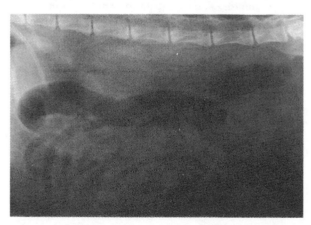

Fig 9—There was thickening of the wall of the entire small intestine with gas accumulation but no evidence of distension in this three-year-old castrated male cat. The cat had a sudden onset of vomiting and anorexia. The clinical and radiographic diagnosis was nonspecific enteritis.

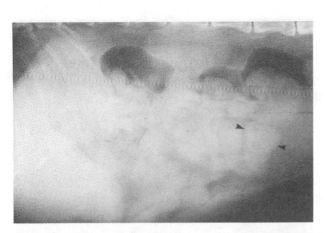

Fig 10—An 11-year-old castrated male cat was presented because of acute blood-stained diarrhea. The major radiographic abnormalities were an enlarged liver and spleen and a turgid small intestine (*arrows*). The biopsy diagnosis was eosinophilic enteritis.

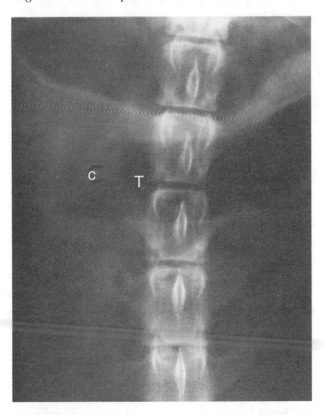

Fig 11—This 4-year-old male Labrador Retriever had several episodes of vomiting and acute abdominal pain. The filling defect (*c*) in the transverse colon (*T*) is the invaginated cecum (cecocolic intussusception).

and colon may produce acute signs of obstruction. Shock may occur due to massive bleeding secondary to ulceration of the free surface of the tumor.

Supporting Structures and Retroperitoneum

Trauma to the abdominal wall is a frequent occurrence in the dog and cat but radiographic findings are usually limited to the recognition of soft tissue swelling due to bruising, or gas accumulation secondary to laceration of the skin and subcutaneous tissue. External hernias or opaque foreign

bodies are easily recognized. Increased opacity of the subcutaneous tissue may be caused by inflammatory soft tissue disease, which simulates an acute abdominal disorder (Fig 1). Fractures of the last few ribs or transverse processes of lumbar vertebrae may be associated with lacerations of the liver, spleen, or kidneys. Bleeding into the abdominal cavity has no distinct diagnostic appearance to differentiate blood from a transudate or exudate. Peritoneal effusion can be due to many abdominal disorders such as pancreatitis; rupture of prostatic abscess; mesenteric abscess; rupture of bile ducts, intestine, or uterus (Fig 12); infectious feline peritonitis; penetrating abdominal wounds; and intestinal obstruction with strangulation. Tumors and abscesses involving the omentum and mesentery are recognized by formation of a mass and stippled opacities in the mid ventral abdomen due to breakdown of fat planes which usually provide contrast between the abdominal viscera. Mesenteric and cecal node enlargement can be the cause of acute abdominal pain (Fig 13).

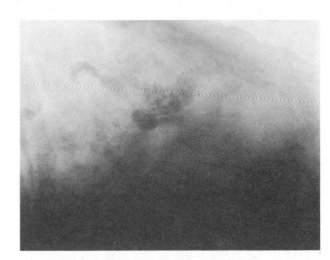

Fig 12—This 13-year-old female, shepherd-cross dog had a persistent purulent vaginal discharge for several weeks, then suddenly developed a distended abdomen and weakness. The abdomen lacked normal definition and there was a tubular, fluid-filled density in the caudal abdomen. The surgical findings were peritonitis secondary to ruptured pyometra.

Trauma to the kidneys and ureters is recognized by increased size and an uneven opacity of the retroperitoneal space. Retroperitoneal hemorrhage, without urinary tract pathology, may produce this same radiographic appearance. Such trauma is often accompanied by fractures of dorsal spinous processes or transverse processes of lumbar vertebrae and fractures of the last few ribs.[5] Retroperitoneal abscesses produce radiographic signs similar to those seen with retroperitoneal hemorrhage or tumor.

Urethra

Perineal swelling, following trauma or associated with anuria, should lead to investigation of the integrity of the urethra by means of positive con-

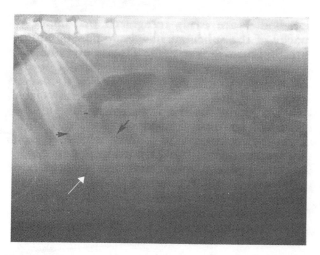

Fig 13—The arrows outline an oval abdominal mass in a 2-year-old male cat that had fever and leucocytosis. The mass was an abscessed ileocecal lymph node.

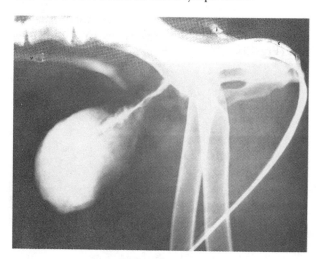

Fig 14—This 6-year-old, male retriever has extravasation of contrast medium into the corpus spongiosum penis* (*c*) The internal pudendal vein (*i*), and the caudal vena cava (*v*) are outlined. The radiographic findings are due to an injury of the urethra in the region of the ischium. Gas can also escape into the venous system when vascular areas are injured, leading to fatal air embolism. (*Editor's note: *Corpus spongiosum penis* is the term that replaces *corpus cavernosum urethrae.* Nomina Anatomica Veterinaria, 1973.)

trast urethrography (Figs 14 and 15). Negative contrast urethrography may also be useful but it carries with it the hazard of air embolism unless carbon dioxide or a soluble gas other than room air is used. In addition to trauma, acute signs may be due to obstructing calculus, urethritis, or post-operative or post-traumatic stricture. Iatrogenic injury may occur with catheters that are too large or inflexible, and occasionally results in tearing of the mucosa with subsequent stricture formation.

Prostate Gland

The prostate gland is generally well-protected by the bony pelvis and is seldom seriously injured by external force. Occasionally, however, a prostatic cyst may be ruptured by external trauma or by passage of a urinary catheter into a cyst which

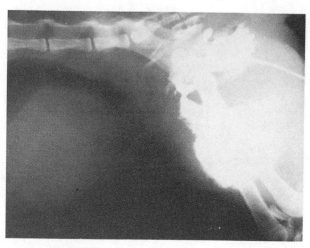

Fig 15—A 2-year-old cat was unable to urinate following an automobile accident. The right ilium and pelvic floor were fractured. The urinary bladder was distended. There was extravasation of contrast medium into an inguinal hernia because of a ruptured urethra.

communicates with the prostatic urethra. When a cyst ruptures, hemorrhage, hematoma formation and necrosis occur. Prostatitis and abscess formation may also cause acute abdominal signs due to pain, dysuria, obstruction, infection or sepsis.

The various types of prostatic enlargement can usually not be distinguished from one another by radiographic means alone. Prostatic enlargement is best recognized by abdominal survey radiography and retrograde cystourethrography. Cysts communicating with the prostatic urethra do not mean that the primary prostatic disease is cystic hyperplasia. Communicating cysts may also be present with prostatitis, abscesses or prostatic tumors. Prostatic neoplasms metastasize to the lumbar spine and pelvis and may produce acute lameness and pain.

Urinary Bladder

Blunt trauma to the urinary bladder in an automobile accident is relatively common.[5] Such lesions include lacerations, contusions, hernias and volvulus of the urinary bladder. When an inflexible catheter is inserted too deeply it can penetrate the wall of the bladder. If a flexible catheter is inserted too deeply it can be knotted. Overinflation during pneumocystography can cause local tears in the mucosa or even complete rupture of the bladder wall. The urinary bladder may be traumatized when the uterine stump is litgated during an ovariohysterectomy.

Volvulus of the urinary bladder may occur following removal of its median ligament in abdominal surgery. In acute cystitis the urinary bladder may be only minimally thickened and the signs of cystitis may be functional (straining and spasm) rather than anatomical changes of thickening and irregularity which are most often seen with chronic cystitis. Granulomas sometimes occur at the bladder neck secondary to an infected uterine stump. Tumors of the urinary bladder may cause obstruction or bleeding thereby producing acute abdominal signs.

Kidneys and Ureters

In trauma to the kidneys and ureters the primary survey radiographic signs are accumulation of fluid in the abdominal cavity or retroperitoneal space or renal enlargement or displacement. These lesions are best evaluated by survey radiography and intravenous urography (Fig 16).

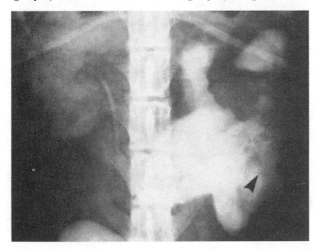

Fig 16—This 5-year-old Cocker Spaniel had been struck by a car several hours before radiographs were made, dislocating its left hip. The black arrow shows the point of rupture of the left renal pelvis in a 30-minute intravenous urogram.

Acute Inflammatory Diseases

Acute inflammatory diseases of the kidneys include pyelitis, pyelonephritis and nephritis. While pyelitis and pyelonephritis are ordinarily caused by infection, nephritis may be either infectious or toxic. The radiographic signs are usually subtle, early and are best recognized by means of intravenous urography. Later in the disease one expects to find distortion of the renal pelvis, a prolonged pyelogram, a variable degree of hydronephrosis, and blunting of the pelvic diverticula. In nephritis there may be enlargement of the parenchymal portion of the kidney with or without hydronephrosis. In some cases of acute nephritis the kidneys may appear more dense than usual.

Calculi Formation

While formation of calculi is not an acute phenomenon, the clinical signs may have a sudden onset due to passage of a renal calculus into a ureter causing obstruction and extreme abdominal pain. Nonradiopaque renal stones cannot be visualized without the aid of intravenous urography.

Tumors

If tumors of the kidneys and ureters rupture, they may cause massive bleeding and the clinical signs will be acute.

Genital Organs
Volvulus of Ovary or Testicle

Volvulus of an ovary or a retained testicle causes

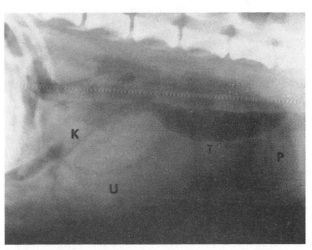

Fig 17—This 6-year-old male dog was presented in acute abdominal pain. The abdominal densities were left kidney (*K*), urinary bladder (*U*), abdominal testicle (*T*), and prostate glad (*P*). There was torsion of the testicle.

abdominal pain due to vascular compromise and swelling of the parenchyma of the organ (Fig 17). A retained testicle or ovary can be recognized radiographically as an oval abdominal mass in the caudal or mid abdomen.

Uterus

The uterus may be traumatized directly by a blunt force such as an automobile accident, causing laceration accompanied by peritoneal bleeding with loss of abdominal contrast. Volvulus of a gravid uterus may occur with vascular compromise, particularly when it enters an inguinal or abdominal hernia. Inflammatory lesions of the uterus are common in both dogs and cats. In endometritis the uterus has a turgid, nodular appearance and is usually two to three times normal size. With pyometra, the uterus is usually not lobulated but instead has a smooth configuration, may be five to eight times its normal diameter and filled with fluid. Both conditions may cause either acute or chronic abdominal signs. Occasionally the infected uterus may rupture, producing radiographic signs of peritoneal effusion and peritonitis (Fig 12).

Dystocia

Dystocia caused by fetal head, maternal pelvis incompatibility, is easily diagnosed radiographically. Fetal death can be recognized by the presence of air within the fetus or uterus or fetal skull fractures (Fig 18).

Other Abdominal Viscera
Liver and Biliary System

Ultrasound examination of the liver and associated viscera is highly effective in evaluation of the acute abdomen. The liver, bile ducts, and gallbladder can be involved in blunt abdominal trauma although they are protected by the rib cage. Laceration and bruising of the liver is usually not clinically significant. Massive laceration with hemorrhage and rupture of the bile ducts or gallbladder results in bile peritonitis. Occasionally

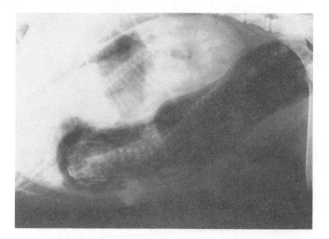

Fig 18—There were clinical signs of septicemia in this 3-year-old female Fox Terrier that had been in labor for 12 hours. Gas surrounds the fetus that is engaged in the pelvic canal in a caudal presentation. The radiographic and clinical findings are those of emphysematous metritis.

traumatic portal vein thrombosis is the cause of an acute abnormality. Hepatitis, cholecystitis, and choledochitis are difficult to diagnose clinically. Oral or intravenous cholegraphic agents may be helpful in differentiating one condition from another or in ruling out the gallbladder as the source of acute abdominal disease. Tumors of the liver, bile ducts, and gallbladder may cause acute abdominal disease by bleeding. Gallstones with bile duct obstruction produce acute abdominal pain and icterus (Fig 19). Emphysematous cholecystitis can be seen as an accompanying lesion of pancreatitis (Fig 20).

Pancreas

The pancreas is afforded protection by the ribs and associated viscera, but when traumatic pancreatitis occurs, the abdominal findings are similar to those described for acute pancreatitis.[4] Pancre-

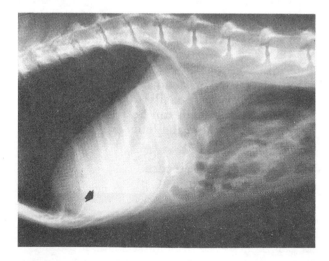

Fig 19—Choleliths are capable of causing cystic duct obstruction and signs of acute pain and jaundice. The arrow points to gallstones in this 7-year-old spayed female cat.

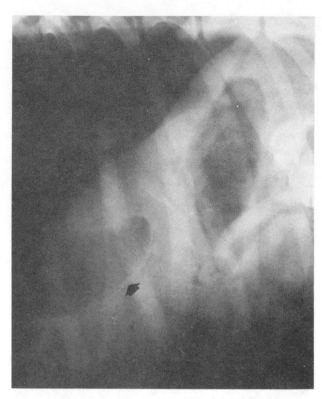

Fig 20—The arrow points to air in the wall of the gallbladder. Intralumenal air was also present in this case of emphysematous cholecystitis in a 6-year-old, male Shepherd-cross dog.

atic neoplasms may produce upper gastrointestinal obstruction when they reach sufficient size or invade the duodenum. Ultrasound examination of the pancreas is often more useful than radiography.

Spleen

The spleen is often involved in abdominal trauma. Lesions that can cause acute abdominal signs include volvulus, infarction, and laceration. Volvulus of the spleen may produce toxemia due to vascular compromise, while lacerations produce either an abdominal mass when a hematoma forms, or, free fluid in the peritoneal cavity in the case of hemorrhage. Infectious disorders of the spleen (splenitis) are an infrequent cause of abdominal pain. Tumors of the spleen may cause acute abdominal signs due to bleeding, especially following vigorous abdominal palpation.

ACKNOWLEDGEMENT
The author gratefully acknowledges the help of Paula Ruel, BSN, RN in the preparation of the manuscript

REFERENCES
1. Dixon JA, et al: Intestinal motility following luminal and vascular occlusion of the small intestine. *Gastroenterology*, 58: 673-678, 1970
2. Donahue JK, Hunter C, Balch HH: Significance of fluid levels in x-ray films of the abdomen. *New Eng J Med* 259: 13-15, 1958
3. Hornbuckle WE, Kleine LL: Obstruction of the small intes-

tine, in Kirk RW, (ed): *Current Veterinary Therapy* VI. Philadelphia, WB Saunders Co., 1977, pp. 952-958.

4. Kleine LJ, Hornbuckle WE: Acute pancreatitis: Radiographic findings in 182 dogs. *J Am Vet Rad Soc* 19: 102-106, 1978.

5. Kleine LJ: Radiographic diagnosis of urinary tract trauma in the dog and cat. *Small Animal Vet Med Update* 7: 1-6, 1978.

6. Kleine LJ: The role of radiography in the diagnosis of intestinal obstruction in dogs and cats. *Compen Contin Educ for Sm An Pract* 1: 44-51, 1979.

7. Laufman H.: Intestinal strangulation fever. *Surg Gynec Obstet* 135: 271-272, 1972.

8. Miller RE, Skucas J.(eds): *Radiographic Contrast Agents*. Baltimore University Park Press, 1977.

9. Osborn D, et al.: The role of angiography in abdominal nonrenal trauma. *Rad Clin No Am* 11: 579-592, 1973.

10. Poole CA, Rowe MI: Clinical evidence of intestinal absorption of gastrografin. *Radiology* 118: 151-153, 1976.

11. Rowe MI, et al. Gastrografin induced hypertonicity: The pathogenesis of neonatal hazard. *Am J Surg* 125: 185-188, 1973.

12. Wolfe DA, Meyer WC: Obstructing intestinal abscess in a dog. *JAVMA* 166: 518-519, 1975.

13. Zheutlin N, Lasser EC, Rigler LG: Clinical studies on effect of barium in the peritoneal cavity following rupture of the colon. *Surg* 32: 967-979, 1952.

Abdominal Trauma[a]

Ronald J. Kolata, DVM
Assistant Professor, Department of Small Animal Medicine
College of Veterinary Medicine
The University of Georgia
Athens, Georgia

Trauma to the abdomen and injury to the intra-abdominal organs is frequently seen in veterinary practice. One survey found that 10% of animals injured in car accidents had trauma to the abdomen, and intra-abdominal injuries were associated with 45% of all deaths. It is therefore important to be aware of the causes of intra-abdominal injuries, their consequences, the methods of diagnosing them and the methods of treating them.

Causes of injury can be divided into two groups, penetrating and nonpenetrating or blunt. Penetrating trauma results in penetration and laceration of the body wall and possibly the abdominal organs. Blunt trauma can result in contusion, laceration, avulsion or rupture of abdominal organs.

Since abdominal trauma can encompass a variety of organ disruptions, it is useful to group specific injuries according to their major consequences to the health of the animal rather than to the type of injury itself. There are four important consequences of abdominal trauma: hemorrhage, peritonitis, uremia and organ function impairment.

Consequences of Abdominal Trauma

Hemorrhage—Bleeding from an injury or injuries can be trivial and not clinically apparent, or can be massive and result in death. It occurs to some degree in all injuries but is most apparent in injuries to the liver, spleen and kidneys, and injuries to major vessels such as the vena cava, the splenic or renal artery and vein, the portal vein and the mesenteric vessels.

In most cases minor or moderate damage to a parenchymous organ occurs and self-limiting bleeding results. By far the most common sources of such bleeding are fractures of the liver. If a large vessel is

---

[a]Editor's note: Abdominal trauma is obviously an immense subject because several organs and systems can be involved. This general article has been selected for publication because it stresses that abdominal trauma tends to be nonspecific and a knowledge of the patterns of injury to all abdominal organs is necessary in the management of a single traumatized animal.

Originally published in Volume 1, Number 6, June 1979

torn, or if a parenchymous organ is massively disrupted, serious and possible fatal hemorrhage will occur. This is seen, for instance, when branches of the splenic artery are avulsed from its hilum.

Peritonitis—Peritonitis, either septic or chemical, results when a hollow viscus is ruptured or the pancreas is injured. In the case of rupture of the biliary tree, pancreas, stomach or bladder there is an initial chemical peritonitis. Later in these cases, and immediately in cases of rupture of the bowel, septic peritonitis develops. The development of septic peritonitis is enhanced by the presence of blood in the peritoneal space.

Uremia—This syndrome develops most commonly when there is leakage of large quantities of urine into the peritoneal space. Bilateral renal injuries, bilateral ureteral injuries and rupture of the bladder or urethra result in uremia. Unilateral renal or ureteral injuries with leakage of urine will not result in uremia if the contralateral organs are functioning but will usually result in peritonitis.

Signs of Abdominal Injury—The most common signs of abdominal injury are those related to hemorrhage. Depression, shock, diffuse abdominal tenderness and accumulation of fluid in the abdomen are seen. If the stomach, gallbladder or urinary bladder are ruptured, leakage of acid stomach contents, hypertonic urine or bile results in chemical peritonitis which causes acute and easily elicited abdominal pain, and often early vomition. In these cases septic peritonitis usually develops in 12 to 48 hours.

In the case of intestinal or colonic rupture septic peritonitis develops within 6 to 24 hours resulting in pyrexia, anorexia, depression, vomition, abdominal tenderness, ileus, intraperitoneal fluid accumulation and hypotension. Signs that are associated with urinary system injury are hematuria, dysuria, anuria, and sublumbar pain as well as signs of uremia.

It is evident that signs of intra-abdominal injuries are largely nonspecific and often subtle. Since such injuries are usually the result of violent trauma where multiple system injury is common, their early signs can often be attributed to other more obvious injuries. Therefore, it is important to actively search for intra-abdominal injuries when signs compatible with their pathophysiological effects are seen and cannot fully be explained on the basis of injuries known to be present.

Methods of Diagnosis

Physical Examination—Careful and repeated physical examination is the most reliable way to detect the early signs of intra-abdominal injury. A definitive diagnosis is then made by one or more specific tests.

To obtain the greatest amount of information a number of facets of the physical examination deserve particular attention. Foremost is gentle and thorough palpation of the abdomen. Areas of tenderness should be determined, the presence or absence of normally palpable structures should be ascertained and ruptures of the abdominal wall should be identified. The abdomen should be ballotted to assist in recognizing the presence of intra-abdominal fluid.

Rectal palpation should be done to detect pelvic fractures, lacerations of the rectum and blood in the feces. The abdomen should also be auscultated at intervals because the persistent absence of normal intestinal sounds is considered a reliable sign of intraperitoneal injury.

Catheterization—If hematuria is seen, or anuria suspected, the urethra and bladder should be gently catheterized. If the catheter meets resistence in the urethra it should be withdrawn slightly and a contrast urethrogram made. If the catheter passes easily into the bladder and no urine is obtained a contrast cystogram should be made. The urine obtained should be measured and a sample submitted for urinalysis in order to detect microscopic hematuria and to determine a base line for evaluating renal function.

Radiography—Radiography of the abdomen is useful in making a diagnosis. Plain films will show the presence or absence of normally expected organ shadows. They will also show the presence of fluid and free gas. Contrast radiographs such as urethrograms, cystograms, excretory urograms, and gastrointestinal studies will provide definitive evidence of rupture of these organs.

Abdominocentesis—Abdominocentesis, when done using a peritoneal dialysis catheter, is an extremely accurate means of obtaining evidence of intra-abdominal injury. The fluid obtained should be examined cytologically and biochemically. These tests will assist in determining if significant injury is present.

In cases of simple hemorrhage a free flow of nonclotting blood having a PCV and WBC count similar to peripheral blood is found. In rupture of a hollow organ the presence of foreign material, bile and creatinine may be found as well as increased numbers of WBCs and, frequently, bacteria. With pancreatic injury the amylase activity of the recovered fluid may be many times greater than that of the serum.

Exploratory Celiotomy—The most direct and expeditious means of confirming the presence of an intra-abdominal injury is by exploratory celiotomy. In the case of persistent hemorrhage it is the diagnostic method of choice and should not be delayed. In cases where signs of intra-abdominal injury are present but such injury cannot be confirmed by other means, exploration is warranted.

Initial Management—The injured animal is managed according to priorities. All immediate life-threatening conditions are dealt with before detailed examination and treatment of nonlife-threatening injuries are undertaken.

A patent and reliable airway and adequate breathing must be assured. Serious external hemorrhage is controlled and blood volume replace-

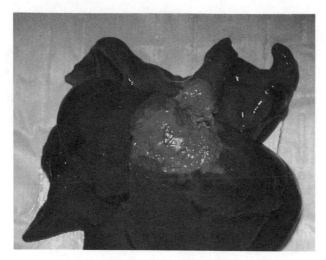

Fig 1—Devitalized area of liver caused by compression and pulping of the parenchyma.

ment is begun as determined by the status of the animal.

If hemorrhage is a consequence of the injury the animal is likely to show signs of hypovolemia. If these signs are persistent, or recur after initial resuscitation and replacement with 40 ml of fluid per kg body weight, continuing hemorrhage must be suspected, its source must be found and the bleeding stopped.

Abdominal and thoracic paracentesis should be done. If nonclotting blood is obtained the cavity of origin should be surgically explored. In most cases of severe internal bleeding the source is in the abdomen and a celiotomy must be done. Although the surgery is done under emergency conditions it should not be undertaken before the above procedures have been carried out.

Prior to anesthesia the animal must have one or more large bore venous catheters in place to facilitate rapid volume replacement. Blood for transfusion should be obtained, but is not necessary until the animal's packed cell volume (PCV) is diluted to 20% by electrolyte solution. If possible the blood should not be administered until the source of hemorrhage is controlled so it will not be wasted. This is especially important where blood reserves are limited.

When a source of bleeding is found it should be clamped off or compressed and the search continued until it is evident that all bleeding is controlled. Once this is accomplished definitive repair is done.

If hemorrhage is self-limiting and if the consequence of the injury is peritonitis or uremia the animal's vital signs will be stable or will stabilize readily after a moderate volume of fluid is given. Under these circumstances a more deliberate approach to the animal's management is indicated.

Methods of Management—The first can be described as the surgical or direct approach. This has been advocated in cases of penetrating injury and in cases where signs of intra-abdominal injury

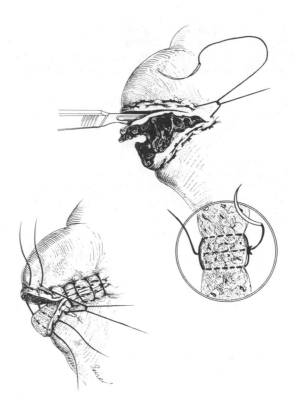

Fig 2—Wedge resection. Through-and-through sutures are placed around the periphery of the arc to be debrided. The wound is closed with additional through-and-through sutures.

are found on initial physical examination. In this approach the animal is taken to surgery as soon as possible. The rationale is that exploratory surgery will not harm a stable animal and early correction of any injury found will lessen the chance of complications. With this approach negative celiotomies are not uncommon.

The second method of management is the expectant approach. In this situation the physical examination is repeated as frequently and in as much detail as necessary until a clear indication of the presence or absence of intra-abdominal injury is detected. In addition to physical examination other diagnostic maneuvers such as radiography, abdominocentesis, hematological and biochemical tests are done.

The expectant approach to the management of the injured animal does not mean the clinician assumes a *wait and see* stance. It is an active, aggressive and controlled diagnostic workup. The advantages of this approach are that it may provide the surgeon a definitive diagnosis prior to surgery, or it may allow avoidance of unnecessary exploratory surgery. It must be pointed out that in cases where the animal has *persistent* and unexplained signs of intra-abdominal injury and its overall condition is deteriorating, exploratory celiotomy is warranted.

Indications for Exploratory Celiotomy— The abdomen is explored for two reasons: It is done to repair injuries known to be present and to diagnose and repair an injury that is suspected but cannot be confirmed by other means. Most indications for celiotomies fall into the following categories.

1. When penetrating wounds of the abdomen are found. These should be explored early unless experienced personnel are available to monitor and reevaluate the animal's condition at frequent intervals until the presence or absence of a significant injury can be established.
2. When hemoperitoneum is found and when the animal cannot be stabilized by moderate volume replacement or when the response to volume replacement is transient.
3. When continuing evidence of peritoneal irritation. (i.e. vomition, ileus or abdominal tenderness) is repeatedly found.
4. When intraperitoneal gas is detected on radiographs.
5. When fluid containing bile, urine, bacterial or foreign material is recovered by abdominocentesis.
6. When a diagnosis of significant intra-abdominal or retroperitoneal injury is made.

Injuries to the Abdomen

Abdominal Wall—Injuries to the abdominal wall consist of contusions, hematomas, punctures, lacerations or ruptures. Diagnosis of these injuries is made by inspection and palpation. Determination of whether or not a laceration or puncture breeches the peritoneum can be made by local exploration through the wound after surgical preparation, or by injection of a soluble organic iodide contrast medium[b] into the wound and then taking a radiograph.

Treatment—Contusions are not treated unless the skin is devitalized and requires debridement and repair. Hematomas are controlled by a compression bandage if feasible. Surgical exploration is reserved for cases where the hematoma continues to expand in the face of compression bandaging and results in a large blood loss.

Punctures and lacerations are treated in a routine manner unless they penetrate the peritoneum. In such cases the abdomen is explored through an appropriate incision and the original wound closed separately. Ruptures are repaired at the earliest opportunity. If abdominal organs are exteriorized through the abdominal wall they are protected by a sterile towel moistened in sterile electrolyte solution until they can be thoroughly cleansed and replaced into the abdomen and the defect closed.

Diaphragm Rupture—Rupture of the diaphragm is caused by a forceful impact to the animal's abdomen when its glottis is open. This injury is dangerous because of the resulting ventilatory impairment. The bellows effect of the diaphragm is lost and abdominal organs enter the thorax and compress the lungs. There is also the possibility of injury to an abdominal organ at initial impact.

Diagnosis of this injury is based on history and physical examination and is confirmed by radiography. Inspection will find the animal to be breathing at a rapid rate and with an altered pattern of breathing. Movements of the chest wall are exaggerated and forceful. Auscultation may find areas of increased, as well as decreased, breath sounds and gut sounds may be heard within the thorax.

Palpation may find the abdomen relatively empty of organs and the apex impulse of the heart displaced. Radiographs will show an absence of the caudal border of the heart and also of the diaphragmatic line. Gas-filled loops of bowel or the stomach may be visualized in the thorax. Small ruptures may not be apparent by any routine diagnostic method, except celiotomy.

Treatment—Early repair should be done and the animal should be taken to surgery as soon as is prudent. If a gas-filled organ is trapped within the thorax it may be kinked so that it cannot empty and consequently it may dilate and severely compress the lungs. The stomach can often be decompressed by passing a stomach tube. The intestines, however, are not so easily controlled without surgery.

Liver—The liver is a large, relatively fixed and friable organ and as a result is the most frequently injured organ in the abdomen. It is subject to contusions, hematomas, fractures, lacerations, punctures, and bursting or pulping of the parenchyma.

Preoperative diagnosis of liver injury is difficult. The most prominent early signs of such injuries are hypovolemia, shock and hemoperitoneum. Devitalization of a significant volume of hepatic tissue can also result in abscessation and peritonitis with signs of sepsis appearing 2 to 4 days after injury.

Treatment—In most cases injury is minor and requires no definitive treatment. Replacement of lost circulating blood volume is sufficient and the animal shows no significant signs of liver injury although SGPT and SAP concentrations are elevated transiently. If signs of intraperitoneal hemorrhage or peritonitis warrant exploratory celiotomy the following principles for treatment of liver injuries should be followed.

1. Shallow fractures and lacerations that are not bleeding are not disturbed.
2. Deep fractures and lacerations are debrided and bleeding vessels and exposed bile ducts are ligated. If feasible the wound edges are apposed with sutures and the area drained through a separate abdominal incision using soft rubber drains. If the wound edges cannot be apposed, omentum or falciform ligament can be used to cover the raw surface.
3. Devitalized parenchyma resulting from bursting or pulping injuries is excised, and the wound created is treated as a fracture or

[b]Gastrografin, E.R. Squibb & Sons, Inc. P.O. Box 4000, Princeton, NJ 08540.

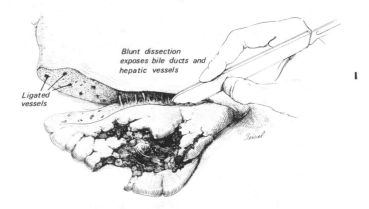

Fig 3—Blunt resection. The devitalized tissue is separated bluntly to allow for identification, and coagulation or ligation of vessels and ducts.

laceration. If the injury is extensive a lobectomy or partial lobectomy may be required (Fig 1).

Methods for Resection of Liver Tissue

1. *Lobectomy*—The blood vessels and bile ducts of the lobe are isolated by blunt dissection as close to the hilum as possible and ligated. The lobe is excised.

2. *Wedge Resection*—The described technique can be used to remove small amounts of devitalized tissue near the periphery of a lobe and to suture lacerations and fractures extending to the periphery (Fig 2). A row of overlapping through-and-through mattress sutures of 0 or 2–0 chromic gut are placed around the perimeter of the wound 3 to 4 mm from its edge. The sutures are tied only tightly enough to slightly compress the liver without lacerating the capsule. The tissue within the boundry of the sutures is excised. Any bleeding points are coagulated or ligated. If feasible the edges of the wound may be approximated using through-and-through sutures placed across the wound. If the defect cannot be closed, omentum can be sutured into the gap.

3. *Blunt Resection*—This technique can be used to make a subtotal lobectomy and debride severe bursting lesions (Fig 3). The capsule and parenchyma are bluntly incised using a scalpel handle. By this means the vessels and ducts are exposed and are ligated before they are severed. The raw surface is covered by omentum.

Biliary Tree—Injury to the gallbladder and bile ducts can occur with blunt or penetrating trauma. Injuries include punctures, lacerations, avulsions, and ruptures. Early signs of bile leakage are nonspecific and are a result of chemical peritonitis. The animal's abdomen may be tense and painful on palpation, and there may be vomition and fluid sequestration into the abdomen.

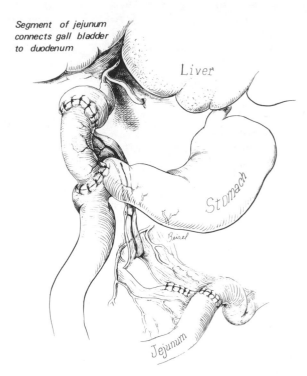

Fig 4—Cholecystoduodenostomy with Roux-en-Y. A segment of jejunum approximately 10 to 15 cm is interposed between the gallbladder and duodenum to replace the damaged common bile duct.

If the bile does not become septic, anorexia, weight loss, ascites, icterus, bile-stained urine and acholic stools become apparent over a period of days to weeks. If the bile becomes infected signs of septic peritonitis are seen. Elevated SGPT, SAP and bilirubin will be found on laboratory examination. Abdominocentesis will recover a muddy brown to black-green fluid containing a high concentration of bile.

Treatment[c]—Lacerated or punctured lobar ducts can be ligated. Injuries of the gallbladder and common duct can be sutured. Meticulous and atraumatic technique is necessary to avoid stricture and wound breakdown. The gallbladder can be removed if it cannot be repaired. Avulsions of the common duct from the duodenum can be reimplanted if the proximal end is long enough to allow reimplantation without tension. If the duct is irreparably damaged a direct cholecystoduodenostomy with or without a segment of jejunum interposed to serve as a duct can be done (Fig 4).

---

[c]Editor's note: Repair of wounds of the gallbladder and bile ducts present many difficulties. Certain repairs will not be successful without supportive complex drainage procedures. In addition, proper selection of the type of suture material is essential. These points will be discussed in subsequent articles.

Spleen—The injuries seen are hematomas, punctures, lacerations, and ruptures. Injuries to the spleen, as with injuries to the liver, can be difficult to diagnose without exploratory surgery.

Treatment—Injuries are treated by partial or total splenectomy. Total splenectomy is warranted

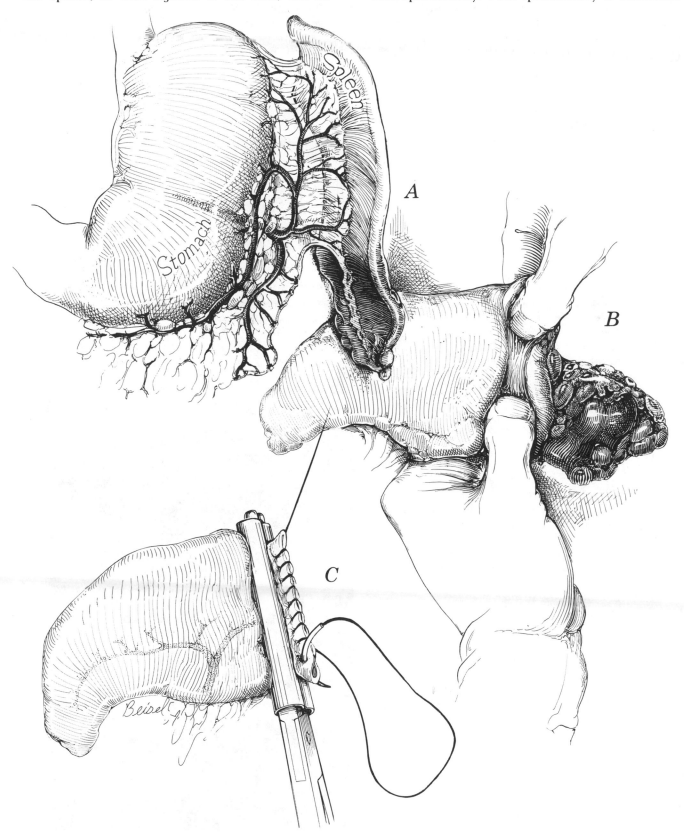

Fig 5—Partial splenectomy. **A**—The vessels feeding and draining the injured area are ligated. **B**—The splenic pulp is squeezed out of an area proximal to the injured tissue leaving the capsule intact. **C**—The area free of pulp is clamped with 1 or 2 intestinal clamps, the injured portion resected, and the capsule oversewn.

only when the majority of the organ is disrupted or has lost its blood supply. Partial splenectomy is usually adequate to control splenic bleeding and avoids the complications of total splenectomy.

Partial Splenectomy—The vessels feeding and draining the portion of the spleen to be removed are ligated and severed if necessary. The spleen is gently but firmly squeezed between the thumb and forefinger along the proposed line of resection (**Fig 5**). Care is taken that the capsule is not ruptured. This procedure results in an area devoid of parenchyma but having the capsule intact.

A rubber-shod intestinal clamp is placed across this area and another placed proximal to it. The capsule is severed distal to the distal clamp and the unwanted portion of spleen removed. The distal clamp is removed and the exposed flap of capsule oversewn with a continuous suture of absorbable material. The proximal clamp is removed and the splenic stump inspected for bleeding.

Pancreas—Injury to the pancreas is rare. It is usually associated with severe crushing or impact injury to the abdomen and is accompanied by other intra-abdominal injuries. The signs of pancreatic injury are those of pancreatitis and peritonitis. Leakage of enzymes causes a chemical peritonitis localized in the area of the pancreas.

Vomition and abdominal tenderness are evident early and increase in severity. The inflammation may become septic and signs of generalized septic peritonitis develop. Depression, dehydration and shock follow. Serum amylase and lipase are elevated. Fluid with a large number of WBC and very high concentrations of amylase will be recovered with abdominocentesis.

Treatment—If signs are mild and not accompanied by fluid accumulation and sepsis medical treatment as for pancreatitis is sufficient. If these signs do appear surgical intervention is warranted. Hematomas should be explored. Debridement and drainage with a soft rubber drain is sufficient if the duct is intact. If the duct is ruptured and if a portion of the pancreas is devitalized a partial pancreatectomy should be done.

Partial Pancreatectomy—By gentle blunt dissection between the lobules, the central duct is exposed and ligated. The distal portion of the pancreas is removed. When working with the right lobe care must be taken to preserve the pancreaticoduodenal vessels as ischemia of the duodenum will result if they are interrupted or dissected from the duodenum. The excretory duct, of which there are one or more entering the duodenum at the junction of the two lobes, should be preserved.

If the pancreatic ducts are ruptured or avulsed the pancreas is debrided and the stump is implanted so that the remaining portion of the pancreas and its duct discharge into the lumen of the duodenum. If necessary a total pancreatectomy can be done. Insulin and pancreatic enzyme supplementation are then necessary for the life of the dog.

Injuries to the Gastrointestinal Tract

Injuries to the stomach, intestines and colon include contusions, intramural and mesenteric hematomas, mucosal and serosal tears, avulsions of the mesentery, ruptures and punctures. The most important consequence of GI injuries is leakage of contents into the peritoneal space and peritonitis. The signs of GI injuries are hematemesis, bloody stool, depression, anorexia, vomition, abdominal tenderness, peritonitis, intraperitoneal accumulation of fluid and shock.

Stomach, Intestines, and Colon—Penetrating injuries due to gunshot are probably the most common. The stomach may also rupture if the animal sustains blunt impact after eating a large meal. The signs associated with injuries to the stomach are abdominal tenderness, unproductive retching and development of peritonitis. Free gas and fluid will be seen on radiographs, and leakage will be seen if contrast studies are done. Abdominocentesis will recover foreign material and fluid, and after sepsis develops bacteria will be found.

Treatment—Wounds of the stomach are debrided and sutured in two layers, the mucosa and submucosa first followed by the muscularis and serosa. Wounds of the intestines and colon are debrided and sutured as an enterotomy or an anastomosis. The peritoneal space is lavaged with copious amounts of warm electrolyte solution containing an antibiotic or a nonirritating antiseptic.

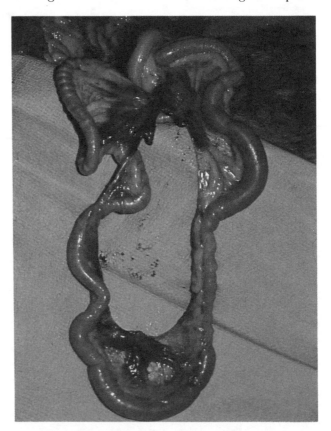

Fig 6—Avulsion of mesentery from jejenum. Severe hemorrhage and bowel infarction may follow such an injury.

Mesentery—Laceration or avulsion of the mesentery is seen with blunt or penetrating trauma. Avulsion of the mesentery is most likely to occur at points of attachment, i.e. the root of the mesentery or distally where it attaches to the bowel (Fig 6). The consequences of mesenteric injury are hemorrhage, and ischemia of the bowel due to thrombosis or avulsion of vessels, or strangulation of a loop of bowel by being incarcerated through a rent in the mesentery.

Early signs depend on the volume of hemorrhage. Subsequently ischemia of the bowel may occur. The segment undergoing infarction will first slough its mucosa and bloody mucoid feces will be seen. As degeneration of the bowel wall progresses, peritonitis develops and its signs become increasingly apparent. Radiographs taken at this time may show a dilated segment of bowel. Contrast studies may show ulcerations and localized ileus. When rupture occurs peritonitis will be apparent and contrast studies may show leakage. Abdominocentesis will recover fluid containing foreign material and bacteria.

Treatment—Treatment consists of ligation of vessels and resection of the affected segment of bowel.

Injuries to the Urinary Tract

Kidney—The kidney is subject to contusions, fractures, lacerations and avulsions. The immediate consequence of renal injury is hemorrhage. It may be subcapsular, retroperitoneal or intraperitoneal and it may be seen macroscopically or microscopically in the urine. Urine may accumulate retro- or intraperitoneally. If the hemorrhage is severe, shock will develop. A painful sublumbar mass may be palpable.

Radiographs may show free peritoneal fluid or a sublumbar mass displacing the colon ventrally. If an excretory urogram is done nonvisualization of a kidney or an abnormally contoured kidney may be seen with or without leakage of contrast media. If there is intraperitoneal leakage of urine abdominocentesis will recover bloody fluid containing a high concentration of creatinine. Unlike the case of bladder rupture, uremia is unlikely to develop unless both kidneys are severely affected.

Treatment—Treatment depends on the severity of injury. Contusions and intracapsular fractures do not require treatment. Lacerations of the capsule and kidney are debrided and the capsule sutured. If the collecting system is lacerated or ruptured it is sutured with fine chromic gut or synthetic absorbable material.

Fragmentation or severe laceration of a pole of the kidney is treated by partial nephrectomy. If more than 50% of the kidney is destroyed or the pedicle is avulsed nephrectomy is indicated. It is vital to know the functional status of the opposite kidney before this is done.

Partial Nephrectomy—The renal pedicle is isolated and controlled with an umbilical tape tourniquet or a vascular clamp (Fig 7). If possible the renal capsule is preserved. The affected portion of

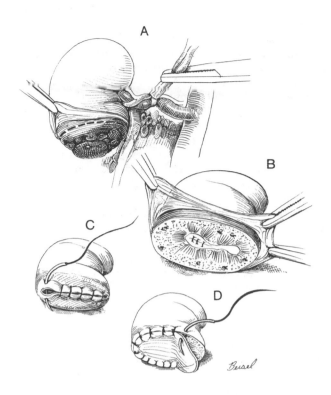

Fig 7—Partial nephrectomy. **A**—After the renal vessels are controlled the injured tissue is debrided. **B**—The capsule is reflected and preserved if possible and the pelvis is closed. **C**—The capsule is sutured over the wound. **D**—Omentum or peritoneum are sutured over the wound to cover the raw surface.

kidney is excised, the vessels ligated and the pelvis sutured. The capsule is then sutured over the wound. If the capsule is unavailable, omentum or peritoneum is used to cover the wound. The kidney is then sutured into its retroperitoneal bed.

Ureter—Ureteral injuries are generally seen at the proximal and distal quarters. Signs of injury are usually those of peritonitis although if bilateral rupture occurs uremia will develop. There is sublumbar or intraperitoneal accumulation of urine. Radiographs will demonstrate fluid in these areas. There will be tenderness in the lumbar area and abdomen on palpation. An excretory urogram will show leakage. Abdominocentesis will recover blood-tinged or turbid fluid with a high concentration of creatinine. If leakage is only retroperitoneal fluid may not be recovered by abdominocentesis. Hematuria is often present.

Treatment—Incomplete tears are debrided and sutured with a fine absorbable material. In transections the ends are debrided, spatulated and anastomosed over a soft rubber catheter using a continuous suture of 5–0 absorbable material (Fig 8). The catheter is exteriorized via the bladder and urethra, and removed in 5–7 days. If the ureter is avulsed from the bladder it can be reimplanted.

Bladder—Common injuries to the bladder include contusion, rupture, puncture, and avulsion.

Signs associated with bladder injury are hematuria, oliguria or anuria and abdominal tenderness. As time passes fluid accumulates in the peritoneal space and uremia develops. The animal becomes increasingly depressed and anorectic, vomition occurs and dehydration develops. Death will occur after about 48 to 72 hours.

Radiographs will show fluid within the peritoneal cavity and the absence of the bladder shadow. A cystogram will show leakage. Abdominocentesis will obtain blood-tinged fluid having a high concentration of creatinine. Hemogram and blood chemistries will find an elevated PCV and serum protein and an elevated BUN and serum creatinine.

Treatment—The wound is debrided and sutured with absorbable material. If the bladder is avulsed from the urethra it can be anastomosed if its blood supply is intact. If the bladder is ischemic the ureters can be implanted into an isolated segment of ileum, one end of which is exteriorized through

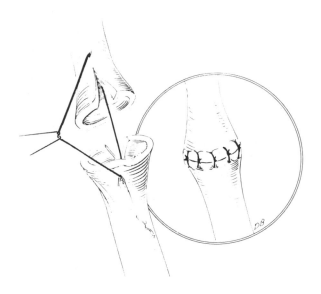

Fig 8—Ureteral anastomosis. The ends are debrided and incised longitudinally for a short distance and then the anastomosis is completed.

the body wall. However, the animal will constantly drip urine and be subject to ascending pyelonephritis.

Prostate and Urethra—These organs may be lacerated or punctured by fragments of the pelvis when it is fractured, and the consequence is leakage of urine. Clinical signs are those of a ruptured bladder. If a catheter is passed it will meet resistance before entering the bladder or it may pass out of the urethra into the peritoneal cavity. If resistance is met or there is question about the integrity of the urethra a contrast urethrogram should be made.

Treatment—If the tear is small and a catheter passes into the bladder the catheter is left in place for 5 to 7 days until the urethra heals. If the tear is large or a catheter cannot pass easily the wound is debrided and the urethra sutured with fine absorbable material. The capsule of the prostate is closed and a urethral catheter is maintained for 7 to 10 days.

Uterus—If the uterus is enlarged due to pregnancy or pyometra it may be injured. The signs of uterine injury are associated with hemorrhage and the development of peritonitis. If the uterus is gravid when ruptured, hemorrhage and displacement of some of the fetuses will occur. The fetuses will usually die and cause peritonitis. If pyometra is present peritonitis develops soon after puncture or rupture.

Treatment—Ovariohysterectomy is generally the treatment of choice. In a valuable brood bitch removal of the affected horn and its ovary is possible.

REFERENCES

1. *Canine Surgery*, 2nd Archibald ed. Santa Barbara, CA, American Veterinary Publications, Inc., 1974.
2. Bojrab MJ (ed): *Current Techniques in Small Animal Surgery*, Philadelphia, Lea & Febiger, 1975.
3. Kolata RJ: Diagnostic abdominal paracentesis and lavage: experimental and clinical evaluations in the dog. *JAVMA* 168:697, 1976.
4. DeHoff WD, Greene RW, Greiner TP: Surgical management of abdominal emergencies, *Vet Clin N Am* 2:301, 1972.

KEY FACTS

- Gastric decompression and vigorous intravenous fluid replacement are initiated simultaneously.
- Successful passage of an orogastric tube does not rule out the presence of gastric volvulus.
- Surgical management is suggested for all large-breed dogs with typical signs of gastric dilatation-volvulus.
- Circumcostal gastropexy provides a strong, permanent gastropexy and is recommended.
- Postoperative ventricular tachycardia is common.

Therapy of Gastric Dilatation-Volvulus in Dogs

Michael S. Leib, DVM, MS
Robert A. Martin, DVM

Department of Small Animal
    Clinical Science
Virginia-Maryland Regional College
    of Veterinary Medicine
Virginia Tech
Blacksburg, Virginia

Gastric dilatation-volvulus is an acute, life-threatening condition that is associated with a high mortality rate. The condition occurs primarily in large, deep-chested canine breeds. Survival depends on prompt diagnosis and vigorous emergency treatment by the veterinarian. In most cases, the correct diagnosis can be made easily. Clinical signs include an abrupt onset of restlessness, discomfort, abdominal pain, excessive salivation, nonproductive retching, and abdominal distention. Physical examination reveals progressive circulatory shock and tachypnea or dyspnea. Simultaneous initiation of gastric decompression and intravenous fluid therapy for hypovolemic shock is indicated to stabilize the patient.

Emergency Therapy

Gastric Decompression

The pathophysiologic changes that occur in acute gastric dilatation-volvulus are related to gastric distention and volvulus.[1-6] Gastric decompression is the primary therapeutic goal of emergency management.[1-6] Ideally, gastric decompression and vigorous intravenous fluid replacement are initiated simultaneously. In most instances, sufficient personnel assistance is unavailable. We first insert an intravenous catheter and initiate fluid therapy and then attempt gastric decompression. Occasionally, gastric decompression receives first priority because the patient is experiencing severe respiratory distress.

Decompression is most commonly achieved by passing a large-bore, well-lubricated orogastric tube through an oral speculum (Figure 1). The authors place a firm roll of adhesive tape behind the patient's incisor teeth and tie the mouth shut with gauze. The orogastric tube should be premeasured from the incisor teeth to the costal arch and properly marked to prevent passage of an excessive length of tube, which can result in gastric trauma or perforation. Resistance is usually met at the esophagogastric junction. Firm, gentle pressure as the tube is rotated slightly will often result in successful passage into the stomach. Gastric gas passes from the distended stomach, resulting in rapid clinical improvement. Fluid and ingesta are removed via gravity and syringe suction. After decompression is achieved, the stomach should be lavaged with warm water to remove remaining ingesta. In the authors' experience, lavage reduces the incidence and severity of immediate recurrence of gastric distention. Successful passage of an orogastric tube does *not* rule out the presence of gastric volvulus.

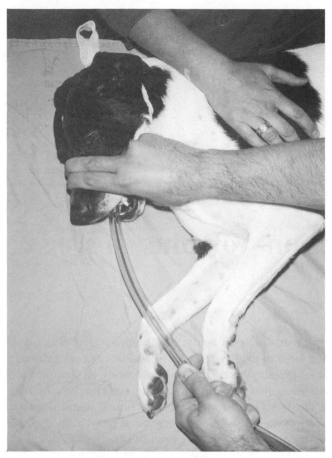

Figure 1—Passage of a large-bore orogastric tube through an oral speculum. The tube has been measured from the incisors to the costal arch. The patient's head is flexed to aid passage into the esophagus.

The orogastric tube can be successfully passed in most cases of gastric dilatation-volvulus. In the event of failure, however, several manipulations can result in successful passage and decompression. The patient should be forced to sit, or its forelegs should be elevated to produce an approximate 45° angle. This reduces the pressure on the esophagogastric junction as gravity forces the abdominal viscera caudally. If successful passage is still not achieved, percutaneous needle decompression should be attempted.[3,6,7] The hair is clipped and a 6 × 6-cm area of skin is prepared sterilely caudal to the costal arch on the right side. This area should be percussed to ensure that the spleen is not along the needle's path. A 16- to 18-gauge, 1- to 1½-inch intravenous needle or a 5- to 6-inch rigid catheter attached to suction is placed through the skin, the abdominal musculature, and the gastric wall, allowing the trapped gastric gas to escape. The partial gastric decompression obtained often allows successful orogastric intubation and gastric lavage by reducing pressure at the esophagogastric junction. Although hemorrhage and leakage of gastric contents and peritonitis are possible sequelae to needle decompression, the authors have not experienced these complications in numerous clinical cases.

Failure to pass the orogastric tube successfully after nee-

dle decompression can be the result of an uncooperative patient excessively resisting restraint and intubation. Gastric distention restricts respiratory tidal volume; this can cause the patient to become agitated and fractious. Narcotic sedation can ease anxiety and improve restraint.[4,7,8] The authors use intravenous oxymorphone hydrochloride (0.05 to 0.10 mg/kg, 3 mg maximum) if sedation is needed. Narcotics should be used with extreme caution because they depress respiration, which is already compromised. Gastric decompression, however, quickly improves respiratory function. A narcotic antagonist, such as naloxone hydrochloride, should be available if respiratory depression occurs before gastric decompression is achieved.

If successful orogastric intubation is still not achieved, temporary gastrostomy might be indicated.[7,8] A larger area caudal to the right costal arch is sterilely prepared. Local anesthesia is provided with 2% lidocaine hydrochloride (without epinephrine) in an inverted L-block pattern. A 5-cm skin incision is made 2 cm caudal and parallel to the costal arch. The stomach is exposed, using a grid incision through the abdominal musculature or a direct incision through all three layers. Care must be exercised not to penetrate the gastric wall because it is pressed tightly against the abdominal musculature. A 3-0 stay suture attaches the stomach to each end of the skin incision. The exposed stomach can be decompressed by needle and suction. The skin is sutured to the stomach in a continuous fashion, producing an oval area of gastric wall sealed from the abdominal cavity (Figure 2). The decompressed stomach is

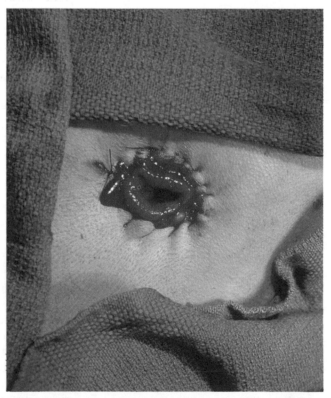

Figure 2—Completed temporary gastrostomy. Gastric decompression has been achieved and can be maintained through the gastrostomy.

opened and gastric lavage is performed via the gastrostomy site.

A major disadvantage of temporary gastrostomy is the additional surgical time necessary to close the incision before exploratory surgery. In addition, performing the procedure too ventrally can result in a disrupted, contaminated body wall in the area in which gastropexy might be performed. Some surgeons perform the procedure on the left side to avoid this potential complication.

Shock Therapy

As soon as orogastric intubation is initiated, vigorous intravenous fluid therapy should be started to combat progressive hypovolemic shock.[9-11] One or two large-bore intravenous catheters are placed, and an isotonic fluid is given rapidly. Approximately 90 ml/kg should be given during the first hour of therapy.[1,3,11-13] The rate of fluid therapy should be carefully adjusted based on monitoring of the following parameters: heart rate, arterial pulse strength, capillary refill time, mucous membrane color, core-extremity temperature differential, mental status, urine output, packed cell volume, and total solids. Successful gastric decompression relieves the obstruction to venous return and greatly improves cardiovascular status.

The use of glucocorticoids in hypovolemic shock remains controversial.[1,3,5,11] Potential benefits include stabilization of lysosomal membranes, increased cardiac output, and improved integrity of the capillary endothelium.[3,12-14] Although the relationship between endotoxemia and gastric dilatation-volvulus has not been established, endotoxins are speculated to be elaborated in gastric dilatation-volvulus. Therefore, corticosteroids might have the additional benefits of reducing serum levels of endotoxin, promoting reticuloendothelial system clearance, and decreasing complement fixation.[3,11-14] The authors routinely give dexamethasone sodium phosphate at 1 to 2 mg/kg intravenously. More rapidly acting agents (prednisolone sodium succinate, 10 mg/kg) have the disadvantage of being more expensive.

The authors routinely give intravenous ampicillin, 22 mg/kg every six hours, during the stabilization period and two to three days postoperatively. Bactericidal antibiotics can potentially benefit the patient by combating sepsis, peritonitis from gastric leakage or necrosis, and postoperative surgical infection.

Temporary Stabilization

Although it is controversial, the authors recommend a prolonged period of temporary stabilization before exploratory surgery.[5-8] The benefits of prolonged temporary stabilization include the following: (1) It allows time for cardiovascular and metabolic stabilization. (2) Exploratory surgery can be performed at a convenient time, with a complete hospital staff and thorough postoperative monitoring available. (3) A preoperative work-up can be performed to gather information that can lead to a rational anesthetic plan and complete postoperative care. Evaluation can include complete blood count, biochemical pro-

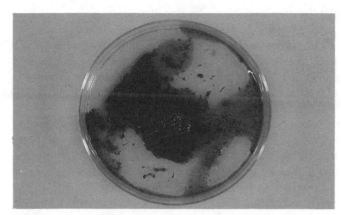

Figure 3—Coffee-grounds gastric lavage solution, suggesting potential gastric-wall devitalization. Prolonged temporary stabilization is not attempted in such a case, and exploratory laparotomy is performed as soon as the patient becomes stable.

file, urinalysis, electrocardiogram, and thoracic or abdominal radiographs. (4) Transport of a stable patient to a referral center for exploratory surgery and postoperative care can be arranged.

Failure to immediately inspect and reposition the stomach is a potential disadvantage of prolonged temporary stabilization. Gastric-wall necrosis, rupture, peritonitis, and sepsis are probably the most common causes of postoperative death in gastric dilatation-volvulus patients.[3,7,15] Immediate inspection of a devitalized stomach allows gastric resection and can prevent gastric rupture and peritonitis. A recent experimental study determined that a 360° gastric volvulus with a nondistended stomach produced reversible gastric-wall edema and hemorrhage.[16] The authors of the study suggested rapid surgical repositioning of the stomach in dogs with gastric dilatation-volvulus. In our experience, however, most cases of gastric dilatation-volvulus do not have 360° volvulus, and it is unknown whether similar pathologic findings occur in these cases.

Another possible disadvantage of prolonged temporary stabilization is that delayed exploratory surgery can permit the development of severe cardiac arrhythmias, which increase the risks of exploratory surgery and anesthesia. Approximately 40% to 50% of dogs with gastric dilatation-volvulus can develop severe cardiac arrhythmias.[3,17,18] Approximately 25% of these arrhythmias are present on admission, however; the other 75% develop within the first 36 hours of hospitalization.[18] Thus, delaying surgery increases the risk that severe cardiac arrhythmias will be present at the time of exploratory surgery.

In our experience, temporary stabilization is successful when the gastric lavage solution does not contain clotted blood or so-called coffee-grounds material (Figure 3). This type of fluid can signify impending gastric-wall devitalization and rupture. Clear lavage fluid does not rule out this possibility, however. Temporary stabilization also is successful after gastric decompression; palpable splenomegaly resolves. Patients with persistent splenomegaly have clinically deteriorated during periods of prolonged temporary stabilization and have developed severe cardiac arrhythmias, increasing anesthetic and surgical risks.

The authors have successfully used prolonged temporary stabilization in treating gastric dilatation-volvulus, apparently with significant benefit to the patients. Temporary stabilization can be maintained for as long as 48 hours without adverse effects.[5,7,8] The length of the period should be based on condition of the patient, time of day of presentation, clinic facilities, and surgical skills of the veterinarian. Some researchers suggest exploratory surgery within one to two hours of gastric decompression.[1]

Gastric decompression can be maintained during the period of stabilization by repeated orogastric intubation, placement of a pharyngostomy tube, temporary gastrostomy, or placement of a nasogastric tube. Repeated orogastric intubation has the disadvantage of being stressful to the patient and potentially causing additional gastric trauma and possible rupture. Using a pharyngostomy tube has the drawback of requiring brief general anesthesia to place the tube through the pharyngeal wall.[19,20] The tube maintains gastric decompression nonstressfully and does not require surgical repair after removal. Temporary gastrostomy should only be used if orogastric intubation cannot be accomplished. As previously stated, a disadvantage of this procedure is the repair time necessary before exploratory surgery.[4,7,8] Recently, the use of a nasogastric tube has been reported to maintain gastric decompression in dogs with gastric dilatation-volvulus.[21] Although we do not have personal experience with this method, it appears to be ideal for maintaining gastric decompression during the temporary stabilization period. Nasogastric tubes were placed with only intranasal anesthesia and minimal restraint, were well tolerated by clinical patients, did not require surgical repair after removal, and were effective in preventing gastric distention.[21]

Once treatment for shock is initiated and gastric decompression is accomplished, a lead II electrocardiogram should be evaluated. Approximately 25% of cardiac arrhythmias in dogs with gastric dilatation-volvulus occur during presentation.[18] Ventricular arrhythmias are the most common arrhythmias seen and usually require aggressive therapy.

Surgical Therapy

The goals of surgical treatment of gastric dilatation-volvulus are gastric repositioning, assessment of gastric and splenic viability, and permanent fixation of the stomach to the body wall in a manner that does not interfere with gastric function yet prevents recurrence. Minimizing anesthetic and surgical time usually will improve survival. The surgeon must be experienced in using techniques for derotating the stomach, judging gastric and splenic viability, and performing permanent gastropexy.

Pyloric sphincter dysfunction has been implicated as a contributing causative factor in gastric dilatation-volvulus[3,6,20,22-25]; procedures to promote increased gastric emptying (pyloromyotomy and pyloroplasty) have been advocated.[23,25-27] The value of such procedures is unknown because no well-controlled clinical studies have documented pyloric dysfunction as a direct causative factor in gastric dilatation-volvulus or have assessed the efficacy of pyloric surgery in preventing recurrence.[3,22] Except in patients with palpably abnormal pyloric sphincters, we do not routinely include pyloric surgery in surgical management.

The authors suggest surgical management for all large-breed dogs with typical signs of gastric dilatation-volvulus. Cases of overeating or foreign-substance engorgement can be successfully managed without surgery. Many cases of gastric dilatation-volvulus that are rapidly stabilized with medical management alone are incorrectly considered as gastric dilatation only and do not receive prophylactic gastropexy. In the authors' experience, these dogs are prone to frequent and often fatal recurrence. Radiography after gastric decompression can be misleading because spontaneous gastric repositioning can occur.[28] Although radiographs taken in right lateral recumbency are effective in distinguishing dilatation from volvulus,[3,28,29] we do not perform routine radiography because this increases cost, causes stress during the stabilization period, and does not alter the protocol for surgical management.

Anesthesia is an important component of surgical management of gastric dilatation-volvulus patients and should be approached with special consideration for the dog's degree of physiologic compromise.[30] If narcotic sedation has been used to assist gastric decompression, we prefer mask induction with isoflurane in oxygen. Intravenous induction with a combination of diazepam and ketamine hydrochloride (0.3 mg/kg and 5.5 mg/kg, respectively) is safe for intubation,[26,31] followed by maintenance with isoflurane in oxygen. Thiobarbiturates should be used cautiously, particularly in severely compromised patients and those with cardiac arrhythmias, because of the agents' ability to reduce myocardial contractility.[3] Thiobarbiturates and halothane have been used successfully in clinical patients, however.[3,32-34] Anesthetic monitoring should include vital signs, electrocardiography, and indirect blood pressure measurements and is critical in maintaining a light surgical plane of anesthesia that avoids further anesthetic depression of myocardial contractility. Assisted ventilation is recommended.

With the patient positioned in dorsal recumbency, a ventral midline celiotomy is performed beginning at the level of the xiphoid cartilage and extending between the umbilicus and the pubis. A partially distended stomach often is seen trapped within a veil of omentum. Gastrocentesis with an 18-gauge needle attached to suction is beneficial in decompressing the stomach through the surgical incision if distention is present.[3,25,35,36] Most often, the stomach rotates and the pylorus shifts from its normal position on the right along the cranioventral abdomen to the left (clockwise rotation as viewed caudally to cranially). The gastric fundus shifts from its normal position in the left dorsal abdomen to the right ventral region of the abdomen. The surgeon, standing on the right side of the patient, should grasp the area of the displaced pylorus near the cardia with the right hand and pull up toward the incision while simultaneously pushing the fundus down into the abdominal cavity and to the left with the other hand.

In most instances, the spleen follows the stomach for almost 270° (being moved from a left dorsocaudal to a right cranial position in the abdomen) and comes to rest against the right diaphragm, folded tightly in a V by its taut gastrosplenic ligament.[37] The spleen often is markedly congested and can twist around its vascular supply.[6] Splenic repositioning usually occurs along with gastric derotation. Congestion often resolves after correct positioning. Splenectomy is not usually necessary and should be reserved for serious changes, such as vessel avulsion and/or infarction with secondary necrosis. Splenectomy does not influence the recurrence of gastric volvulus.[6,20,38-40]

Gastric-wall viability should be assessed next. Gastric rupture, which has a grave prognosis, is usually recognized on entry into the abdomen or during repositioning (Figure 4). Although there are isolated reports of successful management of gastric rupture after gastric dilatation-volvulus,[41] euthanasia should be considered.[3] Gastric-wall necrosis without rupture requires partial gastrectomy; the management of gastric-wall compromise demands surgical judgment. The most frequently involved areas of gastric infarction and necrosis are along the greater curvature of the body and/or the fundic region in the vicinity of the short gastric vessels. Hemoperitoneum can result from avulsion of the short gastric vessels and the epiploic branch of the left gastroepiploic artery.[3,33] Subjective assessment of gastric-wall viability is based on color, perfusion, and vascular patency. Fluorescein dye evaluation of perfusion has been used[33] but is not an accurate indicator of gastric-wall viability when interpreted on the serosal surface.[42] Serosal discoloration and vascular damage are gross visual parameters that help in assessing gastric viability.[3] Avulsion and/or infarction of vessels along the greater curvature of the body and the fundus contribute to the development of gastric necrosis. Black to pale-green to gray serosal areas are highly suggestive of necrosis; dark-red to red-purple or hemorrhagic regions usually indicate compromised regions of the gastric wall.[33]

The areas that are difficult to assess should be reevaluated 10 to 15 minutes after gastric repositioning because vascular and serosal integrity can improve subsequently.[3,25,35] Palpation of discolored areas that reveals marked stretching or thinning of the gastric wall in addition to severe serosal tearing indicates the necessity of gastric resection.[33] When gastric wall necrosis is evident or possible, a partial gastrectomy is performed using 2-0 or 3-0 polyglactin 910 sutures in a two-layer continuous inverting pattern for wound closure. Survival rates are generally poor.

Standard clinical criteria (serosal color and perfusion, condition of the gastric wall, and vascular patency) do not consistently provide accurate assessment of gastric viability.[3,33,42] Many cases might not have devitalized gastric walls and do not require the additional time or risk of abdominal contamination associated with partial gastrectomy. Partial gastric invagination can be performed in such cases.[43] Large inverting sutures (Lembert pattern) of 2-0 polypropylene or monofilament nylon are placed in viable stomach wall to invaginate the compromised area into the gastric lumen while creating serosa-to-serosa contact of healthy stomach wall over the area of compromise. If subsequent gastric-wall necrosis occurs, the inverted portion is sloughed into the gastric lumen without risk of peritonitis. By contrast, a possible area that is inverted and remains viable is not compromised and can continue to function normally.[43] This technique is simple and efficient, does not require opening of the gastric lumen, and can be a beneficial alternative to partial gastrectomy for compromised patients in which gastric-wall viability is difficult to assess and decreased surgical time is essential.[43] Long-term study has not been done in dogs, however, and the safety of this procedure has not been established.

Gastropexy can be a highly effective means of preventing recurrence of gastric dilatation-volvulus and should be performed in all patients during surgical management. In addition, gastropexy is recommended on an elective basis in patients that have survived gastric dilatation-volvulus with medical management alone. We currently recommend four techniques, each involving gastropexy of the pyloric antrum to the right ventrolateral abdominal wall.

Circumcostal gastropexy is proven through follow-up clinical data[15] and mechanical testing[44,45] to provide strong, permanent gastropexy and is the authors' choice in most cases. A single dog in a group of 30 with gastric dilatation-volvulus treated by circumcostal gastropexy and followed-up for a mean of 13.7 months had recurrence (simple dilation). Twenty-seven percent of the patients had multiple episodes (mean 2.75) before circumcostal gastropexy.[15] Advantages of the technique include that it is quick and simple (with experience); it does not enter the gastric lumen; it requires no special postoperative management; and it is reliable the production of a strong, long-lasting attachment.[44,46] The complication of iatrogenic pneumothorax can occur if improper technique is used.

A 5-cm rectangular flap of seromuscularis is created on the parietal surface of the pyloric antrum midway between the greater and lesser curvatures, with its hinge toward the lesser curvature. The most caudal complete rib—usually the eleventh—is palpated, and a 6-cm incision is made through the parietal peritoneum and the transverse abdominal muscle directly overlying the rib and ventral to the costochondral junction. A blunt instrument is passed around the rib and opened to separate the intercostal muscle attachments. The gastric flap is passed in a craniodorsal-to-caudoventral direction around the exposed rib and sutured to its original seromuscular margins on the stomach with 3-0 polyglactin 910. The incised peritoneum and the transverse abdominal muscle fascia adjacent to the exposed rib are brought over the flap and sutured to the seromuscular stomach wall several mm distally (toward the greater curvature) with 3-0 polyglactin 910. This creates a second layer of closure that supports the seromuscular flap while healing occurs (Figure 5).

Traction tube gastrostomy is the accepted means of pro-

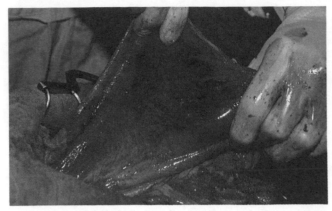

Figure 4—During surgery, gastric contents are evident scattered throughout the abdominal cavity. Gastric rupture and severe gastric-wall devitalization occurred in this four-year-old Irish setter. (From Leib MS, Blass CE: Acute gastric dilatation in the dog: Various clinical presentations. *Compend Contin Educ Pract Vet* 6(8):709, 1984. Used with permission.)

ducing a long-lasting gastropexy that can prevent a recurrence.[22,26,36,47] Potential disadvantages include catheter cost, the postoperative management of complications resulting from a tube placed through the body wall, and the risk of abdominal contamination when the gastric lumen is exposed.[36,48] A large, balloon-tipped Foley catheter (20 to 30 French) is passed through a stab incision in the right ventrolateral body wall 3 to 4 cm caudal to the costal arch and 4 to 10 cm lateral to the ventral midline. The catheter is passed through several layers of omentum and into a stab incision in the parietal surface of the pyloric antrum midway between the greater and lesser curvatures. The stab incision is encircled by a purse-string suture of 2-0 monofilament nylon or polypropylene to maintain catheter placement. The balloon is inflated with 5 ml of saline, and the purse-string suture is drawn tightly and tied. The tube applies traction to the stomach wall to draw it snugly against the right abdominal wall. Balloon positioning should be checked to ensure that it does not obstruct the pyloric outflow region of the stomach. Monofilament nylon or polypropylene sutures are placed between the pyloric antrum and the abdominal wall around the tube to further secure the stomach to the body wall while healing occurs.

Care must be taken to avoid puncturing the balloon within the gastric lumen. This is best prevented by preplacing the gastropexy sutures before the stomach is drawn up against the abdominal wall. The catheter is sutured to the skin with 3-0 monofilament nylon and is capped to prevent loss of gastric fluid unless decompression is needed. A nonconstricting bandage is applied to prevent removal of the tube by the patient. The tube should be left in place for five to seven days or longer while fibrous adhesions form as a result of the gastrocutaneous fistula created by the tube. A potential advantage of tube gastrostomy is that it provides continuous gastric decompression during the postoperative period. Although the consistency of adhesion formation has not been demonstrated, recurrence rates of gastric dilatation-volvulus range from 5% to 11%.[22,36,48]

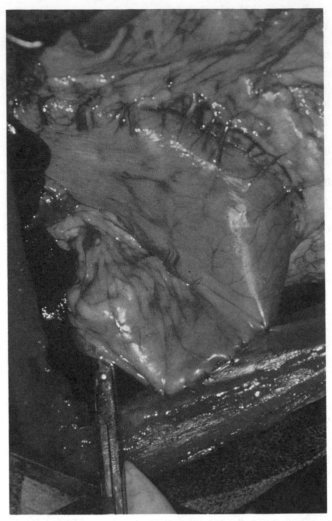

Figure 5—Completed circumcostal gastropexy. (From Leib MS, Blass CE: Gastric dilatation-volvulus in dogs: An update. *Compend Contin Educ Pract Vet* 6(11):966, 1984. Used with permission.)

Incisional gastropexy might be the simplest, quickest means of producing permanent gastropexy.[49] A longitudinal incision is made through the gastric serosa and into the muscularis over the parietal surface of the pyloric antrum, equidistant from the attachments of the greater and lesser omenta. A second incision is made in the peritoneum and the internal fascia of the rectal abdominal muscle or the transverse abdominal muscle of the right ventrolateral abdominal wall adjacent to the incision on the pyloric antrum. The edges of the abdominal wall incision are sutured to the edges of the pyloric incision in a simple continuous pattern with monofilament nylon or polypropylene; first the deeper wound margins then the more superficial margins are apposed, creating an imperforate circular stoma. Deep infiltration of fibrous connective tissue into skeletal and smooth muscles at the gastropexy site occurs when mesothelial surfaces are disrupted.[49] The lack of recurrence of gastric dilatation-volvulus in clinical follow-up of 44 dogs for as long as five years supports experimental evidence of a strong, long-lasting gastropexy.[45,49]

The most recent description of permanent gastropexy involves creating a muscular flap on the abdominal wall in the same area as the incisional gastropexy.[50] The base of the flap is sutured to the seromuscular layers of the parietal surface of the pyloric antrum; the free flap, hinged ventrally, is brought over this attachment and sutured several mm distal to the first attachment, toward the greater curvature. Again, monofilament nylon or polypropylene is used. Long-term follow-up (3 to 33 months in 21 clinical cases, including radiographic and fluoroscopic assessment of the muscular-flap gastropexy in 10 dogs) indicates that the technique is effective in preventing recurrence of gastric dilatation-volvulus and is long-lasting.

Advantages of the technique include its simplicity and the fact that it does not enter the gastric lumen or require specific postoperative management. The incidence of recurrence of gastric dilatation-volvulus after the four gastropexy techniques described is impressive when compared with older techniques. In one study, medical management alone resulted in a 75% recurrence rate within 12 months.[51] Exploratory surgery and gastric repositioning (with or without splenectomy) was associated with a high recurrence rate.[38,39] Supposedly simple gastropexy techniques produce short-lived adhesions and high recurrence rates.[3,5,20,27,39]

The biomechanic strengths of the first three gastropexy techniques described have been evaluated.[45,52] The tensile strength necessary for an effective prophylactic gastropexy is unknown. Circumcostal gastropexy provides the strongest means of attachment of the stomach to the abdominal wall.[45]

Abdominal lavage, using warm isotonic fluids, should be performed before routine three-layer abdominal closure. The surgeon must always be prepared to make sound clinical judgments and to use quick, effective surgical techniques that offer the patient the best chance for survival without surgical sequelae or recurrence of gastric dilatation-volvulus.

Postoperative Management

Diligent postoperative care is an important component of successful management of gastric dilatation-volvulus patients. In the authors' experience, a prolonged period of temporary stabilization leads to decreased postoperative morbidity and mortality. Most dogs that die in the postoperative period do so within the first four days.[38,39]

Oral intake of food and water should be withheld 24 to 48 hours postoperatively. Maintenance of fluid, electrolyte, and acid-base status is critical during this period. Polyionic fluids should be given at a rate of 44 to 66 ml/kg/day to meet maintenance requirements. Continuing losses from vomiting or diarrhea should be immediately replaced.[53]

Although most dogs with gastric dilatation-volvulus maintain normal serum potassium levels (serum levels are not a good indicator of total body content because most potassium is intracellular), a total body potassium deficit probably exists because of nothing-per-os (NPO) status, vomiting, orogastric intubation and removal of gastric secretion, or treatment with potassium-poor fluids.[1,5,46] The authors recommend that 20 mEq of potassium chloride be added to each liter of maintenance fluids to help maintain total body potassium. Potassium-supplemented fluids should be used only after the patient is no longer in shock. Rapid intravenous infusion of potassium supplemented fluids can lead to cardiac arrest. Hypokalemia can contribute to the development of cardiac arrhythmias and gastrointestinal ileus.[17,18,46,53] In the authors' experience, potassium supplementation subjectively decreases the incidence and severity of these postoperative problems. In most cases, maintaining a nothing-per-os status for 24 to 48 hours is sufficient to manage the vomiting and gastritis that normally is present.[5]

If vomiting does not occur, gradual oral alimentation should be initiated by offering ice cubes, followed by small amounts of water, and then small amounts of bland food. The amount of food per meal should be gradually increased and the frequency of feeding gradually decreased over two to four days.

If prolonged postoperative vomiting occurs, oral feeding must be delayed and consideration given to caloric supplementation. A recent clinical report emphasized the benefits of enteral hyperalimentation via needle jejunostomy in postoperative patients, some of which had gastric dilatation-volvulus.[54] Caloric support might diminish some of the problems associated with protein–calorie malnutrition, such as impaired immune response, high prevalence of infection, ineffective wound healing, anemia, hypoproteinemia, muscle weakness, organ dysfunction, decubitus ulcer, and death.[54-56] Alimentation via needle jejunostomy can be used in vomiting patients and can help to reestablish normal intestinal motility after surgery.[54]

Although vomiting usually is self-limiting after surgery, we occasionally use antiemetics. Subcutaneous metoclopramide hydrochloride (0.2 to 0.4 mg/kg every eight hours) not only has central antiemetic effects but also can increase gastric contractions and emptying. In some dogs, it is reasonable to assume that massive gastric distention might temporarily disrupt gastric-muscle function. A short course of treatment with metoclopramide hydrochloride can help to normalize gastric function and stop the vomiting.

Routine postoperative wound management and patient care should be delivered. Patients must be carefully monitored because such complications as peritonitis, intestinal intussusception, gastric rupture, intraabdominal hemorrhage, and shock can occur in postoperative gastric dilatation-volvulus patients.

Electrocardiograms should be assessed two to four times per day because postoperative cardiac arrhythmias are very common.[3,17,18] Approximately 85% of cardiac arrhythmias in dogs with gastric dilatation-volvulus are ventricular in origin, and ventricular tachycardia is the most common.[3,18] The cause of cardiac arrhythmias is multifactorial and includes shock, hypoxia, myocardial ischemia, acid-base and electrolyte disorders, autonomic imbalance, and cardiostimulatory substances.[17,18,57-61] The authors have determined that ventricular tachycardia associated with gastric dilatation-volvulus is a persistent arrhythmia, often refractory to therapy for two to four days. Published studies, however, have indicated that gastric dilatation-volvulus arrhythmias can be responsive to therapy.[17] Treatment for cardiac arrhythmias should be tailored to the individual patient. Antiarrhythmic therapy is indicated if the ventricular arrhythmia significantly decreases cardiac output, if multifocal ventricular premature contractions occur, if long periods of ventricular tachycardia are present with a ventricular rate greater than 140, or if the R wave occurs close to the T wave (R on T phenomenon, a sensitive period in the development of ventricular fibrillation).[1]

The authors have achieved the greatest success with the following protocol.[3,5,17] A slow intravenous bolus of 2% lidocaine hydrochloride (2 to 4 mg/kg; without epinephrine) is given. This can be repeated twice during a 30-minute period if necessary. Additional bolus therapy can lead to toxicity and is not recommended. If conversion of ventricular tachycardia is not maintained after one to three lidocaine hydrochloride boluses, a continuous infusion starting at 50 μg/kg/min should be initiated. This rate should be adjusted based on therapeutic response. Lidocaine hydrochloride toxicity is manifested by vomiting, tremors, and seizures. If toxicity occurs, the continuous infusion should be immediately discontinued. Because lidocaine hydrochloride has a very short half-life in dogs,[62] most signs of toxicity disappear after cessation of the infusion. If neurologic signs continue, 5 to 20 mg of diazepam can be given intravenously. When toxic signs regress, the infusion can be reinstituted at a slower rate. Because most arrthythmias associated with gastric dilatation-volvulus require prolonged therapy, longer-acting antiarrhythmics—such as intramuscular procainamide hydrochloride (6 to 8 mg/kg, four times daily)—should be initiated. If vomiting does not occur, oral procainamide hydrochloride (6 to 20 mg/kg, four times daily) can be used. Toxicity is manifested by vomiting, diarrhea, and prolongation of all electrocardiogram intervals. As the arrhythmia becomes controlled, the lidocaine hydrochloride infusion can be tapered and eventually discontinued; the patient can be maintained on oral procainamide hydrochloride for three to five days after cessation of the arrhythmia. Instead of procainamide hydrochloride, quinidine sulfate can be used at 6 to 8 mg/kg intramuscularly or 6 to 20 mg/kg orally four times daily. Quinidine sulfate has slightly more myocardial depressant effects than procainamide hydrochloride does.

Tocainide, a new, oral, lidocaine-like antiarrhythmic, has recently been approved for use in humans. Although the authors do not have clinical experience with this drug in dogs with gastric dilatation-volvulus, it evidently is an effective antiarrhythmic drug with minimal toxicity. Similar to lidocaine hydrochloride, tocainide minimally depresses cardiac contractility.[62]

The relationship between diet and gastric dilatation-volvulus is disputed, and the authors do not recommend a specific type of diet after surgery; we have not associated any diet type with the development of gastric dilatation-

volvulus. Multiple feedings will reduce gastric volume and can be beneficial in preventing recurrence. Limiting vigorous exercise after feeding can reduce twisting of a distended stomach. In addition, minimizing consumption of large volumes of water after exercise or automobile travel will help reduce gastric distention.

A recent study evaluating the role of diet on gastric emptying in large dogs revealed that dry dog foods did not empty significantly slower than canned foods.[63] This study suggested that dry foods should not be incriminated as a cause of gastric dilatation-volvulus and will not promote excessive gastric distention.

Immediate recognition of gastric dilatation-volvulus by the veterinarian, vigorous emergency management, exploratory surgery with recurrence-preventing techniques, and thorough postoperative care are the effective components for successful management of dogs with gastric dilatation-volvulus. Because of the acute nature of this syndrome and the severe pathophysiologic changes that it produces, however, a significant mortality rate exists. Future research concerning methods of prevention and criteria to identify individual dogs that are at risk will improve the management of this complex syndrome.

Acknowledgments
The authors thank the following emergency clinic veterinarians for their review of the manuscript: Drs. Joe Gaston, Marietta, Georgia; John Holland, Vienna, Virginia; Mark Honeker, Virginia Beach, Virginia; James Thomas, Richmond, Virginia; and Steven Schwartz, Rockville, Maryland.

REFERENCES

1. Orton EC: Gastric dilatation-volvulus, in Kirk RW (ed): *Current Veterinary Therapy IX.* Philadelphia, WB Saunders Co, 1985, pp 856–861.
2. Wingfield WE: Acute gastric dilatation-volvulus syndrome, in Bojrab MJ (ed): *Current Techniques in Small Animal Surgery.* Philadelphia, Lea & Febiger, 1983, pp 149–156.
3. Matthiesen DT: The gastric dilatation-volvulus complex: Medical and surgical considerations. *JAAHA* 19:925–932, 1983.
4. Morgan RV: Acute gastric dilatation-volvulus. *Compend Contin Educ Pract Vet* 4(8):677–686, 1982.
5. Wingfield WE: Acute gastric dilatation-volvulus. *Vet Clin North Am [Small Anim Pract]* 11:147–155, 1981.
6. Todoroff RJ: Gastric dilatation-volvulus. *Compend Contin Educ Pract Vet* I(2):142–148, 1979.
7. Walshaw RW, Johnston DE: Treatment of gastric dilatation-volvulus by gastric decompression and patient stabilization before major surgery. *JAAHA* 12:162–167, 1976.
8. Pass MA, Johnston DE: Treatment of gastric dilatation and torsion in the dog. Gastric decompression by gastrostomy under local analgesia. *J Small Anim Pract* 14:131–142, 1973.
9. Orton EC, Muir WW: Hemodynamics during experimental gastric dilatation-volvulus in dogs. *Am J Vet Res* 44:1512–1515, 1983.
10. Merkley DF, Howard DR, Krehbiel JD, et al: Experimentally induced acute gastric dilatation in the dog: Clinicopathologic findings. *JAAHA* 12:149–153, 1976.
11. Rawlings CA, Wingfield WE, Betts CW: Shock therapy and anesthetic management in gastric dilatation-volvulus. *JAAHA* 12:158–161, 1976.
12. Morgan RV: Shock. *Compend Contin Educ Pract Vet* 3(6):533–541, 1981.

13. Kolata RJ: The clinical management of circulatory shock based on pathophysiological patterns. *Compend Contin Educ Pract Vet* II(4):314-323, 1980.

14. Hardie EM, Rawlings CA: Septic shock. Part II. Prevention, recognition, and treatment. *Compend Contin Educ Pract Vet* 5(6):483-493, 1983.

15. Leib MS, Konde LJ, Wingfield WE, et al: Circumcostal gastropexy for preventing recurrence of gastric dilatation-volvulus in the dog: An evaluation of 30 cases. *JAVMA* 187:245-248, 1985.

16. Lantz GC, Bottoms GD, Carlton WW, et al: The effect of 360° gastric volvulus on the blood supply of the nondistended normal dog stomach. *Vet Surg* 13:189-196, 1984.

17. Muir WW, Bonagura JD: Treatment of cardiac arrhythmias in dogs with gastric distension-volvulus. *JAVMA* 184:1366-1371, 1984.

18. Muir WW: Gastric dilatation-volvulus in the dog, with emphasis on cardiac arrhythmias. *JAVMA* 180:739-742, 1982.

19. Lantz GC: Pharyngostomy tube installation for the administration of nutritional and fluid requirements. *Compend Contin Educ Pract Vet* 3(2):135-142, 1981.

20. DeHoff WD, Greene RW: Gastric dilatation and the gastric and torsion complex. *Vet Clin North Am [Small Anim Pract]* 2:141-153, 1972.

21. Crowe DT: Use of a nasogastric tube for gastric and esophageal decompression in the dog and cat. *JAVMA* 188:1178-1182, 1986.

22. Johnson RG, Barrus J, Greene RW: Gastric dilatation-volvulus: Recurrence rate following tube gastrostomy. *JAAHA* 20:33-37, 1984.

23. Funkquist B, Garmer L: Pathogenic and therapeutic aspects of torsion of the canine stomach. *J Small Anim Pract* 8:523-532, 1967.

24. DeHoff WD, Greene RW, Greimer TP: Surgical management of abdominal emergencies. *Vet Clin North Am [Small Anim Pract]* 2:310-311, 1972.

25. DeHoff WD: Surgical management of gastric dilatation-volvulus. *Proc Kal Kal Symp* 8:33-40, 1985.

26. Parks JL: Surgical management of gastric torsion. *Vet Clin North Am [Small Anim Pract]* 9:259-267, 1979.

27. Betts CW, Wingfield WE, Rosin E: "Permanent" gastropexy as a prophylactic measure against gastric volvulus. *JAAHA* 12:177-181, 1976.

28. Funkquist B: Gastric torsion in the dog—I. Radiological picture during nonsurgical treatment related to the pathological anatomy and to the further clinical course. *J Small Anim Pract* 20:73-91, 1979.

29. Hathcock JT: Radiographic view of choice for the diagnosis of gastric volvulus: The right lateral recumbent view. *JAAHA* 20:967-969, 1984.

30. Harvey RC: Anesthetic management for canine gastric dilatation-volvulus. *Semin Vet Med Surg Small Anim* 1:230-237, 1986.

31. Kolata RJ: Induction of anesthesia using diazepam/ketamine in dogs with complete heart block. A preliminary report. *Vet Surg* 15:339-341, 1986.

32. Funkquist B: Gastric torsion in the dog—III. Fundic gastropexy as a relapse-preventing procedure. *J Small Anim Pract* 20:103-109, 1979.

33. Matthiesen DT: Partial gastrectomy as treatment of gastric volvulus. Results of 30 dogs. *Vet Surg* 14:185-193, 1985.

34. Lanier MW: Safe management and prevention of gastric distention/volvulus in dogs. *VM SAC* 76:683-686, 1981.

35. Wingfield WE, Hoffer RE: Gastric dilatation-torsion complex in the dog, in Bojrab MJ (ed): *Current Techniques in Small Animal Surgery.* Philadelphia, Lea & Febiger, 1975, pp 112-118.

36. Flanders JA, Harvey HJ: Results of tube gastrostomy as treatment for gastric volvulus in the dog. *JAVMA* 185:74-77, 1984.

37. Van Kruiningen HJ, Gregoire K, Meuten DJ: Acute gastric dilatation: A review of comparative aspects, by species, and a study in dogs and monkeys. *JAAHA* 10:294-324, 1974.

38. Wingfield WE, Betts CW, Greene RW: Operative techniques and recurrence rates associated with gastric volvulus in the dog. *J Small Anim Pract* 16:427-432, 1975.

39. Betts CW, Wingfield WE, Greene RW: A retrospective study of gastric dilation-torsion in the dog. *J Small Anim Pract* 15:727-734, 1974.

40. Andrews AH: A study in 10 cases of gastric torsion in the bloodhound. *Vet Rec* 86:689-693, 1970.

41. Dingwall JS, Eger CE: Management of acute gastric dilatation with torsion and rupture: A case report. *JAAHA* 12:23-26, 1976.

42. Wheaton LG, Thacker HL, Caldwell S: Intravenous fluorescein as an indicator of gastric viability in gastric dilatation-volvulus. *JAAHA* 22:197-204, 1986.

43. MacCoy DM, Kneller SK, Sundberg JP, et al: Partial invagination of the canine stomach for treatment of infarction of the gastric wall. *Vet Surg* 15:237-245, 1986.

44. Fallah AM, Lumb WV, Nelson AW, et al: Circumcostal gastropexy in the dog. A preliminary study. *Vet Surg* 11:9-12, 1982.

45. Fox SM, Ellison GW, Miller GJ, et al: Observations on the mechanical failure of three gastropexy techniques. *JAAHA* 21:729-734, 1985.

46. Leib MS, Blass CE: Gastric dilatation-volvulus in dogs: An update. *Compend Contin Educ Pract Vet* 6(11):961-969, 1984.

47. Parks JL, Greene RW: Tube gastrostomy for the treatment of gastric volvulus. *JAAHA* 12:168-172, 1976.

48. Fox SM: Gastric dilatation-volvulus: Results from 31 surgical cases. Circumcostal gastropexy vs. tube gastrostomy. *California Vet* 39:8-11, 1985.

49. MacCoy DM, Sykes GP, Hoffer RE, et al: A gastropexy technique for permanent fixation of the pyloric antrum. *JAAHA* 18:763-768, 1982.

50. Schulman AJ, Lusk R, Lippincott CL, et al: Muscular flap gastropexy: A new surgical technique to prevent recurrences of gastric dilatation-volvulus syndrome. *JAAHA* 22:339-346, 1986.

51. Dann JR: Medical and surgical treatment of canine acute gastric dilatation. *JAAHA* 12:17-22, 1976.

52. Levine SH, Caywood DD: Biomechanical evaluation of gastropexy techniques in the dog. *Vet Surg* 12:166-169, 1983.

53. Twedt DC, Grauer GF: Fluid therapy for gastrointestinal, pancreatic, and hepatic disorders. *Vet Clin North Am [Small Anim Pract]* 12:463-485, 1982.

54. Orton EC: Enteral hyperalimentation administered via needle catheter—Jejunostoma as an adjunct to cranial abdominal surgery in dogs and cats. *JAVMA* 188:1406-1411, 1986.

55. Cunningham-Rundles S: Effects of nutritional status on immunological function. *Am J Clin Nutr* 35:1202-1210, 1982.

56. Sheffy B, Williams AJ: Nutrition and the immune response. *JAVMA* 180:1073-1076, 1982.

57. Horne WA, Gilmore DR, Dietze AE, et al: Effects of gastric distention-volvulus on coronary blood flow and myocardial oxygen consumption in the dog. *Am J Vet Res* 46:98-104, 1985.

58. Orton EC, Muir WW: Isovolumetric indices and humoral cardioactive substance bioassay during clinical and experimentally induced gastric dilatation-volvulus in dogs. *Am J Vet Res* 44:1516-1520, 1983.

59. Muir WW: Acid-base and electrolyte disturbances in dogs with gastric dilatation-volvulus. *JAVMA* 181:229-231, 1982.

60. Muir WW, Weisbrode SE: Myocardial ischemia in dogs with gastric dilatation volvulus. *JAVMA* 181:363-366, 1982.

61. Wingfield WE, Twedt DC, Moore RW, et al: Acid-base and electrolyte values in dogs with acute gastric dilatation-volvulus. *JAVMA* 180:1070-1072, 1982.

62. Novotny MJ, Adams HR: New perspectives in cardiology: Recent advances in antiarrhythmic drug therapy. *JAVMA* 189:533-539, 1986.

63. Burrows CF, Bright RM, Spencer CP: Influence of dietary composition on gastric emptying and motility in dogs: Potential involvement in acute gastric dilatation. *Am J Vet Res* 46:2609-2612, 1985.

Diseases of the Salivary Glands in the Dog

Charles D. Knecht, VMD, MS
Professor and Head
Department of Small Animal Surgery and Medicine
Auburn University School of Veterinary Medicine
Auburn University
Auburn, Alabama

The parotid, mandibular, sublingual, and zygomatic glands are the major paired salivary glands in the dog and cat (Fig 1). Smaller buccal glands are present in the soft palate, lips, tongue, and cheeks. All are lobulated acinar glands that secrete serous- and/or mucous-type saliva.[1-3] Serous saliva contains ptyalin (alpha-amylase), which is useful in digestion of fat. Mucous secretion lubricates food for easy deglutition. The parotid gland secretions are entirely serous, whereas the mandibular gland secretions are mostly serous. Buccal and sublingual secretions are mostly mucous; the zygomatic gland secretion is believed to be mixed.[4,5]

Innervation to the salivary glands is complex. Sympathetic innervation accompanies the arteries. Parasympathetic innervation is by the glossopharyngeal nerve, which supplies the zygomatic and parotid glands. Fibers from the ninth cranial nerve course with the auriculotemporal branch of the trigeminal nerve. The mandibular and sublingual salivary glands receive innervation by the facial nerve via the mandibular division of the trigeminal nerve.

Anatomy

The *parotid* is a lobulated gland located at the base of the auricular cartilage. It has dorsal limbs rostral and caudal to and a deep portion ventral to the cartilage of the external ear canal.[2,5-7] The parotid duct is formed by two or three short radicles. It courses lateral to the masseter muscle and enters the buccal cavity perpendicular to the oral mucosa opposite the upper fourth cheek tooth. Arterial blood is supplied by the parotid artery and other branches of the external carotid artery. Blood and lymph drain to the superficial temporal and great auricular veins and to the retropharyngeal and parotid lymph nodes, respectively.

The ovoid *mandibular* gland is located in the junction of the maxillary and linguofacial veins. It shares a dense capsule with the caudal monostomatic portion of the sublingual gland. The duct leaves the medial surface of the gland and courses rostromedially between the masseter muscle and mandible laterally and the digastricus muscle medially. It continues between the styloglossus and mylohyoideus muscles and empties separately or in common with the accompanying sublingual duct at a papilla(e) lateral to the

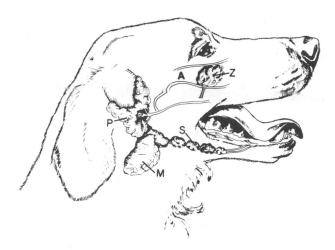

Fig 1—Salivary glands of the dog. M, mandibular; S, sublingual; P parotid; Z, zygomatic; A, zygomatic arch.

rostral end of the frenulum of the tongue. The glandular branch of the facial artery and the branches of the caudal auricular arteries supply the gland. Venous drainage occurs through the lingual, maxillary, and, occasionally, the facial veins.

The *sublingual* gland is multilobed. The caudal monostomatic portion rests on the rostral pole of the mandibular gland lateral to the mandibular duct. Ovoid clusters of the cranial portions lie below the oral mucosa lateral to the tongue. The cranial glands secrete through four to six short excretory ducts into the sublingual duct. The sublingual duct originates at the caudal portion and accompanies the mandibular duct to a common or separate, caudally located sublingual papilla. Six to twelve isolated polystomatic parts lie under the mucosa rostral to the lingual branch of the trigeminal nerve and secrete directly into the oral cavity.

Arterial blood is supplied from the facial and sublingual arteries and is returned through satellite veins. Lymph drainage from the mandibular and sublingual glands reaches the medial retropharyngeal lymph nodes.

The *zygomatic* salivary glands of carnivores are ovoid to pyramidal in shape with the base directed dorsally toward the periorbita. The ventral blunted apex is in the pterygopalatine fossa dorsal and lateral to the roots of the upper last molar tooth. One major duct leaves the apex and enters the buccal cavity at a papilla adjacent to the upper cheek tooth. Several smaller ducts end on a ridge of mucosa caudal to the main duct.

The zygomatic gland is supplied by a branch of the infraorbital artery and is drained by the deep facial vein and medial retropharyngeal lymph nodes.

Treatment of Disease
Inflammation

Sialoadenitis of the parotid, mandibular, and sublingual glands is rare without a sialocele. Inflammation can result from trauma or systemic disease, especially viral disease.[8] The signs of sialoadenitis are swelling, pain, and, rarely, palpable warmth. Fever and neutrophilic leukocytosis are uncommon in the absence of systemic disease.

Zygomatic sialoadenitis is a common cause of retrobulbar abscess. No specific cause has been reported, although foreign body penetration may be suspected.[9,10] The signs are exophthalmos, tearing, divergent strabismus, and reluctance to open the mouth and to eat. Inflammation of the oral mucosa near the papilla and ridge of duct openings is common; mucopurulent discharge from the openings is also common. The discharge may be increased by gentle pressure on the gingiva. Fever and neutrophilic leukocytosis are uncommon.

Treatment includes administration of systemic antibiotics and drainage of the abscess. Drainage is achieved by introducing a mosquito forceps through a small incision in the inflamed oral mucosa. The forceps should be advanced carefully to avoid damage to the maxillary artery and nerve that course across the ventromedial orbit. The draining tract may be flushed with dilute povidone-iodine solution.

Surgical exploration of the orbit is indicated if signs persist and neoplasia or foreign body is suspected. Although a dorsal approach through an incision along the cranial edge of the frontal bone has been described, it is reserved for those cases in which a mass protrudes dorsally.[9] The usual surgical approach is made with the dog in lateral recumbency. Following aseptic preparation, an incision is made ventral to the palpebral fissure along the dorsal edge of the zygomatic arch (Fig 2). The

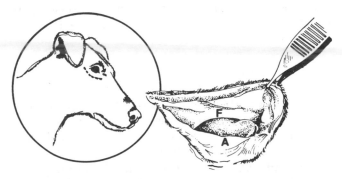

Fig 2—Lateral approach along the dorsal edge of the zygomatic arch of the dog. A, zygomatic arch; F, palpebral fascia.

sparse subcutaneous tissue is dissected and the palpebral fascia is incised. The periosteum is elevated ventrally and the dorsal half of the exposed zygomatic arch is excised with rongeurs. Minimal dissection is necessary to expose the zygomatic gland (Fig 3). The gland can be excised following medial and ventral dissection to expose and clamp

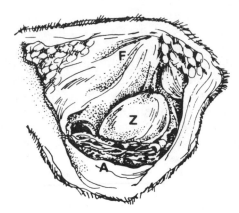

Fig 3—The zygomatic gland is lateral and ventral to the globe. A, zygomatic arch; F, palpebral fascia; Z, zygomatic salivary gland.

the zygomatic branch of the maxillary artery for ligation. The palpebral fascia is apposed with absorbable sutures in a simple interrupted pattern after exploration and excision. The subcutaneous tissue and skin are closed routinely, and a plastic collar is applied to prevent self-mutilation. To detect infectious agents, a direct microscopic examination and culture (anaerobic and aerobic) should be performed on excised tissue.

Fistulae

Fistulae of the mandibular, sublingual, and zygomatic glands are rare. Wounds of the parotid gland occasionally result in draining tracts. The most common causes of fistulae are animal bites and careless excision of the lateral ear canal. Conservative therapy in the form of antibiotics and attempts to cauterize the fistula are rarely successful. Extirpation of the gland, closure over a drain, and appropriate antibiotic therapy is the treatment of choice. Excision of the parotid gland is an exercise in anatomy, patience, and hemostasis. Care is necessary to avoid injury to branches of the trigeminal and facial nerves.

Salivary Mucoceles

Salivary mucoceles (sialoceles) result from damage to the duct or, less often, to the gland, with leakage of saliva into the tissues. The sack of saliva is lined with granulation tissue—not epithelium.[11] Rupture most commonly occurs in the sublingual and mandibular ducts rostral to the angle of the jaw. The nature of the agent that causes damage to the ducts or glands is not known. The damage has been attributed to the use of choke chains. However, in many cases of sialoceles, choke chains have not been used. Obstruction of a salivary duct was once thought to cause sialoceles, but it is now known to produce only a transient swelling followed by atrophy of the gland.[12] The term *salivary cyst* should be abandoned.[1,3,5,7,13-22]

Sialoceles have been most commonly reported in the poodle and German shepherd.[15,16,23] Early signs include a firm, somewhat painful swelling caudal to the angle of the mandible. Pain subsides as the soft, fluctuant mass develops. Most sialoceles occur at the angle of the mandible and caudally in the neck. Respiratory distress occurs rarely as the result of extreme accumulations of saliva. Parotid and zygomatic sialoceles have been observed to produce fluctuant masses on the cheek[7] and in the orbital areas,[24] respectively.

Presumptive diagnosis based on palpation may be confirmed by aspiration of blood-tinged saliva through an 18-gauge needle. Sialography, the radiographic depiction of the glands and ducts with aqueous contrast medium injected with a lacrimal or similar blunted needle in the papillae, is an excellent tool in problem cases.[1,6,14,25] The paucity of nonsalivary cysts in the pharyngeal area, the relative ease of localization by palpation, and the difficulties associated with duct cannulation lessen the usefulness of routine sialography.

A common problem is determining whether the right or left side is involved. With the head and neck in true dorsal recumbency, gentle manual pressure on the sialocele will result in expansion of the sac ventral to the ear on the affected side. In addition, careful palpation will generally reveal that the affected duct and gland are not as clearly defined as the normal duct and gland because of deposition of scar tissue.

Salivary mucoceles occasionally respond to repeated drainage, but the preferred treatment is surgical excision of the contributory glands. In cervical sialocele, the mandibular and sublingual glands are exposed by an incision extending rostrally from the confluence of the maxillary and linguofacial veins medial to the angle of the mandible (Fig 4). The thick common capsule of the mandibular and caudal sublingual glands is incised

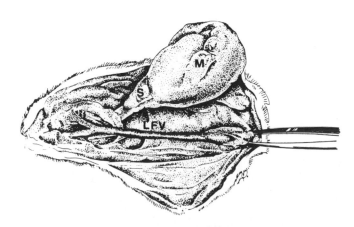

Fig 4—Excision of the mandibular and sublingual salivary glands. The dog is in dorsal recumbency. M, mandibular salivary gland; S, sublingual salivary gland (caudal bundle); LFV, linguofacial vein.

and the glands are excised by blunt dissection. Several small superficial veins and deep arteries are ligated. The rostral bundles of the sublingual gland must be removed by caudal retraction and dissection medial to the digastricus muscle. The rostral stumps of the mandibular and sublingual ducts are ligated with 2-0 chromic gut. The subcutaneous tissue and skin of the original incision are apposed with 2-0 or 3-0 chromic gut and a suitable nonabsorbable suture, respectively.

The sialocele may be ruptured during the dissection. Whether ruptured or not, a stab incision is made ventrally into the sialocele, and the folded middle of a Penrose drain is inserted. The double drain is fixed to the skin opening with a nonabsorbable suture at its cranial and caudal edges and is removed four to five days postoperatively.[5,26]

A sublingual salivary mucocele may also result in an accumulation of saliva along the base of the tongue. This type of sialocele is called a *ranula*. The signs are dysphagia and abnormal tongue movements. Communication with a cervical sialocele is rare. Diagnosis is based on observation, palpation, and aspiration. Although ranulas may result from rupture of the mandibular or sublingual duct, leakage from the rostral monostomatic or polystomatic portions of the sublingual glands is more common. Excision of all potentially contributing glandular tissue is difficult and has been replaced by marsupialization. The oral cavity is thoroughly cleansed, and the ranula is incised longitudinally and explored with hemostats. Membranes that may separate sacs of saliva are removed. The redundant portion of the mucosa and granulation tissue is excised by cutting around the perimeter of the sialocele (Fig 5). The resultant wound in the oral mucosa is allowed to heal as an open wound and is treated by flushing with clear water.[a]

Editor's Note: The above surgical procedure of excision of mucosa and granulation tissue in treatment of ranulas has been used by the Editor in many ranulas and is currently the preferred procedure. Two complications have been encountered. In approximately 10% of cases, the ranula recurs at the same site, and it has occasionally recurred after a second similar operation. The submandibular and sublingual glands and ducts on the affected side are removed if the ranula recurs after two excisions. The second complication, seen in three dogs, is the formation of a cervical sialocele caused not by leakage of saliva from a gland or duct, but by leakage of saliva into an opening in the floor of the mouth at the site of removal of the ranula.

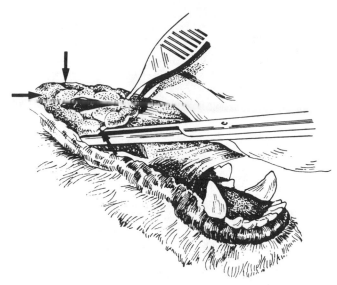

Fig 5—Marsupialization of a ranula. The redundant portion of the mucous membrane and granulation tissue of the ranula is excised with scissors.

Calculi

Sialoliths, which are calcium phosphate or carbonate concretions, are uncommon.[7,27] Inflammation of the gland or duct is the primary predisposing factor. Obstruction without inflammation does not cause sialoliths, but large calculi may cause obstruction of the duct.[28] Calculi can be excised by longitudinal incision of the duct, but excision of the gland and associated duct is more practical.

Neoplasia

Tumors of the salivary glands are uncommon, although adenocarcinomas have been reported.[29-31] Excisional biopsy is the treatment of choice.

Summary

Although salivary glands are subject to inflammation, neoplasia, and calculus formation, a sialocele resulting from rupture of the sublingual or mandibular duct or glandular tissue is the most common disease of the glands. Cervical salivary mucoceles are treated by excision of the contributing glands and drainage of the sialocele. Ranulas are treated by marsupialization.

Acknowledgment

The author is indebted to Rhoda Jeffrey Pidgeon for the illustrations.

REFERENCES

1. Harvey CE, O'Brien JA: Salivary glands, in Ettinger SJ (ed): *Textbook of Veterinary Internal Medicine*. Philadelphia, WB Saunders Co, 1975, p 1083.
2. Spruell JSA, Archibald J: Glands of the head and neck. *Canine Surgery*, ed Archibald 2. Santa Barbara, CA, American Veterinary Publications, Inc, 1974, p 360.
3. Spruell JSA, Head KW: Cervical salivary cyst in the dog. *J Small Anim Pract* 8:17, 1967.
4. Guyton AC: Secretory function of the alimentary tract. *Textbook of Physiology*. Philadelphia, WB Saunders Co, pp 891-894, 1966.
5. Knecht CD: Diagnosis and treatment of diseases of the salivary glands. *Norden News*: 5, 1972.
6. Harvey CE: Canine sialography. *JAVRS* 10:18, 1969.
7. Mulkey C, Knecht CD: Parotid salivary cyst and calculus in a dog. *JAVMA* 159:1174, 1971.
8. Noice F, Bolin FM, Eveleth, DF: Incidence of viral parotitis in the domestic dog. *Am J Dis Child* 98:350, 1959.
9. Knecht CD: Treatment of diseases of the zygomatic salivary gland. *JAAHA* 6:13, 1970.
10. Koch SA: The differential diagnosis of exophthalmos in the dog. *JAAHA* 5:229, 1969.
11. Karbe E, Nielsen SW: Branchial cyst in a dog. *JAVMA* 147:637, 1965.
12. Knecht CD: Salivary glands, in Bojrab MJ (ed): *Pathophysiology of Small Animal Surgery*. Philadelphia, Lea & Febiger, in press.
13. Christopher HJ: Dilation of the salivary glands and ducts in dogs. *Berl Muench Tieraerztl Wochenschr* 69:227, 1956.
14. Glen JB:Salivary cysts in the dog: Identification of sub-lingual defects by sialography. *Vet Rec* 78:488, 1966.
15. Harvey CE: Canine salivary mucocele. *JAVRS* 10:18, 1969.
16. Harvey CE:Canine salivary mucocele. *JAAHA* 5:155, 1969.
17. Hulland TJ: Salivary mucoceles. *Proc AVMA*:152, 1964.
18. Hulland TJ, Archibald J: Salivary mucoceles in dogs. *Can Vet J* 5:109, 1964.
19. Karbe E: Lateral neck cysts in the dog. *Am J Vet Res* 26:717, 1965.
20. Karbe E, Nielsen SW: Canine ranulas, salivary mucoceles and branchial cysts. *J Small Anim Pract* 7:625, 1966.
21. Kealy JK: Salivary cyst in the dog. *Vet Rec* 76:119, 1964.
22. Wallace LJ, Guffy MM, Gray AP, Clifford JH: Anterior cervical sialocele in a domestic cat. *JAAHA* 8:74, 1972.
23. Knecht CD, Phares J: Characteristics of dogs with salivary cyst. *JAVMA* 158:612, 1971.
24. Knecht CD, Slusher R, Guibor EC: Zygomatic salivary cyst in a dog. *JAVMA* 155:625, 1969.
25. Cawley AJ, Sorrell B: The technique of sialography in the dog. *Vet Med* 54:247, 1959.
26. Harvey CE: The salivary glands, in Bojrab MJ: *Current Techniques in Small Animal Surgery I*. Philadelphia, Lea & Febiger, 1975, p 97.
27. Karsner HT: *Human Pathology*. Philadelphia, JB Lippincott Co, 1949, p 91.
28. Irwin DCH, DeVos D: Occlusion of the parotid salivary duct in a dog. *J S Afri Vet Med Assoc* 30:38, 1959.
29. Buyukmihci N, Rubin LF, Harvey CE: Exophthalmos secondary to zygomatic adenocarcinoma in a dog. *JAVMA* 167:162, 1975.
30. Magrane WG: Tumors of the eye and orbit of the dog. *Proc XVII World Vet Congr, Hanover, Germany* 2:1095, 1963.
31. Whitehead JE: Neoplasia in the cat. *Small Anim Clin* 62:357, 1967.

KEY FACTS
- The proximal stomach stores food and has a major role in expulsion of liquids.
- The distal stomach mechanically breaks down and expels solids.
- Gastric pacemaker cells generate slow waves, which control the rate of gastric contractions.
- During fasting, indigestible solids are expelled from the stomach by the migrating myoelectric complex.

Gastric Motility in Dogs. Part I. Normal Gastric Function

Jean A. Hall, DVM, MS
Department of Physiology
College of Veterinary Medicine and
  Biomedical Sciences
Colorado State University
Fort Collins, Colorado

Colin F. Burrows, BVetMed, PhD, MRCVS
Department of Medical Sciences
College of Veterinary Medicine
University of Florida
Gainesville, Florida

David C. Twedt, DVM
Department of Clinical Sciences
College of Veterinary Medicine and
  Biomedical Sciences
Colorado State University
Fort Collins, Colorado

Gastrointestinal signs that can be associated with motility disorders include anorexia, vomiting, diarrhea, constipation, and abdominal pain. Deranged motility is often assumed to be the cause of postsurgical ileus and duodenogastric reflux. Few diagnostic techniques are available to confirm a motility disorder, but motility-enhancing therapeutic agents have made accurate diagnosis and monitoring necessary.

Part I of this two-part presentation focuses on the functional differences between gastric motor regions and on the determinants of gastric emptying in normal dogs. Part II will focus on the diagnosis of gastric motor abnormalities and on specific disorders that alter normal gastric motility.

Gastric motility represents the sum of smooth muscle, neural, and hormonal activity operative at a given time. Specific contractile activities are regulated to perform the following functions[1]:

- When a meal is ingested, the muscles of the proximal stomach relax to accommodate the swallowed material.
- Gastric contractions mix the ingested material with gastric secretions and set up fluid flow patterns that break down and disperse particles.
- Gastric contractions are coordinated with contractions of the pylorus and duodenum so that gastric contents are expelled in a regulated and orderly manner.
- During fasting, forceful periodic contractions sweep mucus and large, undigested particles into the duodenum.

Gastric Anatomic and Motor Regions

The stomach consists of four anatomic regions: the fundus, corpus (also called the body), antrum, and pylorus. In each region, the wall of the stomach has three major layers: the mucosa, which is the epithelial lining of the gastric lumen; the lamina muscularis, which is the smooth muscle coat; and the serosa, which is the thin, membranous outer lining. The lamina muscularis is divided into an outer longitudinal muscle layer and an inner circular muscle layer, which is thickest at the antrum. In some areas of the gastric corpus, there is a third, oblique muscle layer adjacent to the submucosa (Figure 1).[2]

Originally published in Volume 10, Number 11, November 1988

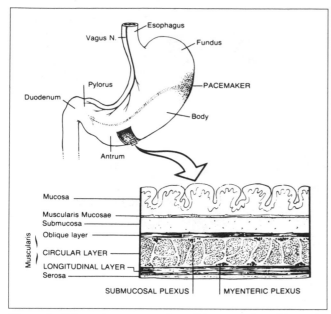

Figure 1—Schematic representation of the stomach and its major regions. The inset shows the major layers of the gastric wall. The origin of the gastric slow waves is indicated by the stippled region on the gastric corpus (*body*). The slow waves are propagated toward the *pylorus* as shown by the *arrow*. (From Stern RM, Koch KL (eds): *Electrogastrography: Methodology, Validation, and Applications*. New York, Praeger Publishers, 1985. Reprinted with permission.)

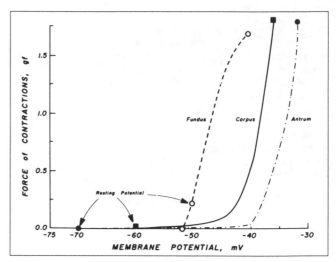

Figure 2—Comparison of voltage-tension curves of *fundus, corpus*, and *antrum* of circular muscle of a canine stomach. The points on the voltage-tension curves that represent the threshold for contraction are at approximately -45 mV for the *corpus* and -40 mV for the *antrum*. Note that the resting membrane potential for the *fundus* is less negative than the threshold for contraction. Thus, tone would be expected. (From Johnson LR (ed): *Physiology of the Gastrointestinal Tract*. New York, Raven Press, 1981. Reprinted with permission.)

The stomach has two distinct motor regions: the proximal stomach and the distal stomach.[1-5] The two motor regions are not distinguished by anatomic divisions. The proximal stomach includes the fundus and the adoral third of the gastric corpus. This region stores food and has a major role in the expulsion of liquids. The distal stomach, which includes the aboral two thirds of the gastric corpus as well as the pylorus, mechanically breaks down (trituration) and expels solids.

Proximal Stomach

The smooth muscles of the proximal stomach interlace and therefore are difficult to separate into distinct layers.[5] Extrinsic innervation is provided by parasympathetic fibers of the vagi and sympathetic fibers of the splanchnic nerves.[6] Preganglionic parasympathetic fibers have synapses on ganglionated plexus within the gut wall. The splanchnic nerves run between the thoracic sympathetic trunk and the celiomesenteric ganglia. Postganglionic sympathetic fibers from these ganglia also have synapses on ganglionated plexus within the enteric wall.

Electrical Activity

The electrical activity of smooth muscle cells can be evaluated in vitro with the use of intracellular electrodes. Cells of the proximal stomach have nonfluctuating transmembrane potentials of approximately –48 mV at rest.[7] This value is usually less negative than the mechanical threshold for contraction (–52 mV in Figure 2). Therefore,

these cells are in a state of slow, sustained contraction and exhibit tone even at rest.[7] Inhibitory neural input causing hyperpolarization decreases tone (the membrane potential moves down the voltage-tension curve), whereas excitatory neural input causing depolarization increases tone (the membrane potential moves up the voltage-tension curve).[7]

Serosal electrodes are used in vivo to record electrical activity. Extracellular recordings represent the net electrical activity from many smooth muscle cells located immediately beneath the electrode. Extracellular recordings of electrical activity of smooth muscle in the proximal stomach have also shown a stable resting potential.[8] Spontaneous fluctuations in membrane potential, which are characteristic of cells in the distal stomach, are not seen in the proximal stomach.[5]

Contractions

Slow, sustained contractions of the proximal stomach regulate intragastric pressure.[5] The amplitude (10 to 50 cm H_2O) and duration (one to three minutes) of these contractions are proportional to the intensity of motor nerve activity.[7] Variations in neural input lead to graded changes in membrane potential and therefore to graded changes in tone.[7] When motor nerve input is interspersed with periods of neural quiescence, phasic contractile activity results.[7] Phasic contractions, with amplitudes of 5 to 15 cm H_2O and durations of 10 to 15 seconds, are usually superimposed on the slow, sustained contractions. A distinct phasic contraction with an amplitude greater than 50 cm H_2O and a duration of approximately one minute has been termed the fundal wave.[5,9]

Regulation of Contractions
Neural

The enteric nervous system coordinates the functions of the gastrointestinal tract.[6,10] Distinct plexus are present within the gut wall. The myenteric (Auerbach's) plexus is located between the longitudinal and circular muscle layers. The submucosal (Meissner's) plexus is located in the submucosa. Interneurons form networks between the plexus. Independent of central nervous system control, interneurons receive feedback from sensory receptors located within the mucosal and muscular layers. This information is integrated within the neural circuitry. Interneurons then control the activity of motor neurons. If activated, motor neurons can initiate, sustain, or inhibit the activity of effector systems. Effector systems include the smooth muscles, secretory and absorptive epithelia, blood vascular system, and endocrine system.[10] Because of the extensive neural circuitry within the gut wall, the various effector systems do not function independently.

The central nervous system monitors information from the gut; but instead of sending commands to individual neurons, it influences programmed circuits of the enteric nervous system. As a result, gastrointestinal functions are more efficiently controlled, and extra space to accommodate the neurons of the enteric nervous system within the spinal cord is not needed. Because the number of neurons in the enteric nervous system is approximately the same as the number present in the spinal cord (1×10^8), conservation of space is important.[10]

In the proximal stomach, extrinsic neural input is needed to regulate contractions because smooth muscle cells in this region cannot undergo spontaneous depolarization.[5] Acetylcholine, a cholinergic neurotransmitter released by certain postganglionic vagal neurons, stimulates gastric contractions. A noncholinergic, nonadrenergic neurotransmitter released by other postganglionic vagal neurons inhibits contraction of proximal gastric smooth muscle cells. Adenosine triphosphate (ATP), which is a purine nucleotide, has been proposed as the transmitter for nonadrenergic inhibitory nerves.[11,12] Sympathetic efferent activity is mediated by the neurotransmitter norepinephrine. Sympathetic discharge also inhibits gastric contractions.

In immunohistochemical studies for neurotransmitters, at least 10 other types of neurons have been identified within the myenteric plexus.[13] Autonomic nerves containing substance P, vasoactive intestinal peptide, enkephalin, neurotensin, somatostatin, bombesin, gastrin, and cholecystokinin have been demonstrated. In addition, there is evidence that serotonin, γ-aminobutyric acid (GABA), dopamine, and bradykinin are autonomic transmitters.[11] The presence of these chemicals in nerve endings within the muscular wall, along with receptors on smooth muscle cells, suggests that these neurotransmitters play a role in coordinating gastric motility.[1]

Hormonal and Paracrine

Various hormones can influence gastric contractions, although cholecystokinin may be the only one that does so at physiologic concentrations.[14-16] Gastrin from antral mucosa, cholecystokinin and motilin from duodenal mucosa, vasoactive intestinal peptide from gastric and intestinal mucosa, and glucagon and somatostatin from the pancreas have all been implicated in the regulation of gastric contractions.[5,17] Motilin stimulates gastric contractions, possibly by enhancing the release of acetylcholine from cholinergic neurons.[18,19] Gastrin inhibits gastric contractions, possibly by facilitating the release of the vagal inhibitory neurotransmitter.[20] Paracrine substances, which act locally on adjacent neurons and smooth muscle cells, may also influence gastric contractions.[1,5]

Consequences of Contractions

Immediately after food is swallowed, the lower esophageal sphincter and the proximal stomach relax to receive the bolus. This short-lasting relaxation of smooth muscle, called receptive relaxation,[5,7] also occurs after a dry swallow (i.e., when there is no bolus). When the stomach is distended by the swallowed bolus, a further and prolonged relaxation of the proximal stomach is produced. This process is called accommodation or adaptive relaxation.[5,7] Receptive and adaptive relaxation, which are mediated by the noncholinergic, nonadrenergic vagal inhibitory neurons, enable the proximal stomach to receive large quantities of food without an appreciable rise in intragastric pressure.[1,5] The proximal stomach thus serves as the gastric reservoir.

The proximal stomach plays a major role in controlling gastric expulsion of liquids. The volume of liquid expelled per unit of time depends on the pressure gradient between the stomach and duodenum and the pyloric resistance to flow.[5,21] The intestine also regulates gastric emptying by increasing resistance to fluid flow.[22] As long as pyloric resistance to flow and intraduodenal pressure remain constant, gastric expulsion of liquid increases in direct proportion to intragastric pressure.[23] To a lesser extent, peristaltic waves of the distal stomach also affect gastric expulsion of liquids because they greatly alter intraluminal pressure.[5]

Distal Stomach

The smooth muscles of the distal stomach are more easily separated into three distinct layers.[5] As in the proximal stomach, extrinsic innervation is provided by vagal excitatory, vagal inhibitory, and sympathetic inhibitory fibers.

Electrical Activity

Intracellular recordings from smooth muscle cells of the distal stomach demonstrate spontaneous fluctuations in membrane potential.[24] In some respects, potentials resemble those seen in the conducting tissue and muscle of the heart. Rapid depolarization from negative to positive is followed by partial repolarization and then a sustained positive potential, which slowly reverts to a more negative potential (Figure 3).[7,25] The sustained positive potential coupled with the slow phase of repolarization is called a plateau potential.

In the gastric corpus, the resting membrane potential (-61 mV) is more negative than the mechanical threshold

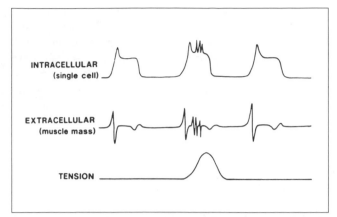

Figure 3—Correlation between *intracellular* and *extracellular* electrical change and *tension* change in intestinal smooth muscle. (From Wingate DL: The electrical and mechanical activity of the small intestine. *Ital J Gastroenterol* 15:262–266, 1983. Reprinted with permission.)

(–45 mV in Figure 2)[7]; but rapid depolarization allows the membrane potential to pass over the mechanical threshold, and activation of the contractile process begins. If the plateau potential after the initial rapid depolarization remains below the mechanical threshold, the subsequent contractile activity is of higher amplitude and sustained.[7] In vivo, this is the gastric peristaltic contraction.[7]

In the antral region, the resting membrane potential (–70 mV) is 30 mV more negative than the mechanical threshold (–40 mV).[7] Contraction depends on depolarization of the membrane to below the mechanical threshold. The amplitude of contraction is affected by the duration of time the plateau potential remains greater than the mechanical threshold.[7] Force of contraction depends on the position of the plateau potential on the voltage tension curve (Figure 2).[7]

Extracellular recordings, which represent the net electrical activity of many smooth muscle cells located beneath the electrode, show that the intracellular changes in potential correspond to slow waves (also called pacesetter potentials, basal electrical rhythm, or electrical control activity).[5,26] Each slow-wave cycle consists of a triphasic complex followed by an isoelectric segment (Figure 3). The end of one cycle occurs when a triphasic complex of the next cycle appears. Action potentials (also called spike potentials, burst potentials, or electrical response activity) may follow a slow-wave complex.[5,25,26]

Slow waves can be recorded from all smooth muscle cells in the distal stomach, but their intrinsic frequencies differ.[1] The highest frequencies are those recorded from cells on the greater curvature on the adoral half of the gastric corpus. This region acts as the dominant gastric pacemaker and is analogous to the sinoatrial node of the heart.[27,28] Frequencies are progressively lower for isolated cells from the gastroduodenal junction and lesser curvature.[5,29] In dogs, the fastest slow waves are generated approximately every 12 seconds, corresponding to a frequency of four to five per minute (0.06 to 0.08 Hz).[5]

Slow waves spread around the stomach and distally, through longitudinal muscle fibers, from the gastric pace-

maker to the pylorus (see Figure 1). The propagation velocity increases as the slow waves approach the pylorus, from 0.1 cm/sec proximally to 4 cm/sec in the terminal antrum.[30] Thus, two or three slow-wave fronts are present simultaneously on the stomach. Slow waves do not spread to the proximal stomach, probably because smooth muscle cells in this region do not have membrane properties capable of supporting them.[7]

Slow waves are always present, regardless of whether gastric contractions occur.[31] Unlike cardiac electrical activity, slow waves are not always associated with contractile activity. If contractions are present, their maximum frequency can never exceed the slow-wave frequency because contractions can only occur during a specific phase of the slow-wave cycle. Action potentials are the electrical events associated with contractions.[5] They appear as rapid changes in electrical potential immediately after the triphasic complex. Usually, the more action potentials present, the greater is the amplitude of contraction.[8] If no action potentials follow the triphasic complex (i.e., an isoelectric segment occurs), no contraction occurs. Extracellular recording techniques demonstrate that the electrical activity of the stomach consists of omnipresent, autonomous, slow waves on which action potentials that coincide with contractions are superimposed. When no action potentials are superimposed on the slow waves, no contraction occurs (Figure 3).

Contractions

Contractions of the distal stomach are called peristaltic waves. Not every slow wave is associated with action potentials and a peristaltic wave. Even if a peristaltic wave is initiated, it may not be propagated the full length of the distal stomach. The waves may also begin distal to the pacemaker region. The degree of muscle tension, the level of stimulation by excitatory nerves, and the amounts of hormones, paracrine, and neurocrine substances present determine whether a contraction follows the slow-wave cycle as it passes over a particular gastric location.[5]

The propagation velocity of peristaltic waves, like that of slow waves, increases as the waves approach the pylorus.[5] As the peristaltic wave approaches the terminal antrum, both the terminal antrum and the pylorus contract together; however, the antral orifice remains larger than the pyloric orifice. Viscous and solid digesta are forced orad during the terminal antral contraction.[4,5]

Regulation of Contractions

To activate contractile proteins, myosin must be phosphorylated by a process that requires calcium. The exact mechanisms for increasing intracellular calcium concentration before activation are not known.[7] Excitatory agents or stimulatory neurotransmitters could increase either voltage-dependent calcium conductance, thus allowing a greater influx of calcium into the cell, or voltage-dependent release of calcium from intracellular storage.[7] The amount of calcium influx during a single action potential is insufficient for maximum contraction. Therefore, multiple action potentials are required.[7] Recordings made by extracellular electrodes show a series of oscillations or action potentials as the muscle contracts.[8]

Neural

Changes in membrane potential and ion conductance of gastric smooth muscle cells are regulated in part by the enteric nervous system.[7,32] Cholinergic parasympathetic activity initiates a contraction when none is present (or increases the amplitude of a contraction) by altering the duration of the plateau potential.[7] Depending on the position of the plateau potential on the voltage-tension curve (Figure 2), a small change in the level of excitatory nerve stimulation can cause a large increase in the force of contraction. Adrenergic sympathetic nervous activity decreases or abolishes contractions.[7] Norepinephrine decreases the amplitude and duration of the plateau potential and similarly affects its associated contraction.

Hormonal and Paracrine

Gastric contractions are also influenced by endocrine and paracrine secretions.[5] Gastrin and cholecystokinin induce contractions similar to those seen during digestion of a meal.[33-35] In addition, gastrin increases the frequency of the pacemaker slow-wave cycle.[36] Motilin also stimulates contraction.[18] Secretin, glucagon, vasoactive intestinal peptide, and somatostatin decrease gastric contractions.[5] The exact physiologic role many specific hormones or combinations of hormones and locally secreted chemicals play in vivo has not been determined.

Consequences of Contractions

Gastric chyme is propelled toward the duodenum as a peristaltic wave passes over the middle of the antrum. Intraluminal pressure may increase to 100 cm H_2O for a duration of one to four seconds. Chyme is not forced into the duodenum. Instead, liquids with small, suspended particles are gently flushed through the pyloric orifice. Solids are retained in the stomach until they have been almost liquefied (i.e., particles are smaller than 2 mm in diameter).[5,37-39]

Selective emptying is possible because of coordinated contractions in the terminal antrum and pylorus, coupled with inhibition of duodenal contractions.[40] Initially, the terminal antral contraction causes the pylorus to close, thus trapping antral contents between the pyloric sphincter and the peristaltic wave; but the peristaltic wave does not occlude the antrum. Rather, a central orifice is formed.[41] Consequently, viscous and solid ingesta are forced orad as the antrum and pylorus continue to contract. Contractions of the terminal antrum and jetlike retropulsion of solid chyme result in thorough mixing of gastric contents with gastric secretions. In addition, repetitive propulsion, mixing, and retropulsion result in trituration of solids.[42,43] Once the solids have been broken into particles smaller than 2 mm in diameter, they can pass with liquids through the gastroduodenal junction into the duodenum.[5,7,37]

Gastroduodenal Junction

The gastroduodenal junction, or pylorus, is the narrowed

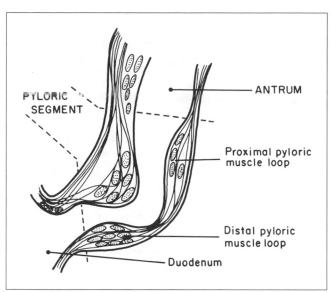

Figure 4—Schematic representation of the muscular anatomy of the gastroduodenal junction. Gastric contents are trapped in the *pyloric segment* after an antral contraction and a constriction of the *pyloric loops*. (From Akkermans LMA, Johnson AG, Read NW (eds): *Gastric and Gastroduodenal Motility*. New York, Praeger Publishers, 1984. Reprinted with permission.)

region between the terminal antrum and the duodenum. Pyloric musculature is thicker than in adjacent regions and is organized into two distinct loops.[44,45] The proximal pyloric loop is a broad muscle band that is not much thicker than the circular muscle layer from which it is derived. The distal pyloric loop is a much thicker muscle bundle that protrudes into the lumen of the gastroduodenal junction (Figure 4). The distal pyloric loop is formed by fusion of circular, longitudinal, and mucosal muscle fibers. This intermingling of gastric muscle layers at the level of the distal pyloric loop is the anatomic basis for the pyloric ring. The pyloric canal is bordered by the proximal and distal pyloric loops. The gastroduodenal junction is innervated by extrinsic autonomic nerves similar to those that innervate the distal stomach.[5]

Electrical Activity

As in the distal stomach, slow waves occur at a frequency of approximately five per minute.[5] Action potentials and contractions are not associated with every slow-wave cycle. Because contractions only occur during a specific phase of the slow-wave cycle, contractile rate never exceeds the slow-wave frequency.

Contractions

Most investigators agree that a distinct pyloric sphincter does not exist.[5] The pyloric canal remains open if the distal stomach is free of peristaltic activity.[5] Pyloric closure occurs only when a peristaltic contraction reaches the terminal antrum and contracts the proximal pyloric loop.[41] Gastric contents that were moved into the pyloric segment by the antral contraction are trapped between the constricted pyloric loops. Only fluids and particles smaller than 2 mm in diameter escape through the narrow pyloric orifice into the duodenum. Larger particles are ground into smaller pieces by the milling action and by the shearing forces that accompany subsequent retropulsion of contents into the proximal antrum.[5,7,42,43]

Regulation of Contractions
Neural
Parasympathetic vagal fibers may either excite or inhibit pyloric contractions. Sympathetic fibers inhibit contractions.[5]

Hormonal
The pyloric sphincter responds differently than the distal stomach to hormonal manipulation.[5,46] Whereas gastrin causes action potentials and contractions in the distal stomach, the pylorus is not affected. Secretin induces contractions of the pylorus but not the distal stomach. Cholecystokinin enhances the contractions of both regions.

Consequences of Contractions
In addition to its role in selective emptying, the pylorus closes to prevent duodenogastric reflux during proximal duodenal contractions.[5,47]

Gastric Emptying
The rate of gastric emptying is ultimately determined by the pressure gradient between the stomach and duodenum and the resistance to flow across the pylorus.[5] Gastric expulsion of liquids depends primarily on the pressure gradient because the pylorus offers little resistance to liquid flow.[5] Because slow tonic contractions of the proximal stomach are the major regulator of intragastric pressure, they also are the major regulator of gastric expulsion of liquids. Conversely, gastric expulsion of solids is primarily determined by resistance to flow of solids across the pylorus.[5] Contractions of the distal stomach and gastroduodenal junction determine pyloric resistance to flow and thus regulate gastric expulsion of solids.

Fed State
Gastric emptying following ingestion of a meal is regulated by factors that affect the gastroduodenal pressure gradient and pyloric resistance to flow. Liquids are expelled more rapidly than solids. The primary determinant of the expulsion rate for inert liquids is volume.[5,48,49] The volume of liquid expelled per unit of time is directly proportional to the volume present in the stomach. The larger the volume of liquid is, the more rapid is its rate of expulsion.

Caloric density determines the gastric emptying rate for solids.[50] Isocaloric quantities of carbohydrate, protein, and fat empty at similar rates.[50] The duration of the fed motility pattern is proportional to the number of calories per kilogram of body weight ingested.[51] The consistency and chemical composition of commercial diets do not alter the gastric emptying rate or the duration of the fed motility pattern.[52] As long as the same number of calories is fed, the duration of the digestive pattern remains constant.[53]

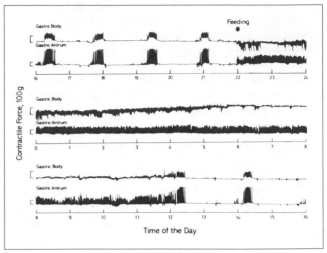

Figure 5—Changes in contractile activity recorded over 24 hours by implanted force tranducers are illustrated. Recordings were made from the gastric corpus (*gastric body*) and *antrum* of a conscious dog. The digestive period ends with a series of strong peristaltic contractions. This series is followed by the migrating myoelectric complex of the fasting period. The time between two consecutive phase III periods is approximately two hours. (From Akkermans LMA, Johnson AG, Read NW (eds): *Gastric and Gastroduodenal Motility*. New York, Praeger Publishers, 1984. Reprinted with permission.)

The rate of gastric emptying is controlled by receptors in the small intestine; these receptors are sensitive to the concentration of acid in and osmolarity of gastric chyme and to fatty acids and tryptophan.[5,54,55] Carbohydrates and amino acids, except for L-tryptophan, retard gastric emptying by stimulating osmoreceptors. Fats slow emptying by acting on fatty-acid receptors.[55] After stimulation, the receptors delay gastric emptying. Hormones and neural reflexes are probably involved in this feedback inhibition.[5]

Fasting State
In the fasting or interdigestive state, a different motor pattern occurs than in the fed state. This pattern, which is specialized for expelling undigested debris from the stomach, is called the migrating myoelectric complex or the interdigestive myoelectric complex.[1,26,56,57] Based on long-term 24-hour studies, time from feeding to appearance of the interdigestive (fasting) pattern ranges from 6.4 to 16 hours in normal dogs (Figure 5).[52,58]

The digestive pattern ends with a series of strong peristaltic contractions involving most of the stomach. This series is followed by a phase of motor quiescence, which lasts approximately 60 to 110 minutes. Gastric contractions then reappear, gradually increase in frequency, and culminate in a 10- to 25-minute phase of intense peristaltic contractions. Quiescence returns and the cycle repeats. Phase I is quiescence, phase II is the period of increasing but irregular contractile activity, and phase III is the period of intense regular contractions (activity front).[56] During phase III, a contraction occurs with almost every slow-wave cycle (four or five contractions per minute).

The migrating myoelectric complex passes from the stomach and small intestine to the colon in approximately two hours.[5] At about the time a phase III front reaches the terminal ileum, another phase III front starts in the stomach.[5] Some investigators have suggested, however, that the migrating myoelectric complex originates in the proximal small intestine rather than in the stomach and moves orad as the postprandial disruption of intestinal motility gives way to the migrating myoelectric complex.[57]

Indigestible solids (e.g., plant fiber) that cannot be broken down into particles smaller than 2 mm in diameter remain in the stomach during the fed state. These particles, along with saliva, basal mucous secretions, and cellular debris, are expelled by the migrating myoelectric complex while the stomach is in the fasting state. In the fasting state, the pylorus remains open as a contraction approaches (in the fed state, the pylorus closes as a contraction approaches). The migrating myoelectric complex empties the stomach completely. Thus, phase III of the migrating myoelectric complex is also called the interdigestive housekeeper.[59]

The duration of the migrating myoelectric complex is probably determined by both neural and hormonal mechanisms. Peak concentrations of motilin occur coincident with phase III of the migrating myoelectric complex in dogs and humans.[60-62] Exogenous infusions of motilin initiate phase III contractions in fasting human subjects[63]; however, the precise cause and effect of endogenous motilin fluctuations have not been determined.

Gastric distention and passage of ingesta into the small intestine inhibit the fasting motility pattern and initiate the fed pattern of contractile activity, through as yet unknown mechanisms.[64] Gastrin inhibits the migrating myoelectric complex[65,66]; however, test meals can disrupt the migrating myoelectric complex without changing serum gastrin levels.[67] Therefore, hormones other than gastrin may inhibit the fasting motility pattern.[68] Neural mechanisms may be another means of regulating the transition from the fasting to the fed motility pattern. Truncal vagotomy delays the onset of gastric contractions after ingestion of a meal.[69] A combination of neural and hormonal mechanisms probably determines the onset of fed and fasting motility patterns.

Summary

Smooth muscle activities in the proximal and distal stomach regions and at the gastroduodenal junction are regulated by neural and hormonal mechanisms. Normal gastric motility patterns are complex and highly coordinated for controlled expulsion of liquids, solids, and nondigestible material. Abnormalities of gastric motility and gastric emptying will be discussed in Part II; the diagnostic approach to gastric motility disorders will be emphasized.

REFERENCES

1. Weisbrodt NW: Basic control mechanisms, in Akkermans LMA, Johnson AG, Read NW (eds): *Gastric and Gastroduodenal Motility.* New York, Praeger Publishers, 1984, pp 3–20.
2. Koch KL: Gastric motility: Electromechanical considerations, in Stern RM, Koch KL (eds): *Electrogastrography: Methodology, Validation, and Applications.* New York, Praeger Publishers, 1985, pp 10–13.
3. Kelly KA: Gastric emptying of liquids and solids: Roles of proximal and distal stomach. *Am J Physiol* 239:G71–G76, 1980.
4. Ehrlein HJ, Akkermans LMA: Gastric emptying, in Akkermans LMA, Johnson AG, Read NW (eds): *Gastric and Gastroduodenal Motility.* New York, Praeger Publishers, 1984, pp 74–84.
5. Kelly KA: Motility of the stomach and gastroduodenal junction, in Johnson LR (ed): *Physiology of the Gastrointestinal Tract.* New York, Raven Press, 1981, pp 393–410.
6. Gabella G: Structure of muscle and nerves in the gastrointestinal tract, in Johnson LR (ed): *Physiology of the Gastrointestinal Tract.* New York, Raven Press, 1981, pp 197–241.
7. Szurszewski JH: Electrical basis for gastrointestinal motility, in Johnson LR (ed): *Physiology of the Gastrointestinal Tract.* New York, Raven Press, 1981, pp 1435–1466.
8. Kelly KA, Code CF, Elveback LR: Patterns of canine gastric electrical activity. *Am J Physiol* 217:461–470, 1969.
9. Lind JF, Duthie HL, Schlegel JF, et al: Motility of the gastric fundus. *Am J Physiol* 201:197–202, 1961.
10. Wood JD: Enteric neurophysiology. *Am J Physiol* 247:G585–G598, 1984.
11. Burnstock G: Purinergic nerves and smooth muscle of the gut, in Chey WY (ed): *Functional Disorders of the Digestive Tract.* New York, Raven Press, 1983, pp 79–85.
12. Burnstock G: Autonomic innervation and transmission. *Br Med Bull* 35:255–262, 1979.
13. Furness JB, Costa M: Types of nerves in the enteric nervous system. *Neuroscience* 5:1–20, 1980.
14. Walsh JH: Endocrine cells of the digestive system, in Johnson LR (ed): *Physiology of the Gastrointestinal Tract.* New York, Raven Press, 1981, pp 59–144.
15. Debas HT, Farooq O, Grossman MI: Inhibition of gastric emptying is a physiological action of cholecystokinin. *Gastroenterology* 68:1211–1217, 1975.
16. Thomas PA, Kelly KA: Hormonal control of interdigestive motor cycles of canine proximal stomach. *Am J Physiol* 277:E192–E197, 1979.
17. Itoh A: Hormones, peptides, opioids and prostaglandins in normal gastric contractions, in Akkermans LMA, Johnson AG, Read NW (eds): *Gastric and Gastroduodenal Motility.* New York, Praeger Publishers, 1984, pp 41–59.
18. Morgan KG, Go VLW, Szurszewski JH: Motilin increases the influence of excitatory myenteric plexus neurons on gastric smooth muscle in vitro, in Christensen J (ed): *Gastrointestinal Motility.* New York, Raven Press, 1980, pp 365–370.
19. Lang IM, Sarna SK, Condon RE: Myoelectric and contractile effects of motilin on dog small intestine in vivo. *Dig Dis Sci* 31:1062–1072, 1986.
20. Morgan KG, Schmalz PF, Szurszewski JH: Action of pentagastrin on nonadrenergic inhibitory intramural nerves of the canine orad stomach. *Gastroenterology* 76:1206, 1979.
21. Minami H, McCallum RW: The physiology and pathophysiology of gastric emptying in humans. *Gastroenterology* 86:1592–1610, 1984.
22. Miller J, Kauffman G, Elashoff J, et al: Search for resistances controlling canine gastric emptying of liquid meals. *Am J Physiol* 241:G403–G415, 1981.
23. Strunz UT, Grossman MI: Effect of intragastric pressure on gastric emptying and secretion. *Am J Physiol* 235:E552–E555, 1978.
24. El-Sharkawy TY, Morgan KG, Szurszewski JH: Intracellular activity of canine and human gastric muscle. *J Physiology* 279:291–307, 1978.
25. Wingate DL: The electrical and mechanical activity of the small intestine. *Ital J Gastroenterol* 15:262–266, 1983.
26. Sarna SK: Gastrointestinal electrical activity: Terminology. *Gastroenterology* 68:1631–1635, 1975.
27. Kelly KA, Code CF: Canine gastric pacemaker. *Am J Physiol* 220:112–118, 1971.
28. Weber J Jr, Kohatsu S: Pacemaker localization and electrical conduction patterns in the canine stomach. *Gastroenterology* 59:717–726, 1970.
29. Sarna SK, Daniel EE, Kingma YJ: Effects of partial cuts on gastric electrical control activity and its computer model. *Am J Physiol* 223:332–340, 1972.
30. Daniel EE, Irwin J: Electrical activity of gastric musculature, in

Code CF, Heidel W (eds): *Handbook of Physiology: Alimentary Canal. Motility*, vol 4. Washington DC, American Physiological Society, 1968, pp 1969–1984.

31. Code CF, Szurszewski JH, Kelly KA, et al: A concept of control of gastrointestinal motility, in Code CF, Heidel W (eds): *Handbook of Physiology: Alimentary Canal: Bile, Digestion, Ruminal Physiology*, vol 5. Washington, DC, American Physiological Society, 1968, pp 2881–2896.

32. Szurszewski JH: Modulation of smooth muscle by nervous activity: A review and a hypothesis. *Fed Proc* 36:2456–2461, 1977.

33. Kelly KA: Effect of gastrin on gastric myoelectric activity. *Am J Dig Dis* 15:399–405, 1970.

34. Morgan KG, Schmalz PF, Go VLW, et al: Effect of pentagastrin, G17, and G34 on the electrical and mechanical activities of canine antral smooth muscle. *Gastroenterology* 75:304–412, 1978.

35. Szurszewski JH: Mechanism of action of pentagastrin and acetylcholine on the longitudinal muscle of the canine antrum. *J Physiol* 252:335–361, 1975.

36. Cooke AR, Chvasta TE, Weisbrodt NW: Effect of pentagastrin on emptying and electrical and motor activity of the dog stomach. *Am J Physiol* 223:934–938, 1972.

37. Hinder RA, Kelly KA: Canine gastric emptying of solids and liquids. *Am J Physiol* 233:E335–E340, 1977.

38. Meyer JH, Thomson JB, Cohen MB, et al: Sieving of solid food by the canine stomach and sieving after gastric surgery. *Gastroenterology* 76:804–813, 1979.

39. Arnold JG, Dubois A: In vitro studies of intragastric digestion. *Dig Dis Sci* 28:737–741, 1983.

40. Hinder RA, San-Garde BA: Individual and combined roles of the pylorus and the antrum in the canine gastric emptying of a liquid and a digestible solid. *Gastroenterology* 84:281–286, 1983.

41. Carlson HC, Code CF, Nelson RA: Motor action of the canine gastroduodenal junction: A cineradiographic, pressure and electric study. *Am J Dig Dis* 11:155–176, 1966.

42. Code CF: The mystique of the gastroduodenal junction. *Rendic Rev Gastroenterol* 2:20–37, 1970.

43. Prove J, Ehrlein HJ: Motor function of gastric antrum and pylorus for evacuation of low and high viscosity meals in dogs. *Gut* 23:150–156, 1982.

44. Torgersen J: The muscular build and movements of the stomach and the duodenal bulb. *Acta Radiol [Suppl] (Stockh)* 45:1–187, 1942.

45. Schulze-Delrieu K, Ehrlein HJ, Blum AL: Mechanics of the pylorus, in Akkermans LMA, Johnson AG, Read NW (eds): *Gastric and Gastroduodenal Motility*. New York, Praeger Publishers, 1984, pp 87–102.

46. Fisher RS, Lipshutz W, Cohen S: The hormonal regulation of pyloric sphincter function. *J Clin Invest* 52:1289–1296, 1973.

47. Muller-Lissner SA, Sonnenberg A, Schaltenmann G, et al: Gastric emptying and postprandial duodenogastric reflux in pylorectomized dogs. *Am J Physiol* 242:G9–G14, 1982.

48. Hunt JN, Spurrell WR: The pattern of emptying of the human stomach. *J Physiol* 113:157–168, 1951.

49. Lieb MS, Wingfield WE, Twedt DC, et al: Gastric emptying of liquids in the dog: Serial test meal and modified emptying-time techniques. *Am J Vet Res* 46:1876–1880, 1985.

50. Hunt JN, Stubbs DF: The volume and energy content of meals as determinants of gastric emptying. *J Physiol* 245:209–225, 1975.

51. Dewever I, Eckhout C, Vantrappen G, et al: Disruptive effect of test meals on interdigestive motor complex in dogs. *Am J Physiol* 235:E661–E665, 1978.

52. Burrows CF, Bright RM, Spencer CP: Influence of dietary composition on gastric emptying and motility in dogs: Potential involvement in acute gastric dilatation. *Am J Vet Res* 46:2609–2612, 1985.

53. McHugh PR, Morgan TH: Calories and gastric emptying: A regulatory capacity with implications for feeding. *Am J Physiol* 236:R254–R260, 1979.

54. Hunt JN, Knox MT: Regulation of gastric emptying, in Code CF, Heidel W (eds): *Handbook of Physiology: Alimentary Canal. Motility*, vol 4. Washington DC, American Physiological Society, 1968, pp 1917–1935.

55. Keinke O, Ehrlein HJ: Effect of oleic acid on canine gastroduodenal motility, pyloric diameter and gastric emptying. *Q J Exp Physiol* 68:675–686, 1983.

56. Code CF, Marlett JA: The interdigestive myoelectric complex of the stomach and small bowel of dogs. *J Physiol (London)* 246:289–309, 1975.

57. Bueno L, Rayner V, Ruckebusch Y: Initiation of the migrating myoelectric complex in dogs. *J Physiol* 316:309–318, 1981.

58. Itoh Z, Aizawai T, Takeuchi S, et al: Diurnal changes in gastric motor activity in conscious dogs. *Dig Dis Sci* 22:117–124, 1977.

59. Code CF, Schlegel JF: The gastrointestinal housekeeper, in Daniel EE (ed): *Gastrointestinal Motility*. Vancouver, Mitchell Press, 1974, pp 631–633.

60. Itoh Z, Takeuchi S, Aizawa I, et al: Changes in plasma motilin concentration and gastrointestinal contractile activity in conscious dogs. *Am J Dig Dis* 23:929–935, 1978.

61. Vantrappen GR, Janssens J, Peeters TL, et al: Motilin and the interdigestive migrating complex in man. *Dig Dis Sci* 24:497–500, 1979.

62. Lee KY, Kim MS, Chey WY: Effects of a meal and gut hormones on plasma motilin and duodenal motility in dogs. *Am J Physiol* 238:G280–G283, 1980.

63. Itoh Z, Takeuchi S, Aizawa I, et al: Effect of synthetic motilin on gastric motor activity in conscious dogs. *Am J Dig Dis* 22:813–819, 1977.

64. Carlson GM, Mathias JR, Bertiger G, Neuron control of the response of the gut to meals, in Brooks FP (ed): *Nerves and the Gut*. Thorofare, NJ, Charles B Slack, Inc, 1977, pp 261–271.

65. Kelly KA: Effect of gastrin on gastric myoelectric activity. *Am J Dig Dis* 15:399–405, 1970.

66. Thomas PA, Schang JC, Kelly KA, et al: Can endogenous gastrin inhibit canine interdigestive gastric motility? *Gastroenterology* 78:16–21, 1980.

67. Eeckhout C, DeWever I, Peeters T, et al: Role of gastrin and insulin in postprandial disruption of migrating complex in dogs. *Am J Physiol* 235:E666–E669, 1978.

68. Schang JC, Kelly KA, Go VLW: Postprandial hormonal inhibition of canine interdigestive gastric motility. *Am J Physiol* 240:G221–G224, 1981.

69. Marik F, Code CF: Control of the interdigestive myoelectric activity in dogs by the vagus nerves and pentagastrin. *Gastroenterology* 69:387–395, 1975.

Gastric Motility in Dogs. Part II. Disorders of Gastric Motility

KEY FACTS

- Vomiting is the clinical sign most frequently associated with delayed gastric emptying.
- Although oral administration of radioisotopes plus external scanning is superior, radiographic contrast studies currently provide the most readily available diagnostic techniques to assess gastric motility.
- Disorders affecting gastric motility are numerous and multisystemic.
- Metoclopramide has revolutionized the therapy of gastric retention because of its prokinetic and antiemetic effects.

Colorado State University
Jean A. Hall, DVM, PhD   David C. Twedt, DVM

University of Florida
Colin F. Burrows, BVetMed, PhD, MRCVS

GASTRIC MOTILITY serves the following three basic functions: storage of ingesta, mixing and dispersion of food particles, and timely expulsion of gastric contents into the duodenum. Disorders of gastric motility result from diseases that, either directly or indirectly, disrupt these functions.[1] Examples of disorders with obstructive lesions that affect gastric emptying directly include chronic hypertrophic gastropathy, pyloric neoplasia, and gastric phycomycosis. In the absence of visible lesions, then functional disorders, or disorders that affect gastric motility indirectly, must be considered. Such disorders are listed on page 248.

The first part of this two-part presentation discussed normal gastric function in dogs. Part II reviews the diagnostic approach for disorders causing gastroparesis and rapid gastric emptying and outlines differentials for specific types of motor abnormalities.

DIAGNOSIS
History and Physical Examination

Delayed gastric emptying often results in gastric distention and vomiting. The differential diagnoses for vomiting are extensive, ranging from Addisonian crisis to Zollinger-Ellison syndrome.[2-5] Although vomiting may occur at varying times after a meal, it usually occurs 10 hours or later with gastric motility disorders, at a time when the stomach should be empty. The character of the vomitus ranges from undigested to partially digested food, depending on the time lapse since the last meal, the degree of gastric trituration, and the amount of gastric secretions. The vomitus is rarely bile stained.

In addition to chronic postprandial vomiting of undigested food, other findings associated with gastric motility disorders include anorexia, nausea, belching, polydipsia, pica, and weight loss. Animals with gastric pain occasionally assume a position of relief known as the praying posture. A thorough history is essential for additional clues of an underlying disease causing abnormal motility.

The physical examination may be normal, or the findings may be related to the primary cause of altered motility. Abdominal auscultation may reveal increased bowel sounds. Tympanites, or distention of the stomach secondary to an obstruction, results in high-pitched bowel sounds. Abdominal palpation may be painful in dogs with gastrointestinal disorders, but this finding is nonspecific. If palpated, abdominal masses are helpful in differentiating vomiting caused by primary gastric disease from a lower intestinal neoplasm, foreign body, or intussusception. Neurologic abnormalities may also be observed in dogs with severe electrolyte or metabolic derangements secondary to vomition from gastric outlet obstruction.

Laboratory Findings

Laboratory findings reflect the underlying cause of the

Originally published in Volume 12, Number 10, October 1990

Classification of Gastric Motility Disorders According to Cause

- Structural or biochemical diseases of the stomach
- Diseases elsewhere in the alimentary tract
- Lesions of the enteric nervous system
- Lesions of the extrinsic nerves supplying the stomach (central nervous system, autonomic nervous system)
- Drugs affecting autonomic or enteric nerves
- Endocrine disorders
- Surgical procedures

gastric motility disorder.[5] Dogs that vomit infrequently usually do not exhibit dehydration, electrolyte losses, or acid-base imbalances. Persistent vomiting can result in severe fluid and electrolyte loss and changes in acid-base balance. Continual vomiting secondary to a gastric outflow obstruction may result in the net loss of fluid rich in hydrogen, chloride, potassium, and sodium ions. Hypokalemia is the most common electrolyte abnormality seen in vomiting patients, resulting from potassium losses in the vomitus and via the kidneys as well as a lack of dietary intake.

Paradoxic aciduria is observed in some dogs with vomiting secondary to a pyloric outflow obstruction. Paradoxic aciduria results when metabolic alkalosis occurs in conjunction with proximal renal tubular bicarbonate reabsorption caused by hypochloremia and with distal renal tubular sodium-hydrogen exchange caused by hypokalemia.

Knowing the pH of the vomitus may be helpful in determining its origin. Gastric vomitus should have an acid pH (<6), whereas regurgitated fluid will have an alkaline pH because of salivary secretions. Duodenogastric reflux of bile and pancreatic juice, however, may neutralize the pH of gastric vomitus.

Tests Used to Evaluate Gastric Motility

Many procedures (see the adjacent box) have been developed to study gastric emptying and motility. This alone indicates that no single technique provides all of the information needed to answer the questions asked by clinicians, "Does this dog's stomach empty normally?" or by researchers, "What is the relationship between contractions of the gastric muscles and forward propulsion of luminal contents?"

Methods used to evaluate gastric emptying include contrast radiography studies, oral administration of radioisotopes plus external scanning, serial sampling of gastric content by intubation, ultrasonography, and computerized tomographic scanning.[6-19] Indirect methods (i.e., measuring the rate at which a substance appears in the bloodstream after absorption from the small intestine) also are used to assess the rate of gastric emptying.[6] Gastric motility can be evaluated using electrophysiologic techniques to record gastric myoelectrical activity.[20] Intragastric pressure also can be monitored by manometry.[13] Despite the various methods available, radiographic techniques are the most definitive means generally available to the practitioner for diagnosing gastric retention in dogs.[3,4]

Liquid barium sulfate has been used to detect gross abnormalities of gastric emptying in routine upper gastrointestinal radiographic studies. Because solids empty differently than liquids,[21] large particles empty differently than small particles,[22] and lipids empty differently than carbohydrate solutions,[23,24] such studies provide inadequate information for assessing emptying of the typical heterogeneous meal. Studies performed with liquid barium are therefore qualitative at best and cannot be expected to provide comprehensive results on gastric emptying.

Other radiopaque materials used in human patients to detect gastric retention include barium burgers and small radiopaque pellets mixed with a standard meal.[6] Barium mixed with food is thought to be a better test of distal gastric function than liquid barium. When solid meals are mixed with barium granules or a barium suspension, however, the barium can dissociate from the food and redistribute in the liquid phase of gastric contents.[7]

The gastric emptying time for a full meal of ground kibble (8 g/kg) mixed with barium sulfate suspension (5 to 7 ml/kg) in a mature, healthy beagle ranged from 5 to 10 hours in one study.[8] In a second study using the same barium meal contrast procedure with mongrels instead of beagles, total gastric emptying time ranged from 7 to 15 hours.[9] Although radiographic techniques are the most rou-

Tests Used to Evaluate Gastric Motility

- Radiographic studies[3,4,6,8,9,12]
    Liquid barium
    Barium mixed with food
    Small radiopaque markers mixed with food
    Fluoroscopy plus positive-contrast material
- Radionuclide emission imaging[6,7,11,13,15,20,25-29]
- Intubative techniques[6,11,14]
    Serial intubations after feeding a test meal
    Double dye dilution technique
- Real-time ultrasonographic techniques[6,17-20]
- Computerized tomographic techniques[16]
- Indirect methods[6,13,20]
    Measurement of blood concentrations of intestinally absorbed drugs
    Electrogastrography
    Manometric techniques

tinely available method used to assess gastric emptying, such a wide range in normal values makes evaluation of clinical patients extremely difficult unless gastric emptying times are markedly prolonged. Similar findings of studies in humans have lead to sweeping conclusions that radiologic measurements using barium are nonquantitative, inadequate, and invalidated by other techniques used to study gastric emptying.[10,11]

Small indigestible particles, one to three millimeters in diameter, have been shown to stimulate a fed-state-like motility pattern. They empty from the stomach slowly, independent of gastric burst activity, which is the motility pattern characteristic of the fasting state.[12] Although these indigestible, radiopaque markers have been used to quantify gastric emptying, they may not accurately represent the emptying of digestible particles.[7]

Gastric motility also can be assessed by fluoroscopy with a positive-contrast material.[3,4] Fluoroscopy may demonstrate antral peristaltic waves of decreased rate and intensity, antral dilatation, delayed entry of gastric contents into the duodenum, or a delay in complete gastric emptying.

R ADIOISOTOPIC methods are the most tolerable and clinically accurate means of evaluating gastric emptying in human patients.[11,13,15] Technetium 99m (^{99m}Tc) is the isotope used most widely because it is safe, simple to use, and nonabsorbable; studies using this nuclide can be repeated without interference from previous studies. Most studies use a gamma camera linked to a computer for precise measurement of gastric emptying. Gamma cameras that are capable of tracking two nuclide markers simultaneously allow solid and liquid emptying to be assessed during the same test period.[11]

Measurement of gastric emptying using radionuclide-labeled test meals has been described in dogs.[25-29] Although wide variations exist in reported values among dogs, the real half-time of gastric emptying is reproducible in the same dog.[25,29] A radioisotope-bound resin (^{99m}Tc-labeled polystyrene triethylenetetramine resin) with particle sizes small enough to empty along with digested food (<0.5 mm), mixed with a test meal (10 kcal/kg), showed the half-time of gastric emptying to range from 0.9 to 4.0 hours in large-breed healthy dogs.[29]

Other techniques used to assess gastric emptying include real-time ultrasonography, recording of gastric myoelectrical activity from the surface of the abdominal wall, and emission computerized tomography. Patient safety and client acceptability are the advantages of these noninvasive techniques. In addition, the ability to conduct repeated studies before and after therapy and the ability to monitor for sustained time periods under normal everyday conditions are major advantages of any of the noninvasive techniques.[20]

Endoscopic and Biopsy Findings

Endoscopic examination of the stomach is helpful for visualizing lesions associated with an underlying cause of altered motility.[3,30] Foreign bodies, antral ulcers, neoplasms, and inflammatory or obstructive lesions (such as hypertrophied antral mucosa) may be observed. Hypertrophic pyloric stenosis, which results from hypertrophy of the circular smooth muscle fibers, may appear as a grossly thickened and closed pyloric sphincter.

The advantages of endoscopy are that it allows both direct examination of the luminal surface and access for diagnostic procedures, such as biopsy, brush cytology, and fluid collection and analysis. In the case of a small foreign body, endoscopy also offers a therapeutic approach. Food must be withheld for at least 24 hours to assure an empty stomach. General anesthesia is required.

Exploratory surgery is indicated as a diagnostic procedure when an extrinsic lesion is suspected of causing obstruction to gastric outflow.[3] The rest of the abdomen should also be evaluated for associated lesions. The stomach can be palpated for infiltrative lesions, and full-thickness biopsies can be taken for definitive diagnosis.

DISORDERS OF GASTRIC MOTILITY

Delayed gastric emptying is often the result of disorders causing gastric-outlet obstruction or disorders causing defective propulsion; however, both conditions may be present and synergistic.

Delayed Transit Caused by Obstruction

Any anatomic lesion of the pylorus or adjacent duodenal segment can impair gastric emptying and cause gastric retention. Pyloric lesions can be categorized as intrinsic, extrinsic, or obstructive (see the box on page 250).[2] Gastric foreign bodies and antral polyps are examples of disorders that can cause pyloric obstruction. Intrinsic lesions include pyloric neoplasia and hypertrophic pyloric gastropathy. Extrinsic lesions, such as hepatic or pancreatic neoplasms, cause gastric-outlet obstruction by encroachment on the pylorus from the exterior.

P YLORIC STENOSIS (the result of *chronic hypertrophic pyloric gastropathy*) is the most common cause of gastric outflow obstruction.[2,4,31-33] Most affected dogs are small breeds, middle-aged, and have a history of chronic intermittent vomiting. Although the cause(s) are unknown, this disorder can be hormonally or neurologically mediated.[2,4] Histopathologic changes include hypertrophy of either the mucosal or muscular layers of the pylorus, or both. Positive-contrast radiographic studies are used to document a gastric outflow obstruction. Surgery, using the least radical procedure to provide adequate gastric outflow, is the treatment of choice for these benign pyloric lesions.[31,33]

Primary *gastric neoplasia*, although uncommon, usually is reported in middle-aged to older dogs.[2,4] Benign tumors include adenomatous polyps and leiomyomas. Adenocarcinomas are the most common malignant gastric tumor in

Gastric Motility Disorders with Transit Delay Caused by Obstruction

- Intrinsic pyloric lesions
    - Chronic hypertrophic pyloric gastropathy
    - Infiltrative pyloric neoplasia
    - Chronic gastritis
        - Chronic hypertrophic gastritis
        - Eosinophilic gastritis
    - Gastric phycomycosis
- Obstructive pyloric lesions
    - Gastric foreign bodies
    - Antral polyps
    - Hypertrophied antral mucosa
    - Scar tissue formation
- Extrinsic pyloric lesions causing external compression
    - Hepatic abscesses
    - Pancreatic abscesses
    - Intraabdominal neoplasia
    - Intraabdominal granulomatous lesions
- Small intestinal obstruction or volvulus

dogs, and metastasis is common. Other primary malignant tumors include lymphosarcoma, leiomyosarcomas, fibrosarcomas, and plasmacytomas.[34] Clinical signs include chronic vomiting, hematemesis, melena, anorexia, and weight loss. Endoscopy or exploratory laparotomy and biopsy are required for definitive diagnosis. The prognosis for malignant gastric neoplasia usually is poor because of the advanced nature at the time of diagnosis and because of complications associated with gastric resection.

Chronic hypertrophic gastritis, which causes diffuse or focal macroscopic thickening of the gastric mucosa, can progress to form obstructive lesions. Lesions are characterized by mucosal hypertrophy and hyperplasia of gastric glands, with inflammatory cells and cystic dilatation of mucous glands.[2] Hypertrophic gastritis is thought to result from chronic mucosal inflammation.

Eosinophilic gastritis also can manifest in obstructive pyloric lesions. These lesions usually consist of a diffuse eosinophilic infiltrate and granulation tissue involving most layers of the stomach wall. Less frequently, it may present as discrete granulomatous nodules.[2] Eosinophilic gastritis may be the result of an allergic or parasitic reaction.[2]

Contrast radiography can demonstrate lesions caused by either chronic hypertrophic gastritis or eosinophilic gastritis, but a definitive diagnosis is based on gastric biopsy. Surgical relief of pyloric obstruction might be required. Changing the diet might benefit hypertrophic gastritis, whereas corticosteroids are the treatment of choice for eosinophilic gastritis.[2]

Gastric phycomycosis[35,36] is a systemic fungal disease reported most commonly in dogs from states bordering the Gulf of Mexico. Dogs are presented for chronic debilitation and vomiting. An abdominal mass is often palpable. Positive-contrast radiographic studies reveal a very thickened gastric wall. The definitive diagnosis is made by identifying the organism in histologic sections or by fungal culture. Surgery is the most effective therapy for localized disease. Intravenous amphotericin B and potassium iodide have been used as treatment for disseminated disease but without reported success.[37]

Obstructive and *extrinsic pyloric lesions* or *objects* usually are demonstrated by plain or contrast radiographic studies. Surgical removal of the foreign object or the affected area is the therapy of choice.

Delayed Transit Caused by Defective Propulsion

Conditions that affect gastric motility in dogs because of defective propulsion are listed on page 251. These are divided according to primary and secondary disorders of the stomach.[1,38] Some of these disease-related motility disorders have been reported only in human patients (see entries marked with asterisks in the list on page 251). Based on clinical experiences and inferences from human studies, many diseases reported to affect motility in human patients also are thought to affect gastric motility in dogs.

Inflammatory *gastritis* and infiltrative lesions, such as those associated with *granulomatous* or *neoplastic disease*, have been documented in dogs in conjunction with gastric stasis.[3] Human gastric ulcer patients have reduced antral motility in both the fasting and fed states.[39,40] *Gastric ulcers* also are considered a cause of defective gastric propulsion in dogs.[41] Endoscopy and biopsy provide the best techniques for identifying these disorders in dogs. Treatment depends on the underlying cause, but antacids and H_2-receptor blocking agents are useful in the management of gastric ulcerations.

HUMAN PATIENTS with atrophic gastritis have delayed emptying of both solids and liquids.[1] Because *chronic atrophic gastritis* predisposes to gastric ulceration,[42] this disorder also can be associated with delayed gastric emptying in dogs. Atrophic gastritis represents the advanced stage of chronic superficial gastritis and is characterized histologically by atrophy of the gastric glands, reduced numbers of chief and parietal cells, and increased numbers of mucous-secreting and inflammatory cells.[2] Gastric biopsies are required for a definitive diagnosis. Reduced parietal cell numbers can result in achlorhydria and hypergastrinemia, as negative feedback from hydrochloric acid on gastrin release is reduced. Most dogs, however, are not completely achlorhydric. Because back diffusion of hydrochloric acid is a perpetuating factor in gastric mucosal damage, treatment consists of H_2-receptor blocking agents to protect against gastric ulceration. Controlled dietary management also can be beneficial.[2,43–45] In addition, corticosteroids may be effective in the treatment of atrophic gastritis by stimulating regeneration of gastric parietal cells.[2]

Acute viral infections in human patients with parvovirus-like agents, such as Norwalk or Hawaii agent, cause significant gastric retention that resolves with recovery.[46] *Canine parvovirus* also is associated with reduced gastric motility.[47]

Intestinal parasites cause abnormal intestinal motility; likewise, *gastric parasites* can cause abnormal gastric motility. The nematode *Physaloptera* was suggested as the cause of chronic gastritis and intermittent vomiting of partially digested food in an otherwise healthy dog.[48] The bloated abdomen commonly seen in puppies infected with ascarids may be the result of altered gastrointestinal motility. Hookworms have been shown to disrupt the fasting-state migrating motility complex in dogs and to decrease motility.[49] Products produced by the parasites are speculated to mediate these changes.[50]

All surgical procedures involving the stomach in human patients alter gastric motility to some extent.[51] Many studies have been performed, often using dogs as models, to determine postoperative sequelae associated with vagotomies and various gastric surgical procedures.[11,51,52]

The effects of *gastric surgery* in dogs may be different from those in humans. Duodenal cannulas were used in one study to assess gastric emptying. Dogs with truncal vagotomy, pyloroplasty, truncal vagotomy plus pyloroplasty, or antrectomy plus gastroduodenostomy all had gastric emptying times similar to those of control dogs.[53] With the exception of dogs with pyloroplasty alone, however, all dogs showed an increase in the size of particles emptied from the stomach. In another study, a two-marker technique was used to show that pylorectomy increased gastric emptying rate and postprandial duodenogastric reflux.[54]

SECONDARY causes of defective gastric propulsion include *acute stress*. Increased sympathetic nervous activity, which would occur with excitement or trauma, decreases or abolishes contractions by decreasing both the amplitude and the duration of the plateau potential in gastric smooth muscle cells.[55]

Transection of the spinal cord above the thoracic region isolates reflex spinal sympathetic control of the stomach from the input of higher centers. In humans, during the stage of spinal shock immediately after cord transection, there is temporary loss of intrinsic sympathetic activity. Gastric dilatation and ileus can develop as a result of imbalanced neural input.[1]

Gastric stasis can result from conditions causing serosal inflammation, such as *peritonitis*.[38] In *pancreatitis*, inflammation often extends from the pancreas to adjacent organs, including the stomach. Hypokalemia and stimulation of the sympathetic nervous system by chemical peritonitis or shock cause altered gastrointestinal motility.[56]

Electrolyte and metabolic disorders also are associated

Gastric Motility Disorders with Transit Delay Caused by Defective Propulsion

- Primary gastric defects
    - Inflammatory gastric lesions
    - Gastric neoplasia
    - Gastric ulcers
        - * Atrophic gastritis[1]
        - * Gastric amyloidosis[1]
    - Viral, bacterial, or parasitic gastroenteritis
        - * Idiopathic gastroparesis[1]
    - After gastric surgery
- Secondary gastric defects
    - Acute stress
        - Increased sympathetic discharge (excitement)
        - Trauma
        - Spinal cord injury or surgery
    - Acute abdominal inflammation
        - Pancreatitis
        - Peritonitis
    - Electrolyte disturbances
        - Hypokalemia
        - Hypercalcemia
        - Hypocalcemia
        - Hypomagnesemia
    - Metabolic disorders
        - * Hyperglycemia[11]
        - * Diabetic gastroneuropathy[1,11,59,60]
        - Acidosis
        - Hypothyroidism
        - Hypoadrenocorticism
        - Hepatic encephalopathy
        - Hypergastrinemia
        - Uremia
    - Drugs
        - Anticholinergics
        - Beta-adrenergic agonists
        - Narcotics
        - Enkephalins
        - L-Dopa
    - Abdominal surgery
    - Total body irradiation
        - * Dermatomyositis[1]
        - * Systemic lupus erythematosus[1]
        - * Brain stem tumor[76]
        - * Chronic pectin ingestion[77,78]

* Reported only in human patients.

with gastric stasis. *Hypokalemia, hypercalcemia, hypocalcemia*, and *hypomagnesemia* often are listed as causes of gastric stasis, although their exact role in delaying gastric emptying needs further study.[11,47] Abnormal sodium and potassium concentrations alter membrane potentials and neuromuscular function.[57] Delayed gastric emptying in disorders with electrolyte imbalances may be the result of abnormal nerve impulses and defective muscle contraction.[57,58]

Diabetes mellitus may cause gastric stasis in dogs because hyperglycemia has been shown experimentally to delay gastric emptying of food.[11] Hyperglycemia may act by augmenting other inhibitory mechanisms of gastric emptying. In humans, diabetic visceral neuropathy is a sequela of poorly controlled insulin-dependent diabetes mellitus. This as yet has not been documented in dogs. *Acidosis* depresses smooth muscle contractile activity in vitro and therefore may contribute to the delayed gastric emptying seen in certain metabolic disorders.[61]

Hypothyroid dogs have decreased electrical and mechanical stomach activity.[62] The manner in which *hypothyroidism* causes these changes and the clinical effects on gastric emptying are not known.

Adrenocortical insufficiency is associated with gastric stasis and vomiting in dogs.[63] In addition to the effects of altered electrolyte concentrations on neuromuscular function, increased corticotropin-releasing factor may promote gastric stasis and vomiting. Intracerebroventricular administration of corticotropin-releasing factor has been shown to suppress gastric contractions during the fasting state in dogs.[64,65] Corticotropin-releasing factor, therefore, acting centrally and independently of corticotropin and cortisol release, may affect fasting gastric motility.

Hepatic encephalopathy, *uremia*, and *hypergastrinemia* also can be associated with gastric stasis.[11] Although elevated gastrin increases the frequency of the pacemaker slow-wave cycle and induces contractions in the distal stomach, gastric emptying is delayed.[66–68]

A considerable number of *drugs*, including anticholinergics, beta-adrenergic agonists, opiate analgesics, enkephalins, and L-dopa, delay gastric emptying.[1,3,11] Prolonged use of *anticholinergic agents* results in severe gastric atony and causes an iatrogenic gastric emptying disorder accompanied by persistent vomiting.[3] The means by which other drugs delay gastric emptying have been hypothesized. Circulating beta-endorphin may mediate the inhibitory effect of stress on gastric motility.[69] The delay in gastric emptying caused by enkephalin may be the result of interaction with central dopaminergic D_2-receptors.[70] Dopamine is an inhibitory neurotransmitter involved in gastric relaxation.[1] Lastly, levodopa is thought to inhibit gastric emptying by stimulating dopamine receptors in the stomach.[11] Caution should be exercised in the administration of these drugs, as delayed gastric emptying might be more detrimental than other beneficial effects.

In addition to gastric surgery, other *abdominal surgeries* in human patients produce gastric atony that can persist for three to five days postoperatively. In dogs, intestinal myoelectrical activity is disrupted for at least two days after laparotomy.[71] Inhibition of myoelectrical activity can be prevented by splanchnicectomy in dogs as well as in humans, suggesting that peripheral reflex pathways control

---

Gastric Motility Disorders with Accelerated Transit

- After gastric surgery–dumping syndrome
    Gastroenterostomy
    Partial gastrectomy
    Proximal gastric vagotomy
    Vagotomy with pyloroplasty
    Vagotomy with antrectomy
- * Exocrine pancreatic insufficiency[11,82,83]
- * Hyperthyroidism[1,84,85]
- * Zollinger-Ellison syndrome[11]
- * Duodenal ulcer disease[11,86]
- * Obesity[1,87]
- Drugs
    Metoclopramide
    Cisapride
    Bethanechol
    Domperidone
    Loperamide

---

* Reported only in human patients.

---

the period of inhibition.[72] Activation of neural reflexes is thought to cause an increase in norepinephrine release by sympathetic neurons in the gastric wall.[51] Delayed gastric emptying of both solids and liquids and loss of fasting-state contractions are transient postoperative problems in human patients. In contrast, postoperative gastric atony is not a significant clinical problem after canine abdominal surgery.

Radiation-induced emesis is associated with suppressed slow-wave frequency and delayed gastric emptying. Increased beta-endorphin release by the pituitary may mediate these transient effects.[73,74]

Gastric Motility Disorders with Accelerated Transit

Disorders of rapid gastric emptying are often iatrogenic.[7] Some dogs experience a postprandial *dumping syndrome* similar to human patients after a gastroenterostomy, partial gastrectomy, proximal gastric vagotomy, or vagotomy with pyloroplasty or antrectomy.[11,51,53,54,75] Patients with dumping syndrome have an increased initial emptying rate for liquids, and some also may have a rapid gastric emptying rate for solids.[79] Human patients with dumping syndrome experience early postprandial vasomotor and cardiovascular symptoms; later symptoms of nausea, vomiting, and diarrhea; and late vasomotor symptoms characteristic of hypoglycemia.[80]

Patients with *pancreatic exocrine insufficiency* theoretically should have increased gastric emptying rates.[11] Fatty acids, by interacting with inhibitory receptors in the small intestine, stimulate the release of cholecystokinin, which in

Gastric Motility Disorders with Retrograde Transit

- Vomiting
- Gastroesophageal reflux
- Duodenogastric reflux
    Bilious vomiting syndrome

turn inhibits proximal gastric contractions and slows gastric emptying.[81] Fatty acids produce more negative feedback on gastric emptying than do undigested fats. The increase in undigested fats associated with pancreatic exocrine insufficiency should therefore increase the gastric emptying rate. Documentation of accelerated transit in human patients with pancreatic exocrine insufficiency, however, remains controversial.[82,83]

Hyperthyroidism is associated with increased gastric myoelectrical activity in human patients.[1] Contrary to what would be expected, however, gastric emptying rates for liquids and solids appear to be normal in hyperthyroid patients.[84,85]

Gastric Motility Disorders with Retrograde Transit

Based on the extent of gastrointestinal tract involved, *vomiting* represents the extreme form of retrograde transit. The gastric motor correlates of vomiting consist of a retrograde peristaltic contraction, which begins in the jejunum; a period in which contractile activity is inhibited; and then a series of phasic contractions.[88] No temporal relationship between the gastric antral contractions and the expulsion of gastric contents exists; therefore, the gastric motor correlates of vomiting are independent of the somatomotor responses. The propulsive forces for expulsion are more likely provided by contractions of the respiratory and/or abdominal muscles. The gastric motor responses can occur without initiating vomiting.[88] If the motility changes are blocked, for example, by domperidone, expulsion fails to occur.[89] This suggests that the parts of the vomiting center controlling gastrointestinal motor responses and somatomotor responses are independent but sequentially activated.[88]

The relationship between delayed gastric emptying and *gastroesophageal reflux* is controversial. A decrease in resting lower esophageal sphincter pressure is considered by some investigators to be the primary factor in the pathogenesis of gastroesophageal reflux.[90,91] Delayed gastric emptying, which may contribute to the symptoms of gastroesophageal reflux, is considered a secondary factor. Abnormalities in liquid and/or solid food emptying, however, and in antral contractility have been observed in patients with gastroesophageal reflux.[11] It is unknown whether delayed gastric emptying precedes gastroesophageal reflux or whether periesophageal inflammation from reflux esopha-

gitis interferes with vagal nerve function and inhibits gastric emptying[92]; therefore, whether delayed gastric emptying associated with gastroesophageal reflux is a primary or a secondary factor remains to be determined.[11,92-94]

Duodenogastric reflux is a normal physiologic event.[95-97] Surgical destruction of the pylorus does not increase duodenogastric reflux in the fasting state, nor does it change the intermittent pattern of reflux.[96] In the postprandial state, however, duodenogastric reflux is increased after pyloroplasty or pylorectomy.[54,96] While acute exposure of the gastric mucosa to bile acids, bile salts, and lysolecithin can damage the gastric mucosal barrier, chronic or repeated exposure appears to have a protective effect.[95,98] No direct evidence for bile reflux as a cause of gastritis or delayed gastric emptying has been presented.[95]

Bilious vomiting syndrome in dogs is an idiopathic disorder associated with duodenogastric reflux of bile.[5] The signs include vomiting of bile early in the morning when the stomach is empty. The dog usually is normal the remainder of the day. Duodenogastric reflux may be an epiphenomenon associated with an undetermined gastric motility disorder, or it may occur secondary to chronic gastritis. Definitive diagnosis is made by symptomatic response to therapy, which includes feeding an additional meal late in the evening. Oral metoclopramide is given at the same time.

DISORDERS OF GASTRIC MOTILITY CONTROL MECHANISMS

The inherent properties of gastric smooth muscle cells and their modification by neurohumoral input ultimately control gastric motility.[99] Disorders of these control mechanisms do not constitute disease entities but may provide the mechanisms by which various disease processes produce similar symptoms of nausea, vomiting, and altered motility.[38,100,101]

Smooth muscle cells in the distal stomach have slow fluctuations in membrane potential. Extracellular recordings from the gastric serosal surface show that these intracellular changes in membrane potential produce the gastric slow waves. The dominant slow waves originate from a group of cells located in the mid-stomach along the greater curvature, called the *gastric pacemaker*. These smooth muscle cells have the highest rate of spontaneous depolarization, and their slow waves propagate distally (approximately five per minute) through the longitudinal muscle layer to the pylorus. Action potentials, which only occur during a specific phase of the slow-wave cycle, are associated with contractions. A cyclically recurring series of electrical events, called the *migrating motility complex*, occurs during the fasting state.[102] This cycle, which repeats every 90 to 120 minutes in dogs, is composed of three phases followed by a transition from Phase 3 back to Phase 1 again (Figure 1).

Disorders Affecting the Fasting State

Abnormalities of the slow-wave rhythm usually occur during the fasting state in Phase 1 and are caused by an

Disorders of Gastric Motility Control Mechanisms Associated with the Fasting State

- Slow-wave dysrhythmias
  Tachygastria
  Bradygastria
  Arrhythmias
    Atropine[105,113]
    Catecholamines[111,112]
    Met-enkephalin[116]
    Glucagon[114,115]
    Prostaglandin E$_2$[104,116]
    After abdominal surgery[105,117,118]
- Increased action potentials
  Cholinergic agonists[112,119]
  Metoclopramide[124]
- Decreased action potentials
  Sympathomimetic agents[119]
  Atropine[119]
- Absence of Phase 3
  * Diabetic gastroneuropathy[38,125]
  * Truncal vagotomy[38]
  * Partial gastric resection[38]
  * Idiopathic gastroparesis[38,126]
  * Bezoars[38]
- Decreased occurrence or disruption of Phase 3
  Gastric ulcers[38,127]
  †Halothane anesthesia[128]
- Retrograde propagation of Phase 3-like activity
    * Nauseating central nervous system stimulation[38]

* Reported only in human patients.
†Reported in rats.

compensatory pause before the normal slow-wave rhythm reappears (Figures 2 and 3). Collectively, these abnormalities are called *dysrhythmias*.

TACHYGASTRIA is caused by an abnormal pacemaker in the antrum.[103] The antrum appears to be more excitable and capable of producing slow waves of higher frequency than the corpus.[107] In addition, the duration of the absolute refractory period is less in the antrum than in the corpus.[108] In vitro studies of gastric smooth muscle have shown that tachygastria is associated with minimal or absent plateau potentials.[109] Because the strength of contraction is related to the size of the plateau potential,[110] tachygastria can be associated with weak or absent contractions and cause gastric retention.

Antral arrhythmias with frequencies of three slow waves per minute or less are called *bradygastria*.[105] Bradygastria usually is detected simultaneously in the corpus and antrum, and slow waves spread aborad.[104] It has been hypothesized that bradygastria represents a selective dysfunction of the corporal pacemaker. A decreasing gradient is known to exist in the intrinsic ability for smooth muscle cells to generate slow waves from mid-corpus to distal antrum.[104] Dysfunction of the normal pacemaker could therefore result in the appearance of a slower more distal pacemaker.

Antral arrhythmias have been observed in healthy dogs.[103-105] In one study, antral arrhythmias occurred during Phase 1 in approximately 50% of dogs considered to be normal when observed over three fasting myoelectric cycles.[105] Similar types of arrhythmias have been induced pharmacologically by such agents as epinephrine,[111,112] levarterenol,[111] atropine,[105,113] glucagon,[114,115] met-enkephalin,[116] and prostaglandin E$_2$.[104,116] Antral arrhythmias also have been reported after surgery[105,117,118] and are associated with disease.[109]

Atropine induces arrhythmias during Phase 1 in approximately 60% of treated dogs.[105] It has been hypothesized that arrhythmias produced after intravenous injections of catecholamines and atropine resulted from a sympathetic dominance or relative absence of acetylcholine on smooth muscle cell receptors.[113] A decrease in the absolute refractory period of antral smooth muscle cells may be responsible for dysrhythmias occurring under sympathetic dominance during Phase 1.[105]

Because the dysrhythmias induced by epinephrine and met-enkephalin are blocked by pretreatment with indomethacin, activation of a prostaglandin-mediated mechanism may occur after alpha-adrenergic and opiate receptors have been activated by their respective agonist drugs.[116] Endogenous prostaglandins increase the frequency of antral slow waves, decrease the amplitude of contractions, and decrease the ability of smooth muscle to respond to excitatory stimuli.[120-122]

Glucagon causes gastric dysrhythmias by a mechanism unrelated to prostaglandin synthesis. Possibly via its effects on the central nervous system, glucagon decreases the

ectopic pacemaker producing extradepolarizations in the antrum.[38,103,104] These premature depolarizations can propagate in both oral and aboral directions.[103-105] If they are accompanied by action potentials, they can produce retrograde contractions. Ingestion of food usually results in reappearance of the normal rhythm.[103] If these arrhythmias were to override the normal slow-wave pacemaker, however, and were not abolished with food, delayed gastric emptying could occur.[105]

Extradepolarizations can be single or occur in runs. If a run persists for a minute or more and is regular, it is called *tachygastria* (≥ 6 slow waves per minute).[105] If the run is made up of a burst of slow waves separated by irregular intervals, it is called an *arrhythmia*.[38,103] These bursts, which can be coupled, tripled, quadrupled, or occur as irregular groups of slow waves, are often followed by a

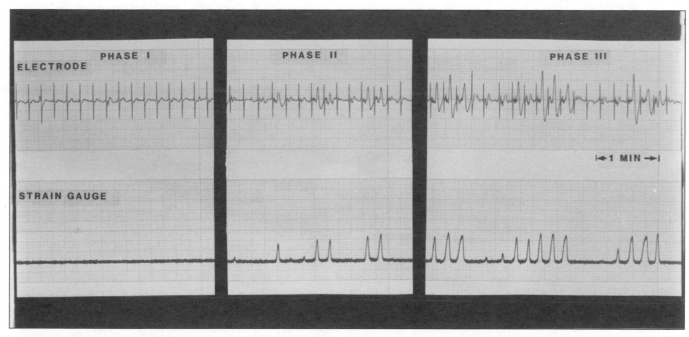

Figure 1—Correlation between normal extracellular myoelectric activity (*top tracings*) and contractile activity (*bottom tracings*) of the canine gastric antrum in the fasting state. The electromechanical activity, called the migrating motility complex, is cyclic and composed of three phases: Phase 1 is characterized by quiescent contractile activity, Phase 2 by increasing but irregular contractile activity, and Phase 3 by intense contractile activity. Phase 3 is associated with antropyloric relaxation, which allows large indigestible particles to empty.

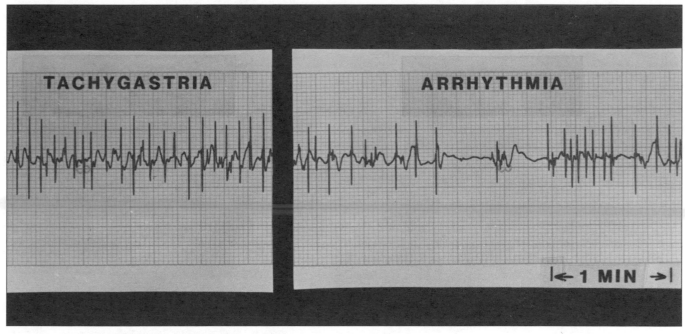

Figure 2—Examples of gastric slow-wave dysrhythmias observed in a dog following surgical treatment (circumcostal gastropexy) and recovery from gastric dilatation-volvulus.

slow-wave frequency and inhibits mechanical activity in dogs, both in the fasting and in the fed states.[115] Anesthesia completely abolishes these effects[115]; therefore, no single unifying mechanism exists for production of gastric dysrhythmias.[116]

In dogs, gastric contractions disappear with gastric dys- rhythmias and remain absent for as long as the dysrhyth- mia persists.[116] Whether this is of functional significance remains to be determined; however, associations between gastric dysrhythmias and motility disorders are being made. Disorders in gastric electrophysiology have been de- scribed in humans with unexplained nausea, vomiting, and

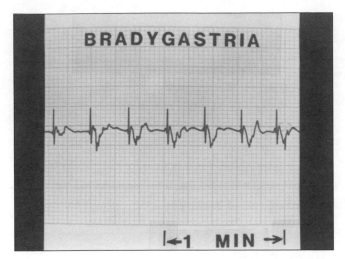

Figure 3—Example of a bradygastric slow-wave dysrhythmia observed in a dog following experimentally induced acute gastric dilatation.

bloating.[100,101] Hypothyroid dogs have gastric slow waves of lower frequency as well as fewer action potentials and less contractile activity after stimulation by pentagastrin, bethanechol, or food.[62] Gastric dilatation-volvulus may be associated with abnormal gastric myoelectrical activity[123] (Figure 2).

Disorders Affecting the Fed State

The disruption of migrating motility complex cycling after a meal may be attributable to neural excitation or to the release of endogenous factors, or both.[129] Although no specific hormone is conclusively implicated, gastrin, cholecystokinin, insulin, pancreatic polypeptide, and secretin increase after a meal and, if administered exogenously, disrupt the migrating motility complex.[129] Persistence of the fasting pattern of gastric motility after a meal has been noted in human patients with unexplained dyspepsia.[38] In humans,[130] as well as dogs,[29] the duration for which the fasting state myoelectrical activity is disrupted after a meal varies widely between individuals.

Antral arrhythmias have been observed in the fed state in dogs after Heineke-Mikulicz pyloroplasty[118] and after surgical removal of the duodenal cap.[105] In the latter procedure, gastric emptying was normal despite abnormalities in myoelectric activity. Altered gastric emptying has been found in association with dysrhythmias in certain human disease states,[109] however, and when antral slow waves were propagated in the reverse direction.[106]

TREATMENT OF DISORDERS OF GASTRIC MOTILITY

Delayed gastric emptying can be a significant clinical problem if an underlying cause cannot be determined; or if determined to be present, the condition cannot be appreciably resolved. Dietary management and drugs that increase gastric emptying time are used to treat delayed gastric emptying disorders, as surgical procedures usually are un-

successful.[7] With surgery, gastroparesis may be supplanted by further motility disturbances. Remedial surgery therefore should be attempted only after dietary and pharmacologic treatments have been exhausted.[11]

Dietary management is attempted initially. Small amounts of a semi-liquid, low-protein, and low-fat diet should be fed at frequent intervals. These recommendations are based on knowledge that liquids are expelled from the stomach faster than solids, carbohydrates faster than protein, and protein faster than fats. Examples of prepared diets would include the canned Prescription Diets® i/d® and d/d® (Hill's Pet Products) blended with water. An equal volume of plain cooked spaghetti noodles, cooked macaroni, or boiled rice is added to these diets.[45] Homemade liquid and carbohydrate-dense diets also are suitable.

Drug therapy has been used successfully in some dogs with delayed gastric emptying. Drugs that increase gastric emptying rate do so by stimulation of postsynaptic muscarinic receptors or by inhibition of peripheral dopaminergic receptors.[132] The effects of acetylcholine on muscarinic receptors are enhanced by cholinesterase inhibition with neostigmine, by muscarinic stimulation with bethanechol, and by facilitation of acetylcholine release with cisapride. Metoclopramide has cholinergic-like properties attributed to facilitation of acetylcholine release or to sensitization of gastric smooth muscle to acetylcholine.[133–136] Dopamine receptor antagonists include domperidone and metoclopramide.

ALTHOUGH several classes of drugs appear promising based on their mechanism of action, side effects (e.g., those associated with neostigmine and its analogues)[132] limit their usefulness. *Bethanechol* stimulates gastric motor activ-

---

Disorders of Gastric Motility Control Mechanisms Associated with the Fed State

- Persistence of fasting pattern after a meal
  - * Unexplained dyspepsia[38]
- Slow-wave dysrhythmias
  - After gastric surgery
- Increased action potentials
  - Domperidone[131]
  - Cholinergic agonists[119]
- Decreased action potentials
  - Hypothyroidism[62]
- Inadequate receptive relaxation
  - * Vagotomy[38]
  - * Lesions of the extrinsic nerves[38]

---

* Reported only in human patients.

ity and reportedly has similar but less severe side effects than neostigmine.[132,136] *Cisapride* enhances antral and duodenal contractions and improves gastroduodenal coordination. Although cisapride is not available at this time, its clinical usefulness appears promising because its activity is restricted to the myenteric nerves, thus avoiding other muscarinic side effects.[132,137]

Because *domperidone* does not easily cross the blood–brain barrier, its antidopaminergic actions are restricted to the periphery.[11] Domperidone accelerates gastric emptying, increases gastric antral contractions, and prevents the abnormal myoelectrical activity associated with retching and/or vomiting.[89,138] Domperidone modifies the gastric myoelectrical pattern to facilitate motility by increasing the frequency of gastric action potentials and by decreasing the slow-wave frequency to a rate similar to that noted with feeding.[139] The lack of extrapyramidal and cholinergic side effects make domperidone an attractive therapeutic alternative; however, dosages have not yet been established.

Metoclopramide has revolutionized the therapy of gastric retention in humans[11] and in dogs[3] because of both its prokinetic and its antiemetic effects. Currently, it is the drug of choice for treatment of delayed gastric emptying disorders. In addition to its central antiemetic action, metoclopramide increases the amplitude of antral contractions; inhibits fundic receptive relaxation; and coordinates gastric, pyloric, and duodenal motility, all of which result in accelerated gastric emptying.[140-143] Metoclopramide is used at a dose of 0.2 to 0.4 mg/kg body weight orally. It is given one-half hour before meals, three to four times a day.

The antiemetic effect of metoclopramide is attributed to its central antidopaminergic activity at the chemoreceptor trigger zone for vomiting.[144] These central effects complement its peripheral effects on gastrointestinal smooth muscle. Peripherally, metoclopramide inhibits vomiting secondary to its effects on motility, most likely by preventing stasis and the retroperistalsis that precedes vomiting. The antiemetic dosage is 1.0 to 2.0 mg/kg body weight per 24 hours given as a continuous intravenous infusion.[145]

Little is known about treatment of hypermotility disorders. Rationally, agents that delay gastric emptying could be used as therapy for rapid gastric emptying disorders. Codeine and other opiates delay both solid and liquid emptying and can reduce symptoms of the dumping syndrome in human patients.[1] Most opiates act centrally to reduce gastric emptying[132]; however, the effects of exogenous opiates on stomach motility depend on the dose given and the predominant site of action of the particular opiate.[1] For example, *loperamide*, an opiate-like drug, acts peripherally to increase gastric emptying.[146]

The response to treatment is variable and depends on the underlying cause of the motility disorder. Failure of delayed gastric emptying to respond to medical management necessitates further investigation to find a mechanical obstruction to gastric emptying.

SUMMARY

The diagnostic approach and some of the major disor-

ders of gastric motility have been summarized in this review. Radiographic techniques, including such newer noninvasive techniques as radionuclide-labeled food markers and scintigraphy, have widespread clinical application for the diagnosis of disorders causing gastric retention and for the assessment of pharmacologic effects on gastric motility. Currently, radiographic contrast studies are the most useful of the diagnostic techniques. Because the mechanical activity of the stomach ultimately is linked to gastric slow waves, any disorder that disrupts the normal slow-wave activity has the potential to disrupt coordination of the mechanical activity. Dysrhythmias may therefore be fundamental in the pathophysiology of disorders affecting gastric motility.

About the Authors

When this article was submitted for publication, Dr. Hall was affiliated with the Department of Physiology, College of Veterinary Medicine and Biomedical Sciences, Colorado State University, Fort Collins, Colorado. She is currently affiliated with the College of Veterinary Medicine, Oregon State University, Corvallis, Oregon. Dr. Twedt is with the Department of Clinical Sciences, College of Veterinary Medicine and Biomedical Sciences, Colorado State University. Dr. Burrows is affiliated with the Department of Medical Sciences, College of Veterinary Medicine, University of Florida, Gainesville, Florida. All three authors are Diplomates of the American College of Veterinary Internal Medicine.

REFERENCES

1. Camilleri M, Malagelada JR: Gastric motility in disease, in Akkermans LMA, Johnson AG, Read NW (eds): *Gastric and Gastroduodenal Motility*. New York, Praeger, 1984, pp 201–232.
2. Twedt DC, Wingfield WW: Diseases of the stomach, in Ettinger SJ (ed): *Textbook of Veterinary Internal Medicine*, ed 2. Philadelphia, WB Saunders Co, 1983, pp 1233–1277.
3. Twedt DC: Disorders of gastric retention, in Kirk RW (ed): *Current Veterinary Therapy. VIII. Small Animal Practice*. Philadelphia, WB Saunders Co, 1983, pp 761–765.
4. Strombeck DR: Chronic gastritis, gastric retention, and gastric neoplasms, in Strombeck DR (ed): *Small Animal Gastroenterology*. Davis, CA, Stonegate Publishing, 1980, pp 110–124.
5. Twedt DC: Differential diagnosis and therapy of vomiting. *Vet Clin North Am [Small Anim Pract]* 13:503–520, 1983.
6. Heading RC: Methods in studying gastric function: Methods based on gastric intubation; x-ray and ultrasound imaging methods; indirect techniques, in Akkermans LMA, Johnson AG, Read NW (eds): *Gastric and Gastroduodenal Motility*. New York, Praeger, 1984, pp 131–147.
7. Horowitz M, Collins PJ, Shearman DJC: Disorders of gastric emptying in humans and the use of radionuclide techniques. *Arch Intern Med* 145:1467–1472, 1985.
8. Miyabayashi T, Morgan JP: Gastric emptying in the normal dog. A contrast radiographic technique. *Vet Radiol* 25:187–191, 1984.
9. Burns J, Fox SM: The use of a barium meal to evaluate total gastric emptying time in the dog. *Vet Radiol* 27:169–172, 1986.
10. Sheiner HJ: Gastric-emptying tests in man. *Gut* 16:235–247, 1975.
11. Minami H, McCallum W: The physiology and pathophysiology of gastric emptying in humans. *Gastroenterology* 86:1592–1610, 1984.
12. Russell J, Bass P: Canine gastric emptying of polycarbophil: An indigestible, particulate substance. *Gastroenterology* 89:307–312, 1985.
13. Bartelsman JFWM: Current techniques in the evaluation of motility disorders. *Scand J Gastroenterol* 19:5–10, 1984.
14. Read NW, Al Janabi MN, Bates TE, et al: Effect of gastrointestinal

intubation on the passage of a solid meal through the stomach and small intestine in humans. *Gastroenterology* 84:1568–1572, 1983.

15. Meyer JH, MacGregor IL, Gueller R, et al: 99mTc-tagged chicken liver as a marker of solid food in the human stomach. *Am J Dig Dis* 21:296–304, 1976.
16. Seide K, Ritman EL: Three-dimensional dynamic x-ray-computed tomography imaging of stomach motility. *Am J Physiol* 247:G574–G581, 1984.
17. Holt S, McDicken WN, Anderson T, et al: Dynamic imaging of the stomach by realtime ultrasound: A method for the study of gastric motility. *Gut* 21:597–601, 1980.
18. Bateman DN, Whittingham TA: Measurement of gastric emptying by real-time ultrasound. *Gut* 23:524–527, 1982.
19. Bolondi L, Bortolotti M, Santi V, et al: Measurement of gastric emptying time by real-time ultrasonography. *Gastroenterology* 89:752–759, 1985.
20. Johnson AG: Non-invasive techniques in the study of gastrointestinal motility, in Wienbeck M (ed): *Motility of the Digestive Tract.* New York, Raven Press, 1982, pp 307–310.
21. Hinder RA, Kelly KA: Canine gastric emptying of solids and liquids. *Am J Physiol* 233(4):E335–E340, 1977.
22. Meyer JH, Dressman J, Fink A, et al: Effect of size and density on canine gastric emptying of nondigestible solids. *Gastroenterology* 89:805–813, 1985.
23. Weisbrodt NW, Wiley JN, Overholt BF, Bass P: A relation between gastroduodenal muscle contractions and gastric emptying. *Gut* 10:543–548, 1969.
24. Keinke O, Schemann M, Ehrlein HJ: Mechanical factors regulating gastric emptying of viscous nutrient meals in dogs. *Q J Exp Physiol* 69:781–795, 1984.
25. van den Brom WE, Happe RP: Gastric emptying of a radionuclide-labeled test meal in healthy dogs: A new mathematical analysis and reference values. *Am J Vet Res* 47:2170–2174, 1986.
26. Akkermans LMA, Jacobs F, Oei Hong-Yoe, et al: A non-invasive method to quantify antral contractile activity in man and dog, in Christensen J (ed): *Gastrointestinal Motility.* New York, Raven Press, 1980, pp 195–202.
27. Theodorakis MC: External scintigraphy in measuring rate of gastric emptying in beagles. *Am J Physiol* 239:G39–G43, 1980.
28. Vogel SB, Brock Vair D, Woodward ER: Alterations in gastrointestinal emptying of 99m-technetium-labeled solids following sequential antrectomy, truncal vagotomy and roux-y gastroenterostomy. *Ann Surg* 198:506–515, 1983.
29. Burrows CF, Bright RM, Spencer CP: Influence of dietary composition on gastric emptying and motility in dogs: Potential involvement in acute gastric dilatation. *Am J Vet Res* 12:2609–2612, 1985.
30. Happe RP, van der Gaag I: Endoscopic examination of esophagus, stomach, and duodenum in the dog. *JAAHA* 19:197–206, 1983.
31. Matthiesen DT, Walter MC: Surgical treatment of chronic hypertrophic pyloric gastropathy in 45 dogs. *JAAHA* 22:241–247, 1986.
32. Walter MC, Goldschmidt MH, Stone EA, et al: Chronic hypertrophic pyloric gastropathy as a cause of pyloric obstruction in the dog. *JAVMA* 186:157–161, 1985.
33. Sikes RI, Birchard S, Patnaik A, et al: Chronic hypertrophic pyloric gastropathy: A review of 16 cases. *JAAHA* 22:99–104, 1986.
34. MacEwen EG, Patnaik AK, Johnson GF, et al: Extramedullary plasmacytoma of the gastrointestinal tract in two dogs. *JAVMA* 184:1396–1398, 1984.
35. Miller RI: Gastrointestinal phycomycosis in 63 dogs. *JAVMA* 186:473–478, 1985.
36. Ader PJ: Phycomycosis in fifteen dogs and two cats. *JAVMA* 174:1216–1223, 1979.
37. Barsanti JA: Miscellaneous fungal infections, in Green CE (ed): *Clinical Microbiology and Infectious Diseases of the Dog and Cat.* Philadelphia, WB Saunders Co, 1984, pp 738–746.
38. Vantrappen G, Janssens J, Coremans G, et al: Gastrointestinal motility disorders. *Dig Dis Sci* 31:5S–25S, 1986.
39. Garret JM, Summerskill WHJ, Code CF: Antral motility in patients with gastric ulcer. *Am J Dig Dis* 11:780–789, 1966.
40. Miller LJ, Malagelada JR, Longstreth GF, et al: Dysfunctions of the stomach with gastric ulceration. *Dig Dis Sci* 25:857–864, 1980.
41. Fioramonti J, Bueno L: Gastrointestinal myoelectric activity disturbances in gastric ulcer disease in rats and dogs. *Dig Dis Sci* 25:575–580, 1980.
42. Sorour VE: The relationship between atrophic gastritis and gastric ulcer. *S Afr J Surg* 14:47–53, 1976.
43. Twedt DC: Gastric ulcers, in Kirk RW (ed): *Current Veterinary*

Therapy. VIII. Small Animal Practice. Philadelphia, WB Saunders Co, 1983, pp 765–770.
44. Twedt DC, Magne ML: Chronic gastritis, in Kirk RW (ed): *Current Veterinary Therapy. IX. Small Animal Practice.* Philadelphia, WB Saunders Co, 1986, pp 852–856.
45. Zimmer JF: Nutritional management of gastrointestinal diseases, in Kirk RW (ed): *Current Veterinary Therapy. IX. Small Animal Practice.* Philadelphia, WB Saunders Co, 1986, pp 909–916.
46. Meeroff JC, Schreiber DS, Trier JS, et al: Abnormal gastric motor function in viral gastroenteritis. *Ann Intern Med* 92:370–373, 1980.
47. Twedt DC: Disorders of gastric motility. *Proc ACVIM*:15–18, 1987.
48. Burrows CF: Infection with the stomach worm *Physaloptera* as a cause of chronic vomiting in the dog. *JAAHA* 19:947–950, 1983.
49. Burrows CF: Disorders of gastrointestinal motility: More common than you think. *Proc ACVIM*:573–575, 1988.
50. Alizadeh H, Castro GA, Weems WA: Intrinsic jejunal propulsion in the guinea pig during parasitism with *Trichinella spiralis*. *Gastroenterology* 93:784–790, 1987.
51. Kelly KA: Effect of gastric surgery on gastric motility and emptying, in Akkermans LMA, Johnson AG, Read NW (eds): *Gastric and Gastroduodenal Motility.* New York, Praeger, 1984, pp 241–262.
52. Bedi BS, Kelly KA, Holley HE: Pathways of propagation of the canine gastric pacesetter potential. *Gastroenterology* 63:288–296, 1972.
53. Meyer JH, Thomson BS, Cohen MB, et al: Sieving of solid food by the canine stomach and sieving after gastric surgery. *Gastroenterology* 76:804–813, 1979.
54. Muller-Lissner SA, Sonnenberg A, Schattenmann G, et al: Gastric emptying and postprandial duodenogastric reflux in pylorectomized dogs. *Am J Physiol* 242:G9–G14, 1982.
55. Szurszewski JH: Electrical basis for gastrointestinal motility, in Johnson LR (ed): *Physiology of the Gastrointestinal Tract.* New York, Raven Press, 1981, pp 1435–1466.
56. Strombeck DR: The pancreas, in Strombeck DR (ed): *Small Animal Gastroenterology.* Davis, CA, Stonegate Publishing, 1979, pp 301–331.
57. Weiner M, Epstein FH: Signs and symptoms of electrolyte disorders. *Yale J Biol Med* 43:76–109, 1970.
58. Burrows CF: Reversible mega-oesophagus in a dog with hypoadrenocorticism. *J Small Anim Pract* 28:1073–1078, 1987.
59. Mearin F, Camilleri M, Malagelada JR: Pyloric dysfunction in diabetics with recurrent nausea and vomiting. *Gastroenterology* 90:1919–1925, 1986.
60. Malagelada JR, Rees WDW, Mazzotta LG, et al: Gastric motor abnormalities in diabetic and postvagotomy gastroparesis: Effect of metoclopramide and bethanechol. *Gastroenterology* 78:286–293, 1980.
61. Schulze-Delrieu K, Lipsien G: Depression of mechanical and electrical activity in muscle strips of opossum stomach and esophagus by acidosis. *Gastroenterology* 82:720–725, 1982.
62. Kowalewski K, Kolodej A: Myoelectrical and mechanical activity of stomach and intestine in hypothyroid dogs. *Am J Dig Dis* 22:235–240, 1977.
63. Willard MD, Schall WD, McCaw DE, Nachreiner RF: Canine hypoadrenocorticism: Report of 37 cases and review of 39 previously reported cases. *JAVMA* 180:59–62, 1982.
64. Bueno L, Fioramonti J: Effects of corticotropin-releasing factor, corticotropin and cortisol on gastrointestinal motility in dogs. *Peptides* 7:73–77, 1986.
65. Bueno L, Fargeas MJ, Gue M, et al: Effects of corticotropin-releasing factor on plasma motilin and somatostatin levels and gastrointestinal motility in dogs. *Gastroenterology* 91:884–889, 1986.
66. Morgan KG, Schmalz PF, Go VLW, et al: Effect of pentagastrin, G17, and G34 on the electrical and mechanical activities of canine antral smooth muscle. *Gastroenterology* 75:304–412, 1978.
67. Cooke AR, Chvasta TE, Weisbrodt NW: Effect of pentagastrin on emptying and electrical and motor activity of the dog stomach. *Am J Physiol* 223:934–938, 1972.
68. Dozois RR, Kelly KA: Effect of a gastrin pentapeptide on canine gastric emptying of liquids. *Am J Physiol* 221:113–117, 1971.
69. Rees MR, Clark RA, Holdsworth CD: The effect of beta-adrenoreceptor agonists and antagonists on gastric emptying in man. *Br J Clin Pharmacol* 10:551–554, 1980.
70. Sullivan SN, Lamki L, Corcoran P: Inhibition of gastric emptying by enkephalin analogue (letter). *Lancet* 2:86–87, 1981.

71. Morris IR, Darby CF, Hammond P, et al: Changes in small bowel myoelectrical activity following laparotomy. *Br J Surg* 70:547-548, 1983.

72. Bueno L, Fioramonti J, Ruckebusch Y: Postoperative intestinal motility in dogs and sheep. *Am J Dig Dis* 23:682-689, 1978.

73. Dubois A, Jacobus JP, Grissom MP, et al: Altered gastric emptying and prevention of radiation-induced vomiting in dogs. *Gastroenterology* 86:444-448, 1984.

74. Dorval ED, Mueller GP, Eng RR, et al: Effect of ionizing radiation on gastric secretion and gastric motility in monkeys. *Gastroenterology* 89:374-380, 1985.

75. Hinder RA, San-Garde BA: Individual and combined roles of the pylorus and the antrum in the canine gastric emptying of a liquid and a digestible solid. *Gastroenterology* 84:281-286, 1983.

76. Wood JR, Camilleri M, Low PA, et al: Brainstem tumor presenting as an upper gut motility disorder. *Gastroenterology* 89:1411-1414, 1985.

77. Levine RA, Schwartz SE, Singh A: Chronic pectin ingestion delays gastric emptying, in Wienbeck M (ed): *Motility of the Digestive Tract.* New York, Raven Press, 1982, p 379.

78. Leeds AR, Ralphs DNL, Ebied F, et al: Pectin in the dumping syndrome: Reduction of symptoms and plasma volume changes. *Lancet* 1:1075-1078, 1981.

79. MacGregor IL, Martin P, Meyer JH: Gastric emptying of solid food in normal man and after subtotal gastrectomy and truncal vagotomy with pyloroplasty. *Gastroenterology* 72:206-211, 1977.

80. Becker HD: Dumping syndrome and hormones, in Akkermans LMA, Johnson AG, Read NW (eds): *Gastric and Gastroduodenal Motility.* New York, Praeger, 1984, pp 263-281.

81. Kelly KA: Motility of the stomach and gastroduodenal junction, in Johnson LR (ed): *Physiology of the Gastrointestinal Tract.* New York, Raven Press, 1981, pp 393-410.

82. Regan PT, Malagelada JR, Dimagno EP, et al: Postprandial gastric function in pancreatic insufficiency. *Gut* 20:249-254, 1979.

83. Long WB, Weiss JB: Rapid gastric emptying of fatty meals in pancreatic insufficiency. *Gastroenterology* 67:920-925, 1974.

84. Wiley ZD, Lavigne ME, Liu KM, et al: The effect of hyperthyroidism on gastric emptying rates and pancreatic exocrine and biliary secretion in man. *Am J Dig Dis* 23:1003-1008, 1978.

85. Miller LJ, Owyang C, Malagelada JR, et al: Gastric, pancreatic, and biliary responses to meals in hyperthyroidism. *Gut* 21:695-700, 1980.

86. Lam SK, Isenberg JI, Grossman MI, et al: Rapid gastric emptying in duodenal ulcer patients. *Dig Dis Sci* 27:598-604, 1982.

87. Dubois A: Obesity and gastric emptying (editorial). *Gastroenterology* 84:875-876, 1983.

88. Lang IM, Sarna SK, Condon RE: Gastrointestinal motor correlates of vomiting in the dog: Quantification and characterization as an independent phenomenon. *Gastroenterology* 90:40-47, 1986.

89. Lee KY, Park HJ, Chey WY: Studies on mechanism of retching and vomiting in dogs: Effect of peripheral dopamine blocker on myoelectric changes in antrum and upper small intestine. *Dig Dis Sci* 30:22-28, 1985.

90. Behar J: The role of the lower esophageal sphincter in reflux prevention. *J Clin Gastroenterol* 8:2-4, 1986.

91. Cohen S, Merio A: Gastroesophageal reflux: Evaluation and current treatment. *Postgrad Med* 81:203-218, 1987.

92. Skinner DB: Pathophysiology of gastroesophageal reflux. *Ann Surg* 202:546-556, 1985.

93. Richter JE, Castell DO: Gastroesophageal reflux: Pathogenesis, diagnosis, and therapy. *Ann Intern Med* 97:93-103, 1982.

94. Navab F, Texter C: Gastroesophageal reflux: Pathophysiologic concepts. *Arch Intern Med* 145:329-333, 1985.

95. Muller-Lissner SA, Fimmel CJ, Blum AL: Is there a relationship between duodenogastric reflux, gastric ulcer and gastritis? in Akkermans LMA, Johnson AG, Read NW (eds): *Gastric and Gastroduodenal Motility.* New York, Praeger, 1984, pp 282-291.

96. Muller-Lissner SA, Schattenmann G, Schenker G, et al: Duodenogastric reflux in the fasting dog: Role of pylorus and duodenal motility. *Am J Physiol* 241:G159-G162, 1981.

97. Sonnenberg A, Muller-Lissner SA: Duodenogastric reflux in the dog. *Am J Physiol* 242:G603-G607, 1982.

98. Chaudhury TK, Robert A: Prevention by mild irritants of gastric necrosis produced in rats by sodium taurocholate. *Dig Dis Sci* 25:830-836, 1980.

99. Weisbrodt NW: Basic control mechanisms, in Akkermans LMA, Johnson AG, Read NW (eds): *Gastric and Gastroduodenal Motility.* New York, Praeger, 1984, pp 3-20.

100. You CH, Lee KY, Chey WY, et al: Electrogastrographic study of patients with unexplained nausea, bloating and vomiting. *Gastroenterology* 79:311-314, 1980.

101. Hanson JS, McCallum RW: The diagnosis and management of nausea and vomiting: A review. *Am J Gastroenterol* 80:210-218, 1985.

102. Code CF, Marlett JA: The interdigestive myoelectric complex of the stomach and small bowel of dogs. *J Physiol* (London) 246:289-309, 1975.

103. Code CF, Marlett JA: Modern medical physiology: Canine tachygastria. *Mayo Clin Proc* 49:325-332, 1974.

104. Kim CH, Azpiroz F, Malagelada JR: Characteristics of spontaneous and drug-induced gastric dysrhythmias in a chronic canine model. *Gastroenterology* 90:421-427, 1986.

105. Gullikson GW, Okuda H, Shimizu M, et al: Electrical arrhythmias in gastric antrum of the dog. *Am J Physiol* 239:G59-G68, 1980.

106. Sarna SK, Bowes KL, Daniel EE: Gastric pacemakers. *Gastroenterology* 70:225-231, 1976.

107. Kelly KA, La Force RC: Pacing the canine stomach with electric stimulation. *Am J Physiol* 222:588-594, 1972.

108. Sarna SK, Daniel EE: Threshold curves and refractoriness properties of gastric relaxation oscillators. *Am J Physiol* 226:749-755, 1974.

109. Telander RL, Morgan KG, Kreulen DL, et al: Human gastric atony with tachygastria and gastric retention. *Gastroenterology* 75:497-501, 1978.

110. Szurszewski JH: Mechanism of action of pentagastrin and acetylcholine on the longitudinal muscle of the canine antrum. *J Physiol* 252:335-361, 1975.

111. McCoy EJ, Bass P: Chronic electrical activity of gastroduodenal area: Effects of food and certain catecholamines. *Am J Physiol* 205:439-445, 1963.

112. You CH, Chey WY: Study of electromechanical activity of the stomach in humans and in dogs with particular attention to tachygastria. *Gastroenterology* 86:1460-1468, 1984.

113. Daniel EE: Electrical and contractile responses of the pyloric region to adrenergic and cholinergic drugs. *Can J Physiol Pharmacol* 44:951-979, 1966.

114. Abell T, Tucker R, Malagelada JR: Glucagon-evoked gastric dysrhythmias in healthy humans demonstrated by an improved electrogastrographic method. *Gastroenterology* 88:1932-1940, 1985.

115. Watanabe O, Atobe Y, Akagi M, et al: Effects of glucagon on myoelectrical activity of the stomach of conscious and anesthetized dogs. *Eur J Pharmacol* 79:31-41, 1982.

116. Kim CH, Zinsmeister AR, Malagelada JR: Mechanisms of canine gastric dysrhythmia. *Gastroenterology* 92:993-999, 1987.

117. Dauchel J, Schang JC, Kachelhoffer J, et al: Gastrointestinal myoelectrical activity during the postoperative period in man. *Digestion* 14:294-303, 1976.

118. Ormsbee HS, III, Mason GR, Bass P: Effects of pyloroplasty on the electrical activity of the canine gastroduodenal junction, in Vantrappen G (ed): *Proceedings of the Fifth International Symposium on Gastrointestinal Motility.* Herentals, Belgium, Typoff, 1975, pp 293-299.

119. Daniel EE: The electrical and contractile activity of the pyloric region in dogs and the effects of drugs. *Gastroenterology* 40:403-418, 1965.

120. Sanders KM: Role of prostaglandins in regulating gastric motility. *Am J Physiol* 247:G17-G126, 1984.

121. Kowalewski K, Kolodej A: Effect of prostaglandin E$_2$ on myoelectrical and mechanical activity of totally isolated, ex vivo perfused, canine stomach. *Pharmacology* 13:325-339, 1975.

122. Sanders KM, Szurszewski JH: Does endogenous prostaglandin affect gastric antral motility? *Am J Physiol* 241:G191-G195, 1981.

123. Burrows CF, Stampley A, Ellison G: Gastric myoelectrical activity in experimental canine gastric dilatation volvulus. *Proc 67th Annu Meet Conf Res Anim Dis*:A293, 1986.

124. Wingate D, Pearce E, Hutton M, et al: Effect of metoclopramide on interdigestive myoelectric activity in the conscious dog. *Dig Dis Sci* 25:15-21, 1980.

125. Achem-Karam SR, Funakoshi A, Vinik AI, et al: Plasma motilin concentration and interdigestive migrating motor complex in diabetic gastroparesis: Effect of metoclopramide. *Gastroenterology* 88:492-499, 1985.

126. Labo G, Bortolotti M, Vezzadini P, et al: Interdigestive gastroduodenal motility and serum motilin levels in patients with idiopathic delay in gastric emptying. *Gastroenterology* 90:20–26, 1986.

127. Fioramonti J, Bueno L: Gastrointestinal myoelectric activity disturbances in gastric ulcer disease in rats and dogs. *Dig Dis Sci* 25:575–580, 1980.

128. Wright JW, Healy TEJ, Balfour TW, et al: Effects of inhalation anaesthetic agents on the electrical and mechanical activity of the rat duodenum. *Br J Anaesth* 54:1223–1229, 1982.

129. Sarna SK: Cyclic motor activity, migrating motor complex: 1985. *Gastroenterology* 89:894–913, 1985.

130. Kellow JE, Borody TJ, Phillips SF, et al: Human interdigestive motility: Variations in patterns from esophagus to colon. *Gastroenterology* 91:386–395, 1986.

131. Hinder RA, San-Garde BA: Gastroduodenal motility—A comparison between domperidone and metoclopramide. *S Afr Med J* 63:270–273, 1983.

132. Lake-Bakaar G, Teblick M: Drugs and gut motility, in Akkermans LMA, Johnson AG, Read NW (eds): *Gastric and Gastroduodenal Motility*. New York, Praeger, 1984, pp 299–313.

133. Hay AM, Man WK: Effect of metoclopramide on guinea pig stomach: Critical dependence on intrinsic stores of acetylcholine. *Gastroenterology* 76:492–496, 1979.

134. Jacoby HI, Brodie DA: Gastrointestinal actions of metoclopramide: An experimental study. *Gastroenterology* 52:676–684, 1967.

135. Eisner M: Gastrointestinal effects of metoclopramide in man: In vitro experiments with human smooth muscle preparations. *Br Med J* 4:679–680, 1968.

136. You CH, Chey WY: Study of electromechanical activity of the stomach in humans and in dogs with particular attention to tachygastria. *Gastroenterology* 86:1460–1468, 1984.

137. Schuurkes JAJ, Verlinden M, Akkermans LMA, et al: Stimulating effects of R 51 619 on antroduodenal motility in the conscious dog. *Gastroenterol Clin Biol* 7:704–706, 1983.

138. Broekart A: Effect of domperidone on gastric emptying and secretion. *Postgrad Med J* 55:11–14, 1979.

139. Hinder RA, San-Garde BA: Gastroduodenal motility—A comparison between domperidone and metoclopramide. *S Afr Med J* 63:270–273, 1983.

140. Pinder RM, Brogden RN, Sawyer PR, et al: Metoclopramide: A review of its pharmacological properties and clinical use. *Drugs* 12:81–131, 1976.

141. Johnson AG: The actions of metoclopramide on human gastroduodenal motility. *Gut* 12:421–426, 1971.

142. Eisner M: Effect of metoclopramide on gastrointestinal motility in man. *Am J Dig Dis* 16:409–419, 1971.

143. Valenzuela JE: Dopamine as a possible neurotransmitter in gastric relaxation. *Gastroenterology* 71:1019–1022, 1976.

144. McCallum RW, Albibi R: Metoclopramide: Pharmacology and clinical application. *Ann Intern Med* 98:86–95, 1983.

145. Burrows CF: Metoclopramide. *JAVMA* 183:1341–1343, 1983.

146. Cann PA, Read NW, Holdsworth CD: Loperamide improves dyspeptic symptoms and accelerates gastric emptying in patients with irritable bowel syndrome. *Gut* 25:A437, 1982.

UPDATE

In humans, cisapride has been used to treat gastrointestinal disorders, such as abdominal pain, dyspepsia, irritable bowel syndrome, and postoperative ileus.[1] For dogs, cisapride may be useful for treating gastrointestinal disorders, including delayed gastric emptying of meals and gastroesophageal reflux.

Cisapride—a benzamide—exerts its effect via facilitation of cholinergic neurotransmission.[2] It enhances both amplitude and coordination of antral, pyloric, and duodenal contractions. Gastric secretion is not affected. In one study, cisapride (0.16 to 1.25 mg/kg PO) accelerated the gastric emptying of a liquid and solid test meal in dogs that had been given oleic acid either intragastrically or intraduodenally to delay gastric emptying.[2] In another study, the solid and liquid phases of gastric emptying in dogs fed a standard canned food meal were measured using a double radiolabeled technique. In these dogs, cisapride (5 mg/kg PO) increased emptying of the solid and liquid phases by 41% and 73%, respectively, at one hour. Metoclopramide (1 mg/kg PO) and domperidone (5 mg/kg PO) increased emptying of the liquid phase one hour after eating by 106% and 59%, respectively, but did not modify that of the solid phase.[3]

In a third study,[1] cisapride was found to be eight times more potent as a gastric prokinetic agent than metoclopramide. At twenty times its gastrokinetic dose, cisapride was unable to antagonize apomorphine, the dopamine D_2-receptor agonist. With metoclopramide, antiemetic activity against apomorphine is present at a gastrokinetic dose. Thus, cisapride does not produce the unwanted side effects of other gastric prokinetic compounds, such as enhanced gastric secretion (expected after stimulation of muscarinic acetylcholine receptors with bethanechol), enhanced prolactin release (expected after blockade of peripheral dopamine receptors with metoclopramide), and extrapyramidal side effects (expected after blockade of central dopamine receptors with metoclopramide).[1]

Prokinetic drugs like cisapride clearly stimulate gastric and intestinal contractions in normal healthy dogs and humans. To demonstrate potential usefulness of prokinetic drugs in animals with gastrointestinal motility disorders, however, the prokinetic activity must correlate with improved gastric emptying. Of concern is whether or not an enhanced flow of nutrients into the small intestine may intensify the intestinal brake mechanism on gastric motility and emptying.[4] In normal dogs, the control mechanisms that regulate gastric emptying provide an optimal emptying rate that cannot be increased markedly by cisapride.[4] If the emptying rate is below its maximal capacity either in pathologic states, by a small volume of the meal, or toward the end of the emptying process, however, the motor-stimulating drugs may accelerate gastric emptying without interference by the normal control mechanisms.[4] Thus, it is necessary to induce gastroparesis pharmacologically in dogs to demonstrate clearly the effects of prokinetic benzamides on gastric emptying.

Cisapride at 0.1 mg/kg intravenously increases the gastric emptying rate in dogs not by increasing the number of antral contractions but by increasing the volume of flow at each pulse.[5] When administered intravenously, cisapride will reduce the transpyloric passage of liquid for five to seven minutes. This effect occurs when antral and pyloric motility are most vigorous, a finding indicative of increased antroduodenal resistance. Cisapride increases gastric emptying after 10 minutes because increased antroduodenal resistance is brief compared with the sustained increase in the amplitude of gastric contractions. Thus, when injected intravenously, cisapride initially inhibits gastric emptying of liquid in the conscious dog. During the first 10 minutes, the stroke volume of each pulse is reduced, probably as a consequence of a 1500% increase in antroduodenal resistance. Stroke volume increases as soon as resistance is reduced and while gastric motility is still enhanced.[5]

Although doses for cisapride in dogs and cats have not yet been established, one of the authors (DCT) has used cisapride in dogs at 2.5 to 10 mg every 8 hours PO and in cats at 2.5 to 5 mg every 8 hours PO. The dose is decreased if there are abnormal gastrointestinal signs or abdominal pain.

Nizatidine and ranitidine are two other agents with gastroprokinetic activity. Nizatidine—a new H_2-receptor antagonist—stimulates gastrointestinal contractions and accelerates gastric emptying at gastric antisecretory doses. These effects are thought to be caused by the drug's anti-acetylcholinesterase (anti-AChE) activity.[6] Ranitidine also inhibits AChE activity with a potency equal to that of nizatidine and facilitates gastrointestinal motor activity by stimulating cholinergic excitation through anti-AChE ac-

tivity.[7] Thus, in stimulating gastrointestinal motility, nizatidine and ranitidine may have efficacies not found with the other H_2-receptor antagonists.

REFERENCES

1. Megens AA, Awouters FH, Niemegeers CJ: General pharmacology of the four gastrointestinal motility stimulants bethanechol, metoclopramide, trimebutine, and cisapride. *Arzneimittelforschung* 41:631–634, 1991.
2. Schuurkes J: Effect of cisapride on gastric motility. *Z Gastroenterol* 28:27–30, 1990.
3. Gue M, Fioramonti J, Bueno L: A simple double radiolabeled technique to evaluate gastric emptying of canned food meal in dogs. Application to pharmacological tests. *Gastroenterol Clin Biol* 12:425–430, 1988.
4. Wulschke S, Ehrlein HJ, Tsiamitas C: The control mechanisms of gastric emptying are not overridden by motor stimulants. *Am J Physiol* 251:G744–G751, 1986.
5. Malbert CH, Serthelon JP, Dent J: Changes in antroduodenal resistance induced by cisapride in conscious dogs. *Am J Physiol* 263:G202–G208, 1992.
6. Ueki S, Seiki M, Yonita T, et al: Gastroprokinetic activity of nizatidine, a new H_2-receptor antagonist, and its possible mechanism of action in dogs and rats. *J Pharmacol Exp Ther* 264:152–157, 1993.
7. Mizumoto A, Fujimura M, Iwanaga Y, et al: Anticholinesterase activity of histamine H_2-receptor antagonists in the dog: Their possible role in gastric motor activity. *J Gastrointest Motility* 2:273–280, 1990.

KEY FACTS

- Ulceration of the upper gastrointestinal tract in small animals occurs secondary to liver disease, neurologic disease, uremia, tumors, or the administration of ulcerogenic drugs.
- Ulcers result from an imbalance between the acid-secreting mechanisms and the mucosal defense mechanisms.
- Vomiting and pain in the cranial abdomen are the most common clinical findings.
- Diagnosis is based on clinical findings, contrast radiography, and endoscopy.
- Treatment with antisecretory drugs, cytoprotective agents, and antacids is rewarding. In refractory cases or severe hemorrhage, surgery is indicated.

Ulcer Disease of the Upper Gastrointestinal Tract in Small Animals: Pathophysiology, Diagnosis, and Management

Karen J. Moreland, DVM*
Department of Small Animal
  Medicine and Surgery
College of Veterinary Medicine
Texas A&M University
College Station, Texas

Ulcer disease of the gastrointestinal tract occurs in domestic and laboratory animals but is recognized as a primary condition only in cows and pigs.[1] Ulcer disease in companion animals is infrequently reported and is usually secondary to another disease process (e.g., mast cell neoplasia, liver disease, or uremia) or to ulcerogenic drug administration. Although such complications of ulcer disease as hemorrhage and perforation are frequently life-threatening, ulcers are often masked by the signs of the primary condition or misdiagnosed entirely because of vague clinical signs, lack of a complete diagnostic workup, or the veterinarian's lack of awareness of ulcer disease. Definitive diagnosis of ulcer disease is challenging, but improved prognosis and increased survival times make aggressive diagnostic and therapeutic strategies rewarding.

Anatomy and Physiology

Medical and surgical therapy of duodenal and gastric ulcer disease are based on an understanding of gastric anatomy, physiology, and pathophysiology.[2] The stomach stores food and liquids, mixes and grinds solid food to decrease particle size and enhance absorption, and controls emptying of its contents into the duodenum. The stomach is divided into five anatomic regions: the cardia, which joins the esophagus; the fundus, which is the dome-shaped portion that extends to the left of and cranial to the cardia; the body, which is the portion that extends from the fundus to the angularis (the notch on the lesser curvature); the antrum, which is the segment that extends from the angularis to the pylorus; and the pyloris, which is the most tubular part and which joins the stomach to the proximal duodenum. The stomach secretes many substances, including hydrochloric acid, bicarbonate, pepsinogen, mucus, intrinsic factor, and various hormones. The body and fundus (i.e., the oxyntic or parietal portion) contain acid-secreting parietal cells, pepsinogen-secreting chief cells, and mucous neck cells. Mucous neck cells

*Dr. Moreland is now with the Department of Small Animal Medicine, Surgery, and Radiology, School of Veterinary Medicine, Tuskegee University, Tuskegee Institute, Alabama.

secrete mucus and pepsinogen and are the progenitor cells of the gastric epithelium. The mucosa of the gastric antrum has few parietal cells but contains pyloric cells, which secrete gastrin. Bicarbonate is produced by the oxyntic, pyloric, and duodenal mucosae.[2-6]

Hydrochloric acid, which is secreted by the parietal cells, converts pepsinogen to pepsin, which partially hydrolyzes ingested proteins. Hydrochloric acid also maintains an acid environment to prevent invasion of viable bacteria, viruses, and parasites into the gut. Secretion of hydrochloric acid occurs against a concentration gradient and thus requires energy. Hydrogen-potassium adenosinetriphosphatase is the enzyme responsible for hydrolyzing adenosinetriphosphate (ATP) to provide energy for the active transport of hydrogen ions to the gastric lumen in exchange for potassium ions; several drugs are under investigation for their inhibitory effect on this enzyme as therapy in gastric ulcers.[3] Acid secretion by the oxyntic cells is modulated by gastrin, acetylcholine, and histamine. Gastrin, which is released by the antral G cells in response to vagal stimulation, gastric distention, and the chemical constituents of food (especially amino acids), is a potent stimulator of gastric acid secretion.

When the antral pH decreases below approximately 2.5, antral gastrin release is inhibited by a negative feedback mechanism. The decrease in duodenal pH after a meal also stimulates secretin release, which contributes to gastrin suppression. Acetylcholine is released by postganglionic vagal neurons near the parietal cells, and its secretion is stimulated by the presence of food in the stomach and by the sight, smell, and taste of food.

Histamine is released by mast cells in the lamina propria mucosae of the stomach and stimulates gastric acid secretion in much the same way as gastrin; however, its potency as an acid secretagogue is only about 80% of that of gastrin.[5] The histamines and acetylcholine are continually released and partially account for the basal acid output. The basal acid output varies from hour to hour in the same individual but tends to follow a circadian rhythm; the lowest secretory rates occur in the morning and the highest rates in the evening. The cause of this circadian pattern is unknown.[2,4] The basal acid output is considerably higher in men than in women. Such data for dogs and cats are unavailable. The exact role of many hormones in the gastrointestinal tract has not been determined.

In vitro and in vivo studies have shown a strong synergism between secretagogues: the secretory response to submaximum doses of two secretagogues is often greater than the sum of the response to the same agents given independently. Thus, in a complex interaction, the combined mechanisms of the major secretagogues potentiate the gastric acid stimulatory effect.[2,4,5] Several other substances, such as calcium, bombesin, and enkephalins, play a lesser role in stimulating gastric acid production. Other inhibitors of gastric acid secretion include somatostatin, calcitonin, glucagon, dopamine, vasoactive intestinal peptide, epinephrine, and prostaglandins. The physiologic role of these agonists and antagonists is still under investigation.

Gastric acid secretion occurs in three phases: a cephalic phase, a gastric phase, and an intestinal phase. Although the phases are considered separately in this article, they do overlap. The cephalic phase results from the sight, smell, taste, or thought of food and is mediated through neurogenic stimuli arising from the brain. The vagus stimulates the parietal cells directly by releasing acetylcholine and indirectly by stimulating the release of gastrin. The gastric phase results from stimuli within the stomach, such as gastric distention and the chemical constituents of food. Gastric distention causes local reflexes in the myenteric plexus and vagovagal reflexes that pass from the brain stem to the stomach. Proteins, amino acids, and peptides in the gastric lumen are strong stimulants of gastric acid secretion, primarily through stimulation of gastrin release. Carbohydrates and fats, whether infused into the gastrointestinal lumen or into the veins, inhibit secretion of gastric acid. The mechanism of inhibition is unknown.[2] Two thirds of the total gastric acid secretion occurs in the gastric phase. In the intestinal phase, which is initiated by the presence of food in the proximal small bowel (especially the duodenum), the stomach secretes small amounts of gastric juice. An increase in gastrin release results from distention and the presence of food constituents in the duodenum as well as in the stomach.

Mucus, another important secretion of the gastric mucosa, is produced by mucous cells and by superficial epithelial cells throughout the stomach. Gastric mucus is a viscous gel consisting of glycoprotein (5%) and water (95%); it adheres to and covers the entire surface of the mucosa. Mucus lubricates foods, thus protecting the mucosa against mechanical abrasion, and provides an undisturbed layer that maintains bicarbonate at the surface to allow the neutralization of acid. The regulatory mechanisms for mucus secretion are not well understood. Prostaglandins stimulate mucus secretion, and nonsteroidal antiinflammatory drugs inhibit it. Bicarbonate, along with mucus, functions in gastric mucosal defense by neutralizing acid near the gastric lumen. Stimulants for bicarbonate secretion include prostaglandins, cholinergic agents, and glucagon.[2,4,5] Inhibitors include nonsteroidal antiinflammatory drugs, α-adrenergic agonists, and bile salts.

Intrinsic factor, a glycoprotein secreted by parietal cells, is required for absorption of vitamin B_{12}. Secretion of intrinsic factor normally exceeds the amount necessary for vitamin B_{12} absorption. A small amount of intrinsic factor prevents signs of deficiency; but in humans, complete lack of intrinsic factor leads to pernicious anemia.

Pepsinogen is secreted by the chief cells and is converted to pepsin by acid. Pepsin is the proteolytic enzyme in gastric juice. The stimulants for pepsinogen release are the same as those for acid. Humans with a hereditary low serum concentration of pepsinogen are predisposed to duodenal ulcers.[4] No similar disease has been reported in animals.

Pathogenesis and Pathophysiology

The pathogenesis of ulcer disease in humans and animals

results from a complex interplay of reactions between the acid-secreting mechanisms and defense mechanisms of the upper gastrointestinal tract. An ulcer is a mucosal defect extending through the lamina muscularis mucosae into the submucosa or deeper, whereas an erosion does not penetrate the lamina muscularis mucosae. The term *peptic ulcer* is inappropriately used as a synonym for ulcer disease; pepsin plays a role in mucosal damage only when the pH of luminal contents is between 1.3 and 3.2. The term *corrosive ulcer* is used for an ulcer that develops in the presence of increased amounts of acid and pepsin (a true peptic ulcer). In the gastrointestinal tract, ulcer disease can occur anywhere that acid contacts the mucosa. In humans and animals, duodenal ulcers considerably outnumber gastric ulcers.[3,7,8] The most common location for ulcer formation is the upper duodenum. In one study of 22 dogs with ulcers, 17 had duodenal ulcers.[8] As in humans, the principal sites of ulceration of the canine gastric mucosa are in the non–acid-producing areas, such as the fundus and the pyloric antrum. The reason for the susceptibility of the non–acid-secreting mucosa to injury is unknown, but the vasculature or gastric muscles might be responsible.[3,4,9,10]

Canine peptic ulcers usually occur in dogs 2½ to 12 years of age. In reported cases, females had a higher incidence than males; but there is no breed predisposition.[8] In dogs, ulcer disease is generally associated with other diseases. In a study of 22 dogs with ulcer disease, only six had no complicating disease.[8] The diseases most commonly associated with gastrointestinal ulceration in humans and in small animals include mast cell neoplasia, liver disease, and uremia.[8] The following conditions are also associated with ulcers in small animals[11-15]:

- Zollinger-Ellison syndrome
- Gastroduodenal neoplasia
- Recurrent pancreatitis
- Intervertebral disk disease or other neurologic disease
- Gastrinoma
- Mastocytosis
- Chronic renal failure
- Gastric adenocarcinoma
- Shock
- Trauma
- Bile acid reflux
- Severe illness
- Major surgery
- Psychologic stress.

Drugs (e.g., aspirin, steroids, and nonsteroidal antiinflammatory agents) are also incriminated in the production of ulcers in dogs and cats.

Regardless of the causative factors, the basic pathogenic mechanism for ulcer formation remains the same. None of the several theories that explain how ulcers are formed and why the generalized changes that occur in ulcer disease usually lead to single, discrete lesions rather than widespread mucosal damage can explain the complex pathogenesis and pathophysiology of ulcer disease.

No acid, no ulcer is the basis of all theorized mechanisms of ulcer formation. Hydrogen ions but not necessarily hypersecretion of acid are required for duodenal ulcer to occur.[3] Several reported cases of gastric ulcers in humans were associated with hypochlorhydria.[16] The integrity of the gastric mucosa depends on a delicate balance between destructive and defensive factors. An ulcer that develops in the presence of mucosal defense failure is called a trophic ulcer. As mentioned, an ulcer that develops in the presence of increased amounts of acid and pepsin is called a corrosive ulcer. If both increased amounts of acid and pepsin and impaired defenses are present but it is not clear which factor predominates, the ulcer is called a mixed ulcer. Because mixed ulcers usually appear in areas of the gastrointestinal tract where normal mucosa has been replaced by dysplastic epithelium, they are also called dysplastic ulcers.

Mucosal damage usually does not occur when the luminal pH is greater than 7. Some ulcers are produced when the normal defensive forces are overwhelmed by hypersecretion of acid or pepsin, as occurs in Zollinger-Ellison syndrome. Other ulcers form when normal or reduced acid secretion occurs in the presence of severely impaired mucosal defenses. Destructive factors acting on the mucosa include the caustic properties of gastric acid, the proteolytic enzymes (e.g., pepsin), the necrotizing properties of certain pharmacologic agents (e.g., aspirin or indomethacin) or such organic secretions as bile and pancreatic juice, and the irritating action of gross food particles as well as of microorganisms and their toxins.

The gastrointestinal mucosa has the following defenses: (1) thick, viscous, alkaline mucus that slows the inward infiltration of hydrogen ions and traps them for neutralization; (2) the production of bicarbonate, which neutralizes acid at the gastric lumen; (3) the gastric barrier to hydrogen ion diffusion, which is composed of active phospholipids, hydrophobic lipoprotein cell membrane, and tight junctional complexes; (4) the ability of the mucosa to increase local blood flow to facilitate rapid access of nutrients and bicarbonate and to facilitate the removal of toxic and caustic products from the area; and (5) the rapid cellular replication rate of the mucosa.[3] The last two defense mechanisms are much stronger than the first three. When all five mechanisms are functioning optimally, they present an effective barrier to potentially ulcerogenic factors.

Once erosion occurs, the damaged tissue stimulates production and release of agents that increase local blood supply and stimulate the growth of mucous cells and the rapid replication and maturation of primitive epithelial cells. Erosions generally heal in one or two days. If cell replication cannot keep up with the destructive processes, the lesion expands into the submucosa and forms a chronic ulcer. Complete healing of ulcers requires several days to several weeks, and damaged epithelium is replaced by scar tissue. Scar tissue is more resistant to peptic and acid degradation than normal mucosa is. Ulcers are usually single, discrete mucosal craters because destruction overcomes defense only in areas of vulnerability. Vulnerable areas of mucosa generally have the following characteristics: transitional epithelium, which occurs at the boundary between two types of mucosa (i.e., the antral and oxyntic mucosae); changes in the arrangement of muscle bundles; and poor vascularization attributable to absent submucosal capillary plexus or to arteriovenous communications.[3]

Ulcer pain results from the exposure of sensitive nerve endings to acid and from changes in the motility of the affected area. In human ulcer patients, there is no association between abdominal pain and the activity of the ulcer crater.[9] Ulcer healing does not guarantee disappearance of pain, and relief of symptoms does not mean that the crater has healed.[9]

Bleeding is caused by the erosion of superficial capillaries and venules. Blood loss at this stage is acid dependent: the more acid, the more bleeding. Severe hemorrhage occurs secondary to arterial erosion deep in the ulcer crater. At this stage, blood loss is independent of the intraluminal concentration of hydrogen ions.[3]

Predisposing Factors and Associated Conditions

The equilibrium between the destructive and defensive factors is affected by predisposing or determining factors.[3]

Stress

Stress ulcers occur in acutely and critically ill human and animal patients. The lesions can occur in the gastric, duodenal, or colonic mucosa and are usually superficial to the lamina muscularis mucosae. Occasionally, a penetrating ulcer surrounded by erosions occurs. Stress ulcers in dogs are infrequently reported but are associated with high mortality.[14,15] In dogs, small mucosal erosions are frequently associated with trauma, shock, surgery, and severe illness.[17]

Stress ulcers secondary to surgical and medical management of intervertebral disk disease have been reported.[14,15] The association of spinal cord injury with gastrointestinal bleeding is also documented in the human medical literature.[18] Some investigators believe that injury to the spinal cord results in vagotonia secondary to an altered equilibrium between the sympathetic and parasympathetic pathways. Paralytic vasodilation follows loss of sympathetic inhibitor effects and leads to decreased mucosal blood flow and increased production of gastric acid and pepsin. The decrease in blood flow and increased acid secretion may cause erosions, hemorrhage, and necrosis.[14-16,18,19] This deterioration is exacerbated by the added stress of a surgical procedure, hospitalization, and frequent administration of exogenous corticosteroids. Such complications as perforation of a colonic ulcer or severe gastrointestinal hemorrhage occasionally occur; the associated mortality is high. One study suggested that 2% of all dogs with intervertebral disk disease die of gastrointestinal complications.[15] Administration of intestinal protectants in conjunction with antacids and histamine$_2$ antagonists, along with a decrease in the duration of corticosteroid administration, may help reduce the prevalence of the disease in high-risk individuals.

The ulcerogenic potential of corticosteroids has been documented.[18,20,21] Chronic steroid administration increases acid output in dogs and may do so in humans.[17,20,21] This effect is not dramatic, and few investigators believe that it is the major link between steroid administration and gastrointestinal ulceration. Steroid administration leads to decreased mucus production by the stomach and to disturbances in the carbohydrate moiety of the mucus. Mucosal cell renewal is modified by steroids. In dogs, administration of adrenocorticotropic hormone leads to increased exfoliation of surface cells and decreased mitotic activity.[20,21] Thus, evidence strongly suggests that steroids exert their ulcerogenic effect by altering mucosal defense mechanisms rather than by potentiating the effects of the destructive factors.

Drugs

Aspirin and other nonsteroidal antiinflammatory drugs, such as phenylbutazone and indomethacin, damage the gastric mucosa and may precipitate upper gastrointestinal bleeding from mucosal ulceration.[7,17,22,23] Aspirin has both a topical irritating effect on the mucosa and a systemic effect following absorption.[4] Evidence suggests that the major mechanism responsible for ulcer formation is aspirin's inhibitory effect on prostaglandin synthesis. In laboratory animals, the prophylactic administration of exogenous prostaglandins or the stimulation of endogenous prostaglandin synthesis prevented aspirin-induced ulcers.[4] The protective effect of prostaglandins on the gastric mucosa has already been discussed. Most of the nonsteroidal antiinflammatory drugs act by inhibiting prostaglandins; chronic administration of these agents produces mucosal lesions that may progress to ulcer formation.

Liver Disease

Acute and chronic liver disease can damage the gastrointestinal mucosa.[24,25] In acute hepatitis or liver failure, the lesions are attributable mostly to bleeding disorders. The mucosal lesions are secondary to decreased blood flow, usually as a result of thrombosis caused by disseminated intravascular coagulation. In acute hepatic necrosis, thromboplastin is released and initiates widespread intravascular coagulation and thrombosis. In addition, the impaired synthesis of blood clotting factors and removal of fibrin degradation products and circulating anticoagulants by the liver contribute to gastrointestinal bleeding.[24]

Chronic liver disease can also cause gastric lesions. Both the incidence and the prevalence of duodenal ulcers are apparently increased in patients with hepatic cirrhosis.[7] Proposed mechanisms of mucosal injury include failure of the liver to remove gastrin and histamine from the portal circulation; elevated circulating bile acids, which stimulate gastrin production; portal hypertension, which decreases mucosal blood flow; and negative nitrogen balance (hypoalbuminemia), which results in an altered gastric mucosal barrier and reduced cell turnover.[25] In the only major study of canine ulcer disease to date, 16 of the 22 reported patients had severe liver abnormalities, including fatty degeneration, tumor involvement, cirrhosis, or severe necrosis.[8] These results suggest that liver disease plays a prominent role in secondary ulcerative disease in dogs.

Pancreatitis

In humans, the prevalence of ulcer disease in persons with chronic pancreatitis is about 20%.[26] The reasons for the association are unclear, but it may be attributable to the decreased availability of bicarbonate in pancreatic juice. Gastrointestinal bleeding during acute pancreatitis may result from diffuse bleeding from duodenal and antral erosions caused by inflammation spreading from the head of the pancreas. Gastric irritation from regurgitated pancreatic juice has already been discussed and may play a role in mucosal ulceration. In necropsies of dogs, I have found that chronic pancreatitis and gastroduodenal ulceration often coexist.

Uremia

In humans and animals, gastrointestinal bleeding is often associated with uremia.[7,24,27,28] The pathogenesis of uremic gastric ulceration is unknown; but popular theories include local irritation by ammonia produced from urea, alteration of the mucous protective coating, uremic vasculitis, and coagulopathies. Release of histamine from mast cells, acidosis, hypergastrinemia, and alterations in plasma concentrations of calcium, phosphorus, and magnesium are apparently involved in the pathogenesis of uremic ulcers.[24,27]

Mast Cell Disease

Mast cell tumors are common cutaneous neoplasms in dogs and cats.[29-32] Primary mastocytomas in the spleen and other hematopoietic tissues have resulted in mastocythemia.[32] The metachromatic cytoplasmic granules that characterize the mast cell contain varying amounts of vasoactive amines and heparin. Histamine is the most potent vasoactive amine stored in these granules; its rapid release can result in hypotensive shock,[29] urticaria, and pruritus.

Gastrointestinal ulceration is a common complication of massive mast cell degranulation and histaminemia. The elevated blood histamine concentration produces gastric hyperacidity and hypermotility, which predispose the patient to ulceration.[8,29,30] Histamine also dilates small veins and capillaries in the gastrointestinal tract. The resultant increase in blood flow in the gastrointestinal vasculature results in altered endothelial permeability. The resultant leakage of plasma components promotes intravascular thrombosis and ischemic necrosis of the gastrointestinal mucosa. In one series of necropsies of 24 dogs with mastocytomas and concurrent gastroduodenal ulceration[29], small vascular thrombi were found in the gastric submucosa more often than in the duodenal submucosa. Systemic mastocytosis also occurs in humans and has similar gastrointestinal complications.[33] Any animal with possible ulcer disease and no other obvious predisposing conditions should be examined for mast cell tumors.

Motility Disorders

Gastric hypermotility is believed to contribute to duode-

nal ulcers in humans and animals. Rapid gastric emptying and gastric hypersecretion are reportedly more common in patients with a duodenal ulcer than in normal subjects.[4,7] Accelerated emptying of gastric contents into the duodenum causes an increased acid load in the duodenum and a lower duodenal pH. This alteration in gastric motility does not allow sufficient time for bicarbonate to neutralize the hydrochloric acid in the pyloric antrum.

Gastric hypomotility or delayed gastric emptying has been associated with gastric ulceration in humans.[3,4,9] Gastric stasis may contribute to ulcer disease by one of several proposed mechanisms. If gastric emptying is delayed, food remaining in the stomach for prolonged periods may stimulate gastric hypersecretion. Retention of the duodenal contents, including pancreatic juice and bile, normally regurgitated into the stomach results in prolonged mucosal contact with these irritating substances, thus leading to gastritis and ulceration. Pyloric sphincter abnormalities have been identified in some gastric ulcer patients. Sphincter incompetence allows excessive amounts of the duodenal contents to be regurgitated into the stomach. Bile acids, lysolecithin, and pancreatic secretions are the substances in duodenal juice that are believed to be most damaging to the gastric mucosa.[4,9,34] Of the bile acids, deoxycholic acid is apparently the most irritating.[3,4,9,34] The exact mechanism by which duodenal contents damage gastric mucosa is unknown; hypotheses include alteration of the protective mucus layer or damage to the gastric mucosal barrier; these changes make the barrier more permeable to hydrogen ions.[4]

Gastric motility disorders in small animals have had little documentation. Delayed gastric emptying secondary to primary gastrointestinal disorders or other disease processes may play a role in errosive gastritis.

Tumors

Gastritis and ulceration are frequently associated with malignant neoplasms of the stomach. Gastric cancer may present as an ulcer; and in those cases in which gastric cancer is found in a chronic ulcer, the neoplasm was probably missed on previous presentations. Evidence suggests that benign ulcers do not become malignant.[35] Adenocarcinoma and lymphoma are the two most common types of gastric cancer in humans and animals.[13,35]

Gastrinomas are gastrin-secreting tumors of the alimentary tract. Most gastrinomas are primary pancreatic tumors that involve the non-β islet cells. These tumors release gastrin and cause severe corrosive ulceration attributable to chronic hyperacidity.[36] Zollinger-Ellison syndrome (hypersecretion of acid, severe ulcer disease, and non-β islet cell pancreatic tumor) in dogs and cats has been reported.[11,12] Intractable ulcer disease should prompt investigation into the possibility of a gastrin-secreting tumor.

Clinical Findings

Vomiting is the clinical sign most often associated with upper gastrointestinal ulceration in dogs and cats.[8,17,28] The vomitus may contain partially digested blood (which looks like coffee grounds) or fresh blood and clots.[17] Blood in the vomitus generally signifies gastric ulceration or erosion but is not always grossly evident. Vomiting associated with eating is a variable finding.[8,17] The animal may have an acute episode of severe vomiting, or vomiting may have been sporadic for months or years.[37] Other signs of ulcer disease include anemia, melena, nausea, weight loss, variable appetite, and abdominal pain. Some animals have no clinical signs; in others, perforation and peritonitis have occurred and rapidly result in death.[8,10,17,24,28]

Pain in the cranial abdomen is the most common sign on physical examination.[8,17,37] The patient with possible gastric ulcers should be examined for cutaneous mast cell tumors. There are no consistent hematologic or biochemical abnormalities in an ulcer patient. A regenerative (or nonregenerative if chronic) anemia should prompt an investigation of the gastrointestinal tract as a possible route of blood loss. In cases of severe anemia, signs referable to blood loss (e.g., weakness, syncope, or cardiac murmur) may be the primary reason for presentation. Biochemical profiles and urinalysis should be performed to exclude metabolic disease from the differential diagnosis and to determine the primary condition.[37]

Diagnosis

A diagnosis of gastrointestinal ulcers should be considered when the factors that potentiate ulcer formation are present.[21] Diagnosis is rarely based on a single parameter but instead relies on a combination of history, clinical findings, radiology, and endoscopy. Necropsy is still a common method of confirming diagnosis.

Routine radiographs are rarely helpful in diagnosing ulcer disease. Single-contrast radiography is also associated with a low diagnostic yield in human and veterinary medicine.[38,39] Studies comparing single-contrast studies with endoscopy have reported false-negative radiographic determinations of up to 77%.[38] The use of double-contrast technique has resulted in a decrease in false-negative determinations to 17%.

Barium is the contrast agent most commonly used in an upper gastrointestinal study and is the best medium for routine use.[38,39] In cases in which perforation, laceration, or rupture of the gastrointestinal tract is possible, an oral organic iodine preparation (e.g., Gastrografin®—E. R. Squibb & Sons, or Hypaque®—Winthrop) is the medium of choice for contrast radiography. Unlike barium, organic iodine preparations are innocuous in body cavities. A double-contrast gastrogram (instillation of barium and then air through a stomach tube to distend the stomach) is indicated for detailed examination of the gastric mucosa. Radiographs of the distended stomach in several positions should be taken to complete the study. A large ulcer appears as a collection of contrast material that extends beyond the gastric wall. Multiple superficial erosions are manifested by small, shallow barium collections that are often surrounded by a radiolucent halo that represents elevated edematous mucosa. Even if double-contrast techniques are used, single, discrete lesions may be difficult to find.

Endoscopy

Endoscopy is the most effective method of diagnosing gastric ulcers.[17] An experienced endoscopist can help differentiate benign from malignant, chronic from acute, and active from healing ulcers by visual examination. Endoscopy may also help in establishing the diagnosis of drug-induced lesions, in which the edges are often sharply defined and the surrounding mucosa is often apparently undamaged.[3] Endoscopy has an advantage over radiography because small, discrete lesions and superficial erosions that may be missed by barium-contrast evaluation can be visualized. It is also a safe method by which the clinician can obtain mucosal biopsies, brush cytology, or aspiration of fluid for analysis. One disadvantage of endoscopy is that in veterinary medicine it requires general anesthesia. Duodenal ulcers may be more difficult to detect because expertise is required to pass the fiber-optic endoscope into the pylorus.

On endoscopy, active ulcers appear as round or oval niches and craters with radiating mucosal folds and are surrounded by a smooth mound of edema and covered by mucus or debris.[3] The mucosal lesion may be bleeding or pale and yellowish. Acute ulcers have little or no connective tissue in the margin or floor. Chronic ulcers have a fibrin-filled crater and wrinkled mucosa peripheral to the ulcer and may show minimal inflammatory response. Stress ulcers appear as small, punctate submucosal hemorrhages. Small, punctate erosions can be identified later along the crests of the rugae gastricae.[17]

Gastric fluid analysis plays a limited role in the diagnosis and management of ulcer disease. It may be useful, however, for identifying gastric hypersecretion of hydrochloric acid. Measurement of serum gastrin levels is useful for confirming the diagnosis of gastrinomas, which should be suspected in patients with multiple ulcers and thin, watery diarrhea.[3]

Treatment

Rational medical and surgical treatment of ulcer disease have received widespread attention in human medicine, and the methods for treating ulcers have changed dramatically in the past 10 years. Because clinical signs of gastrointestinal ulcers are uncommon in veterinary medicine, therapy in companion animals has been based on extrapolation from human literature. Double-blind, randomized clinical trials that use fiber-optic endoscopy to document the status of an ulcer crater during the therapeutic period have begun to provide a basis for rational decisions regarding the management of gastric and duodenal ulcers.

The goals of treatment should include alleviation of clinical signs, avoidance of complications, prevention of recurrence, and eventual cure. Because ulcer disease in animals is generally secondary to other conditions, the primary condition should also be treated. The therapeutic agents used for treating ulcers, including anticholinergics, antacids, agents that inhibit the secretion of acid (i.e., histamine$_2$ blockers), and agents that enhance mucosal resistance to acid or peptic injury (e.g., prostaglandins and su-

TABLE I
Drugs Used in the Treatment of Ulcer Disease

Drug	Mechanism of Action	Suggested Dosage	Common Side Effects
Antacids (magnesium antacids, aluminum antacids, bicarbonate antacids, and calcium antacids)	Neutralize hydrochloric acid	0.5–1.0 ml/kg every 2–4 hours; dosage varies by product	Diarrhea (magnesium antacids); constipation, phosphate depletion (aluminum antacids); hypercalcemia (calcium antacids), rebound acid hypersecretion, alkalosis (all antacids)
Cimetidine (Tagamet®—Smith Kline & French Laboratories)	Decreases hydrochloric acid secretion (histamine₂ antagonist)	5 mg/kg intravenously or orally four times daily	Mental confusion; gynecomastia; inhibition of microsomal enzymes; rarely granulocytopenia or decreased libido[a]
Isopropamide iodide (Darbid®—Smith Kline & French Laboratories)	Decreases hydrochloric acid secretion (anticholinergic)	0.2–1.0 mg/kg orally twice daily	Should not be used for more than three days; gastric distention, increased intraocular pressure
Propantheline (Pro-Banthine®—Searle &	Decreases hydrochloric acid secretion (anticholinergic)	0.25 mg/kg orally three times a day	Same as for isopropamide iodide
Metoclopramide (Reglan®—Danbury Pharmacal)	Enhances gastric emptying	0.5–1.0 mg/kg orally or subcutaneously ½ hour before meals	Restlessness, fatigue, drowsiness; contraindicated in duodenal ulcers, perforating ulcers
Prostaglandins	Stimulate mucus secretion, inhibit acid secretion, stimulate bicarbonate secretion	None established for use in dogs and cats	Diarrhea, nausea, abdominal cramping
Ranitidine (Zantac®—Glaxo)	Decreases hydrochloric acid secretion (histamine₂ antagonist)	0.5 mg/kg orally twice daily	None to date
Sucralfate (Carafate®—Marion Laboratories)	Forms protective complex with protein in ulcer base	1.0 g/30 kg orally four times daily	Constipation

[a]These side effects are associated with a long duration of treatment and have not been documented in small animals.

cralfate) (Table I). Dietary management and avoidance of ulcerogenic drugs also play a role in an effective therapeutic and prophylactic program.

Antacids

Antacids used in the proper dose regimens are effective in the treatment of ulcer disease. Antacids neutralize secreted acid and thus reduce peptic activity, stimulate the release of endogenous prostaglandins, and bind bile salts, which some believe play an important role in the pathogenesis of gastric ulcers.[3] Antacids are not believed to have an important mucosal coating effect.[40] All antacids react with gastric acid to form a neutral salt and water. The most commonly used antacids are sodium bicarbonate, calcium carbonate, magnesium hydroxide, and aluminum hydroxide; simethicone is sometimes added as a defoaming agent (Table II). Variations in the chemical formulation of antacids account for differences in neutralizing capacity, rapidity of action, and side effects.[40]

Liquid antacids are apparently more effective than antacid tablets, but this conclusion is controversial.[3,40] In vitro studies have shown that several antacid tablets are required

to equal the neutralizing capacity of a small dose of liquid antacid.

Antacid therapy in dogs and cats has many drawbacks. The therapeutic dosage is empirical because no specific dosage is defined for use in animals. In humans, the ideal daily dose for aluminum hydroxide and magnesium hydroxide is up to 1000 mEq of neutralizing capacity, or 80 to 160 mEq of acid neutralizing capacity (30 to 60 ml) one and three hours after each meal and at bedtime. This regimen poses an additional problem because antacids must be given at least six times daily to be effective; if an inadequate amount of antacid is given too infrequently, it causes an acid rebound that can exacerbate the existing condition. Poor palatability of liquid antacids and poor owner compliance attributable to the frequent dose are other problems encountered in veterinary medicine. Daily treatment should be given for four to six weeks for maximum effectiveness.

Antacids are less expensive than the histamine₂ antagonists and are fairly safe, although they are not totally free from side effects. The most common side effects are diarrhea (with magnesium-containing products), constipation

TABLE II
Commonly Used Antacids[a]

Trade Name	Active Ingredients	Acid-Neutralizing Capacity (mEq/5ml)[b]	Sodium Content (mg/5ml)[b,c]
Liquid preparations			
ALternaGEL®—Stuart Pharmaceuticals	Aluminum hydroxide	16	2.0
Aludrox®—Wyeth Laboratories	Aluminum hydroxide, magnesium hydroxide	14	1.5
Amphojel®—Wyeth Laboratories	Aluminum hydroxide	7	7.0
Basaljel® Extra Strength—Wyeth Laboratories	Aluminum hydroxide	22 (14.5)	23.0
Camalox®—Rorer Consumer Pharmaceuticals	Aluminum hydroxide, calcium carbonate, magnesium hydroxide	18 (16)	2.5
Gelusil-M®—Parke-Davis	Aluminum hydroxide, magnesium hydroxide, simethicone	24 (12)	1.3
Kolantyl®—Lakeside Pharmaceuticals	Aluminum hydroxide, magnesium hydroxide	11	5.0
Maalox® TC—Rorer Consumer Pharmaceuticals	Aluminum hydroxide, magnesium hydroxide	23 (21)	0.8
Mylanta®-II—Stuart Pharmaceuticals	Aluminum hydroxide, magnesium hydroxide, simethicone	25 (18)	1.1
Riopan®—Ayerst Laboratories	Magaldrate	13.5 (9)	0.3
Titralac®—3M	Calcium carbonate	19 (21)	11.0
Tablets			
Aludrox®—Wyeth Laboratories	Aluminum hydroxide, magnesium hydroxide	12	1.6
Amphojel®—Wyeth Laboratories	Aluminum hydroxide	9 (2)	7.0
Basaljel®—Wyeth Laboratories	Aluminum hydroxide	14 (15)	2.1
Camalox®—Rorer Consumer Pharmaceuticals	Aluminum hydroxide, calcium carbonate, magnesium hydroxide	18 (15)	1.5
Gelusil-II®—Parke-Davis	Aluminum hydroxide, magnesium hydroxide simethicone	21 (8.2)	2.1
Kolantyl®—Lakeside Pharmaceuticals	Aluminum hydroxide, magnesium hydroxide	11	15.0
Maalox® TC—Rorer Consumer Pharmaceuticals	Magnesium hydroxide, aluminum hydroxide	18	1.9
Mylanta®-II—Stuart Pharmaceuticals	Aluminum hydroxide, magnesium hydroxide, simethicone	23 (11)	1.3
Riopan®—Ayerst Laboratories	Magaldrate	13.5 (10)	0.3
Titralac®—3M	Calcium carbonate	7.3 (9.5)	0.3

[a]From Meeroff JC: Ulcer disease of the upper gastrointestinal tract. *Hosp Pract*:223, 1984. Modified with permission.
[b]Data derived from information provided by the manufacturers. Values in parentheses represent data obtained in an independent study (Drake D, Hollander D: Neutralizing capacity and cost effectiveness of antacids. *Ann Intern Med* 94:215, 1981.). Sodium values corrected according to another independent study (McCoy LK: Antacids tabulation [letter]. *Ann Intern* 95:394, 1981.)
[c]To convert milligrams of sodium into milliequivalents of sodium, divide milligrams of sodium by 23 (atomic weight of sodium).

(with aluminum preparations), acid rebound, alkalosis (particularly at the high recommended doses), intestinal bacterial overgrowth, hypernatremia, magnesium toxicity or hypercalcemia (either of which is rare except in renal dysfunction), and hypophosphatemia (with phosphate-binding aluminum-containing gels). Antacids may also interfere with the absorption of such drugs as tetracycline, digoxin, and cimetidine.

Histamine₂ Antagonists

Black's development of histamine$_2$ antagonists revolutionized the treatment of ulcer disease.[41] In most clinical trials in humans and dogs, cimetidine (Tagamet®—Smith, Kline & French Laboratories) caused healing of benign duodenal ulcers in four to six weeks. Histamine$_2$ antagonists block the histamine receptors on gastric parietal cells. These drugs are potent inhibitors of both secretory volume and hydrogen ion concentration in normal subjects and in patients with duodenal ulcers.[3,42]

Clinical assessment of such histamine$_2$ antagonist drugs as cimetidine is lacking in the veterinary literature, although cimetidine was reportedly effective in one dog with a naturally occurring gastric ulcer.[37] The cimetidine dosage for dogs is 5 mg/kg orally or subcutaneously every six hours.[25] The maximum duration of treatment for an acute ulcer is eight weeks.[40] In an experiment in dogs, cimetidine had an insignificant effect on the healing of gastric ulcers but did promote healing of duodenal ulcers.[40] Cimetidine is less effective than antacids in the treatment and prophylaxis of acute gastrointestinal bleeding attributable to stress ulcers, perhaps because cimetidine impairs the secretory capacity of the gastric mucosa, thereby decreasing bicarbonate concentrations.[43]

Cimetidine's advantages over antacids include ease of administration (it is available in injectable and oral tablet form), longer dose intervals, better palatability, and fewer side effects at the recommended dose. Although cimetidine is more expensive than antacids, improved patient and owner compliance make it a worthwhile alternative. The veterinary use of cimetidine in the routine therapy of uremic gastropathy, acute pancreatitis, gastrinomas, and gastroduodenal ulcers in mast cell disease is becoming more popular. Doses used to treat gastrinomas (e.g., Zollinger-Ellison syndrome) may be much higher than those required for other ulcer-related conditions.[36]

Side effects of cimetidine in conventional doses are rare and are usually associated with treatment of several months duration. In humans, the most significant side effect is gynecomastia.[3,40] Table I lists conditions commonly associated with cimetidine treatment in humans and experimental animals. Cimetidine administration evidently leads to general inhibition of hepatic microsomal enzymes and may impair the elimination of drugs undergoing metabolism by these enzymes.[3] Cimetidine delays the metabolism of warfarin, theophylline, and propranolol.[40]

Ranitidine (Zantac®—Glaxo), another histamine$_2$ antagonist used for the treatment of ulcer disease, is more potent and has a longer duration of action than cimetidine. Several advantages over cimetidine make ranitidine particularly attractive for use in veterinary medicine. Because of its longer duration of action, oral ranitidine given twice daily provides effective control of gastric acid secretion. Preliminary studies suggest that it has fewer side effects than cimetidine[40] and that it does not inhibit hepatic microsomal enzymes.[3] Ranitidine is no more effective than cimetidine in the treatment of ulcer disease.[44,45] The use of ranitidine in dogs or cats has not been documented, although recent veterinary literature does recommend ranitidine as an alternative to cimetidine.[25] Neither cimetidine nor ranitidine affects pancreatic secretion or gastric motility.

Anticholinergics

The rationale for the use of anticholinergic antimuscarinic agents is that they reduce basal and stimulated acid secretion by 70% to 80% and 30% to 40%, respectively, and inhibit gastrointestinal motility.[3] The anticholinergic drugs occupy the muscarinic receptors and prevent the action of acetylcholine on glands and smooth muscle. Atropine and glycopyrrolate, which are commonly used anticholinergics, are not suitable agents for use in ulcer therapy because of their other antimuscarinic effects, such as decreased salivation, increased smooth muscle contraction in the bladder and ileum, and increased heart rate.

Anticholinergics are often used in combination with antacids and histamine$_2$ blockers. The use of an anticholinergic agent along with a histamine$_2$ antagonist is more effective than the use of cimetidine alone.[40] Anticholinergics should not be prescribed for patients with severe pulmonary disease, delayed gastric emptying, or glaucoma.[40] Three days has been suggested as a maximum duration for the administration of anticholinergics in small animals because prolonged use results in gastric atony and ileus. Common anticholinergic agents include atropine, methscopolamine bromide, isopropamide iodide, and propantheline bromide.[17]

Motility Modifiers

Metoclopramide (Reglan®—A. H. Robins) enhances gastrointestinal motility without affecting the secretion of acid or gastrin. Metoclopramide in combination with other therapeutic agents may be useful for enhancing gastric ulcer healing but may be contraindicated in duodenal ulcer disease.[3] Stimulation of gastric emptying may cause rapid delivery of acidic gastric contents to the duodenum before adequate time has elapsed for effective neutralization by bicarbonate. Such enhanced gastric motility worsens a preexisting duodenal ulcer.

Coating Agents

Sucralfate (Carafate®—Marion Laboratories) is a complex of sulfated sucrose and aluminum hydroxide and is the only cytoprotective agent available in the United States.[7,40,46-48] When ingested sucralfate reacts with acid, it forms an adherent and protective complex with proteins in the ulcer base. Sucralfate protects the ulcer against pepsin, acid, and bile. Sucralfate is used primarily for the short-term treatment of duodenal ulcers, but it also effectively enhances the healing of gastric ulcers.[3,40,46,47] Oral use of this drug (1 g for a 30-kg animal four times daily) has been recommended for the treatment of ulcers in dogs and cats.[25,49] Constipation is the only significant side effect of sucralfate administration in humans and dogs, and its effectiveness in promoting ulcer healing is comparable with and sometimes superior to that of cimetidine.[40,48,50] At present, evidence does not suggest that concurrent use of sucralfate and other ulcer therapy is contraindicated. The usefulness of this drug in veterinary medicine needs further investigation.

Prostaglandins

Prostaglandins are naturally occurring derivatives of arachidonic acid[40,51,52] and are distributed throughout the gastrointestinal tract. In humans and animals, the experimental administration of the methylated derivative of prostaglandin E$_2$ prevents mucosal damage from acid, bile, and other gastric irritants.[40,46,47,51,52] Several mechanisms for the prevention of mucosal injury by synthetic prostaglandins are possible, including inhibition of acid secretion, stimulation of bicarbonate secretion, and stimulation of mucus production.[40] Diarrhea sometimes occurs when prostaglandins are given in doses that inhibit the secretion of acid; however, when smaller, cytoprotective doses are used, diarrhea does not occur.[40] Prostaglandins are currently being investigated for clinical use in the United States.

Combination Therapy

Various combination therapies can be used to meet the special requirements of an individual patient. A combination of anticholinergics with histamine$_2$ antagonists is more effective than histamine$_2$ antagonists used alone in inhibiting acid secretion.[40,47] Other patients may benefit from the combination of cimetidine with sucralfate if marked ulcer penetration is possible.[48] Because antacids may interfere with the bioavailability of other drugs used in the treatment of ulcer disease, they should not be administered concurrently.

Other Therapeutic Considerations

In humans, dietary restrictions neither enhance the healing of ulcers nor prevent ulcer recurrence.[1,46] The traditional ulcer diet of bland, soft foods has been largely replaced by the recommendation that the patient eat three well-balanced meals daily.[46] Dietary management does play a role in the care of patients with gastric ulceration secondary to chronic gastritis caused by food allergies. In veterinary medicine, homemade bland diets consisting mainly of cottage cheese and rice or specially formulated commercial diets (e.g., Prescription Diet® Canine i/d® — Hill's Pet Products) have been recommended. Quantity and frequency of feeding depend on individual responses. In general, owners should avoid giving their pets bedtime snacks. Food in the stomach during the night stimulates nocturnal hypersecretion of acid.

Milk, which was originally believed to be an effective antacid, is often given by well-intentioned owners as a remedy for gastrointestinal problems. Although milk does have some neutralizing ability and contains large amounts of prostaglandins and other protective substances, calcium and milk proteins are potent stimulators of acid secretion.[3,7,46] In general, adult dogs and cats do not tolerate large amounts of milk in the diet; diarrhea is a common result of its administration.

Drugs known to be ulcerogenic (e.g., aspirin, nonsteroidal antiinflammatory drugs, or steroids) should be used with caution and avoided when possible. Especially in ulcer patients, only an enteric-coated brand of aspirin should be used. Buffered aspirin does not prevent the corrosive effects of aspirin on the gastric mucosa.

Role of Surgery

Surgical treatment of ulcer disease should be recommended if a proved or possible malignant neoplasm is found on initial or follow-up histologic or radiographic examination, an ulcer fails to heal completely by 12 to 15 weeks, or a serious complication (e.g., uncontrollable bleeding or perforation) develops.[46] In dogs, partial gastrectomy, pyloromyotomy, and vagotomy have been successful alone and in combination.[17]

Emergency Treatment

Severe gastric hemorrhage is an emergency; immediate control of gastric bleeding and correction of blood and fluid loss are required. Control of bleeding by intragastric lavage with ice water should be attempted.[17,24] The low temperature promotes vasoconstriction, thus reducing blood flow and bleeding. Norepinephrine bitartrate (8 mg/500 ml) can be added to the ice water.[17,24] As an alternative, it can be given intraperitoneally (8 mg/100 ml cold saline). This treatment in animals with experimental bleeding ulcers saves animals that would otherwise die of exsanguination.[24] The potent α-adrenergic effect of nor-

epinephrine bitartrate enhances vasoconstriction but has little cardiovascular effect, as it is rapidly metabolized in the liver.[17,24] The lavage solution should be instilled into the stomach via a nasogastric tube, which should remain there for 30 minutes and then be removed. The lavage is repeated until gastric bleeding has ceased.

Gastric hemorrhage should be treated by the replacement of blood losses. Stored whole blood is used unless disseminated intravascular coagulation is determined to be the cause of the bleeding. In this situation, transfusions only worsen the condition. If the disseminated intravascular coagulation is caused by hepatic disease, however, transfusion of fresh whole blood to replace deficient clotting factors is indicated.[24] Gastric hemorrhage resulting from ulceration caused by thrombosis is difficult to treat. If all medical therapy fails to control gastric bleeding, surgery is indicated.[24]

Perforation of an ulcer with resultant peritonitis is a complication of chronic ulcer disease and requires immediate and aggressive medical and surgical management. Perforating ulcers are always associated with a poor prognosis.

Prognosis

In the past, the long-term prognosis for dogs and cats with gastroduodenal ulcers was poor. With the introduction of new drugs, better awareness of the incidence of the disease in pets, and more sophisticated diagnostic techniques, survival rates should improve. Because ulcer disease in animals generally occurs secondary to other conditions, every attempt should be made to control the initiating process.

Patients at high risk for developing secondary ulcers might benefit from the conservative medical prophylaxis commonly used for human patients. The incidence of ulcer disease in dogs and cats that have no clinical signs of ulcer disease or that have clinical signs only intermittently is probably high. These cases are often diagnosed only at necropsy. In one study, 7 of 14 dogs suddenly collapsed and died of a perforating ulcer. Only one of these patients had clinical signs of ulcer disease before the fatal crisis.[8] Such cases will continue to contribute significantly to the high mortality associated with ulcer disease; however, early diagnosis and aggressive therapy make ulcer disease a considerably more manageable condition than it has been.

REFERENCES

1. Barker IK, van Dreumel AA: Alimentary system, in Jubb KVF, Kennedy PC, Palmer N (eds): *Pathology of Domestic Animals*, ed 3. Orlando, FL, Academic Press, 1985, pp 44–49.
2. Feldman M: Gastric secretion, in Sleisenger MH, Fordtran JS (eds): *Gastrointestinal Disease: Pathophysiology, Diagnosis, Management.* Philadelphia, WB Saunders Co, 1983, pp 541–558.
3. Meeroff JC: Ulcer disease of the upper gastrointestinal tract. *Hosp Pract*:177–248, 1984.
4. Holt KM, Isenberg JI: Peptic ulcer disease: Physiology and pathophysiology. *Hosp Pract*:89–106, 1985.
5. Guyton AC: Secretory functions of the alimentary tract, in *Textbook*

of Medical Physiology. Philadelphia, WB Saunders Co, 1976, pp 867–880.

6. Murray M, McKeating FJ, Lauder IM: Peptic ulceration in the dog: A clinicopathological study. *Vet Rec* 91(19):441–447, 1972.
7. Soll AH, Isenberg JI: Duodenal ulcer diseases, in Sleisenger MH, Fordtran JS (eds): *Gastrointestinal Disease: Pathophysiology, Diagnosis, Management.* Philadelphia, WB Saunders Co, 1983, pp 624–672.
8. McGuigan JE, Ament ME: Anatomy, embryology, and developmental anomalies, in Sleisenger MH, Fordtran JS (eds): *Gastrointestinal Disease: Pathophysiology, Diagnosis, Management.* Philadelphia, WB Saunders Co, 1983, pp 505–511.
9. Richardson CT: Gastric ulcer, in Sleisenger MH, Fordtran JS (eds): *Gastrointestinal Disease: Pathophysiology, Diagnosis, Management.* Philadelphia, WB Saunders Co, 1983, pp 672–693.
10. Ader P: Penetrating gastric ulceration in a dog. *JAVMA* 175(7):710–713, 1979.
11. Happe RP, van der Gaag I, Lamers CB, et al: Zollinger-Ellison syndrome in three dogs. *Vet Pathol* 17:177–182, 1980.
12. Middleton DJ, Watson ADJ, Vasack E, et al: Duodenal ulceration associated with gastrin-secreting pancreatic tumor in a cat. *JAVMA* 183:461–462, 1983.
13. Wright RP: Malignant gastric ulcer associated with adenocarcinoma of gastric fundus in a dog. *VM SAC* 6:845–848, 1981.
14. Thoombs JP, Caywood DD, Lipowitz AJ, et al: Colonic perforation following neurosurgical procedures and corticosteroid therapy in four dogs. *JAVMA* 177(1):68–72, 1980.
15. Moore RW, Withrow SJ: Gastrointestinal hemorrhage and pancreatitis associated with intervertebral disk disease in the dog. *JAVMA* 180:1443–1447, 1982.
16. Sagge MR, Butler ML: Reassessment of the management of benign gastric ulcer with achlorhydria. *Clin Gastroenterol* 3:13–15, 1981.
17. Twedt DC: Gastric ulcers, in Kirk RW (ed): *Current Veterinary Therapy VIII.* Philadelphia, WB Saunders Co, 1983, pp 765–770.
18. Kewaeramani LS: Neurogenic gastroduodenal ulceration and bleeding associated with spinal cord injury. *J Trauma* 9:259–265, 1979.
19. Robert A, Kauffman GL: Stress ulcers, in Sleisenger MH, Fordtran JS (eds): *Gastrointestinal Disease: Pathophysiology, Diagnosis, Management.* Philadelphia, WB Saunders Co, 1983, pp 612–623.
20. Fenster LF: The ulcerogenic potential of glucocorticoids and possible prophylactic measures. *Med Clin North Am* 57:1289–1294, 1973.
21. Max MH, Menguy RB: Influence of ACTH on rate of gastric mucosal cell turnover. *Surg Forum* 20:331–332, 1969.
22. Cameron AJ: Aspirin and gastric ulcer. *Mayo Clin Proc* 50:565, 1975.
23. Ewing GO: Indomethacin-associated gastrointestinal hemorrhage in a dog. *JAVMA* 161:1665–1668, 1972.
24. Strombeck DR: *Small Animal Gastroenterology.* Davis, CA, Stonegate Publishing, 1979, pp 99–109.
25. Twedt DC: Cirrhosis: A consequence of chronic liver disease. *Vet Clin North Am [Small Anim Pract]* 15:166–167, 1985.
26. Grendell JH, Cello JP: Chronic pancreatitis, in Sleisenger MH, Fordtran JS (eds): *Gastrointestinal Disease: Pathophysiology, Diagnosis, Management.* Philadelphia, WB Saunders Co, 1983, p 1503.
27. Twedt DC, Wingfield WE: Diseases of the stomach, in Ettinger SJ (ed): *Textbook of Veterinary Internal Medicine.* Philadelphia, WB Saunders Co, 1983, pp 1259–1262.
28. Wingfield WE: Small animal gastric diseases, in Anderson NV (ed): *Veterinary Gastroenterology.* Philadelphia, Lea & Febiger, 1980, pp 438–440.
29. Howard EB, Sawa TR, Nielsen SW, et al: Mastocytoma and gastroduodenal ulceration. *Path Vet* 6:146–158, 1969.

30. Zontine WJ, Meierhenry EF, Hicks RF: Perforated duodenal ulcer associated with mastocytoma in a dog: A case report. *J Am Vet Radiol Soc* 18:162–165, 1977.
31. Tams TR, Macy DW: Canine mast cell tumors. *Compend Contin Educ Pract Vet* 3(10):869–882, 1981.
32. Liska WD: Feline systemic mastocytosis: A review and results of splenectomy in seven cases. *JAAHA* 15:589–597, 1981.
33. Webb TA, Chin-Yang L, Lung TY: Systemic mast cell disease: A clinical and hematopathological study of 26 cases. *Cancer* 49:927–938, 1982.
34. Duane WC, Wiegard DM: Mechanism by which bile salts disrupt the gastric mucosal barrier in the dog. *J Clin Invest* 66:1044, 1980.
35. Davis GR: Neoplasms of the stomach, in Sleisenger MH, Fordtran JS (eds): *Gastrointestinal Disease: Pathophysiology, Diagnosis, Management.* Philadelphia, WB Saunders Co, 1983, p 581.
36. McGuigan JE: The Zollinger-Ellison syndrome, in Sleisenger MH, Fordtran JS (eds): *Gastrointestinal Disease: Pathophysiology, Diagnosis, Management.* Philadelphia, WB Saunders Co, 1983, pp 693–707.
37. Schulman J: Control of gastric ulcers in a dog using cimetidine. *Canine Pract* 6:42–43, 1979.
38. Federle MP, Goldberg HI: Conventional radiography of the alimentary tract, in Sleisenger MH, Fordtran JS (eds): *Gastrointestinal Disease: Pathophysiology, Diagnosis, Management.* Philadelphia, WB Saunders Co, 1983, pp 1635–1652.
39. Brawner WR, Bartels JE: Contrast radiography of the digestive tract: Indications, techniques, and complications. *Vet Clin North Am [Small Anim Pract]* 13:599–626, 1983.
40. Peterson WL, Richardson CT: Pharmacology and side effects of drugs used to treat peptic ulcer, in Sleisenger MH, Fordtran JS (eds): *Gastrointestinal Disease: Pathophysiology, Diagnosis, Management.* Philadelphia, WB Saunders Co, 1983, pp 708–725.
41. Fleshler B: The impact of cimetidine on the treatment of acid-peptic disease. *Primary Care* 8:195–203, 1981.
42. Thomas JM, Misiewicz G: Histamine H$_2$-receptor antagonists in the short- and long-term treatment of duodenal ulcer. *Clin Gastroenterol* 13:447–472, 1984.
43. Priebe HJ, Skillman JJ, Bushnell LS, et al: Antacid versus cimetidine in preventing acute gastrointestinal bleeding. *N Engl J Med* 302:426–430, 1980.
44. Quatrini M, Basilisco G, Bianchi PA: Treatment of "cimetidine-resistant" chronic duodenal ulcers with ranitidine or cimetidine: A randomised multicentric study. *Gut* 25:1113–1117, 1984.
45. The Belgian Peptic Ulcer Study Group: Single-blind comparative study of ranitidine and cimetidine in patients with gastric ulcer. *Gut* 25:999–1002, 1984.
46. Lewis JH: Treatment of gastric ulcer: What is old and what is new. *Arch Intern Med* 143:264–272, 1983.
47. Marks IN: Current therapy in peptic ulcer. *Drugs* 20:283–299, 1980.
48. Brogden RN, Heel RC, Speight TM, et al: Sucralfate: A review of its pharmacodynamic properties and therapeutic use in peptic ulcer disease. *Drugs* 27:194–209, 1984.
49. Twedt DC: Differential diagnosis and therapy of vomiting. *Vet Clin North Am [Small Anim Pract]* 13:519, 1983.
50. Goldfarb JP, Craja MJ: A comparison of cimetidine and sucralfate in the treatment of bleeding peptic ulcers. *Am J Gastroenterol* 80:5–7, 1985.
51. Konturek SJ, Radecki T, Brzozowski T, et al: Aspirin-induced gastric ulcers in cats: Prevention by prostacyclin. *Dig Dis Sci* 26:1003–1012, 1981.
52. Wilson DE, Kaymakcalan H: Prostaglandins: Gastrointestinal effects and peptic ulcer disease. *Med Clin North Am* 65:773–787, 1981.

The Use of Enteral Nutrition in Small Animal Medicine*

The University of Liverpool
Bryn Tennant, BVSc, PhD, MRCVS
Kim Willoughby, BVMS, MRCVS

KEY FACTS

❏ Nutritional support is an essential therapeutic tool in the support and maintenance of the critically ill patient.

❏ Malnutrition results in poorer survival, poor wound healing, and metabolic dysfunction of critically ill patients.

❏ Enteral nutritional support using orogastric, nasal feeding, pharyngostomy, or gastrostomy tubes is the most practical method of providing nutrition to the small animal patient.

❏ Nutritional support needs to be provided early in the course of disease.

The importance of providing adequate nutritional support in the management of critically ill patients has been a significant part of human medicine for many years. Malnutrition is a major cause of increased morbidity and mortality.[1-6] Following severe trauma and the provision of immediate emergency treatment, survival is subsequently dependent upon the prevention of malnutrition, sepsis, and organ failure.[7-10] The commonest type of malnutrition seen in hospitalized human patients is that of protein-energy malnutrition (PEM), the incidence of which varies from 25% to 65%.[11-14] Although figures are unavailable for veterinary medicine, it is probable that similar, if not greater, proportions of animals with severe illnesses also suffer from protein-energy malnutrition.

AETIOLOGY OF MALNUTRITION

Protein-energy malnutrition results from inadequate food intake, nutrient imbalances, and alterations in a patient's metabolism, generally as a consequence of the disease processes present or treatment modalities used. However, iatrogenic malnutrition does occur and is a major concern in human medicine. The term *the skeleton in the hospital closet* was coined by Butterworth in 1974 to emphasize iatrogenic malnutrition.[15] Butterworth considered physician-induced malnutrition to be one of the most serious nutritional problems at that time. The extent of iatrogenic malnutrition in veterinary medicine is not clear, although in the opinion of Crowe, bacterial infections are often blamed for the death of a patient when the real cause, malnutrition, was not addressed by the clinician.[16] It is important to remember that malnutrition, if not present on admission, may become apparent during hospitalization for a variety of reasons, often because of a combination of several factors (see Practices Adversely Affecting the Nutritional Status of a Hospitalized Animal).

Three types of protein-energy malnutrition are described in human

Editor's Note: In keeping with the international scope of the *Compendium®* subscription base, readers will note that the integrity of British English has been preserved in this review article.

Practices Adversely Affecting the Nutritional Status of a Hospitalized Animal

Failure to record daily weight

Failure to observe, measure, and record the amount of food consumed

Delay of nutritional support until the patient is in an irreversible state of depletion

Withholding food because of diagnostic tests

Failure to recognize and treat increased nutritional needs brought about by injury or illness

Failure to appreciate the role of nutrition in the prevention of and recovery from infection; unwarranted reliance on drugs

Prolonged administration of glucose and electrolyte solutions

Rotation of staff at frequent intervals and diffusion of responsibility for patient care

Inadequate post-operative nutritional support

Limited availability of laboratory tests to assess nutritional status

medicine: kwashiorkor, marasmus, and mixed marasmus and kwashiorkor (marasmic kwashiorkor).[17] Kwashiorkor develops acutely and is associated with low serum proteins in the absence of loss of skeletal muscle and fat stores. Kwashiorkor arises as a consequence of inadequate protein intake, increased protein catabolism, imbalance in protein and carbohydrate intake, or a combination of factors and often results in immunoincompetence. Marasmus is associated with general wasting of skeletal muscle and fat stores as a consequence of chronic undernutrition associated with chronic wasting diseases. Serum protein levels may be maintained within normal limits. Mixed marasmus–kwashiorkor is the most severe form of protein-energy malnutrition and arises from stress or trauma in chronically malnourished animals. Mixed marasmus–kwashiorkor is characterized by depletion of skeletal muscle mass, fat stores, and serum protein concentrations.

The provision of adequate nutrition in medical and surgical patients is essential to avoid protein-energy malnutrition and thus to maximize the effectiveness of other treatments. The consequences of malnutrition include immunoincompetence, depletion of en-

ergy stores, weakness, delayed wound healing, and organ failure.[16,18] These changes may occur within three to five days of anorexia and will increase a patient's susceptibility to infection and shock.

Previously well-nourished patients with acute medical or surgical problems of anticipated short duration and that generally resume eating upon resolution of disease are usually not candidates for nutritional support. On the other hand, chronically debilitated patients that face a situation in which food intake is likely to be reduced for an extended period of time or that are anorectic and have an increased metabolic rate (hypermetabolic) should be considered for nutritional support. In small animal medicine, failure to appreciate the importance of providing adequate nutrition to the chronically ill patient is probably the most important type of malnutrition that is seen.

NUTRITIONAL ASSESSMENT

The clinical indices of nutritional status have been reviewed recently.[19] In general, some form of support is needed whenever a patient is unable or unwilling to eat.

The approximate basal energy requirement (BER) of small animal patients can be calculated using the following formulae (KJ = kilojoule; 4.2 KJ = 1 kilocalorie [kcal]):

For all patients,
$$\text{BER (KJ)} = 70 \times (\text{body weight [kg]})^{0.75} \times 4.18$$

or

For patients weighing between 2 and 40 kg,
$$\text{BER (KJ)} = 70 + (30 \times \text{body weight [kg]}) \times 4.18$$

To calculate the illness-energy requirement (IER), the basal energy requirement must be multiplied by an illness factor of between 1.3 and 2 for dogs, with the higher number used for animals with greater nutrient requirements, and 1.4 for cats. For example, the illness factor for a dog resting in a cage would be 1.3; for a dog with severe trauma, this factor would be increased to 1.6; and for a patient with serious burns, the factor would be 2. The illness-energy requirement is calculated as:

$$\text{Volume of food (ml/day)} = \frac{\text{IER (KJ)}}{\text{energy density of the food (KJ/ml)}}$$

The protein requirement of a normal dog is approximately 1 g/100 KJ/day and of a cat approximately 1.5 g/100 KJ/day.[20] If renal or liver disease is present, these requirements may need to be reduced to 0.5 g/100 KJ/day and 1 g/100 KJ/day, respectively. For

Possible Indications for Enteral Nutritional Support

Recent weight loss of more than 10% of the body weight

Recent severe trauma or major surgery

Poor body condition (e.g., easily depilated hair, cracked and split nails, non-healing wounds, oedema, ascites, and muscle atrophy)

Decreased food intake or anorexia for more than three days

Increased nutrient losses from diarrhoea, wounds, or burns

Increased needs due to trauma, infection, pyrexia, or neoplasia

Chronic disease processes

Low serum albumin, anaemia, and/or lymphopenia

Use of drugs that promote catabolism (e.g., corticosteroids) or anorexia (e.g., digoxin, chemotherapeutic drugs)

Routes Available for Enteral Nutrition[27]

Force-feeding with a syringe
Orogastric intubation
Nasogastric/nasooesophageal intubation
Pharyngostomy tube feeding
Oesophagostomy tube feeding
Gastrostomy tube feeding
Gastroduodenostomy tube feeding
Jejunostomy tube feeding

chronically ill patients with marked protein malnutrition (i.e., patients with muscle wastage or hypoalbuminaemia), the protein requirements will be higher than normal.

Prior to the provision of nutritional support, pre-existing fluid or acid-base deficits should be corrected. Subsequently, the route of support and the nature of the nutrients to be provided should be established. Two routes of nutritional support may be used in small animal medicine. Enteral nutrition, which is the provision of a patient's nutritional requirements via a functional gastrointestinal tract, is the commonest method of nutritional support. Some of the criteria for the use of enteral nutrition are listed in Possible Indications for Enteral Nutritional Support. Parenteral nutrition, which is the provision of nutrients by the intravenous route, requires specialized equipment and on-site laboratory facilities. The indications for parenteral nutrition are limited to patients with gastrointestinal failure (e.g., protracted vomiting, inflammatory bowel disease, pancreatitis, severe burns, and peritonitis). Parenteral nutrition is rarely used in general practice (outside specialist referral centres).

ENTERAL NUTRITIONAL SUPPORT

Several routes are available for the provision of nu-

trients enterally (see Routes Available for Enteral Nutrition). Force-feeding with a syringe, orogastric intubation, or surgical placement of a pharyngostomy tube have been the commonest methods used. However, more recently these methods have been superseded by the increased use of nasal feeding and gastrostomy tubes.[16] Oesophagostomy tubes have been used[16] but offer little advantage over pharyngostomy tubes and may increase the risk of oesophageal stricture formation. The indications for gastroduodenostomy and jejunostomy tubes are limited to cases of intractable vomiting and are therefore rarely used.

Syringe Feeding and Orogastric Intubation

Syringe feeding of liquid or canned food can be used for a few days on patients either in a hospital or home environment. However, liquids in particular should be administered slowly to reduce the risk of laryngotracheal aspiration of food.[21] Orogastric intubation can be used to deliver food into the stomach of hospitalized patients for two to three days.[21] However, for both methods, a cooperative patient is required. If a patient is uncooperative or nutritional support is intended to be prolonged, other enteral techniques should be considered.

Nasogastric/Nasooesophageal Intubation

The nasogastric/nasooesophageal route is probably the route of choice if endoscopic facilities are unavailable. Human infant feeding tubes may be passed through the external nares and oropharynx into the oesophagus or stomach. Such tubes are often called nasogastric or nasooesophageal tubes. However, in many cases, the exact position of the tube tip is not determined and therefore these tubes would be better referred to solely as nasal feeding tubes.

Prior to tube placement, the nostril is anaesthetized with lidocaine or proxymetacaine hydrochloride

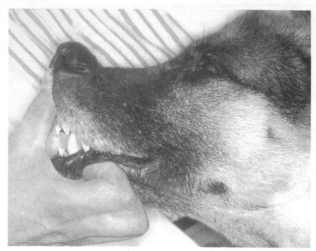

Figure 1—Placement of a nasal feeding tube in a dog. The nose is pushed dorsally to facilitate passage of the nasogastric tube into the ventral meatus.

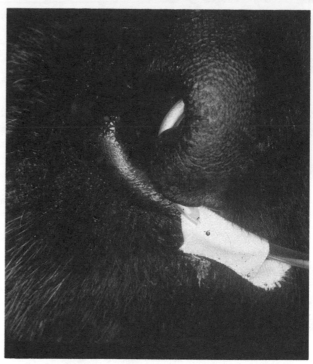

Figure 2—The nasal feeding tube is tucked under the alar fold to reduce the risk of being dislodged by the patient.

(proparacaine) drops. The tube is lubricated with a water-soluble lubricant and passed in a caudoventral medial direction into the ventrolateral aspect of the external nares. A wire stylet may occasionally be needed to facilitate passage of the tube. The patient's head should be in a normal position. In cats, the tube is then advanced into the ventral meatus and subsequently into the pharynx. In dogs, placing digital pressure on the nose so that the external nares are deviated dorsally facilitates passage of the tube into the ventral rather than medial meatus[22] (Figure 1). Advancement of the tube into the pharynx should elicit a swallowing reflex, thereby allowing its passage into the oesophagus and subsequent placement in the distal oesophagus (the preferred location) or in the stomach. If the tube enters the trachea, then air will be aspirated and the infusion of a sterile saline solution will induce coughing. The tube should be withdrawn and replaced. Once in place, zinc oxide tape should be wrapped around the tube and secured with permanent adhesive to the hair to ensure that the tube is tightly tucked into the alar fold (Figure 2). The tube can then be taken over the top of the head (Figure 3) or round the side of the face.

As a general rule, the widest tube that the patient can accommodate should be used. Five or 6 French tubes are suitable in most cases, although in large-breed dogs 8 French or wider tubes may be placed. An Elizabethan collar may be required to prevent the patient from dislodging the tube. The tube can remain in position for several weeks and is usually well tolerated by the patient. For the smaller diameter tubes (5 and 6 French), commercial liquid diets are used; whereas liquidized canned food can be successfully used in tubes of 8 French or larger.

Pharyngostomy Tube Feeding

Pharyngostomy tubes should be placed through the lateral aspect of the oropharynx into the oesophagus while the patient is under general anaesthesia[16] (Figure 4). In the cat, an 8 to 14 French tube may be used; and in the dog, a 12 to 28 French tube can be placed. The tube can remain in place for several days. Feeding can be accomplished through the larger-bore tubing by administering liquidized canned food. Pharyngostomy tubes placed according to the original Bohning technique may be associated with gagging, partial airway obstruction (particularly in cats and brachycephalic dogs), and aspiration pneumonia. A modified technique has been reported whereby the pharyngostomy tube is placed distal to the hyoid apparatus and immediately rostral to the start of the oesophagus.[23] This modification reduces tube interference with the airway. However, the popularity of the pharyngostomy tube has declined in favour of other forms of feeding.

Gastrostomy Tube Feeding

The use of gastrostomy tubes is increasing in small animal medicine because of the development of techniques which allow tube placement percutaneously without the need for a laparotomy.[24] The materials needed for the placement of percutaneous endoscopic gastrostomy (PEG) tubes are:

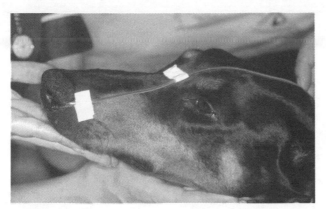

Figure 3—A nasal feeding tube positioned over the top of a dog's head.

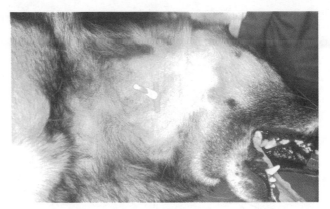

Figure 4—A pharyngostomy tube in a dog.

- Flexible endoscope with biopsy or foreign body retrieval forceps
- Scalpel blade
- Two strands of monofilament nylon (1 metric)
- Cutting needle
- An 18-gauge intravenous catheter
- A 0.1-ml disposable pipette tip
- A de Pezzer (mushroom tip) urological catheter.

Gastrostomy tubes for use in humans are available but expensive.

Prior to placement of a percutaneous endoscopic gastrostomy tube, the animal should be fasted for 12 hours. The de Pezzer catheter is modified by discarding the wide end of the catheter. Two 2-cm flanges are cut from the end of the tube, and a stab incision is made through the centre of each flange. One flange is then slipped over the tube until it rests adjacent to the mushroom tip. The nipple tip of the mushroom is then removed (Figure 5). The anaesthetized patient is placed in right lateral recumbency. The area extending approximately 15 cm behind the last rib on the left flank should be clipped and surgically prepared. The endoscope is passed down the oesophagus into the stomach, which is then inflated by insufflation of air. The endoscope light should be visible through the left flank, and a small skin incision is then made caudal to the last rib in the dorsal two thirds of the flank. An intravenous catheter is passed through the skin into the lumen of the stomach. It may be necessary to push the transilluminated spleen out of the path of the intravenous catheter. The stylet is removed, and the nylon suture material is threaded through the catheter into the stomach and grasped by the biopsy forceps (Figure 6). It is necessary to place a finger over the catheter to prevent deflation of the stomach.

The endoscope, biopsy forceps, and suture material are pulled from the mouth as one unit; and the catheter is removed from the stomach. The nylon is

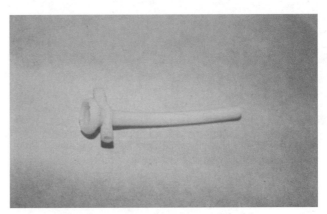

Figure 5—The de Pezzer catheter is modified by removing and discarding the wider end of the tube. Two flanges are cut from the end of the tube, and a small incision is made through each of them. One is slid over the tube to lie against the mushroom tip. The nipple part of the catheter head is removed.

passed through the narrow end of the pipette tip and sutured securely to the gastrostomy tube (Figure 7). The second piece of nylon is sutured as a loop through the mushroom tip, but not tied. If any difficulty is encountered during placement, the tube can be removed through the mouth by applying traction on the suture material. After successful placement, the suture material can be removed by pulling on one end. As the nylon exiting through the abdominal wall is pulled steadily, the tube passes down the oesophagus into the stomach. As the pipette tip abutts the stomach wall, resistance will be encountered. Firm application of digital counterpressure to the abdominal wall and the exertion of steady traction on the suture are required to pull the pipette tip out through the stomach and body wall (Figure 8). The pipette tip may be grasped with a pair of artery forceps to make it easier to pull the tube out. The skin incision may need to be carefully extended (by 2 to 3 mm) to assist this procedure. The gastrostomy tube is posi-

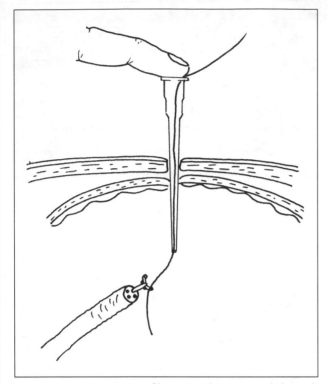

Figure 6—A 1-metric monofilament nylon is passed through the catheter into the stomach, and a finger is placed over the catheter to prevent deflation of the stomach. The suture material is then grasped using the biopsy forceps.

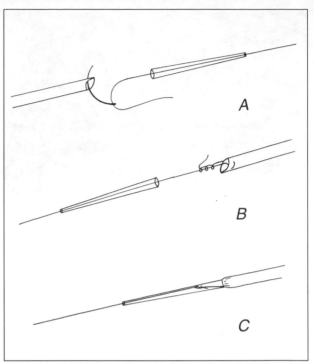

Figure 7—(*A*) The monofilament nylon is passed through the pipette tip and is sutured to the percutaneous endoscopic gastrostomy tube. (*B*) The monofilament nylon is tied to the tube. (*C*) The tube is pulled into the wider end of the pipette tip.

tioned so that the internal flange gently abutts the mucosa. The second flange is slid over the tube until it lies on the skin (Figure 9). The endoscope can be re-introduced into the stomach to ensure correct placement, but the stomach should not be further insufflated. Air can then be aspirated from the stomach and the tube capped with a catheter bung.

To prevent flange removal or tube migration, a piece of zinc oxide tape can be wrapped around the tube distal to the external flange; there is no need to suture the tube in place. Antimicrobial ointment on a gauze swab may be applied to the exit site, and a conforming stretch bandage can be used to protect the tube. This may need to be changed within the first three days but subsequently only if soiled or dislodged.

Alternatively, a Foley catheter can be placed at laparotomy into the stomach and used as a gastrostomy tube.[25] This tube can be sutured to the abdominal wall to prevent migration.

Gastrostomy tubes should remain in place for at least five days before removal. To remove a percutaneous endoscopic gastrostomy tube, firm traction should be exerted on the tube whilst counterpressure is being applied to skin around the ostomy site. The mushroom tip will collapse as it is pulled through the skin, whilst the flange only remains in the stomach. In dogs heavier than 10 kg, gentle traction may be applied to the tube which can then be cut off flush with the skin to allow the mushroom tip to drop into the gastric lumen and eventually be passed in the faeces. The Foley catheter is removed by deflating the balloon and pulling the catheter out.

Food should be withheld for 12 hours after gastrostomy tube removal. The gastrocutaneous fistula which is present heals rapidly. These tubes may remain in place for several months with few complications. Liquidized canned food or commercial liquid diets can be administered with relative ease through a gastrostomy tube.

METHODS OF FEEDING

Irrespective of the type of tube used, certain guidelines should be followed for enteral nutrition to be successful. With nasal feeding tubes, prior to the administration of each meal a test injection of a small bolus of air should produce bubbling sounds if placed in the stomach whilst an injection of 2 ml of sterile saline solution will produce coughing if incorrectly placed in the trachea. The animal should be standing in an upright position (Figure 10) or placed in sternal or right lateral recumbency for feeding.

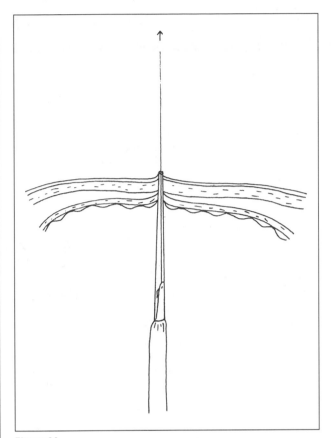

Figure 8A

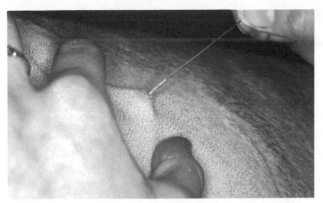

Figure 8B

Figure 8—(**A**) The pipette tip acts as a guide to facilitate the passage of the tube through the stomach and body wall. (**B**) Traction is applied to the suture material in order to pull the tube through the skin.

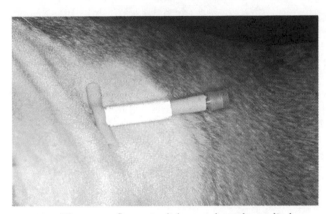

Figure 9—The outer flange is slid over the tube to lie loosely on the skin. Zinc oxide tape is wrapped around the tube to prevent the flange from slipping off the tube.

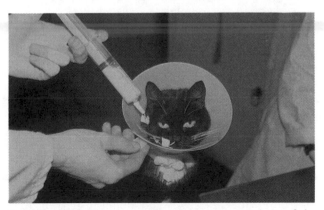

Figure 10—While in an upright position, a cat is being fed a liquidized canned food through a feeding tube.

Tube feeding may be administered continuously by gravity or with an enteral pump or, more commonly, by intermittent boluses. In critically ill patients, continuous infusion is recommended at an initial flow rate of 1 ml/kg/hr and increased gradually over 48 hours until the total daily volume can be given over a 12- to 18-hour period.[16] However, if overfilling of the stomach occurs, the rate should be reduced.

With bolus feeding, the required volume of food should be divided into six feeds initially and given every four hours. The volume given at each feed can be increased up to a maximum of 90 ml/kg of body weight for dogs and 50 ml/kg of body weight for cats, as tolerance allows. However, no more than one third of the total daily volume should be given at any one time. The volume to be fed should be given at room temperature and over a 5- to 10-minute period to reduce the incidence of vomiting or regurgitation. If either of these should occur, feeding should be stopped immediately and the mouth cleared of food to reduce the risk of inhalation of the food. After feeding, the tube should be flushed with 5 ml of water and capped. Water is left in the tube in order to keep the tube patent.

The patient should be observed for a few minutes after feeding for signs of discomfort or vomiting. It is essential that all feedings are recorded on the patient's case record, along with any problems encountered. All patients receiving enteral nutrition should be weighed daily.

Animals with feeding tubes are usually able to eat voluntarily and should, as they respond to treatment, be offered food. The feeding tube can be removed once the patient voluntarily consumes 75% of its daily caloric intake. Hospitalization is necessary during the initial stages of nutritional support. However, many patients can be discharged with the feeding tube in place, as most owners are able to accept the presence of the tube and to manage it successfully.

COMPLICATIONS

Complications of enteral feeding include mechanical, gastrointestinal, metabolic, or infectious problems. The most common mechanical problem is tube occlusion, which should be an infrequent problem as long as liquid diets are used with fine-bore tubes and liquidized canned diets are sieved through a pharyngostomy or gastrostomy tube prior to administration through pharyngostomy or gastrostomy tubes. If occlusion does occur, the tube should be flushed with water or replaced if this is unsuccessful. Pharyngostomy and occasionally nasal feeding tubes may compromise oropharyngeal function; such patients may present with gagging, regurgitation, airway occlusion, or aspiration pneumonia. Susceptible patients, cats and brachycephalic dogs in particular, should be monitored regularly for any signs of oropharyngeal discomfort. Regurgitation of nasooesophageal tubes is occasionally seen in dogs and more frequently in cats. The use of tubes with weighted ends may help to prevent this.

Gastrointestinal complications include vomiting and bloat due to rapid administration of food or obstruction of the pylorus by the mushroom tip if the tube should migrate into the stomach. Diarrhoea may also be seen, possibly associated with the use of hyperosmolar solutions, a low-fibre intake, lactose intolerance, too rapid delivery, or (most likely) administration of drugs.

Metabolic, fluid, and electrolyte abnormalities are uncommon with uncomplicated cases in which a food formulated specifically for dogs or cats is used. However, careful attention to the dietary make-up is necessary where organ dysfunction, such as renal or hepatic failure, is present.

Infectious complications are generally restricted to ostomy sites associated with pharyngostomy or gastrostomy tubes. Necrosis and cellulitis at an ostomy site may occur if there is excessive pressure on or too large an incision in the skin. With percutaneous endoscopic gastrostomy tubes in particular, some discharge from the ostomy site is commonly encountered for up to seven days after tube placement. This discharge is usually self-limiting but may occasionally develop into a more serious diffuse cellulitis. Cellulitis may also develop as a result of the leakage of gastric contents if the exit site for gastrostomy tubes are too far ventral in the body wall.

CONCLUSION

In conclusion, enteral nutrition is an essential therapeutic tool in the support and maintenance of the critically ill patient. For it to be successful requires careful management of the patient, the avoidance of factors which will compromise an animal's nutrition, and the provision of nutrition at an early stage of the disease process.

ACKNOWLEDGMENTS

The authors are grateful to Hill's Pet Products Limited for its funding of the clinical nutrition residency and to Intervet Laboratories UN for their funding of the feline residency at The University of Liverpool.

About the Authors

Drs. Tennant and Willoughby are affiliated with the Department of Veterinary Clinical Science and Animal Husbandry, Faculty of Veterinary Science, The University of Liverpool, Liverpool, United Kingdom.

REFERENCES

1. Studley HO: Percentage of weight loss: A basic indicator of surgical risk in patients with chronic peptic ulcer. *JAMA* 106:458–460, 1936.
2. Seltzer MH, Bastidas JA, Cooper DM, et al: Instant nutritional assessment. *J Parenter Enteral Nutr* 3:157–159, 1979.
3. McLaren DS, Meguid MM: Nutritional assessment at the crossroads. *J Parenter Enteral Nutr* 7:575–579, 1983.
4. Long CL: Nutritional assessment of the critically ill patient, in Wright RA, Heymslfield S (ed): *Nutritional Assessment.* Boston, Blackwell Scientific Publications, 1984.
5. Mughal NM, Meguid MM: The effect of nutritional status on morbidity after elective surgery for benign gastrointestinal disease. *J Parenter Enteral Nutr* 11:140–143, 1987.
6. Curtas S, Chapman G, Meguid MM: Evaluation of nutritional status. *Nurs Clin North Am* 24:301–313, 1989.
7. Border JR, Chenier R, McMenamy RH, et al: Multiple systems organ failure: Muscle fuel deficit with visceral protein malnutrition. *Surg Clin North Am* 56:1147–1167, 1976.
8. Baker CC, Oppenheimer L, Stephens B, et al: Epidemiology of trauma deaths. *Am J Surg* 140:144–148, 1980.
9. Fry DE, Pearlstein L, Fulton RL, Polk HC: Multiple system organ failure. *Arch Surg* 115:136–140, 1980.
10. Goris RJA, Draaisma J: Causes of death after blunt trauma. *J Trauma* 22:141–146, 1982.
11. Bistrian BR, Blackburn GL, Hallowell E, et al: Protein status of general surgical patients. *JAMA* 230:858–860, 1974.
12. Bistrian BR, Blackburn GL, Vitale J, et al: Prevalence of malnutrition in general medical patients. *JAMA* 235:1567–1570, 1976.
13. Hill GL, Blackett RL, Pickford I, et al: Malnutrition in surgical patients. An unrecognised problem. *Lancet* 1:689–692, 1977.
14. Wilcutts HD: Nutritional assessment of 1000 surgical pa-

tients in an affluent suburban community hospital. *J Parenter Enteral Nutr* 1:25, 1977.

15. Butterworth CE: The skeleton in the hospital closet. *Nutr Today*:4–8, 1974.

16. Crowe DT: Nutritional support for the hospitalized patient: An introduction to tube feeding. *Compend Contin Educ Pract Vet* 12(12):1711–1720, 1990.

17. Haider M, Haider SQ: Assessment of protein-calorie malnutrition. *Clin Chim Acta* 3:1286–1299, 1984.

18. Remillard RL: Gastrointestinal disease. Nutritional dietary management. *Vet Med Report* 1:418–430, 1989.

19. Carnevale JM, Kallfelz FA, Chapman G, Meguid MM: Nutritional assessment: Guidelines to selecting patients for nutritional support. *Compend Contin Educ Pract Vet [European Edition]* 13(2):115–122, 1991.

20. Donoghue S: Nutritional support of hospitalized patients. *Vet Clin North Am* 19:475–495, 1989.

21. Lewis LD, Morris ML, Hand MS: Anorexia, in *Small Animal Clinical Nutrition. III.* Topeka, KS, Mark Morris Associates, 1987, pp 5-20 to 5-21.

22. Abood SA, Buffington CA: Improved nasogastric intubation technique for administration of nutritional support in dogs. *JAVMA* 199:577–579, 1991.

23. Crowe DT, Downs MD: Pharyngostomy complications in dogs and cats and recommended technical modifications: Experimental and clinical investigations. *JAAHA* 22:493–503, 1986.

24. Armstrong PJ, Hardie EM: Percutaneous endoscopic gastrostomy. *Vet Med Report* 1:404–411, 1989.

25. DeHoff WD: Right-side tube gastrostomy, in Bojrab MJ (ed): *Current Techniques in Small Animal Surgery.* London, Lea & Febiger, 1990, pp 218–221.

26. Mobarhan S, Trumbore LS: Enteral tube feeding: A clinical perspective on recent advances. *Nutr Rev* 49:129–140, 1991.

Partial Hepatectomy *(continued from page 199)*

20. Cromheecke M, Wijffels RT, Meijer D, et al: Hepatic resection: Haemostatic control by means of compression sutures: A new method. *Neth J Surg* 43:95–98, 1991.

21. Lee KS, Kim BR: The banding method as a simplified technique for resection of the liver. *Surg Gynecol Obstet* 167:77–78, 1988.

22. Mies S, Raia S: A simple method for controlling hemorrhage during hepatectomy. *Surg Gynecol Obstet* 168:265–266, 1989.

23. Ivatury RR, Nallathambi M, Gunduz Y, et al: Liver packing for uncontrolled hemorrhage: A reappraisal. *J Trauma* 26:744–753, 1986.

KEY FACTS

- Aspiration pneumonia is seen with certain esophageal disorders.
- Many animals with cases of myasthenia gravis do not present with a history of peripheral weakness or collapsing episodes, but rather regurgitation secondary to megaesophagus.
- The diagnosis of esophagitis is usually made by endoscopic visualization of the esophageal mucosa.
- The advantages of balloon dilation over bougienage for treatment of esophageal stricture include decreased risk of perforation, longer period free of signs between procedures, and decreased number of procedures required.
- Foreign bodies typically lodge in the thoracic inlet, the base of the heart, or cranial to the gastroesophageal junction.

Medical Diseases of the Esophagus

Dennis A. Zawie, DVM
Diplomate, ACVIM
Farmingville Animal Hospital
Farmingville, New York

Anatomy of the Esophagus

The esophagus has four distinct microscopic layers: (1) the mucosa, which is lined by stratified squamous epithelium; (2) the submucosa, which contains glands, nerves, and blood vessels; (3) the muscle layer; and (4) the fibrous outercoat. In dogs, the muscle layer of the esophagus is composed entirely of striated muscle. In cats, the cranial two thirds of the esophagus is striated muscle and the distal one third is smooth muscle.[1] Branches of the thyroid arteries supply blood to the cervical esophagus; the bronchoesophageal arteries supply the cranial portion of the thoracic esophagus; and branches of the aorta, intercostals, and gastric arteries supply the remaining portion.

Two primary sphincters of physiologic importance are present in the esophagus. The cricopharyngeal, or upper esophageal, sphincter is composed of fibers from both the cricopharyngeus and thyropharyngeus muscles. This area between the oropharynx and esophagus remains closed except when a bolus of ingesta passes. The upper esophageal sphincter is an important aspect of the swallowing mechanism and necessary for the initiation of synchronous esophageal function.[1] The gastroesophageal, or lower esophageal, sphincter is located at the gastroesophageal junction. This is a true physiologic sphincter.[1] It is functionally important because it prevents reflux of gastric contents into the esophagus.

Physiology of Swallowing and Esophageal Motility

The sensory pathway of swallowing begins in the pharynx when a bolus of ingesta is first encountered. Afferent nerve fibers (sensory fibers) from the pharynx course their way to the tractus solitarius and ultimately to the swallowing center located in the lateral reticular formation.[1,2] During swallowing, respiration is temporarily inhibited. Motor fibers (efferent nerves) from the swallowing center travel to the cell bodies of the lower motor neurons located in the nucleus ambiguus.[1,2] The lower motor neurons arrive at the esophagus via the vagus nerve. Once stimulated, regional muscular contractions are initiated and transport the bolus of ingesta aborally. This first wave of esophageal muscular contraction initiated by the swallowing reflex is called primary peristalsis.

Secondary peristalsis is identical to primary peristalsis, but it is initiated by distention of the esophagus with food. As food approaches the stomach, sensory information is sent to the lower esophageal sphincter, which then relaxes and allows the ingesta to pass from the esophagus to the stomach. As previously stated, the distal portion of the feline esophagus is made up of smooth muscle. Innervation is under control of parasympathetic fibers of the vagus nerve and the dorsal motor nucleus.[1,2]

Clinical Signs of Esophageal Disease

Regurgitation shortly after a meal is the classic clinical sign of esophageal disorders. Clinical signs can vary greatly, however, depending on the specific disease process present in the animal. For example, dysphagia, excessive salivation, and anorexia resulting from intense pain or discomfort are often associated with severe esophagitis or esophageal foreign bodies. In contrast, dogs and cats with megaesophagus, esophageal stricture, or vascular ring anomalies may have ravenous appetites accompanied by regurgitation of food. Aspiration pneumonia is seen with certain esophageal disorders; and coughing, lethargy, depression, dyspnea, and fever may be present.

Diseases of the Esophagus
Persistent Right Aortic Arch

Although a number of congenital vascular ring anomalies can occur in both dogs and cats, persistent right aortic arch is the most common.[3,4] In this condition, the right fourth aortic arch instead of the left aortic arch forms the aorta. The esophagus, therefore, becomes entrapped between the aorta on the right, the pulmonary artery on the left, the ligamentum arteriosum dorsally, and the trachea ventrally. This anatomic derangement results in obstruction and dilation of the esophagus cranial to the base of the heart. Affected puppies or kittens usually begin regurgitating as soon as they are placed on solid food. In addition, clinically affected animals are smaller than their normal littermates. Severe illness can occur if aspiration pneumonia develops. Although reported in several breeds, practitioners most frequently encounter this disorder in German shepherds. Diagnosis is based on survey radiographs of the thorax or a positive-contrast study of the esophagus (Figure 1). Surgical ligation and division of the ligamentum arteriosum should be performed as early in the clinical course as possible, before extensive esophageal fibrosis occurs or peristaltic activity is lost.

Megaesophagus

Megaesophagus refers to a disease syndrome characterized by a loss of esophageal motor function. Although megaesophagus is a commonly diagnosed esophageal disorder, the cause remains unknown. Results of direct nerve stimulation and electromyography in cases of mega-

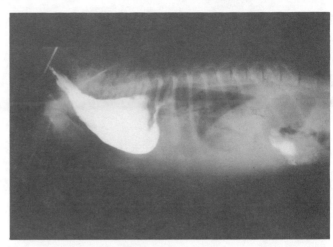

Figure 1—Lateral-view esophagram depicting a persistent right aortic arch. Note the characteristic dilation cranial to the heart base. Severe pneumonia is also evident in this animal.

esophagus have been normal; therefore, motor-unit disease is not considered to be the cause.[1,5] Currently, most investigators believe the lesion is located in either the sensory receptors, the afferent vagal fibers, or between the tractus solitarius and the swallowing centers.[2] The term *esophageal achalasia* has been used from time to time in the veterinary literature. In humans, achalasia is defined as a high-pressure area at the lower esophageal sphincter resulting in dilation and aperistalsis of the esophagus. Achalasia has not been reported in dogs.[2] Lower esophageal sphincter pressures in dogs with megaesophagus are normal; therefore, the term *achalasia* should not be used to describe canine megaesophagus.[5]

In the veterinary literature, megaesophagus is most frequently reported in young puppies; however, in my practice, the majority of cases are adult-onset. The disorder is inherited in the wirehaired terrier and schnauzer, and there is a high incidence in Great Danes, Irish setters, German shepherds, and golden retrievers.[1,2,4]

The history and clinical signs of canine megaesophagus vary dramatically. Classically affected dogs regurgitate food and water shortly after ingestion. Many dogs gag or retch tenacious, white foam many times per day. Some dogs consistently make a gurgling or rattling noise. This sound occurs when air enters the esophagus during respiration and flows through fluid and saliva retained in the esophageal lumen. Although difficult to comprehend, in a significant number of cases of megaesophagus (approximately 15%),[3] dogs exhibit no gastrointestinal signs. The majority of dogs with megaesophagus have normal physical examinations; however, in spite of ravenous appetites, they are thin as a result of the decreased caloric intake associated with chronic regurgitation. If aspiration pneumonia is present, such signs as fever, lethargy, anorexia, cough, dyspnea, and nasal discharge can be seen.

Megaesophagus has been reported in myasthenia gravis, polymyositis, hypoadrenocorticism, lead poisoning, and systemic lupus erythematosus.[4] The clinical signs and

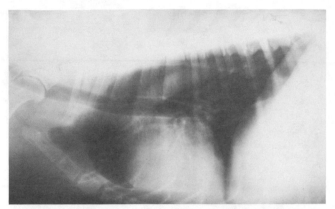

Figure 2—Lateral thoracic radiograph of a dog with a large, dilated, air-filled esophagus characteristic of megaesophagus.

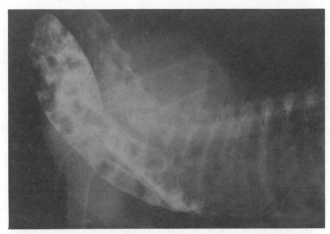

Figure 3—Lateral thoracic radiograph of a dog with megaesophagus filled with food and barium.

physical findings in these instances can reflect a more systemic illness. Myasthenia gravis is of particular interest. Many animals with cases of myasthenia gravis do not present with a history of peripheral weakness or collapsing episodes, but rather they present for regurgitation secondary to megaesophagus. Further examination generally reveals a bilaterally absent blink response. The eventual diagnosis is based on electromyography, a Tensilon® test, the presence of serum antireceptor antibodies, and special stains of muscle receptors.

Diagnosis of megaesophagus is usually based on routine thoracic radiographs (Figure 2). Esophagrams and esophagoscopy can be performed but are often unnecessary (Figure 3). Animals with megaesophagus should be fed in an upright position. It is sometimes helpful for the owner to keep an animal with megaesophagus in an upright position for 10 to 15 minutes after the meal has been completed to allow gravity to aid in the transport of food to the stomach. The animal can be fed either a gruel or small boluses of canned dog food. Animals must be considered as individuals; the form of diet fed may vary from case to case. Parenteral administration of broad-spectrum antibiotics is indicated if aspiration pneumonia is present. Chloramphenicol, trimethoprim-sulfa, and the cephalosporins are commonly used. Ideally, culture and sensitivity tests are done on a tracheal wash so that the appropriate antibiotic can be administered. If the animal is seriously ill, intravenous fluids are often necessary to maintain hydration and proper electrolyte balance.

In general, the prognosis for megaesophagus is poor. Because aspiration pneumonia is so commonly seen with the condition and because medical management is difficult for the majority of owners, most animals are euthanatized shortly after the diagnosis is made.[2]

Megaesophagus rarely occurs in cats.[2,3] It must be remembered that the anatomy and physiology of the feline esophagus are entirely different from those of the dog; as a result, the pathogenesis of feline and canine idiopathic megaesophagus is not the same.[2] Esophageal dilation has been reported in cats (especially Siamese) with pyloric obstruction. Pyloromyotomy has been successful in some

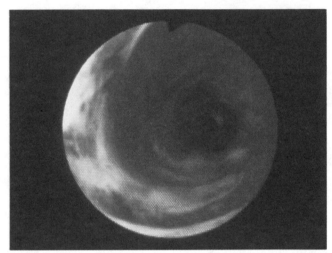

Figure 4—Endoscopic view of severe esophagitis following routine ovariohysterectomy in a dog.

cases.[3] Megaesophagus has been seen in cases of feline myasthenia gravis.[3] In addition, megaesophagus may be both clinical and physical findings in feline dysautonomia (Key-Gaskell syndrome). Dilated, nonresponsive pupils, constipation, and dry mucous membranes are other common features of this disease.[6]

Esophagitis

Esophagitis can result from the ingestion of a strong acid or alkali, thermal burns, trauma caused by foreign bodies, or reflux of gastric fluid into the esophagus (Figure 4). Acute, ulcerative esophagitis can occur in cats with upper respiratory infections caused by calicivirus, but that finding is rarc.[3] Reflux is the most common cause of esophagitis in dogs and cats and is most frequently encountered after general anesthesia.[7] Preanesthetic and anesthetic agents cause the lower esophageal sphincter to relax and suppress normal esophageal motility, predisposing the esophagus to gastric reflux. Hydrochloric acid can reduce esophageal pH to 2.0 and cause protein denaturation of the esophageal mucosa.[8]

In addition, pepsinogen is activated to pepsin at a low pH. Because of pepsin's proteolytic properties, further tissue destruction occurs.[8] Bile salts and pancreatic enzymes also play a role in the formation of esophageal inflammation.[8] Once esophagitis is present, the lower esophageal sphincter becomes incompetent and predisposes the esophagus to further reflux of gastric juice, thereby perpetuating the inflammation.[8] Contact time between esophageal mucosa and destructive elements within gastric fluid plays an important role in the formation of esophagitis. In addition to the anesthetic agents used, tilting of the surgery table and poor patient preparation (food-filled stomach) before surgery predispose animals to reflux esophagitis.[4] The clinical signs of esophagitis vary depending on the degree of inflammation present. In mild cases of esophagitis, repeated attempts at swallowing as well as decreased appetite are sometimes seen. In more severe cases, intense pain can result and lead to total anorexia, dysphagia, and excessive salivation.

The diagnosis of esophagitis is usually made by endoscopic visualization of the esophageal mucosa. Plain radiographs and esophagrams are unrewarding. Rarely is a biopsy necessary to make an accurate diagnosis. In many cases, esophagitis is suggested by the history alone, especially if signs of esophageal dysfunction begin shortly after an anesthetic procedure.

Mild esophagitis generally resolves without therapy; however, in severe cases cimetidine (Tagamet®—Smith Kline & French) is routinely used to increase gastric pH and allow time for esophageal healing. The drug is given orally or parenterally at a dose of 5 mg/kg three times a day.[3,4] Viscous xylocaine can be administered to decrease pain. Some veterinary gastroenterologists add metaclopramide (Reglan®— A. H. Robins) to the treatment regimen. This drug increases lower esophageal pressure and increases the strength of esophageal contractions. The drug is given either orally or by subcutaneous injection at a dose of 0.2 to 0.5 mg/kg three times a day. It is often helpful to give metaclopramide 30 minutes before meals and before bedtime. Occasionally, esophageal damage is so extensive that corticosteroids are used to decrease the chance of stricture formation. Small, frequent feedings of soft foods are recommended in the early stages of therapy.

Esophageal Stricture

When esophagitis is severe and extends into the deeper layers of the esophagus, fibroblastic proliferation takes

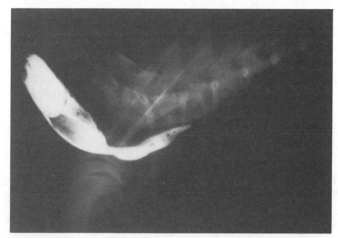

Figure 6A

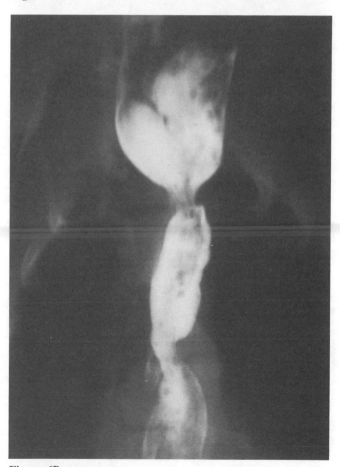

Figure 6B

Figure 6—(A) Lateral view of an esophagram showing an esophageal stricture at the thoracic inlet. (B) Ventrodorsal view.

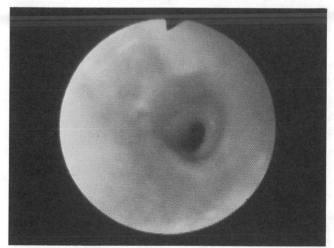

Figure 5—Endoscopic view of esophageal stricture that developed after gastrotomy to remove a Superball® in a one-year-old miniature poodle.

place and forms intraluminal scar tissue.[1,4] Animals with esophageal strictures exhibit signs of regurgitation and dysphagia. The onset of clinical signs may range from a few days to several weeks after the initial insult to the esophagus. Pain is not a hallmark of the disease process, and affected animals are often hungry but can only handle gruels or liquids.

Although endoscopic examination can be useful, most strictures are less than the diameter of the endoscope (approximately 9 mm). Thus, in the majority of cases the endoscope cannot be advanced through the stricture, so the extent of stricture formation cannot be assessed (Figure 5). Contrast radiography of the esophagus remains the best method of evaluating esophageal strictures (Figure 6).

Appropriate therapy for esophageal stricture depends on the length and the location of the stricture, the amount of scar tissue, and the extent of mucosal damage. Dilation of the esophagus can be established. Dilation is accomplished by passing graduated dilators or bougies through the fibrous band(s). It is imperative that proper equipment be used. This procedure (bougienage) must sometimes be repeated on several occasions before the desired effect is achieved and has a highly variable success rate.

Recently, a new technique using balloon catheters has been described for the treatment of esophageal strictures.[7]

A specially treated polyethylene catheter[a] is advanced to the stricture under fluoroscopic control. Once positioned properly, the catheter is inflated with dilute contrast medium (Figure 7). Luminal pressure is monitored with a manometer (Figure 8).[b] When adequate distention occurs, the

[a]Rigiflex Dilator—Microvasive Inc., 31 Maple St., Milford, MA 01757.
[b]Rigiflex Dilation Monitor—Microvasive Inc., 31 Maple St., Milford, MA 01757.

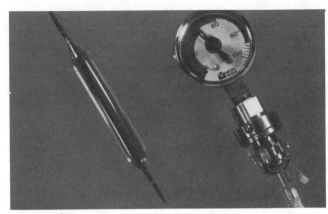

Figure 8—Shown are the polyethylene catheter, balloon inflated with contrast medium, and manometer used to measure balloon pressure.

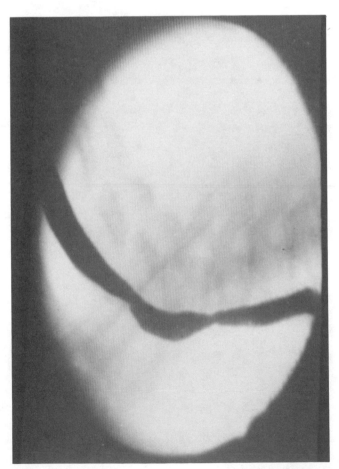

Figure 7—Lateral fluoroscopic view showing the polyethylene catheter in place and the balloon partially filled with contrast medium. The strictures can be seen as indentations in the balloon.

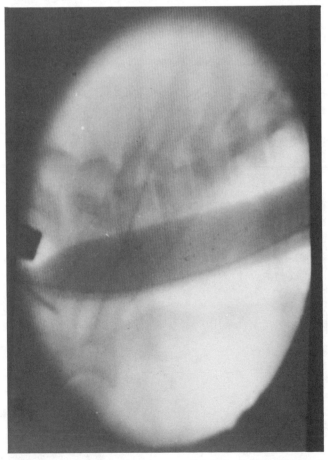

Figure 9—Lateral fluoroscopic view with balloon fully distended. No strictures are evident.

stricture visibly dilates (Figure 9). Balloon catheter dilation is superior to bougienage because greater force can be achieved to expand the stricture. The advantages of balloon dilation over bougienage include a decreased risk of esophageal perforation, a longer period free of clinical signs between procedures, and a decrease in the total number of procedures required.' General anesthesia is used to perform either bougienage or balloon dilation. Routine therapy for esophagitis is administered for two to three weeks after both balloon dilation and bougienage. Corticosteroids are always given to treat this disorder in hope of preventing further stricture formation. Generally, 1 to 2 mg/kg of prednisone or prednisolone divided to twice daily and slowly tapered over a 10-day to 14-day period is recommended.

Esophageal Foreign Bodies

Bones are the esophageal foreign bodies most commonly seen in dogs and cats; but other objects, such as pins, fishhooks, and bottle caps, can be encountered (Figures 10 and 11).[9] Animals usually present with an acute history of salivation and regurgitation; in some cases, there is forceful retching. Foreign bodies typically lodge in one of three places: (1) the thoracic inlet, (2) the base of the heart, or (3) cranial to the gastroesophageal junction.[9] Foreign objects in the esophagus are best evaluated and removed by endoscopy. Using an endoscope, the foreign body can be evaluated and removed with a forceps or gently pushed into the stomach (Figure 12).

Sequelae of esophageal foreign bodies would include intraluminal stricture, pulsion diverticula, or perforation. Animals that present with a perforated esophagus are seriously ill. Most are dehydrated, febrile, and septic. Pleural effusion is usually noted on thoracic radiographs. Fluid analysis reveals a septic exudate. An emergency thoracotomy is absolutely necessary for the patient's survival. It is obvious that the prognosis in such cases is extremely guarded.

Esophageal Neoplasms

Neoplasms of the esophagus are rare.[3,4,9] Squamous cell carcinoma would be the most common primary malignant tumor seen in both dogs and cats (Figure 13). Leiomyomas and carcinomas can also occur. Fibrosarcomas associated with the parasite *Spirocerca lupi* are seen in the southern United States. In addition, metastatic neoplasms are known to occur. In one study, metastatic thyroid neoplasms were the most common esophageal tumor seen.[10] Little can be done for patients with esophageal tumors. Surgical excision can be considered, but the prognosis is poor.

Esophageal Diverticula

Diverticula are saclike evaginations of one or more layers of the esophageal wall. Traction diverticula arise from extraluminal forces.[9] At one time, this type of diverticulum was common in humans infected with tuberculosis. Hilar lymph nodes often became abscessed and adhered to the esophageal wall. These extraluminal adhesions would then

contract, and a diverticulum would form. Traction diverticula are not reported in veterinary medicine. Pulsion diverticula arise from intraluminal forces and can result from

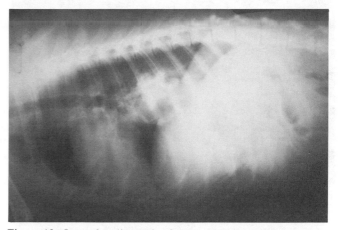

Figure 10—Lateral radiograph of dog with bone lodged near the gastroesophageal junction.

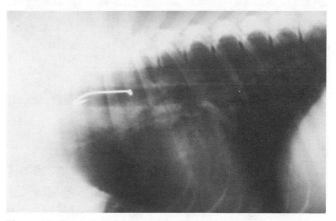

Figure 11—Lateral radiograph of a dog with a fishhook imbedded in its esophagus.

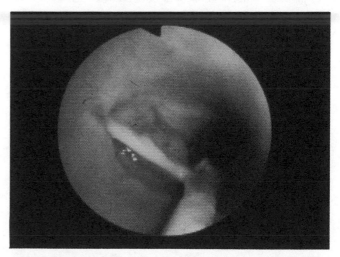

Figure 12—Endoscopic view of a small chicken rib bone lodged in the esophagus. The bone had been in the esophagus for 30 days.

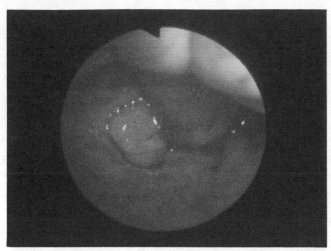

Figure 13—Endoscopic view of cat with an esophageal tumor. Histologic diagnosis was squamous cell carcinoma.

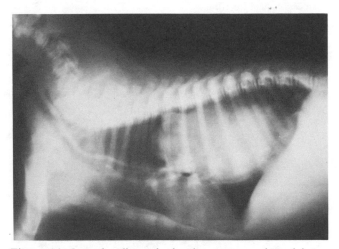

Figure 14—Lateral radiograph showing gastroesophageal intussusception.

foreign bodies and endoscopic procedures.[9] Diagnosis is based on survey radiographs, contrast studies, or endoscopy.

Periesophageal Masses

Heart-base tumors, rib tumors, cranial mediastinal masses, intrathoracic abscesses, and lung tumors can cause extraluminal compression of the esophagus resulting in clinical signs of esophageal disease.[3,4,9] Routine thoracic radiographs and contrast studies of the esophagus are helpful in establishing a diagnosis.

Miscellaneous Esophageal Disorders

Hiatal hernias, gastroesophageal intussusceptions, and bronchoesophageal fistulas have been reported in veterinary medicine but are uncommon findings (Figure 14).[3,4,9] Diagnosis is based on routine thoracic radiographs or contrast studies of the esophagus. All of these disorders can be treated surgically, and in some cases the outcome is favorable.

REFERENCES

1. Strombeck DR: Diseases of swallowing, in: *Small Animal Gastroenterology*. Davis, CA, Stonegate Publishing, 1979, pp 50-67.
2. Leib MS: Megaesophagus in the dog, in: Kirk RW (ed), *Current Veterinary Therapy IX*. Philadelphia, WB Saunders Co, 1986, pp 848-852.
3. Tams TR: Disorders causing regurgitation and vomiting in cats, in: *AAHA 1985 Scientific Proceedings* 52:229-235, 1985.
4. Zawie DA: Medical diseases of the esophagus, in: *AAHA 1980 Scientific Proceedings* 52:267-269, 1980.
5. Rogers WA, Fenner WR, Sherding RG: Electromyographic and esophagomanometric findings in clinically normal dogs and in dogs with idiopathic megaesophagus. *JAVMA* 173:181-183, 1979.
6. Sharp NJH, Nash AS: Feline dysautonomia, in: Kirk RW (ed): *Current Veterinary Therapy IX*. Philadelphia, WB Saunders Co, 1986, pp 802-804.
7. Burke RL, Zawie DA, Garvey MS: Balloon catheter dilation of intramural esophageal strictures in the dog and cat: A description of the procedure and a report of 6 cases. *Semin Vet Med Surg*, accepted for publication, 1987.
8. Pope CE: Gastroesophageal reflux disease, in: *Gastrointestinal Disease*, ed 3. Sleisenger MH, Fordtran JS (eds): Philadelphia, WB Saunders Co, 1983, pp 449-475.
9. Jones B: Esophageal diseases, in: *AAHA 1980 Scientific Proceedings* 47:259-265, 1980.
10. Ridgeway RL, Suter PF: Clinical and radiographic signs in primary and metastatic esophageal neoplasms of the dog. *JAVMA* 174:700-704, 1979.

Canine Parvovirus Infection: Effects on the Immune System and Factors That Predispose to Severe Disease

Cindy J. Brunner, PhD, DVM
Assistant Professor of Immunology

Larry J. Swango, DVM, PhD
Associate Professor of Virology

Department of Microbiology
College of Veterinary Medicine
Auburn University, Alabama

Canine parvovirus (CPV) disease emerged in 1978 as epizootic gastroenteritis of dogs often characterized by depression, inappetence, vomiting, diarrhea, and leukopenia.[1,2] The diarrhea was mucoid to hemorrhagic in more severe cases. The case-fatality ratio was high, although serologic surveys and limited epidemiologic studies revealed that most infections with CPV were subclinical.[3-5] CPV particles were observed in the feces of dogs with diarrhea in fall 1977[6]; however, it was not until spring 1978 that CPV was recognized as a canine pathogen.[1,2] Within a period of a few months in 1978, CPV disease had been recognized and confirmed on three continents—Australia, Europe, and North America.[1,2,7-9]—and soon thereafter it was confirmed on two more continents.[10,11]

The emergence of CPV on three continents almost simultaneously suggested a probable common source. Theories have been offered about the origin of CPV, but it has not been established. CPV is antigenically related to feline panleukopenia virus (FPV) and mink enteritis virus (MEV).[7,12,13] Restriction enzyme analyses have revealed that all strains of CPV examined are similar and are different from FPV and MEV.[14] This suggests that CPV probably did not arise from either FPV or MEV, although such a possibility exists.[14] CPV is distinctly different from a previously described nonpathogenic parvovirus isolated from dogs.[15] The nonpathogenic parvovirus from dogs is appropriately referred to as *canine parvovirus Type 1 (CPV-1)*, and the pathogenic CPV that emerged in 1978 is regarded as *CPV-2*.[16,17] Because CPV-1 is not easily isolated or readily detected and it is nonpathogenic, common usage of the abbreviations *parvo* and *CPV* refers to CPV-2; this terminology is used in this article without the Type 2 designation.

Numerous publications have been issued about CPV, CPV disease, and CPV vaccines since the virus was recognized as a canine pathogen in 1978. The properties of CPV and antigenic relatedness to FPV and MEV have been characterized.[13,14] The clinical, pathologic, and epizootiologic features of CPV disease have been described,[1,2] and the pathogenesis of CPV disease has been elucidated for the most part.[6,7,10-13,18,19] There still is a lack of understanding about the varied clinical responses of dogs to infection with virulent strains of CPV and the effects of CPV on the immune system. Much has been learned about the immunology of CPV infections and immunologic responses to CPV vaccines.[20-23]

Vaccine development progressed from the initial use of killed and attenuated FPV vaccines, through the MEV vaccine, to killed and attenuated CPV vaccines.[20-24] There are several good CPV vaccines now available that are safe and effective. Vaccination does not always result in immunization, though, primarily because of maternally derived antibody.[23-25] The occurrence of CPV disease in vaccinated pups and young dogs has resulted in misunderstanding about the safety and efficacy of CPV vaccines.[17,26] The idiosyncrasy of pups becoming susceptible to infection with virulent CPV when levels of maternally derived antibody are sufficient to interfere with immunization by vaccination is a factor in understanding so-called vaccine failures. Also, vaccination during the incubation period after infection with CPV may not prevent disease from occurring; this should not be regarded as "vaccine failure" or lack of safety of the vaccine. Concern has been expressed about the possible immunosuppressive effects of both virulent and attenuated strains of CPV on the immune system of dogs.[26,27] There is lack of definitive evidence in published reports to resolve the issue of immunosuppression by CPV.

The primary objectives of this article are to address factors that predispose dogs to severe disease and to discuss immunosuppression by CPV. Results of experimental studies are presented and related to published reports pertaining to these aspects of the virus–host interactions of CPV infections in dogs. Readers are encouraged to review selected references for more detailed discussions of other aspects of CPV and CPV disease.

Factors that Predispose to Severe CPV Disease

Caution must be exercised in drawing hard conclusions from clinical observations that are not confirmed by controlled studies. At times it is difficult to confirm experimentally certain observations that suggest disease patterns, and the lack of disease reporting precludes accurate assessment of conditions encountered in veterinary practice. Early attempts to experimentally reproduce severe, fatal CPV disease were generally unsuccessful.[11,28-30] The disease observed in the field by veterinarians was not reproducible. Serologic surveys indicated that severe clinical disease with high mortality was the exception rather than the rule for the outcome of CPV infections.[3-5,11,31,32] Most naturally occurring infections with CPV were subclinical or resulted in mild signs of disease that did not require veterinary care. It was concluded that the morbidity was less than 20%, and the mortality was less than 5%—perhaps no more than 1%.[31,32] These findings were disparate from experiences in some kennels, pet stores, and animal shelters where morbidity in pups exceeded 90% and mortality was greater than 50%. Additional factors apparently affected the pathophysiologic consequences of infection with CPV.

Age

The consequences of gastroenteritis are severer in the young of any species because of the effects of electrolyte imbalance and dehydration from vomiting and diarrhea in neonates.[33] The target cells for CPV enteritis are the crypt cells of the small intestine. Crypt cells normally have a high mitotic index, and it is even higher in rapidly growing puppies. Therefore, CPV would replicate more efficiently in young pups and would be expected to cause severer disease. The severity of clinical disease has been shown to correlate with the extent of CPV replication.[19] In addition to the normally higher mitotic activity of crypt cells in the small intestine, the ubiquitous presence of intestinal parasites in puppies may enhance further the severity of CPV infection by stimulating increased mitotic activity of cells in response to tissue and cellular injury induced by the parasites, e.g., hookworms, coccidia, and *Giardia* (see the subsequent appropriate section for data on the effect of intestinal parasites).

The immune system and other host defenses are not fully developed in young pups. Fetal pups begin to respond immunologically to certain antigens about the sixth week of gestation, but the magnitude of the immune response of pups does not approximate that of adult dogs until about three months of age.[34-37] The hyporesponsive immune system of young pups renders them more susceptible to severe consequences of CPV infection because it is unable to respond efficiently to CPV and suppress viral replication. It has been shown that cessation of CPV replication in dogs coincides with demonstrable immune response.[19,31] Vaccination of pups less than four weeks of age may stimulate suppressor T lymphocytes and prolong the hyporesponsiveness of the immature immune system. This must be considered in evaluating the benefits and risks when vaccinating pups less than five weeks of age.

If pups are orphaned and colostrum deprived or are from a dam known to have a low titer of antibody to CPV, passive immunity can be provided by administering serum that has a high titer of antibody to CPV.[25] A single injection of high-titered serum at the rate of 2.2 ml/kg (1 ml/lb) body weight at two to three weeks of age will protect pups against CPV until about five weeks of age. Discretion must be used in selecting a donor for the serum because there are inherent risks associated with serum injection. A dog that has recovered from known CPV infection or disease will have a high-titer serum. The titer of antibody to CPV in serum can be determined to ensure that adequate protection is provided.

Infection of young pups with CPV may result in acute death caused by myocarditis.[10,38,39] The myocardial form of CPV disease usually occurs in pups less than eight weeks of age at the time of infection. The myocardium of the pup has a high mitotic index because of the rapid growth and dynamic pressure changes that occur in the heart associated with closure of the foramen ovale at about six to eight weeks of age. The myocardial form of CPV disease occurred more frequently when CPV first emerged than it does currently because most female dogs now are immune to CPV and provide passive immunity via colostral transfer that protects pups to an age at which myocardial cells do not facilitate extensive CPV replication.

Stress

It is common knowledge that stress increases susceptibility to infections and enhances disease severity. Inadequate nutrition, concurrent infections with viral or bacterial infections, parasitism, extreme environmental temperature (hot and humid or cold and damp), and unsanitary environment are commonly encountered conditions that contribute to stress. The impact of stress factors on CPV disease appears to be inversely related to socioeconomic conditions. Observations in urban areas suggest that CPV disease in the canine population at large is a greater problem in environments of lower socioeconomic status. Lack of health maintenance and pet care in general are undoubtedly contributing factors.

Injuries and surgical procedures are stressful and may contribute to increased susceptibility to infections. A frequently reported problem is the occurrence of CPV disease in young dogs following surgical treatment of injuries from an accident or following elective surgery. The latter has occurred too often following ear-trim surgery in Doberman pinschers. Administration of high-titered serum at the rate of 1.1 to 2.2 ml/kg (0.5 to 1.0 ml/lb) body weight has resulted in a marked decrease in the frequency of postsurgical CPV disease in Doberman pups.

Breed or Genetics

All breeds of dogs are susceptible to infection with CPV, and severe disease and death can occur in any dog infected with CPV. Observations by veterinarians, clinical records at veterinary schools, and records of complaints of CPV with high morbidity and mortality indicate that severe CPV disease with high mortality occurs more frequently in some breeds than in others. Rottweilers and Doberman pinschers seem to be more severely affected by CPV than other breeds. CPV disease commonly occurs in Labrador retrievers, greyhounds, Siberian huskies, and German shepherds. Observations by the authors suggest that black Labrador retrievers are more severely affected by CPV than are yellow-colored Labrador retrievers. Trends are less evident among other breeds for rank order of susceptibility to severe parvovirus disease.

The reasons for the increased susceptibility to parvovirus infection by rottweilers and Dobermans are unknown. They have a common ancestry, which could indicate a common genetically determined factor (or factors). Dobermans have an inherited bleeding disorder, von Willebrand's disease, with a prevalence of more than 60%.[40,41] The bleeding in von Willebrand's disease involves diathesis of mucosal surfaces. Clinical signs vary, with many affected dogs showing no signs of von Willebrand's disease until they are stressed by infectious diseases, traumatic injury, surgery, etc.[40,41] Occurrence of the disease in Doberman pinschers may be a contributing factor to severe CPV disease. It has been suggested that rottweilers may have a hereditary immunodeficiency. There is not enough data to substantiate either of these suggestions as primary factors in enhanced severity of CPV infections in these breeds. Results from limited studies in the authors' laboratory indicate that rottweilers develop expected serum titers of antibody to CPV vaccines, and that CPV infection can result in mild signs of disease that clinically may be considered as something else. High titers of antibody were present in sera from rottweiler pups that recovered from mild signs of parvovirus infection. Veterinarians in the field have observed that severe CPV disease with high mortality occurs more often in rottweiler litters that are concurrently infected with intestinal parasites, especially those with giardiasis and coccidiosis. Published reports on the influence of protozoan infections on the severity of CPV disease are limited, and the findings are inconsistent.[18,19,28,31] Observations in three kennels in Alabama revealed that the original puppy mortality rate of 60% to 75% decreased to less than 5% after implementation of procedures to decrease the prevalence of giardiasis. An example of such a procedure would be to treat all dogs in the kennels with quinacrine hydrochloride (9 mg/kg/day in two to three divided doses for five days) or metronidazole (65 mg/kg/day for five days) and to decontaminate the premises and improve sanitation. Controlled studies are in progress in attempts to validate the field observations on the role of giardiasis in predisposing young dogs to severe viral enteritis.

Intestinal Parasites and Concurrent Infections

Field observations by practicing veterinarians suggested that intestinal parasites were an important factor in the socioeconomic influence on severe CPV disease. Preliminary studies in the authors' laboratory tend to corroborate the field observations and suggest that intestinal parasites and/or concurrent infection with a mildly virulent strain of canine distemper virus (CDV) enhanced the severity of CPV disease.[31] Unpublished data from further studies with the same strain of CPV resulted in mild signs of disease in 14 of 31 seronegative, parasite-free dogs, with no deaths; all 14 recovered without treatment after illness of one to three days duration (Table I).[42] In contrast, severer CPV disease occurred in 23 of 26 seronegative, parasitized dogs, and 9 died.

Concurrent infection with a mildly virulent strain of CDV enhanced the severity of experimentally induced CPV disease (Table I).[42] The mildly virulent strain of CDV used in the authors' studies was derived from a modified live virus (MLV) canine distemper vaccine that is virulent in gray foxes.[43] Reversion to a mildly

TABLE I
Enhancement of CPV Disease by Concurrent Infection with Intestinal Parasites and a Mildly Virulent Strain of CDV

Combination of Infections in Groups of Dogs[a]	Number of Dogs in Group	Results of CPV Disease	
		Morbidity	Mortality
CPV only	31	14/31 (45%)	0
CPV + parasites	26	23/26 (88%)	9/26 (35%)
CPV + CDV	20	17/20 (85%)	5/20 (25%)
CPV + CDV + parasites	26	26/26 (100%)	22/26 (85%)

[a]Infections with CPV and CDV were experimentally induced; infections with parasites were naturally acquired. Dogs in groups without parasites had been treated to obliterate parasitic infections before experimental infection with CPV and/or CDV.

virulent status for dogs occurred during a single passage in a gray fox that died of vaccine-induced distemper. Although MLV distemper vaccines are generally safe in young dogs and pups over six weeks of age, vaccine-induced distemper has been reported in pups vaccinated at three weeks of age.[27] With many breeders and some veterinarians vaccinating puppies beginning at two weeks of age, the possibility exists that vaccine-induced distemper can occur in very young seronegative pups with reversion of virulence resulting in transmission of mildly virulent CDV among young dogs. This could contribute to the apparent differences in CPV disease severity observed in different areas. Concurrent infections with CPV and CDV have been reported and may be more frequent than anticipated.[44] The clinical manifestations of the mildly virulent distemper would likely be masked by the signs of CPV disease, as was noted in the authors' studies. Signs of central nervous system disease were observed occasionally and may have resulted from either the mildly virulent distemper or the CPV that has been isolated from the brains of infected pups.[45]

It has been stated that concurrent infections with bacteria contribute to severe CPV disease.[46,47] It has also been reported that *Campylobacter jejuni* alone may cause signs of enteritis that resemble parvovirus clinically in pups.[48] Disruption of the integrity of the intestinal mucosa by CPV allows for bacterial invasion and septicemia to occur with otherwise normal flora of the gut.[46] Bacterial endotoxemia is believed to be an important factor in the terminal acute shock in fatal cases of parvovirus disease. Incorporation of corticosteroids and/or flunixin meglumine (Banamine®—Schering) are indicated in the therapeutic regimen to combat endotoxic shock in CPV disease.

The Safety of Modified Live Virus Vaccines

The safety of MLV CPV vaccines has been questioned from the time of their development and licensed use in dogs. Most concerns have focused on two factors: lymphopenia following vaccination and shedding of vaccine virus in the feces of vaccinated dogs.[26]

The concern over vaccine virus shedding involves the question of possible reversion of virulence of attenuated CPV. There are biologic differences among attenuated strains of CPV used in MLV vaccines, including differences in the shedding of vaccine virus.[17] The amount of vaccine virus shed following vaccination with some MLV CPV vaccines is very limited and does not always result in transmission to seronegative contact dogs.[21] Other modified live virus CPV vaccine viruses are shed to such an extent that vaccination of only one seronegative puppy in a litter will result in immunization of the entire litter. Testing for evidence of virulence reversion by back-passage studies in seronegative dogs is a requirement for licensing of MLV CPV vaccines. All licensed MLV CPV vaccines have been found to be safe with no evidence of virulence reversion after five serial back passages. Vaccination of seronegative pups with up to 50 times a normal field dose of MLV CPV vaccine did not cause illness.[21,23] Vaccine-induced CPV disease has not been documented in either field or uncomplicated laboratory situations.

Lymphopenia is a consistent finding in dogs infected with virulent CPV.[2,17-19,28,29] Lymphopenia may occur following vaccination with some MLV CPV vaccines.[49] This observation has resulted in impressions that MLV CPV vaccines are immunosuppressive and that vaccines with MLV CPV in combination with MLV distemper, adenovirus, and parainfluenza virus are not safe.[26,50,51] Controlled studies using MLV CPV vaccines alone or in combination have not verified allegations of immunosuppression by CPV or of vaccine-induced disease.[21,23,31] The authors examined five different MLV CPV vaccines in seronegative pups in their laboratory. All five vaccines induced high titers of antibody and protected pups against challenge with virulent CPV; there were no signs of CPV disease, and CPV was not detected in feces by hemagglutination assay after challenge. Two of the MLV CPV vaccines consistently induced lymphopenia of one to two days duration, one of the vaccines induced lymphopenia in 6 of 10 pups, and the other two vaccines rarely induced lymphopenia. Extensive vaccine virus shedding in feces occurred with the two vaccines that consistently induced lymphopenia. There was moderate vaccine virus shedding with the vaccine that caused lymphopenia in 6 of 10 pups. Vaccine virus was not detected in the feces of dogs vaccinated with the two vaccines that rarely caused lymphopenia. The transient lymphopenia occurred when the humoral antibody response was becoming detectable, and virus shedding ceased within two to three days after the lymphopenia (Table II). The transient lymphopenia that occurs following vaccination with MLV CPV may be indicative of active immune response to the vaccine and may represent changes in the dynamics of circulation and migration of sensitized lymphocytes in response to the replication of vaccine virus in the dog. Similar to the findings of others,[17] there were no overt changes in the blastogenic response of peripheral blood lymphocytes from six dogs vaccinated with modified live virus CPV in a limited study.

Immunologic Effects of Canine Parvovirus Infection and Disease

Several published articles have emphasized the immunosuppressive properties of virulent CPV and have attributed certain findings to these properties.[26,27,50,51] The basis for the assumption that CPV is immunosuppressive has been the common occurrence of lymphopenia[2,17-19,28-30,52] and the depletion of lymphocytes from the lymph nodes and thymus of dogs infected with virulent CPV.[18,19,52] Canine parvovirus can produce severe lymphoid necrosis,[18,19,30,52] similar to the lesions produced in cats by FPV.[53] There is a lack of definitive data, though, to justify the conclusion that CPV is immunosuppressive.

The authors have investigated the immunosuppressive effects of CPV by quantitating changes in leukocyte concentrations, by measuring in vitro blastogenic responses of lymphocytes to mitogens, and by determining the humoral antibody response to components of combination modified live virus vaccines in dogs infected with virulent CPV.

Humoral Immune Response

Clinical signs of CPV disease usually occur in four to seven days following experimental infection by the oral route of inoculation (Figure 1).[19,28,30,52] Primary virus replication takes place in lymph nodes, followed by viremia from about Day 2 to Day 5.[18,19,28] Virus disappears from the blood as the titer of humoral antibody increases rapidly between Days 4 and 7, and fecal virus shedding declines markedly between Days 7 and 10.[18,19,31,52] Viremia is essential in the pathogenesis of CPV disease, and it precedes the onset of clinical signs and fecal virus shedding. Inoculation of virulent CPV intravenously shortens the incubation period by about two days.[19] The cessation of viral replication and shedding of CPV in feces and recovery from clinical signs of disease are closely correlated with development of humoral antibody to CPV.[19,31]

Secretory antibody of the IgA class appears in the intestinal tract and feces by Day 4 after infection with CPV, and it is reported to affect the severity of disease and the duration of virus shedding.[54,55] Some dogs have been found to develop high titers of humoral antibody but have little or no secretory antibody in the intestinal lumen.[55] It has been postulated that these dogs are more likely to have severe disease and prolonged virus shedding.[55] This could explain the periodic shedding of CPV by some dogs for a month or more.[31] The absence of secretory antibody in the intestine may or may not represent immune dysfunction or specific immunosuppression by CPV; however, the fact that almost all dogs develop high titers of humoral antibody during the course of disease suggests that CPV may not be as immunosuppressive as has been assumed.

Unpublished data from a series of studies in the authors' laboratory indicated that virulent CPV did not affect the humoral antibody response to other MLV canine vaccines.[56] The studies involved a total of 62

TABLE II
Differences Among Modified Live Virus CPV Vaccines with Respect to Fecal Shedding of Vaccine Virus, Humoral Antibody Response, and Lymphopenia

Number of Dogs in Group[a]	Fecal Virus[b]	Number of Lymphopenic Dogs[c]	Correlation of Antibody Titer and Lymphopenia on Postvaccination Days				
			Day 3	Day 5	Day 7	Day 10	Day 14
10	++++[d]	9/10	8[e] +	256 +	2048 −	8192 −	8192 −
10	++	6/10	0 −	0 −	8 +	1024 +	8192 −
13	±	1/13	0 −	16 ±	256 −	1024 −	2048 −

[a]Each group of dogs was vaccinated with a given modified live virus CPV vaccine.
[b]Relative shedding of virus in feces by hemagglutination titer.
[c]Lymphopenia was defined as >40% reduction in lymphocytes from mean absolute lymphocytes for each dog before vaccination.
[d]+ indicates days of lymphopenia; − indicates days of normal lymphocyte count.
[e]Reciprocal titer of serum-virus neutralizing antibody on day indicated.

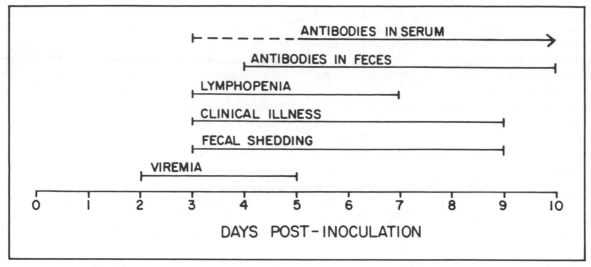

Figure 1—Timetable of events following oronasal inoculation of pups with virulent canine parvovirus.

seronegative, young dogs, including controls. Groups of the dogs were vaccinated with MLV distemper, adenovirus$_2$, parainfluenza, leptospirosis (DA$_2$P-L) at time intervals ranging from one week before experimental infection with virulent CPV to two weeks after experimental infection. There were no overt differences in serum-virus neutralizing antibody titers to canine distemper virus among the groups compared with uninfected controls except for the group vaccinated one week before infection with virulent CPV. This group was sick with signs of parvovirus disease from about Day 11 to Day 14 after vaccination with MLV DA$_2$P-L. Antibody titers were slightly lower in sera collected on Days 14 and 18 postvaccination, but titers on Day 21 were equal to those of vaccinated controls not infected with CPV. The authors hypothesize that the slightly lower response resulted from the constitutional effects of acute gastroenteritis occurring at a time 10 to 14 days postvaccination, when the response to MLV distemper vaccine is increasing rapidly,[57] rather than from specific immunosuppressive effects of CPV. In other words, sick dogs do not respond as well immunologically as do healthy dogs. This could also explain the slight delay in antibody response to CPV reported in symptomatic dogs compared with asymptomatic dogs.[19] Antibody responses to the canine adenovirus Type 2 component of the MLV DA$_2$P-L vaccine were essentially the same for all groups of dogs.

In addition to data suggesting the lack of immunosuppressive effect by virulent CPV on the humoral antibody response to DA$_2$P-L vaccine, there were no signs of vaccine-induced distemper in dogs vaccinated before, after, or concurrent with infection with virulent CPV, as have been reported by others.[27,50,51] The seronegative dogs used in the authors' studies were from three to four months of age at the time of vaccination and infection with CPV, compared with three-week-old puppies used in studies with apparent vaccine-induced

distemper attributed to immunosuppressive effects of CPV.[27] The virulence of the strain of CPV used in the authors' studies was illustrated by six deaths and clinical signs of parvovirus disease in 29 of 32 infected dogs.

Changes in Blood and Bone Marrow

The most consistent hematologic change in CPV infection is transient lymphopenia, observed as early as three days after oral exposure[28,52] but occurring in most dogs within five days of infection.[19,28,30,49,52] The decrease in lymphocyte concentration is more marked in severely affected or symptomatic dogs than in dogs with subclinical infections.[19] Lymphopenia from CPV infection is much shorter in duration than the lymphopenia that occurs following infection with virulent distemper virus. Distemper-associated lymphopenia lasts up to eight weeks,[58] whereas the lymphocyte concentration usually returns to normal within seven to nine days after infection with virulent CPV.[19,21,28,30,49]

Lymphocytosis has been reported during recovery from CPV infection.[30,49,52] As early as seven days after infection, but usually by Day 11, the concentration of lymphocytes increases and large, atypical lymphocytes are found in the blood.[52] The bone marrow may also contain reactive, activated lymphocytes even in terminal cases,[59] though changes in bone marrow lymphocytes are not usually noted.[30]

Neutropenia associated with CPV infection usually is restricted to dogs with severe or terminal illness.[30,52] The onset of neutropenia six to seven days after infection coincides with signs of intestinal damage, such as hemorrhagic diarrhea and sloughing of mucosal epithelium.[30,52] Depletion of mature granulocytes from the bone marrow storage pool also is associated with severe CPV disease[19,30,52,59] and is observed during clinical illness rather than during incubation or recovery periods.[52] Neutropenia with accompanying depletion of the bone marrow storage pool may be the result of accumulation and exudation of neutrophils at the intestinal mucosa.[30,52] In mild CPV infection, the concentration of mature neutrophils in the blood actually may increase, and immature (band) neutrophils may appear five to seven days after infection (Figure 2). A statistically significant decrease in neutrophil bactericidal ability has been observed during the second week after experimental CPV infection.[49] Many immature neutrophils and marked toxic changes in mature and band neutrophils often are seen in the blood during severe natural CPV infections.[32] The effect of CPV on neutrophil precursors in the bone marrow is inconsistent. There may be an increase in blast cells and hyperplasia of granulocyte precursors[30,52] or there may be toxic, degenerative changes[59] and depletion of precursor cells.[19] Toxic changes in neutrophils probably reflect the loss of integrity of the mucosal epithelium, with subsequent absorption of bacterial endotoxins[17,19,32,59] and entry of bacteria into the bloodstream.[46] Hematologic effects of endotoxemia depend upon the concentration of endotoxin; they range from leukocytosis (neutrophilia) from low concentrations to neutropenia and even pancytopenia from high doses.[60]

CPV seldom causes leukopenia and rarely induces pancytopenia in dogs in the absence of concurrent infections or parasitism. There is a decrease in total leukocyte concentration, usually because of a decrease in neutrophil concentration, in severely affected dogs.[30,52]

Leukopenia and neutropenia should be associated with poor prognosis and the need for aggressive (some say heroic) treatment.[19,30,32,52,59]

Effect of CPV Infection on Lymphoid Tissues

Thymic atrophy is the most frequently observed and striking change in lymphoid tissues at necropsy following infection with virulent CPV.[18,19,52] The thymus is edematous and depleted of mature cortical thymocytes only two days after oral infection with CPV.[52] Some cytolysis may be evident. CPV can be detected in or isolated from thymocytes on Day 3 and perhaps earlier,[18,19] which indicates that the thymocyte depletion is caused at least partly by virus replication and probable cytocidal effects. The changes progress to marked depletion of cortical thymocytes by Days 5 to 7[18,19,52]; this is especially severe in symptomatic dogs, compared with dogs with subclinical infection.[19] Regeneration of the thymus during recovery occurs more slowly than regeneration of other lymphoid tissues. In some dogs, the thymus appears normal 12 to 13 days after infection[18]; in others the thymus is still small and hypocellular at that time[52] despite full repopulation of other lymphoid tissues. Whether the thymus ever regenerates completely in these dogs has not been reported.

Some reports indicate that lymphoid tissues filtering the gastrointestinal tract, including tonsil, Peyer's patches, and mesenteric lymph nodes, are selectively

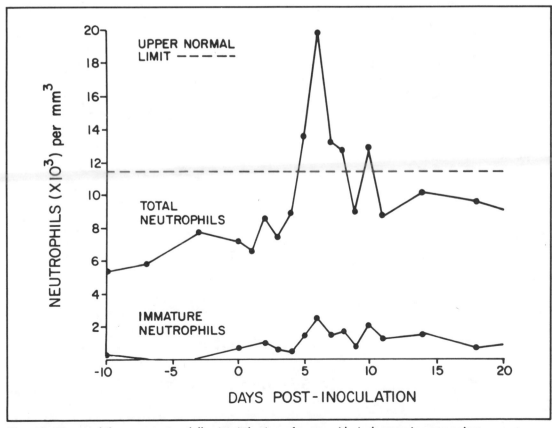

Figure 2—Neutrophil concentration following infection of a pup with virulent canine parvovirus.

affected by CPV.[18,30] Cytolysis is evident in lymph nodes only two days after oral infection[52]; necrosis is widespread by Days 4 to 5.[18,52] CPV can be isolated from lymphoid tissues or detected by immunofluorescence at this time,[18,19] again suggesting local viral replication in rapidly dividing lymphocytes. Germinal centers are particularly affected by CPV[19,52]; the paracortex also may be involved.[19] Lymphoid cell depletion is severest in symptomatic dogs; it is only mild to moderate in dogs with subclinical infections.[19] Whether the degree of lymphoid cell depletion and severity of clinical signs are related causally or simply reflect the amount of virus disseminated through the body is unknown. By Day 7, lymph nodes from dogs with terminal illness are hypocellular, whereas nodes from recovering dogs are repopulated and have expanding germinal centers.[52] Regeneration of lymph nodes is clearly evident by Day 9[19]; by Days 12 to 13, lymph nodes are enlarged and lymphoid hyperplasia is marked.[18,52]

The Effect of CPV Infection on Leukocyte Function

Despite the striking lesions that develop in lymphoid tissues during CPV infection, little is known of the effect of the virus on the function of lymphocytes and granulocytes. In vitro lymphocyte blastogenesis, a laboratory test used to detect deficiencies in lymphocyte function, was abnormal in shelter dogs shedding CPV in their feces compared with dogs not shedding the virus.[61] Although the authors did not rule out the possibility of concurrent infection with canine distemper virus, their study did demonstrate significant impairment of lymphocyte function in CPV-infected dogs. The authors have been unable to detect a similar degree of suppression of lymphocyte blastogenesis in dogs infected experimentally with virulent CPV under controlled conditions.[49] Mild, transient suppression sometimes occurs (Figure 3)[17] but has not always been reproducible in the laboratory. In dogs with fatal experimental CPV infection, however, the lymphocyte blastogenic response decreases dramatically within one or two days of death (Figure 3). It is unclear whether this is a direct effect of CPV or is due instead to the secondary effects of severe damage to the intestinal mucosa, electrolyte imbalance, and dehydration typically seen in severe CPV disease.

Is Canine Parvovirus Immunosuppressive?

A paradox of the virus-host interactions of virulent CPV is the rapid antibody response that occurs in the presence of lymphopenia, severe necrosis of lymph nodes, and thymic atrophy in dogs infected with virulent CPV.[19,28,31] The antibody response of symptomatic dogs is delayed slightly compared with that of asymptomatic dogs, but by Day 7 postinfection the titers are essentially the same.[19] If CPV were significantly immunosuppres-

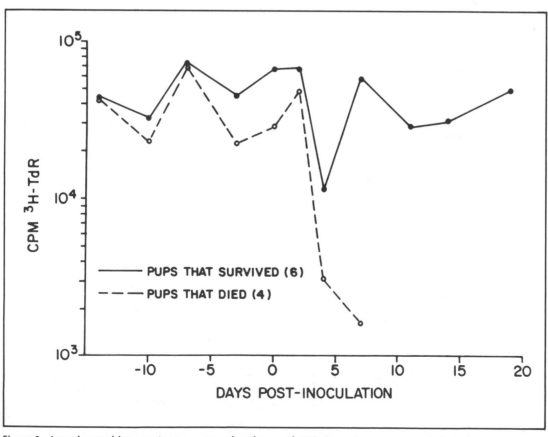

Figure 3—Lymphocyte blastogenic response to phytohemagglutinin in canine parvovirus–infected pups.

sive, a marked decrease in antibody response would be expected to occur in symptomatic dogs similar to that which occurs in dogs infected with virulent canine distemper virus.[57,58,62] Transient lymphopenia and depletion of lymphocytes from lymph nodes and thymus apparently are not categorical indicators of immunosuppression. The transient, slight decrease in blastogenic response of lymphocytes from dogs infected with CPV that occurred at the onset of the humoral response[17] was similar to the occurrence of lymphopenia following vaccination of dogs with MLV CPV vaccines reported in this article (Table II). Both may have been the result of dynamic changes in populations of circulating lymphocytes at the time of lymphocyte response to antigenic stimulation. The reported failure of dogs to respond to an MLV CDV used in combination with MLV CPV vaccine[26] is enigmatic, because others have reported that MLV CPV vaccine has no effect on the antibody response

to MLV canine CDV vaccines.[21,23,24] The putative potentiation of vaccine-induced distemper by infection with CPV[27] may have been influenced more by the age of the colostrum-deprived puppies at the time of vaccination (three weeks) than by immunosuppressive effects of CPV.

Confusion has resulted from widely publicized claims of immunosuppression by CPV in both professional and lay publications without definitive data from controlled studies to substantiate those claims. It is suggested that there is as much evidence to indicate that CPV is not immunosuppressive as there is supporting claims of immunosuppression by CPV. Further studies are needed to resolve the question about immunosuppressive properties of CPV. Conclusions should be based on data demonstrating that dogs infected with virulent strains of CPV or vaccinated with attenuated strains have impaired immune responses to other antigens.

REFERENCES

1. Eugster AK, Bendele RA, Jones LP: Parvovirus infection in dogs. *JAVMA* 173:1340-1341, 1978.
2. Appel MJG, Cooper MJ, Greisen H, et al: Status report: Canine viral enteritis. *JAVMA* 173:1516-1518, 1978.
3. Helfer-Baker C, Evermann JF, McKeiran AJ, et al: Serologic studies on the incidence of canine enteritis viruses. *Canine Pract* 7:37-42, 1980.
4. Meunier PC, Glickman LT, Appel MJG, et al: Canine parvovirus in a commercial kennel: Epidemiologic and pathologic findings. *Cornell Vet* 71:96-110, 1981.
5. Walker ST, Feilen CP, Sabine M, et al: A serologic survey of canine parvovirus infection in New South Wales, Australia. *Vet Rec* 106:324-325, 1980.
6. Eugster AK, Nairn C: Diarrhea in puppies: Parvovirus-like particles demonstrated in their feces. *Southwest Vet* 30:59-60, 1977.
7. Johnson RH, Spradbrow PB: Isolation from dogs with severe enteritis of a parvovirus related to feline panleukopenia virus. *Aust Vet J* 55:151, 1979.
8. Kelley WR: An enteric disease of dogs resembling feline panleukopenia. *Aust Vet J* 54:593, 1978.
9. Burtonboy G, Coignoul F, Delferriere N, et al: Canine hemorrhagic enteritis—Detection of viral particles by electron microscopy. *Arch Virol* 61:1-11, 1979.
10. Van Rensburgh IBJ, Botha WS, Lange AL, et al: Parvovirus as a cause of enteritis and myocarditis in puppies. *J S Afr Vet Assoc* 30:249-253, 1979.
11. Azetaka M, Kirasawa T, Konishi S, et al: Studies on canine parvovirus isolation, experimental infection and serologic survey. *Jpn J Vet Sci* 43:243-255, 1981.
12. Appel M, Scott FW, Carmichael LE: Isolation and immunization studies of a canine parvo-like virus in dogs with haemorrhagic enteritis. *Vet Rec* 105:151-159, 1979.
13. Parrish CR, Carmichael LE, Antczak DF: Antigenic relationships between canine parvovirus type 2, feline panleukopenia virus and mink enteritis virus using conventional antisera and monoclonal antibodies. *Arch Virol* 72:267-278, 1982.
14. Tratschin J-D, McMaster GK, Kronauer G, et al: Canine parvovirus: Relationship to wild-type and vaccine strains of feline panleukopenia virus and mink enteritis virus. *J Gen Virol* 61:33-41, 1982.
15. Binn LN, Lazar EC, Eddy GA, et al: Recover and characterization of a minute virus from canines. *Infect Immunol* 1:503-508, 1970.
16. Carmichael LE, Binn LN: New enteric viruses in the dog. *Adv Vet Sci Comp Med* 25:1-37, 1981.
17. Carmichael LE: Immunization strategies in puppies—Why failures? *Compend Contin Educ Pract Vet* 5:1043-1051, 1983.
18. O'Sullivan G, Durham PJK, Smith JR, et al: Experimentally induced severe canine parvoviral enteritis. *Aust Vet J* 61:1-4, 1984.
19. Meunier PC, Cooper BJ, Appel MJG, et al: Pathogenesis of canine parvoviral enteritis: The importance of viremia. *Vet Pathol* 22:60-71, 1985.
20. Pollock RVH, Carmichael LE: Dog response to inactivated canine parvovirus and feline panleukopenia virus vaccine. *Cornell Vet* 72:16-35, 1982.
21. Kahn DE, Emery JB, Smith MJ, et al: Safety and efficacy of modified-live canine parvovirus vaccine. *VM SAC* 78:1739-1746, 1983.
22. Wallace BL, Salsbury DL, McMillen JK: An inactivated canine parvovirus vaccine: Protection against virulent challenge. *Vet Med* 80:41-48, 1985.
23. Carmichael LE, Joubert JC, Pollock RVH: A modified live canine parvovirus vaccine. II. Immune response. *Cornell Vet* 73:13-29, 1983.
24. O'Brien SE, Roth JA, Hill BL: Response of pups to modified live virus canine parvovirus vaccine. *JAVMA,* in press.
25. Pollock RVH, Carmichael LE: Maternally derived immunity to canine parvovirus infection: Transfer, decline and interference with vaccination. *JAVMA* 180:37-42, 1982.
26. Kesel ML, Neil DH: Combined MLV canine parvovirus vaccine: Immunosuppression with infective shedding. *VM SAC* 78:687-691, 1983.
27. Krakowka S, Olsen RG, Axthelm MK, et al: Canine parvovirus infection potentiates canine distemper encephalitis attributable to modified live-virus vaccine. *JAVMA* 180:137-139, 1982.
28. Pollock RVH: Experimental canine parvovirus infection in dogs. *Cornell Vet* 72:103-119, 1982.
29. Eugster AK: Studies on canine parvovirus infections: Development of an inactivated vaccine. *Am J Vet Res* 41:2020-2024, 1980.
30. Potgieter LND, Jones JB, Patton CS, et al: Experimental parvovirus infection in dogs. *Can J Comp Med* 45:212-216, 1981.
31. Swango LJ: Frequently asked questions about CPV disease. *Norden News* 58:4-10, 1983.
32. Woods CB, Pollock RVH, Carmichael LE: Canine parvoviral enteritis. *JAAHA* 16:171-179, 1980.
33. Council on Biologic and Therapeutic Agents, AVMA: Colloquium on selected diarrheal diseases of the young. *JAVMA* 173:509-676, 1978.
34. Shifrine M, Smith JB, Bulgin MS: Response of canine fetus and

neonates to antigenic stimulation. *J Immunol* 107:965-970, 1971.

35. Lewis RM, Smith CA, Garfield L: Kinetics of antibody synthesis to particulate and soluble antigen in newborn pups and adult dogs. *Am J Vet Res* 34:235-240, 1973.
36. Krakowka S, Koestner A: Age-related susceptibility to infection with canine distemper virus in gnotobiotic dogs. *J Infect Dis* 134:629-632, 1976.
37. Gerber JD, Brown AL: Effect of development and aging on the response of canine lymphocytes to phytohemagglutinin. *Infect Immunol* 10:695-699, 1974.
38. Hayes MA, Russel RG, Babiuk LA: Sudden death in young dogs with myocarditis caused by parvovirus. *JAVMA* 174:1197-1203, 1979.
39. Carpenter JL, Roberts RM, Harpster NK, et al: Intestinal and cardiopulmonary forms of parvovirus infection in a litter of pups. *JAVMA* 176:1269-1273, 1980.
40. Dodds WJ, Moynehan AC, Fisher TM, et al: The frequencies of blood and eye diseases as determined by genetic screening programs. *JAAHA* 17:697-704, 1981.
41. Johnstone IB, Crane S: Von Willebrand's disease in two families of Doberman pinschers. *Can Vet J* 22:239-243, 1981.
42. Swango LJ, Barbery R: Unpublished data, College of Veterinary Medicine, Auburn University, 1983.
43. Halbrooks RD, Swango LJ, Schnurrenberger PR, et al: Response of gray foxes to modified live-virus canine distemper vaccines. *JAVMA* 179:1170-1174, 1981.
44. Ducatelle R, Burtonboy G, Coussement W, et al: Concurrent parvovirus and distemper virus infections in a dog. *Vet Rec* 108:310-311, 1981.
45. Johnson BJ, Castro AE: Isolation of canine parvovirus from a dog brain with severe necrotizing vasculitis and encephalomalacia. *JAVMA* 184:1398-1399, 1984.
46. Kreeger TJ, Jeraj KP, Manning PJ: Bacteremia concomitant with parvovirus infection in a pup. *JAVMA* 184:196-197, 1984.
47. Sandstedt K, Wierup M: Concomitant occurrence of *Campylobacter* and parvoviruses in dogs with gastroenteritis. *Vet Res Commun* 4:271-273, 1980.
48. Fox JG, Moore R, Ackerman JI: *Campylobacter jejuni*-associated diarrhea in dogs. *JAVMA* 183:1430-1433, 1983.
49. Brunner CJ, Swango LJ, Nusbaum KE: Unpublished data, College of Veterinary Medicine, Auburn University, 1984.
50. Ritter J: Immunosuppression with combined vaccines (letter to the editor). *JAVMA* 182:1160-1161, 1983.
51. Henry SC: Immunosuppression by parvovirus (letter to the editor). *JAVMA* 183:492-493, 1983.
52. Macartney L, McCandlish IAP, Thompson H, et al: Canine parvovirus enteritis I: Clinical, haematological and pathological features of experimental infection. *Vet Rec* 115:201-210, 1984.
53. Kahn DE: Pathogenesis of feline panleukopenia. *JAVMA* 173:628-630, 1978.
54. Nara PL, Winters K, Rice JB, et al: Systemic and local intestinal antibody response in dogs given both infective and inactivated canine parvovirus. *Am J Vet Res* 44:1989-1995, 1983.
55. Rice JB, Winters KA, Krakowka S, et al: Comparison of systemic and local immunity in dogs with canine parvovirus gastroenteritis. *Infect Immunol* 38:1003-1009, 1982.
56. Swango LJ, Brunner CJ, Nusbaum KE: Unpublished data, College of Veterinary Medicine, Auburn University, 1984.
57. Krakowka S, Cockerell G, Koestner A: Effects of canine distemper virus on lymphoid function *in vitro* and *in vivo*. *Infect Immunol* 11:1069-1078, 1975.
58. Krakowka S, Higgins RJ, Koestner A: Canine distemper virus: Review of structural and functional modulations in lymphoid tissues. *Am J Vet Res* 41:284-292, 1980.
59. Boosinger TR, Rebar AH, DeNicola DB, et al: Bone marrow alterations associated with canine parvoviral enteritis. *Vet Pathol* 19:558-561, 1982.
60. Schalm OW, Jain NC, Carroll EJ: *Veterinary Hematology*, ed 3. Philadelphia, Lea & Febiger, 1975, pp 524-525.
61. Olsen CG, Stiff MI, Olsen RG: Comparison of the blastogenic response of peripheral blood lymphocytes from canine parvovirus-positive and -negative outbred dogs. *Vet Immunol Immunopathol* 6:285-290, 1984.
62. Appel MJG: Pathogenesis of canine distemper. *Am J Vet Res* 30:1167-1182, 1969.

KEY FACTS

- *Campylobacter jejuni* is a common cause of enteritis in humans and is commonly isolated from domestic and pet animals.
- *C. jejuni* is microaerophilic with special culture and handling requirements; thus "rectal swabs" for routine laboratory cultures are inadequate.
- Differences in strains of both spontaneous and experimental isolates probably account for the inconsistent clinical disease induced by this organism.
- Exposure of both pet and owner to a common source rather than pet-to-owner contamination is a likely scenario if both should develop campylobacter enteritis.

Campylobacter Enteritis in Dogs and Cats

A. R. Dillon, DVM, MS
Diplomate, ACVIM
Department of Small Animal
  Surgery and Medicine
Scott-Ritchey Research Program
College of Veterinary Medicine

T. R. Boosinger, DVM, PhD
Diplomate, ACVP
Department of Pathology
College of Veterinary Medicine

W. T. Blevins, BS, MS, PhD
Department of Botany
  and Microbiology
College of Science
  and Mathematics

Auburn University
Auburn, Alabama

Nonculturable spiral-form gram-negative bacteria were noted in 1886 by Theodor Escherich in stool specimens and intestinal mucus from human neonates with diarrhea and from adult cats. Later, similar organisms that would not grow on solid media were found mainly in the colon or associated with mucus in diarrhea stool specimens were described as "spirilla." These spirilla were reported in cases of "choleralike" and "dysenteric" disease. Growth on solid media was unsuccessful, although bacteria remained viable in liquid culture media for a few days. Based on the morphologic description, the association with enteritis in neonates and infants, the failure to grow on solid media, and the fact that no other bacteria with comparable morphology had been associated with human enteric infections,[1] this initial description of the microorganism probably describes *Campylobacter* species. "In less than a decade, *Campylobacter jejuni* has emerged from obscurity as a veterinary pathogen to recognition as a leading cause of enteritis in human beings. When proper culture techniques are used, *C. jejuni* is isolated in North America and Europe from patients with diarrhea at least as often as *Salmonella* or *Shigella* species. Moreover, *C. jejuni* has been found in virtually every country in which it has been sought."[2]

The genus *Campylobacter*, previously named *Vibrio fetus*, was recognized in 1909 as a cause of abortion in cattle and sheep. It was not until 1977 that it was generally recognized that *Campylobacter* was a common cause of acute diarrhea in humans. The genus *Campylobacter* (*campylo* meaning curved and *bacter* meaning rod) was proposed, separating it from *Vibrio* species initially on the basis of the variation of serologic and biochemical characteristics of the human isolates and ultimately on the DNA composition.[3,4]

The species that in the past was classified as "related vibrios" and *C. fetus* subsp. *jejuni* is now known as *Campylobacter jejuni*. The other *Campylobacter* species are listed in Table I according to the host(s) that each infects and their zoonotic potential. Under the present classification, *C. fetus* subsp. *venerealis* causes infertility and abortions in cattle; *C. fetus* subsp. *fetus* causes abortions in sheep and is a potential human pathogen; *C. sputorum* subsp. *sputorum* is a commensal oral microbe in humans; *C. sputorum* subsp. *bubulus* and *C. fecalis* are commensals of the bovine reproductive and ovine intestinal tract; and *C. sputorum* subsp. *mucosalis* and *C. hyointestinalis* have been associated with porcine proliferative enteritis.[3,4] *Campylobac-*

TABLE I
Campylobacter Species as Potential Pathogens

Campylobacter	Host	Disease	Human Disease
C. fetus subsp. venerealis	Cattle	Infertility, abortion	Rare
C. intestinalis	Cattle, sheep		Opportunistic
C. jejuni/coli	Many species	Enteritis	Enteritis
C. laridis	Sea gulls	?	Rare
C. pyloridis	Humans, others?	?	Gastritis
C. fetus	Sheep	Abortion	Rare
C. sputorum subsp. sputorum	Humans	Commensal, oral	?
C. sputorum subsp. bubulus	Cattle	Commensal, reproductive	?
C. fecalis	Sheep	Commensal, gastrointestinal	?
C. mucosalis	Pigs	Enteritis	?
C. hypointestinalis	Pigs	Enteritis	?

ter coli, which at one time was believed to be the cause of swine dysentery,[5] and *C. jejuni* differ only slightly and are often discussed together as potential human pathogens.[3] A recently recognized species, *C. laridis*, is prevalent in sea gulls and has caused infection in humans; another species, *C. pyloridis*, is associated with peptic ulcers and chronic gastritis in humans but has unknown potential in animals.[6]

Campylobacter jejuni is a curved, motile, gram-negative rod that requires some oxygen for growth but cannot tolerate normal oxygen concentrations in room air.[7] Special culture techniques are needed, therefore, for its isolation; and that may explain its relatively late discovery. The organism is typical of gram-negative bacteria with its endotoxic properties of the lipopolysaccharide cell wall.[7] *Campylobacter* has also been implicated as releasing an enterotoxin that is cytotoxic. In veterinary medicine, *C. jejuni* has generated additional interest because animals might represent an important reservoir for the organism.[3,5,7,8]

Campylobacter Enteritis in Humans

Campylobacter jejuni is a major cause of acute diarrhea in children and adults.[3,9-14] Recently, *C. jejuni* has rivaled *Salmonella* as a cause of enteritis and might actually be present more often than *Shigella* or *Salmonella*.[7,14] The usual incubation period of 24 to 72 hours after ingestion can extend up to 10 days. The disease in humans is usually accompanied by fever and diarrhea (in 90% of cases), abdominal pain (70%), myalgia, malaise, anorexia, and occasionally vomiting. Feces are loose, usually becoming watery; mucus and blood (in 50% of cases) may be present. The disease usually is self-limiting; recovery is complete in one to two weeks. Deaths have been reported, however, in severe cases of *C. jejuni* enterocolitis.[10,11]

The disease can vary and bacteremia, meningitis, and abortions have been reported. In addition to direct tissue invasion of the bowel, the release of endotoxins or enterotoxins has been implicated and may be strain-specific.[3,4,7,15] The pathology is most common in the jejunum and ileum; but the colon, extending to the rectum, may be involved.[2,7,12,14]

After oral ingestion, bacteria that survive the gastric acid barrier reach the bile-rich, microaerobic small intestine, where multiplication enables diarrheic patients to shed 10^6 to 10^9 bacteria per gram of stool. The pathology is consistent with a nonspecific colitis with acute inflammation of the lamina propria, degeneration and atrophy in the goblet cells and epithelium, crypt abscesses, and mucosal ulceration.[3] Administration of erythromycin, the drug of choice in *C. jejuni* infections in humans, results in disappearance of the organism in the stool.[10,16]

Reservoirs for *Campylobacter jejuni*

Transmission appears to be by a fecal-oral route through contaminated food and water or by direct contact with fecal material from infected animals or humans. In general, person-to-person spread of the organism is believed to be rare.[17] Untreated humans can be carriers for six weeks during convalescence, and shedding can occur for up to one year in some cases.[3,18]

For the veterinarian, the zoonotic potential of pet–owner contact is important. In domestic animals, the organism is almost ubiquitous. In mammals, *C. jejuni* has been isolated from healthy cattle, sheep, horse, pigs, goats, dogs, cats, rodents, and monkeys and from diarrheic calves, lambs, dogs, cats, and monkeys. In avian species, *C. jejuni* has been isolated from 30% to 100% of fecal samples. Once fecal contamination has occurred, viable organisms can be present up to four weeks. The organism also has been isolated from fresh and salt water and has survived up to five weeks in fresh, untreated water.[3,5,7,9,14,16,17,19,20]

Because campylobacter enteritis in humans is clearly a zoonosis with animals as an important reservoir, both dogs and cats are sources of infection.[14,21,22] How important they are as sources is still uncertain. Skirrow and Benjamin stated that in Britain no more than 5% of cases of campylobacter enteritis in humans have been associated with dogs and cats, and those zoonoses were associated with newly acquired puppies.[23] Recently, *C. jejuni* infection in a young woman was associated with infection in an apparently healthy adult cat.[9]

Despite the ubiquitous nature of the organism, the epidemiologic associations of *C. jejuni* are not well established. Outbreaks with water and milk as the vehicles of transmission have been confirmed.[22] The evidence for ill-cooked chicken as a source is interesting but not conclusive.[18]

Based on matched controlled studies of sporadic human *C. jejuni* enteritis in Colorado, the odds ratios of increased risk factors were noted for drinking raw water (10.7), drinking raw milk (6.9), eating undercooked chicken (2.8), and living in a household with a cat (3.2).[24]

In a study of human cases of diarrhea in Japan, 188 of 881 cases had *C. jejuni* isolated from the stool and the rates of positive stool cultures of animals in the area were cattle (12%), chickens (45%), dogs (5%), and cats (10%). The strains found in chickens most closely resembled the human isolates.[25]

Studies on heat-stable antigens using unabsorbed antisera of human isolates compared with domestic farm isolates indicated a high similarity index for, in decreasing order, poultry, wild birds, flies, and pigs. The predominant porcine strain was never isolated from humans, and the strains found in flies closely resembled those from animals in the area.[26] Serotyping also showed a close relationship between isolates of human and chicken origin but little relationship between human and pig strains.[27]

Although the sources of human infection are usually poultry, unpasteurized milk, contaminated water, and direct contact with animals with enteritis, food poisoning caused by campylobacter appears to be uncommon, unlike the situation with *Salmonella*. *Campylobacter* dies during cooling of pork and beef carcasses because of drying effects of ventilation. Furthermore, the inability of the organism to grow at temperatures below 30°C (86°F) and its microaerophilic nature would make contamination of most foods, except for chicken and vacuum-packed processed meats, uncommon for *Campylobacter*.[28]

Typing of *Campylobacter jejuni*

With the increasing interest in the zoonotic potential of *C. jejuni*, several methods of distinguishing strains have been developed. Criteria for classification of *C. jejuni* are summarized in the box on this page. Serotyping, biotyping, and phage-typing techniques have helped differentiate pathogenicity of different strains but have not clearly discerned the role of the small pet animal in the epidemiology. Most of the methods are technically difficult and expensive, and reliance on only one can be confusing.[22,29]

In a human outbreak of *C. jejuni* associated with dogs, a litter of 11 puppies was given to local residents of a community. All but 1 of the puppies died with enteritis, and people in most of the households with puppies developed diarrhea. *Campylobacter jejuni* was diagnosed in nine households involving 16 human cases. Use of 2 serologic methods and 1 biotyping scheme, however, revealed that 3 different strains were involved in the outbreak.[22]

Even with the use of hemagglutination methods of serotyping,[30] a slide agglutination method,[31] and the biotyping scheme of Preston,[22] confusion exists as to the best methods for strain classification. Serology involves the separation of strains by the tolerance to heat of the somatic, flagellar, and capsular antigens (O, H, and K). Evaluation of data suggests that heterogenicity within apparently similar

---

Classification of *Campylobacter*

Gram stain, morphology:
  Dark-field or phase-contrast microscopy
  Curved, motile, gram-negative
  "Sea gull–shaped," with tapered ends
  0.2 to 0.4 µm × 1.5 to 3.5 µm
Microaerophilic growth at 25°C vs. 37°C vs. 42°C
Heat-labile toxin
Enzyme activity:
  Catalase, hippurate, hydrogen sulfide production
Serotyping
Biotyping
Phage typing
Plasmid profile (band and base-pair)
Pathogenesis
  Invasive
  Enterotoxin production
  Cytotoxic

---

strains exists. Strains that are of similar serotypes may be of different biotypes, or strains by the same biotype may be of the same serotype according to one but not another serologic method. Further confusion is inherent in the ability of the strains of *Campylobacter* to change antigenicity with serial passage in vivo and in vitro.[22,29,31,32] Thus, it has been suggested that a serotyping scheme should always be combined with a biotyping scheme to document an epidemiologic study of an outbreak when human, animal, and environmental isolates are involved.[22]

Plasmids in *Campylobacter* Isolates

The rate of occurrence of plasmids in *Campylobacter* isolates in diarrheic humans (9.5%), pigs (83.3%), and poultry (0% to 100% depending on flock; mean 58%) indicates variability and probably adaptability of the organism.[33]

Animal isolates of *Campylobacter* species frequently have plasmids of various molecular weights. For plasmids that act as R factors, the high frequency of plasmid DNA may result from the exposure of the organisms to antibiotics present in animal feeds. Under normal conditions, plasmids can be superfluous and tend to be lost; when plasmid function becomes essential for survival, cells containing the appropriate plasmid will be selected. These genetic loci may be transient and unstable and lost or gained based on necessity. In addition to antibiotic resistance, plasmids may encode for phenotypic traits involved in virulence, toxicity, and hydrocarbon catabolism. The pathogenic potential of *C. jejuni* to invade and produce enterotoxin has been confirmed.[14,36,37,63] The possibility exists, as in *Escherichia coli*, that there might be a separate plasmid-induced property of either invasiveness or enterotoxigenicity.[49,50] Several researchers have identified a choleralike enterotoxin produced by strains of *C. jejuni*.[63]

Screening of *C. coli* and *C. jejuni* strains from domestic animals revealed plasmid profiles that varied according to the health status of the animal host. The frequency of plasmids in diarrheic cattle with *C. jejuni* was higher than in normal cattle. Isolates showing resistance to ampicillin, tetracycline, and gentamicin were more likely to contain plasmids, suggesting a probable plasmid-mediated resistant for tetracycline and perhaps gentamicin.[34] A tetracycline-resistant plasmid has not been associated with enterotoxin or cytotoxic activity.

Plasmid profiles have indicated homology between DNA-encoding tetracycline resistance in *Campylobacter* species and tetracycline resistance from *Streptococcus* species indicating a transfer of genetic information between a gram-negative and a gram-positive coccus. Tetracycline resistance could not be transferred to *E. coli* by conjugation or transformation, suggesting that transfer between *Campylobacter* and unrelated gram-negative organisms is unlikely.[38]

Campylobacter jejuni in Dogs and Cats

The interest in *C. jejuni* in dogs and cats has been directed at documentation of the prevalence of the organism in diarrheic and healthy dogs and cats. Attempts have also been made experimentally to induce infestation or infection.

Clinical Evidence

Although it is clear that *C. jejuni* can cause enteric disease in humans with relatively few organisms (500 bacteria per os), the pathogenicity is unclear in dogs and cats. *Campylobacter* species have been isolated from both normal and diarrheic dogs at about the same frequency, suggesting that *Campylobacter* species are not primary pathogens of dogs.[19] Reported canine isolates indicate that *C. jejuni* may be a cause of diarrhea in dogs and can be found more frequently in diarrheic dogs.

Conditions associated with increased frequency of isolation of *C. jejuni* in dogs and cats are summarized in the box below. Differences in the animals' ages, degree of sanitation, and environment of the survey populations might explain the discrepancies in the reported rate of infection. The histories of the dogs surveyed often are not documented. The young puppy in a concentrated population with poor sanitation, such as an ill-kept kennel, has the greatest potential for exposure. Isolation frequency ranges from less than 5% to as high as 90% in puppies.[6,7,39]

In reported spontaneous *Campylobacter*-associated diar-

Conditions Associated with Increased Frequency of Isolation of *Campylobacter jejuni* in Dogs and Cats

Diarrheic animals
Young animals
Concentrated housing or poor sanitation
Stressful conditions
  New arrivals in kennel
  Pregnancy, surgery
  Other illness
Other enteric pathogens
  Parvovirus, *Salmonella*, *Giardia*, parasites

---

rhea, dogs developed a mucous, watery, and occasionally bloody stool of 5 to 15 days duration. Anorexia, vomiting, and a febrile response have been noted. In that these are nonspecific signs and the disease reportedly is most common in the young, the differential diagnosis would include all causes of acute enteritis in dogs. The higher incidence of disease in the young, in poor kennel conditions, in stressed adult dogs, and concomitant with other intestinal disease agents would indicate that the organism may be synergistic or opportunistic in the mechanism of disease. The synergistic role of *C. jejuni* in parvovirus infections has been documented, and there has been speculation on a potential role for other viral agents. *Campylobacter jejuni*-associated disease in adult dogs can clinically and histopathologically mimic parvovirus infection and should be considered in dogs developing diarrhea after environmental, physiologic, or surgical stress.[40-44]

In one study, *Campylobacter jejuni* was isolated from 29% of dogs and 21% of cats with diarrhea as compared with 4% of normal dogs and cats. *Campylobacter coli* was isolated from dogs (8%) and cats (5%) with diarrhea but rarely from normal dogs (2%) or cats (0%).[45] The rate of occurrence of *C. jejuni* in positive stools from laboratory beagles was higher in diarrheic (90%) than in normal (63%) dogs.[39] The occurrence in privately owned healthy dogs would generally appear to be low (3.8%) compared with dogs in public kennels (12.8%).[47]

In young (less than six months old) dogs, the influence of stress is supported by finding *C. jejuni* in 3.1% of healthy dogs, 21.7% of dogs with diarrhea, and 6.7% of dogs without diarrhea but sick from other causes.[42] In a production colony of beagles with a 14.7% infection rate (25% in the young and 3.9% in adults), the rate of infection in recently acquired dogs was 32%.[46] Evaluation of age and stress demonstrated that on arrival at the kennels there was no difference in the rate of isolation among dogs less than or over six months of age; however, a significant increase in the rate of isolation by Days 5 to 7 compared with Day 1 was noted, suggesting that while dogs may acquire campylobacter infection in kennels, excretion of the organism may be intermittent and precipitated by stress.[48]

The incidence in cats is less well described than in dogs. *Campylobacter jejuni* has been isolated from feces of up to 45% of nondiarrheic cats.[7,17,49,50] The infection rate seems to be low, however, in most cat populations in which good hygiene is practiced. No correlation between the environment or age of animal and incidence of infection was noted in a population of cats, 1% of which had campylobacter isolates. Contact of uninfected cats with cats shedding the organism caused a transient diarrhea in the previously healthy cats, and the sporadic pattern of excretion of organisms tends to make diagnosis based on one culture difficult.[51] Clinical signs in another cat with seroconversion abated when treated, and the organism could not be recultured from the stool.[52] In another report, *C. jejuni* was isolated from 21% of diarrheic cats compared with 4% of normal cats, similar to the rates in dogs (29% of diarrheic dogs versus 4% of normal dogs).[45]

Experimental Evidence

The incidence of positive stool cultures for *C. jejuni* provides serious confusion and consternation for the veterinarian. Given the fact that the organism can be found in normal, adult dogs but is isolated more frequently in young, diarrheic, stressed dogs, the diagnosis can be elusive as far as a cause and effect relationship.

Variables associated with experimental infection of dogs with *C. jejuni* include the following:

- Selection of pathogenic strain
- Serial passage of strains versus frozen ($-70°$ C)
- Number of organisms for inoculation
- Route of delivery of infective dose
- Animal host conditioning
- Concomitant diseases.

Although initially unsuccessful in producing diarrhea in puppies with *Campylobacter* species of human origin,[53] a mild diarrhea was produced in gnotobiotic beagle puppies using either human or canine isolates of *C. jejuni*.[54] A moderate, superficial, erosive colitis was noted. Feces from infected puppies became increasingly fluid at the peak of the illness. Other signs were tenesmus, lassitude, and mild anorexia. In contrast with the disease in humans, the clinical disease in dogs appears to be less severe and to require more infective organisms. Reports of induction of enteritis in conventional puppies[55] and fieldwork with natural cases indicate that a 7- to 10-day course of semiformed to watery stools with mucus and occasional blood, tenesmus, and ileus, as in humans, occurs in conventional dogs rather than just a colitis as in the gnotobiotic dogs.[55]

Inconsistencies in the experimental induction of the disease obviously center on the source and method of inoculation of the organism. Given the multiple strains and the ability of the organism to change both in vivo and in vitro, laboratory manipulation before inoculation may influence the pathogenicity of the *C. jejuni* to be tested. The difficulty in inducing the disease in gnotobiotic beagles must also be viewed in reference to the synergistic role of other enteric pathogens. Oral inoculation of up to 8.8×10^9 organisms from diarrheic dogs to puppies did not induce disease, but the organism multiplied in 60% of the cases and was excreted for two to seven weeks.[5]

Organisms that are pathogenic in humans can reproduce, shed, and cause seroconversion in dogs. Although this is of public health concern, the role of the bacteria as a primary pathogen is still in doubt. The higher incidence in the young, in animals under stress, and in animals with diarrhea is too compelling to allow veterinarians to ignore the role of *C. jejuni* as at least a secondary pathogen. Careful challenge with an endotoxin-producing strain with known human pathogenesis would illuminate the role of *C. jejuni* as a primary pathogen in dogs and cats.

The histologic pattern may depend on the strain of the organism but the ileum, cecum, and colon are primarily involved. Mucosal hyperplasia, blunting of intestinal villi, inflammatory cell infiltrates of the lamina propria, and Peyer's patches have been described in dogs.[39] *Campylobacter jejuni* can be found, however, in the stools of dogs with diarrhea even when none of the above histologic changes are observed. In one study of 32 strains isolated, 43% were from the rectum, 75% from the colon, and 81% were from the cecum.[56]

In Sweden, thermotolerant, catalase-negative, hippurate-positive *Campylobacter* species have been isolated from diarrheic humans[57] and dogs that have been considered non-enteropathogenic. Based on DNA studies, this "Swedish catalase-negative or weak strain" closely resembles *C. jejuni*.[57] Clinical signs ascribed to a similar *Campylobacter* species in a dog that responded to antibiotics have been described.[58]

Identification of Campylobacter jejuni

Examination of diarrheic feces by dark-field or phase-contrast microscopy can permit a presumptive diagnosis and suggest whether fecal cultures are indicated. The finding by the untrained observer of motile curved rods darting across a microscopic field is nonspecific and not definitive.[21] The use of Gram stain on human stool specimens for early presumptive diagnosis has been reported.[59]

Campylobacter jejuni are gram-negative, slender, curved (vibrio), S-shaped, or "sea gull–shaped" bacteria with tapered ends. They are 0.2 to 0.4 μm in width and vary from 1.5 to 3.5 μm in length, depending on the shape of the particular bacterium. The organism is microaerophilic with an optimal growth temperature from $37°$ to $42°$ C ($98.6°$ to $107.6°$ F). *Campylobacter jejuni* will not grow at $25°$ C ($77°$ F) nor does it tolerate atmospheric concentrations of oxygen,[10,17,18,45,60] thus it is very important that fecal specimens or swabs be processed soon after collection. The specimens should be kept chilled ($4°$ C [$39.2°$ F]); if the sample is a swab it should be placed in an anaerobic transport medium.[45,60]

Isolation of *C. jejuni* from stool specimens can be difficult and requires from two to five days. Special requirements include selective techniques to reduce the growth of competing organisms and microaerophilic (not anaerobic) incubation conditions (5% oxygen, 10% carbon dioxide, and 85% nitrogen). The use of a selective campylobacter-specific medium (commonly known as "Campy-BAP") gives better recovery than other direct-plating media. Excellent discussions of the isolation and identification of campylobacters have been published.[7,17,18,45,60,61]

Antibody titer techniques being developed will augment the current knowledge and provide a clearer prospective of the clinical importance of campylobacters in dogs and cats. The isolation of *Campylobacter jejuni* does not confirm the organism as the causative agent in dogs and cats with diarrhea. Specific serum antibodies in humans can be detected after *C. jejuni* infections using tube agglutination, bactericidal assays, and indirect immunofluorescence.[3,22]

Therapy

Antibiotic therapy for *C. jejuni* enteritis in dogs or cats has not been experimentally evaluated. Therapy of spontaneous cases has resulted in elimination of the organism from the stools. In that the disease is usually self-limiting and rarely disseminated, therapy may not affect the clinical course of the disease[61,62] but might decrease the duration of bacterial shedding.

Based on a series of experiments of antibiotic sensitivity patterns of *C. jejuni*, high concentrations of ampicillin, penicillin, tetracycline, and metronidazole[61] were required to inhibit growth. Because *Campylobacter* is believed to produce β-lactamase, most strains are relatively resistant to ampicillin and other related antibiotics. More isolates containing plasmids were resistant to tetracycline, gentamicin, and ampicillin than were isolates not carrying plasmids. This tendency has been shown especially for tetracycline and gentamicin. In general, most isolates were susceptible to gentamicin, kanamycin, neomycin, erythromycin, and sulfonamide. Erythromycin is the drug of choice for therapy in humans, although resistant strains have been noted in human and animal isolates.[64-67] In a prospective trial in children with campylobacter enteritis, erythromycin did not alter the course of the disease but did decrease the duration of bacterial shedding.[68,69] The use of erythromycin in dogs with campylobacter enteritis did not change the clinical signs when compared with fluid therapy alone.[62] Furazolidone was effective at low minimum inhibiting concentrations (MIC), and resistance to the antibiotic apparently is rare. Chloramphenicol and doxycycline were effective, but canine isolates resistant to both antibiotics have been reported.[61] The use of chloramphenicol for one week in a dog with campylobacter enteritis (the organism was catalase-negative and sodium hippurate-negative but was not *C. jejuni*) did result in abatement of clinical signs and in the elimination of the organism from the stool.[58] Resistance to sulfamethoxazole and trimethoprim was high (60.2%) in isolates of *C. jejuni* and *C. coli*.[33]

With the increased incidence of transmission of antibiotic-resistant *Salmonella* to humans and the apparent increase in plasmid-mediated resistance in other enteric bacteria in response to the widespread use of antibiotics, the zoonotic potential of campylobacters is obvious. It would appear, however, that transmission of plasmid-mediated resistance among strains of *E. coli* and *C. jejuni* does not occur.[33] Comparison of the antibiotic sensitivity of *C. jejuni/C. coli* strains isolated from dogs and cats with acute enteritis in 1986 versus 1981 confirms the concern.[70] In that report from Germany, resistance to all antibiotics increased from 1981 to 1986 with the exception of chloramphenicol, which did show, however, an increase in isolates that were only moderately sensitive. Increases in percentages of antibiotic-resistant isolates from 1981 to 1986 included 56.4% to 85.7% for benzylpenicillin, 17.9% to 41.3% for ampicillin, 0% to 9.5% for tetracycline, 0% to 8% for erythromycin, 10.3% to 65.1% for streptomycin, 2.6% to 4.8% for gentamicin, 0% to 4.8% for kanamycin, 0% to 9.5% for neomycin, and 7.7% to 14.3% for polymyxin B. All of these antibiotics had been used in the area of Germany in the years examined and the increases in resistance may reflect the bacterial response to the antibiotic pressure.[70]

From the data, erythromycin or chloramphenicol would appear to be the therapeutic drug of choice; however, *C. jejuni* susceptibility can be variable. In vitro antibiotic testing should be performed before therapy is instituted. The isolation of the causative organism and determination of antibiotic sensitivity are of increased importance because of the zoonotic potential of *C. jejuni*.

The Role of the Small Animal Practitioner

A *C. jejuni* infection in dogs or cats cannot be clinically distinguished at this time. Furthermore, isolation of the organism from healthy or diseased dogs or cats is not sufficient to warrant a diagnosis of enteritis. With the increased awareness of the organism, however, pets should be considered a potential reservoir for human infection and child–puppy contact may be questioned in the future. Although less than 5% of human *C. jejuni* enteritis cases are reportedly acquired from dogs,[23] the history of development of diarrhea in the owner(s) after a previous bout of diarrhea in a puppy is suggestive. This implication would be strengthened if the pet were newly acquired or had been recently stressed or if poor sanitation were suspected.

Small numbers (500) of *C. jejuni* potentially can cause infection in humans; therefore, the possibility of acquiring an infection from contact with feces from an infected or carrier pet animal is real. This hazard would appear to be more likely than with *Salmonella* species in which large numbers (10^5 to 10^7) usually are required for human infection.[10] The zoonotic potential of campylobacter enteritis is compared with that of *Salmonella* enteritis in Table II. The large reservoir and multiple modes and vehicles of transmission would dictate that clients developing *C. jejuni* enteritis should examine water, meats and foodstuffs, and milk for contamination before the pet dog or cat is incriminated as the source. If both pet and owner are affected, the most likely scenario would be the exposure of both pet and owner to a common source.

For both pet owners and veterinarians, the basics of good hygiene and the necessity for hand-washing after contact with diarrheic animals or feces are reinforced by this disease. For the practitioner, the isolation of hospitalized puppies with enteric disease and the careful handling of

TABLE II
Comparisons of Zoonotic Potential of Bacterial Enteritis

	Salmonella	Campylobacter
Growth	Easy	Special
Typing	Established	Developing
Identification	Easy	Easy
Growth in meat	+++	?
Growth in milk	+++	No
Normal flora	+	+++
Infective dose	++++	+
Dissemination	++	?
Person-to-person contact	+++	+?
Carriage	3 months	+?

their feces is recommended for the benefit of both the animal handlers and other hospitalized pets. When it is determined that a diarrheic pet is shedding *C. jejuni*, antibiotic sensitivity testing and the initiation of erythromycin therapy are indicated. Good client education and professional awareness should avoid potential problems until more answers are available.

REFERENCES

1. Kist M: Wer entdeckte *Campylobacter jejuni/coli?* Eine Zusammenfassung bisher unberucksichtigter Literaturquellen. *Zentralbl Bakteriol Mikrobiol Hyg [A]* 261(2):177-186, 1986.
2. Ahnen DJ, Brown WR: Campylobacter enteritis in immune-deficient patients. *Ann Intern Med* 96:187-188, 1982.
3. Blaser MJ, Reller LB: Medical progress: Campylobacter enteritis. *N Engl J Med* 305:1444-1452, 1981.
4. Smibert RM: The genus *Campylobacter. Annu Rev Microbiol* 32:674-709, 1978.
5. Blaser MJ, LaForce FM, Wilson NA, et al: Reservoirs for human campylobacteriosis. *J Infect Dis* 141:665-669, 1980.
6. New faces among the campylobacters. *Lancet* 2:662, 1983.
7. Prescott JF, Munroe DL: *Campylobacter jejuni* enteritis in man and domestic animals. *JAVMA* 181:1524-1530, 1982.
8. Fox JG, Moore R, Ackerman JI: Canine and feline campylobacteriosis: Epizootiology and clinical and public health features. *JAVMA* 183:1420-1424, 1983.
9. Blaser MJ, Weiss SH, Barrett TJ: Campylobacter enteritis associated with a healthy cat. *JAMA* 247:816, 1982.
10. Butzler JP, Skirrow MB: Campylobacter enteritis. *Clin Gastroenterol* 8:737-765, 1979.
11. Coffin CM, L'Heureaux P, Dehner LP: Campylobacter-associated enterocolitis in childhood. *Am J Clin Pathol* 78:117-123, 1982.
12. Colgan T, Lambert JR, Newman A, et al: *Campylobacter jejuni* enterocolitis. *Arch Pathol Lab Med* 104:571-574, 1980.
13. Shane SM, Montrose MS, Harrington KS: Transmission of *Campylobacter jejuni* by the housefly *(Musca domestica). Avian Dis* 29:384-391, 1985.
14. Skirrow MB: Campylobacter enteritis: The first five years. *J Hyg [Camb]* 89:175-184, 1984.
15. Klipstein FA, Engert RF: Immunological relationship of the B subunits of *Campylobacter jejuni* and *Escherichia coli* heat-labile enterotoxins. *JAVMA* 187:629, 1985.
16. Holt PE: The role of dogs and cats in the epidemiology of human campylobacter enterocolitis. *J Small Anim Pract* 22:681-685, 1981.
17. Bruce D, Zochowski W, Fleming GA: Campylobacter infections in cats and dogs. *Vet Rec* 197:200-201, 1980.
18. Cruckshank JG: *Salmonella* and *Campylobacter* infections—An update. *J Small Anim Pract* 27(10):673-681, 1986.
19. Hosie BD, Nicolson DB, Henderson DB: Campylobacter infections in normal and diarrhoeic dogs. *Vet Rec* 105:80, 1979.
20. Skirrow MB, Benjamin J: "1001" Campylobacters: Cultural characteristics of intestinal campylobacters from man and animals. *J Hyg [Camb]* 85:427-442, 1980.
21. Dillon AR, Wilt GR: Campylobacter species in the dog and cat. A cause for concern? *Vet Clin North Am [Small Anim Pract]* 13:647-652, 1983.
22. Hutchinson DN, Bolton FJ, Jones DM, et al: Application of three typing schemes (Penner, Lior, Preston) to strains of *Campylobacter* spp. isolated from three outbreaks. *Epidemiol Infect* 98(2):139-144, 1987.
23. Skirrow MB, Benjamin J: The classification of 'thermophilic' campylobacters and their distribution in man and domestic animals, in Newell DG (ed): *Campylobacter: Epidemiology, Pathogenesis and Biochemistry.* Hingham, MA, MTP Press, 1981, pp 40-44.
24. Hopkins RS, Olmsted R, Istre GR: Endemic *Campylobacter jejuni* infection in Colorado: Identified risk factors. *Am J Public Health* 74:249-250, 1984.
25. Tanaka H: Isolation of campylobacter from human patients with sporadic diarrhoea and from animals, and the serovars isolated. *J Jpn Vet Med Assoc* 39(12):791-795, 1986.
26. Rosef O, Kapperud G, Lauwers S, Gondrosen B: Serotyping of *Campylobacter jejuni, Campylobacter coli,* and *Campylobacter laridis* from domestic and wild animals. *Appl Environ Microbiol* 49(6):1507-1510, 1985.
27. Oosterom J, Banffer JRJ, Lauwers S, Busschbach AE: Serotyping of and hippurate hydrolysis by *Campylobacter jejuni* isolates from human patients, poultry and pigs in the Netherlands. *Antonie Van Leeuwenhoek* 51:65-70, 1985.
28. Oosterom J: *Campylobacter jejuni:* An important causative agent of food infection in man. An overview. *Tijdschr Diergeneeskd* 109(11):446-455, 1984.
29. Patton CM, Barrett TJ, Morris OK: Comparison of the Penner and Lior methods for serotyping *Campylobacter* spp. *J Clin Microbiol* 22:558-565, 1985.
30. Penner JL, Hennessy JN: Passive haemagglutination technique for serotyping *Campylobacter fetus* subsp. *jejuni* on the basis of soluble heat-stable antigens. *J Clin Microbiol* 12:732-737, 1980.
31. Lior H, Woodward DL, Edgar JA, et al: Serotyping of *Campylobacter jejuni* by slide agglutination based on heat-labile antigenic factors. *J Clin Microbiol* 15:761-768, 1982.
32. Kazmi SU, Roberson BS, Stern NJ: Animal-passed, virulence-enhanced *Campylobacter jejuni* causes enteritis in neonatal mice. *Curr Microbiol* 11:159-164, 1984.
33. Treschnak E, Moser I, Hellmann E: Identification of species, plasmid pattern and drug resistance of *Campylobacter* strains isolated from faecal samples of domestic animals and humans. *Tierarztl Umschau* 42(2):133-136, 139-144, 1987.
34. Bradbury WC, Marko MA, Hennessy JN, Barrett TJ: Occurrence of plasmid DNA in serologically defined strains of *Campylobacter jejuni* and *Campylobacter coli. Infect Imun* 40:460-463, 1983.
35. Bradbury WC, Marko MA, Congi RV, Penner JL: Investigation of a *Campylobacter jejuni* outbreak by serotyping and chromosomal restriction endonuclease analysis. *J Clin Microbiol* 19:342-346, 1984.
36. Klipstein FA, Engert RF: Properties of crude *Campylobacter jejuni* heat-labile enterotoxin. *Infect Immun* 45:314-319, 1984.
37. Ruiz-Palacios GM, Torres J, Escamilla E, et al: Cholera-like enterotoxin produced by *Campylobacter jejuni. Lancet* 2:250-253, 1983.
38. Taylor DE: Plasmid-mediated tetracycline resistance in *Campylobacter jejuni:* Expression in *Escherichia coli* and identification of homology with streptococcal class M determinant. *J Bacteriol* 165:1037-1039, 1986.
39. Fox JG, Maxwell KO, Ackerman JI: *Campylobacter jejuni*-associated diarrhea in commercially reared beagles. *Lab Anim Sci* 34:151-155, 1984.
40. Fox JG, Krakowka S, Taylor NS: Acute-onset campylobacter-associated gastroenteritis in adult beagles. *JAVMA* 187:1268-1270, 1985.
41. Gruber A, Nascimento Mos E, Durigon EL, Noronha AM: Prevalence of *Campylobacter jejuni* and *C. coli* in normal and diarrhoeic faeces of dogs in Sao Paulo. *Rev Microbiol* 16(4):287-289, 1985.
42. Nair GB, Sarkar RK, Chowdhury S, Pal SC: Campylobacter infection in domestic dogs. *Vet Rec* 116(9):237-238, 1985.
43. Boscato U, Crotti D: *Campylobacter jejuni:* A major cause of enterocolitis in kennelled dogs. *Clin Vet* 53(5):303-308, 1985.
44. Sihvonen L, Hedlund M: *Campylobacter jejuni* in dogs and its association with enteritis. *Suomen Elainlaakarilehti* 93(2):51-53, 1987.
45. Rubsamen S: Detection of *Campylobacter jejuni* and *C. coli* from several animal species with and without enteritis using various media supplements. *Tierarztl Umschau* 10(2):131, 136-140, 1980.
46. Yoshimura M, Ebukuro M, Kagiyama N, et al: Isolation of *Campylobacter jejuni* from experimental dogs and monkeys in Japan. *Jikken Dobutsu* 33(2):209-212, 1984.
47. Romagnoli G, Pastoni F, Coccini T, Manidi AM: *Campylobacter jejuni* attraverso feci di animali domestici. *Riv Ital Igiene* 46(1/2):17-21, 1986.
48. Burnie AG, Simpson JW, Lindsay D, Miles RS: The excretion of campylobacter, salmonellae and *Giardia lamblia* in the faeces of stray dogs. *Vet Res Commun* 6(2):133-138, 1983.
49. Skirrow MB: Campylobacter enteritis in dogs and cats: A "new" zoonosis. *Vet Res Commun* 5:13-19, 1981.
50. Fleming MP: Association of *Campylobacter jejuni* with enteritis in dogs and cats. *Vet Rec* 113(16):372-374, 1983.
51. Gifford DH, Shane SM, Smith RE: Prevalence of *Campylobacter jejuni* in felidae in Baton Rouge, Louisiana. *Int J Zoonoses* 12(1):67-73, 1985.
52. Fox JG, Claps M, Beaucage CM: Chronic diarrhea associated with *Campylobacter jejuni* infection in a cat. *JAVMA* 189(4):455-456, 1986.
53. Prescott JF, Karmali MA: Attempts to transmit campylobacter enteritis to dogs and cats. *Can Med Assoc J* 119:1001-1002, 1978.

54. Prescott JF, Barker IK, Manninen KI, et al: *Campylobacter jejuni* colitis in gnotobiotic dogs. *Can J Comp Med* 45:377–383, 1981.
55. Macartney L, McCandlesh AP, Al-Mashat RR, et al: Natural and experimental enteric infections with *Campylobacter fetus* ssp. *jejuni* in dogs, in Newell DG (ed): *Campylobacter: Epidemiology, Pathogenesis, and Biochemistry*. Hingham, MA, MTP Press, 1981.
56. Pellerin JL, Milon A, Humbert E, et al: Campylobacter infection of the dog and cat: A "new" zoonosis. *Rev Med Vet* 135(11):675–689, 1984.
57. Steele TW, Sangster N, Lanser JA: DNA relatedness and biochemical features of *Campylobacter* spp. isolated in central and south Australia. *J Clin Microbiol* 22(1):71–74, 1985.
58. Davies AP, Gebhart, Meric SA: Campylobacter-associated chronic diarrhea in a dog. *JAVMA* 184:469–471, 1984.
59. Ho DD, Ault MJ, Ault MA, et al: Campylobacter enteritis. Early diagnosis with Gram's stain. *Arch Intern Med* 142:1858–1960, 1982.
60. Fox JG, Moore R, Ackerman JI: *Campylobacter jejuni*–associated diarrhea in dogs. *JAVMA* 183:1430–1433, 1983.
61. Fox JG, Dzink JL, Ackerman JI: Antibiotic sensitivity patterns of *Campylobacter jejuni/coli* isolated from laboratory animals and pets. *Lab Anim Sci* 34(3):264–267, 1984.
62. Boscato U, Cellie P, Rossi E, Crotti D: Il Campylobacter nel cane e in altri animali domestici: Suo possible ruolo eziopatogenetico in enteriti acute emorragiche e aspetti epidemiologici delle campylobacteriosi. *Malat Infet Parrassit* 36(9):990–997, 1984.
63. Walker RI, Caldwell MB, Lee EC, et al: Pathophysiology of campylobacter enteritis. *Microbiol Rev* 50:81–94, 1986.
64. Vanhoof R, Vanderlinden MP, Dierickx R, et al: Susceptibility of *Campylobacter fetus* subsp. *jejuni* to twenty-nine antimicrobial agents. *Antimicrob Agents Chemother* 14:553–556, 1978.
65. Walder N: Susceptibility of *Campylobacter fetus* subsp. *jejuni* to twenty antimicrobial agents. *Antimicrob Agents Chemother* 16:37–39, 1979.
66. Telfer-Brunton WA, Wilson AMM, Macrae RM: Erythromycin-resistant campylobacters. *Lancet* 2:1201, 1978.
67. Karmali MA, Bannatyn PM, Leers W, et al: *Campylobacter jejuni*. *Can Med Assoc J* 123:263–264, 1980.
68. Pai CH, Gillis G, Toumanen E, et al: Erythromycin in treatment of campylobacter enteritis in children. *Am J Dis Child* 137:286–288, 1983.
69. Robins-Browne RM, Mahandra KR, MacKenjee MB, et al: Treatment of campylobacter-associated enteritis with erythromycin. *Am J Dis Child* 137:282–285, 1983.
70. Rubsamen S, Rubsamen S: Comparison of the antibiotic sensitivity of thermophilic *Campylobacter* species in 1981 and 1986. *Tierarztl Umschau* 41(12):965–971, 1986.

Giardiasis

KEY FACTS

- *Giardia* is a common protozoan parasite of the gastrointestinal tract of dogs, cats, and humans.
- Transmission of *Giardia* occurs after ingestion of the parasite cyst.
- Clinical signs in small animals are variable, ranging from no detectable signs to chronic diarrhea.
- Zinc sulfate flotation of feces is recommended for diagnosis of *Giardia* cysts.
- The importance of dogs and cats as reservoirs for human infection is unknown, but many parasitologists believe that some strains have zoonotic potential.

Virginia Tech
Anne M. Zajac, DVM, PhD

GIARDIA, a flagellate protozoan parasite of the intestinal tract, is found in many host species throughout the world. Surveys of dogs reveal considerable variation in prevalence, with the highest infection rates observed in puppies. In one recent study in the United States, 36% of puppies that were privately owned or housed in animal shelters were infected.[1] In cats, rates of infection are lower, usually ranging from 1% to 11%.[2] Despite the frequency of giardiasis in small animals, much remains unknown about the biology and pathogenesis of *Giardia* infection. Currently, even the zoonotic potential of infections in dogs and cats is not completely understood.

BIOLOGY

There are two forms of *Giardia*. The motile trophozoite, which is approximately 12 to 17 micrometers long and 7 to 10 micrometers wide, is found in the intestinal lumen. The parasite attaches to the surface of epithelial cells by means of a ventral disk, although the exact mechanism of attachment is controversial. The presence of a ventral disk gives the organism a distinct concave appearance when seen from a side view or in cross section. There are no intracellular stages in the life cycle of *Giardia*, and *Giardia* normally does not penetrate the mucosal epithelium or appear in other tissues. Reproduction is by binary fission.[3-6] Under appropriate conditions, which may be affected by fluctuations in pH and concentrations of bile salts and fatty acids, the trophozoite is transformed into the cyst form, which then reaches the environment in the feces.[7]

The cyst of *Giardia* is a nonfeeding structure surrounded by a distinct wall. The cyst is approximately 9 to 13 micrometers long, and it is the form of the parasite specialized for transmission. Although the cyst is very susceptible to desiccation, it can survive outside the host in cool water for a period of several months. After ingestion of the cyst by an appropriate host, excystation of the cyst occurs in the small intestine and trophozoites become established. The prepatent period of the parasite is approximately one to two weeks.[3-6]

The specific location of *Giardia* in the intestinal tract of small animals has been investigated in a limited number of studies. Trophozoites were found principally in the jejunum of an experimentally infected cat eight days after infection,[8] although *Giardia* was observed throughout the length of the intestinal tract in an infected kitten.[9] In a series of naturally infected dogs, *Giardia* was found in the small intestine but the location of the maximum number of trophozoites varied with the individual and ranged from the ileum to the duodenum.[10] Diet has also been shown to affect the distribution of *Giardia* in dogs.[11] The influence of factors, such as diet, duration of infection, or immunity, may be important in explaining the various clinical signs associated with *Giardia* infections.

GIARDIA INFECTION IN DOGS AND CATS

Most infections of dogs and cats with *Giardia* are probably not associated with clinical signs, and varying numbers of cysts may be present in feces of animals with no histories of gastrointestinal disease. In animals that develop clinical giardiasis, the most common sign is diarrhea. Feces are soft, pale, and foul smelling. Levels of split and unsplit fecal fats were detected in five cats with giardiasis,[12] and feces of clinically affected animals may have a greasy appearance suggestive of steatorrhea. The course of diarrhea caused by *Giardia* may be acute and self-limiting or chronic. Intermittent diarrhea caused by the parasite may also be encountered.

Giardia has been associated with weight loss and poor condition. Very watery or melenic feces are unlikely to be caused by *Giardia* alone. Fever and other systemic signs are also rarely associated with giardiasis, although some animals may become depressed.[3–5] Diarrhea caused by *Giardia* is usually characteristic of small intestinal maldigestion and malabsorption. Occasionally, animals are presented, however, with signs indicative of large bowel disease (e.g., feces containing large amounts of mucus or frank blood); these animals respond to treatment for *Giardia*.[13] Because the parasite is usually not present in the large intestine, it is difficult to explain the pathogenesis of large bowel diarrhea.

PATHOGENESIS

The pathogenesis of giardiasis in dogs and cats has not been thoroughly examined, but infected humans and laboratory animals have shown reduced digestion and absorption of several nutrients, including disaccharides, fats, and vitamins. Decreased levels of intestinal disaccharidases and lipases have been recorded.[14,15] Enterocyte production and turnover are increased in the small intestine. Biopsy samples often show no histologic changes, but villous atrophy may occur in severe infections. The alterations in epithelial cell turnover and structure of the villus appear to be associated with development of the host immune response.[16,17]

CURRENTLY, very little information is available to explain the wide variation in the pathogenicity of *Giardia* infection. In some cases, the status of the host immune response is clearly important. Clinical disease appears to be more common in humans with hypogammaglobulinemia.[18,19] Giardiasis oftens occurs, however, in healthy humans and animals with no evidence of immunologic deficiency. Other factors, such as host nutritional status or strain variation in the parasite, may contribute to the development of clinical signs, but there is limited experimental evidence to support these speculations.

IMMUNITY

Experimentation with *Giardia* infections in laboratory animals indicates that both antibody (especially immunoglobulin A) and T lymphocytes are required for development of immunity to the parasite.[20] The importance of immunity in influencing the status and course of infection in dogs and cats has not been experimentally evaluated, but the higher prevalence of infection in young animals suggests that some degree of protective immunity develops.[4] In one study, the prevalence of infection was higher in a colony of immunoglobulin A–deficient beagles than in normal animals.[21] Immunity, however, may not eliminate existing infection or provide absolute protection against reinfection. Experimentally infected dogs have been found to shed cysts over long periods[22] and to shed cysts repeatedly despite treatment for the parasite.[23]

DIAGNOSIS

Identification of *Giardia* in fecal samples is the simplest and most inexpensive procedure for diagnosing infection. Although recovery from feces and recognition of *Giardia* are not difficult, it is important to use the most effective procedure.

Direct Smears and Zinc Sulfate Flotation

Fecal samples may be examined for trophozoites by direct smear. If direct smears alone are relied on for diagnosis, however, many cases of *Giardia* infection will be missed. Trophozoites may be present if the feces are very loose, but in feces that are formed or semiformed, identification of trophozoites can rarely be accomplished. Samples should then be examined for cysts by a concentration technique.

TO PERFORM a direct smear, a very small amount of feces is mixed with physiologic saline on a glass slide and examined microscopically after adding a coverslip. The general rule of thumb is that newsprint should be readable through the smear. Trophozoites are usually recognized by their characteristic rapid motion and concave ventral surface. The parasites are recognized more easily if the slide is examined with a reduced light level. For example, keeping the condenser in its lowest position or partially closing the condenser diaphragm can effectively increase contrast. Addition of Lugol's iodine kills the organisms but enhances recognition of characteristic internal structures. Because *Giardia* is most readily found in a direct smear by detecting movement, a fresh fecal sample should be used. A refrigerated sample or one examined several hours after collection probably contains no living organisms. Cysts may be present but are difficult to identify in the midst of the fecal debris because of their immobility and small size.[5,24]

The only other motile organisms that are approximately the same size as *Giardia* and that may be present in fecal smears are intestinal trichomonads. The pathogenic significance of these flagellates is controversial, but they can be distinguished from *Giardia* by a more rolling form of motion, the presence of an undulating membrane, and the absence of a distinct concave surface on profile.[24]

Examination of fecal samples for the presence of *Giardia* cysts should always be performed if trophozoites are not

Zinc Sulfate Flotation Technique[5,23,24]

1. Thoroughly mix approximately 2 grams of feces with approximately 15 milliliters of 33% zinc sulfate solution (33 grams zinc sulfate made up to 100 milliliters with distilled water; specific gravity 1.18).
2. Strain the solution through cheesecloth or a tea strainer.
3. Pour the strained suspension into a 15-milliliter centrifuge tube; polypropylene tubes are preferable to polystyrene tubes.
4. Place the tube in a centrifuge (a standard bench top centrifuge can be used). If the tubes hang vertically in the centrifuge, flotation solution can be added until a reverse meniscus forms. A coverslip is added and spun in place on top of the tube. If the tubes are placed in the centrifuge at an angle, the surface layer is harvested after spinning.
5. Spin the tube at approximately 1500 rpm for three to five minutes.
6. Remove the coverslip and the adhering drop of fluid and place them on a microscope slide. When a coverslip is not used, collect the surface layer of fluid by touching a glass rod (a 3-milliliter blood collection tube makes a convenient substitute) or bacteriologic loop to the surface of the centrifuge tube. Deposit the collected fluid on a slide, add a coverslip, and examine. Lugol's iodine may be added, if desired, to stain organisms.

Some of the debris in the fecal sample can be removed by initially mixing the sample with water and centrifuging it. Resultant supernatant is discarded, and zinc sulfate solution is added to the pellet and centrifuged as described above. I have not found this initial water wash to be necessary on a routine basis. When steatorrhea is present, large amounts of fat float with the *Giardia* cysts and may complicate reading of the slide. In these situations, an ethyl acetate sedimentation technique can be used; the sample is mixed with water, filtered, and placed in a centrifuge tube with two to three milliliters of ethyl acetate or ether. After centrifuging, the supernatant, including a distinct layer containing the organic solvent and fat, is discarded. The pellet is then resuspended, and a drop is stained with Lugol's iodine and examined.

found in a direct smear. In general, the best technique for identifying cysts is the zinc sulfate flotation test.[25] Routine flotation tests that use saturated salt solutions (e.g., sodium nitrate or sodium chloride) are more hypertonic than the zinc sulfate solution and destroy the fragile parasite cysts. The cysts will float without distortion when a 33% solution of zinc sulfate (specific gravity 1.18) is used; however, cysts prepared by this technique eventually collapse if the slide is allowed to sit for more than 15 to 20 minutes. Because the 33% zinc sulfate solution also floats other common parasite eggs, it can be used as the routine flotation solution in small animal practice.[24] Instructions for the zinc sulfate flotation test are provided in the box entitled Zinc Sulfate Flotation Technique. In feces, cysts are most often confused with

yeast but *Giardia* cysts have distinct internal structures and are usually readily distinguishable from yeast (Figure 1).

Because *Giardia* is known to produce cysts only intermittently, it is usually recommended that at least three samples be examined over a period of about one week before excluding the possibility of *Giardia*.[3,5] If a fecal sample cannot be examined immediately, it can be stored in the refrigerator for several days. The sample should not be frozen. While addition of 10% formalin to fecal samples satisfactorily preserves most helminth eggs, it is not effective for *Giardia* cysts.[4]

Duodenal Aspirates

Examination of duodenal aspirates for trophozoites has also been recommended for the diagnosis of *Giardia* infections in small animals (Figure 2). A duodenal aspirate was found to be more effective than a single fecal sample in diagnosing clinical giardiasis in one series of 47 dogs.[26] In another study of subclinically infected dogs, however, a single fecal sample was as effective as a duodenal aspirate for diagnosis of parasites.[23]

A DUODENAL aspirate can be easily collected during duodenoscopy by attaching a syringe containing saline to polyethylene tubing passed through the endoscope channel, injecting the fluid, and then aspirating back immediately. As much of the original saline as possible should be recovered. The sample is then centrifuged at approximately 1500 rpm for several minutes, and the sediment is examined. As is the case with direct smears, motility of the trophozoite is important for identification, particularly if only a few organisms are present. Consequently, it is important to examine an aspirate immediately after collection. An alternative method of examination is to prepare a dried and Giemsa-stained smear of the aspirate.[5]

ELISA Kits

Recently, commercial enzyme-linked immunosorbent assay (ELISA) kits have become available for the diagnosis of *Giardia*. These kits have been developed for human *Giardia* infections but can also be used for small animals. The kits are based on the detection of trophozoite antigens in fecal samples (Figure 3). Frozen feces can be used if the samples are not preserved with fixative. In a limited study performed at the Virginia-Maryland Regional College of Veterinary Medicine,[27] one of these tests was found to be slightly more effective than a single zinc sulfate flotation in diagnosing experimental canine *Giardia* infection. The ELISA kits are more expensive and technically more difficult than the zinc sulfate flotation test. At this time, there does not seem to be any substantial benefit in replacing microscopic examination of feces with an ELISA kit for diagnosis of *Giardia* in veterinary practice.

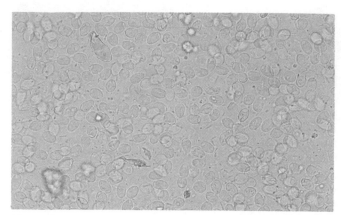

Figure 1—A zinc sulfate flotation test reveals *Giardia* cysts. Without special staining, internal structures of the cysts can be seen. (×400)

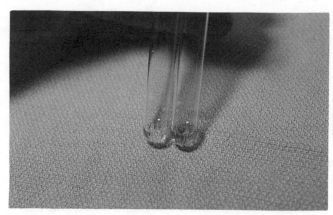

Figure 3—Commercial ELISA kits detect parasite antigen in fecal samples. The positive sample produces a distinct change in color.

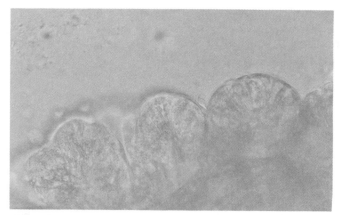

Figure 2—Diagnosis of *Giardia* infection by examination of a duodenal aspirate. A trophozoite is present between two villi dislodged by the procedure. The motility of the parasite permits rapid detection, even if very few organisms are present. (×400)

TREATMENT

The drug most commonly used in the United States for treatment of *Giardia* in small animals is metronidazole. A standard recommended dosage is 25 mg/kg orally twice daily for five days in dogs and 10 or 25 mg/kg orally twice daily for five days in cats. Metronidazole tablets have a very bitter taste and should not be crushed before use, especially when given to cats.[5,8] Although metronidazole is not associated with side effects in most animals, vomiting and diarrhea may occur. In a recent report, five dogs given daily doses as low as 63 mg/kg for 10 days had neurologic signs, including ataxia and nystagmus.[28] Metronidazole has been found to have some mutagenic effect in laboratory tests and should not be used in pregnant animals.[5]

Quinacrine may also be used to treat giardiasis. A dosage of 6.6 mg/kg orally twice daily for five days can be used for dogs; 2.3 mg/kg/day for 12 days controlled clinical signs but did not eliminate cyst shedding in a series of five cats.[12] Side effects associated with the use of quinacrine in-

clude vomiting, fever, anorexia, lethargy, and altered behavior (e.g., increased barking and fly biting).[5,29] In one study of dogs, quinacrine was found to be more effective than metronidazole in treating giardiasis; however, side effects occurred only in dogs treated with quinacrine.[29] Quinacrine is not recommended during pregnancy in humans because it readily crosses the placenta[30]; quinacrine should probably also be avoided in pregnant animals.

A third compound used in the treatment of giardiasis is furazolidone. Although evidence from human trials indicates that furazolidone may be less effective than metronidazole and quinacrine,[30] it has been used effectively to treat cats. Furazolidone is available in sweet-tasting liquid preparations for swine and children and is used in cats at a dosage of 4 mg/kg twice daily for seven days. Side effects include vomiting and diarrhea. Furazolidone has been reported to be mutagenic in laboratory animals; its use should be avoided during pregnancy.[8]

RECENTLY, other compounds have also been investigated for their activity against *Giardia*. Paromomycin, an aminoglycoside antibiotic, has been used to treat human giardiasis. Reports of use in humans suggest that paromomycin is less effective than other antigiardial drugs, but because of the limited absorption of paromomycin from the gastrointestinal tract, it has been used in pregnant women. Currently, there are no reports on the use of paromomycin in small animals.

Benzimidazole anthelmintics have also been recently investigated for activity against *Giardia*. Albendazole and mebendazole have been found to be effective in vitro against the parasite,[31] and albendazole was used successfully in treating mice infected with *Giardia*.[32] Although there are no reported studies on the use of benzimidazole anthelmintics in small animals, these compounds may represent useful alternatives for *Giardia* treatment.

Treatment should be repeated if clinical signs do not resolve. A combination of quinacrine (6.6 mg/kg twice daily for five days) and metronidazole (22 mg/kg twice daily for five days) was more effective in dogs than either drug alone[29] and may be useful in persistent cases of giardiasis. Because disease caused by *Giardia* is usually not severe, it is probably best to delay treatment of pregnant animals until after parturition.

Establishing the efficacy of treatment is difficult because of the intermittent production of cysts by the parasite. It has not been determined whether the drugs described here eliminate the parasite from the intestinal tract or merely reduce the number of organisms to a level that can then be effectively controlled by the host. Because it is impractical in many circumstances to perform several fecal examinations after treatment, it should probably be assumed that some animals continue to shed *Giardia* cysts despite resolution of clinical signs.

EPIDEMIOLOGY AND CONTROL

Because many of the dramatic outbreaks of giardiasis occurring in humans have been traced to contaminated water supplies, there is a widespread perception that *Giardia* infection is most often acquired from contaminated water. The high rates of infection in children in day care centers and dogs in animal shelters, however, demonstrate how easily infection can occur in the absence of contaminated water.[1,33]

TROPHOZOITES passed in diarrheic feces die quickly and are unlikely to infect another animal. The cyst is responsible for transmission to new hosts and should be considered infective as soon as it is passed in the feces. Because cysts are very susceptible to desiccation, thorough drying and exposure to sunlight are very important in attempts to control *Giardia*. Common disinfectants at dilutions recommended by the manufacturer can also be used to kill cysts. Dilutions of quaternary ammonium disinfectants appropriate for kennel situations inactivated cysts within 1 minute at 20°C (68°F). Bleach and phenolic compounds were also effective but required longer contact times. Colder temperatures increased the length of time required for inactivation.[34] Cysts do not survive boiling or freezing[35] but may live for several months in cool water and are usually resistant to chlorination procedures at water treatment facilities.[36]

At this time, it is not known how many distinct species of *Giardia* occur in animals. Parasites from various mammalian hosts and humans are morphologically identical and are now identified by many authorities as a single species, *Giardia intestinalis* (also referred to as *duodenalis* or *lamblia*). Many attempts have been made to identify the relationships between *Giardia* isolates from different hosts and locations using DNA and enzyme analysis, but these tests have yet to show consistent similarities or differences.[37]

Understanding the taxonomy of *Giardia* would be helpful in establishing the relationship between human and small animal *Giardia* infections. A number of animals, including dogs and cats, have been proposed as sources of infection for humans. Strong evidence of zoonotic infection from small animals, however, is lacking. Experimental attempts to infect dogs with cysts derived from human infections have provided contradictory results. Also, canine and human *Giardia* appear to be very different in their ability to establish in culture in the laboratory. These differences have led to the suggestion that dogs may not play an important role in the transmission of *Giardia* to humans.[37,38] Similarly, *Giardia* isolated from humans did not show great infectivity for cats. In one study, only one of six cats became infected; and in another study, two of eight cats briefly excreted cysts.[8]

ALTHOUGH the described results do not suggest a major role for small animals in human infection, definitive conclusions cannot be drawn from the limited number of *Giardia* isolates examined. Some parasite strains may have broader host preferences than the few strains used in these studies. Infection of humans with animal strains of the parasite may also occur more readily than animal infection with human strains.[37] Because the significance of dogs and cats as sources of human infection is still controversial, treatment of all infections diagnosed in small animals, whether or not clinical signs are apparent, is appropriate.

About the Author

Dr. Zajac is affiliated with the Department of Pathobiology at the Virginia-Maryland Regional College of Veterinary Medicine, Virginia Tech, Blacksburg, Virginia.

REFERENCES

1. Hahn NE, Glaser CA, Hird DW, Hirsch DC: Prevalence of *Giardia* in the feces of pups. *JAVMA* 192:1128–1129, 1988.
2. Kirkpatrick CE: Feline giardiasis: A review. *J Small Anim Pract* 27:69–80, 1986.
3. Barlough JE: Canine giardiasis: A review. *J Small Anim Pract* 20:613–623, 1979.
4. Kirkpatrick CE, Farrell JP: Giardiasis. *Compend Contin Educ Pract Vet* 5(4):367–378, 1982.
5. Kirkpatrick CE: Giardiasis. *Vet Clin North Am [Small Anim Pract]* 17:1377–1387, 1987.
6. Feely DE, Holberton DV, Erlandsen DL: The biology of *Giardia*, in Meyer EA (ed): *Giardiasis*. New York, Elsevier, 1990, pp 11–50.
7. Schupp DF, Reiner DS, Gillin FD, Erlandsen SL: In vitro encystation of *Giardia*, in Meyer EA (ed): *Giardiasis*. New York, Elsevier, 1990, pp 137–155.
8. Kirkpatrick CE, Farrell JP: Feline giardiasis: Observations on natural and induced infections. *Am J Vet Res* 45:2182–2188, 1984.
9. Hitchcock DJ, Malewitz TD: Habitat of *Giardia* in the kitten. *J Parasitol* 42:286, 1956.
10. Douglas H, Reiner DS, Gault MJ, Gillin FD: Location of *Giardia* trophozoites in the small intestine of naturally infected dogs in San

Diego, in Wallis PM, Hammond BR (eds): *Advances in Giardia Research.* Calgary, University of Calgary Press, 1988, pp 65–69.

11. Tsuchiya H: The localization of *Giardia canis* (Hegner, 1922) as affected by diet. *J Parasitol* 18:232–246, 1931.

12. Brightman AH II, Slonka GF: A review of five clinical cases of giardiasis in cats. *JAAHA* 12:492–497, 1976.

13. Ewing GO, Aldrete A: Canine giardiasis presenting as chronic ulcerative colitis: A case report. *JAAHA* 9:52–55, 1973.

14. Hartong WA, Gourley WK, Arvanitakis C: Giardiasis: Clinical spectrum and functional-structural abnormalities of the small intestinal mucosa. *Gastroenterology* 77:61–69, 1979.

15. Buret A, Gall DG, Olsen ME: Effects of murine giardiasis on growth, intestinal morphology, and disaccharidase activity. *J Parasitol* 76:403–409, 1990.

16. Ferguson A, Gillon J, Munro G: Pathology and pathogenesis of the intestinal mucosal damage in giardiasis, in Meyer EA (ed): *Giardiasis.* New York, Elsevier, 1990, pp 155–174.

17. Oberhuber G, Stolte M: Giardiasis: Analysis of histological changes in biopsy specimens of 80 patients. *J Clin Pathol* 43:641–643, 1990.

18. Ament ME, Rubin CE: Relation of giardiasis to abnormal intestinal structure and function in gastrointestinal immunodeficiency syndromes. *Gastroenterology* 62:216–226, 1972.

19. Vinayak VK, Kum K, Venkateswariu K, et al: Hypogammaglobulinaemia in children with persistent giardiasis. *J Trop Ped* 33:140–142, 1987.

20. Janoff EN, Smith PD: The role of immunity in *Giardia* infections, in Meyer EA (ed): *Giardiasis.* New York, Elsevier, 1990, pp 215–233.

21. Felsburg PJ, Glickman LT, Shofer F, et al: Clinical, immunologic and epidemiologic characteristics of canine selective IgA deficiency, in McGhee JR, Mestecky J, Ogra PL, Bienenstock J (eds): *Recent Advances in Mucosal Immunology.* New York, Plenum Press, 1987, pp 1460–1470.

22. Bemrick WJ: Observations on dogs infected with *Giardia. J Parasitol* 49:1031–1032, 1963.

23. Zajac AM, Leib MS, Burkholder WJ: Comparison of diagnostic tests for *Giardia* infection and effect of corticosteroids on naturally infected dogs. *J Small Anim Pract* (in press, 1992).

24. Williams JF, Zajac A: *Diagnosis of Gastrointestinal Parasitism in Dogs and Cats.* St. Louis, Ralston Purina Company, 1980.

25. Zimmer JF, Burrington DB: Comparison of four techniques of fecal

examination for detecting canine giardiasis. *JAAHA* 22:161–167, 1986.

26. Pitts RP, Twedt DC, Mallie KA: Comparison of duodenal aspiration with fecal flotation for diagnosis of giardiasis in dogs. *JAVMA* 182:1210–1211, 1983.

27. Zajac AM, Leib ML, Saunders G, et al: Experimental infection of dogs with *Giardia* (Abstract). Accepted for publication, *Proc Annu Meet Am Assoc Vet Parasitol*:August 1992.

28. Dow SW, LeCouteur RA, Poss ML, Beadleston D: Central nervous system toxicosis associated with metronidazole treatment of dogs: Five cases (1984–1987). *JAVMA* 195:365–368, 1989.

29. Zimmer JF, Burrington DB: Comparison of four protocols for the treatment of canine giardiasis. *JAAHA* 22:168–172, 1986.

30. Davidson RA: Treatment of giardiasis: The North American perspective, in Meyer EA (ed): *Giardiasis.* New York, Elsevier, 1990, pp 325–334.

31. Edlind TD, Hang TL, Chakraborty PR: Activity of the anthelmintic benzimidazoles against *Giardia lamblia* in vitro. *J Infect Dis* 162:1408–1411, 1990.

32. Meloni BP, Thompson RCA, Reynoldson JA, et al: Albendazole: A highly effective antigiardial agent. *Bull Soc Francaise Parasitol* (Abstracts of the VII International Congress of Parasitology, Paris, France) 8:1054, 1990.

33. Bartlett AV, Endlender MD, Jarvis BA, et al: Controlled trial of *giardia lamblia*: Control strategies in day care centers. *Am J Public Health* 81:1001–1006, 1991.

34. Zimmer JF, Miller JJ, Lindmark DG: Evaluation of the efficacy of selected commercial disinfectants in inactivating *Giardia muris* cysts. *JAAHA* 24:379–385, 1988.

35. Jarroll EL, Hoff JC, Meyer EA: Resistance of cysts to disinfection agents, in Erlandsen SL, Meyer EA (eds): *Giardia and Giardiasis.* New York, Plenum Press, 1984, pp 311–328.

36. Craun GF: Waterborne giardiasis, in Meyer EA (ed): *Giardiasis.* New York, Elsevier, 1990, pp 267–293.

37. Thompson RCA, Lymbery AJ, Meloni BP: Genetic variation in *Giardia* Kunstler, 1882: Taxonomic and epidemiological significance. *Protozool Abstracts* 14:1–28, 1990.

38. Healy GR: Giardiasis in perspective: The evidence of animals as a source of human *Giardia*, in Meyer EA (ed): *Giardiasis.* New York, Elsevier, 1990, pp 305–314.

UPDATE

A recent study[1] has demonstrated the efficacy of albendazole, a benzimidazole anthelmintic, against *Giardia* infection in dogs. In this study, albendazole at 25 mg/kg PO twice a day for a total of four doses eliminated *Giardia* cysts from the feces of 18 of 20 dogs. No signs of toxicity were observed in the dogs. A similar dose was not effective in eliminating cysts from the feces of *Giardia*-infected cats.[2]

REFERENCES

1. Barr SC, Bowman DD, Heller RL, Erb HN: Efficacy of albendazole against giardiasis in dogs. *Am J Vet Res* 54:926–928, 1993.
2. Barr SC, Bowman DD, Heller RL, et al: Efficacy of albendazole against *Giardia* sp in dogs and cats. *Proc 38th Annu Mtg Am Assoc Vet Parasitol* 83, 1993.

REFERENCES

1. Barr SC, Bowman DD, Heller RL, Erb HN: Efficacy of albendazole against giardiasis in dogs. *Am J Vet Res* 54:926–928, 1993.
2. Barr SC, Bowman DD, Heller RL, et al: Efficacy of albendazole against *Giardia* sp in dogs and cats. *Proc 38th Annu Mtg Am Assoc Vet Parasitol* 83, 1993.

Ascites

KEY FACTS

- Ascites is the accumulation of fluid in the peritoneal cavity.
- The accumulation of ascitic fluid always indicates an underlying disease process.
- The physical presence of peritoneal fluid may lead to systemic problems by causing cardiovascular collapse.
- Samples of fluid may be obtained by abdominal paracentesis and/or peritoneal lavage.
- Fluid analysis can provide important clues concerning the underlying disease and can help to guide therapy.

University of Pennsylvania

Lesley G. King, MVB, MRCVS   Hans C. J. Gelens, DVM

ASCITES is the accumulation of fluid in the peritoneal cavity. This definition classically applies to exudative and transudative fluids[1] but has been used to refer to accumulations of blood, chyle, urine, or bile.[2] Ascites is a sign of disease rather than a diagnosis. The historical findings thus vary depending on the underlying cause in each case.

HISTORY

In a patient with apparent peritoneal effusion, historical information can provide vital clues to assist the practitioner in determining the probable cause of the underlying disease process and in formulating a plan for further diagnostic efforts. For example, a history of trauma may suggest rupture of the urinary bladder, diaphragmatic hernia, hemoperitoneum, or septic peritonitis; cough, respiratory distress, or exercise intolerance may indicate cardiovascular disease; and disorientation, neurologic signs, or weight loss may suggest hepatic failure.

Similarly, the signalment may suggest the underlying cause of peritoneal effusion. For example, neoplasia is more common in old dogs, and spayed females are unlikely to have septic peritonitis caused by a ruptured pyometra.

PHYSICAL EXAMINATION

Fluid in the peritoneal cavity is typically recognized by the presence of abdominal distention (Figure 1). This distention also may be caused by such other disorders as intraabdominal masses or neoplasms, organomegaly, weakness of the abdominal musculature, gas-filled organs (e.g.,

gastric dilatation and volvulus), or an obstructed and/or atonic urinary bladder.[3]

Dogs with hyperadrenocorticism may be erroneously assumed to have ascites because of hepatomegaly, intraabdominal fat deposition, and weakened abdominal wall musculature. In such instances, owners might not recognize that abdominal distention is abnormal and might assume that the dog is simply gaining weight. In clinical patients with chronic disease, the clinician may recognize generalized muscle wasting associated with the abnormal abdominal distention.

Other physical examination findings that may be recognized depend on the underlying cause of the peritoneal effusion. For example, a heart murmur, jugular venous distention, and weak pulses may suggest the presence of heart failure; hepatomegaly may suggest liver disease or hepatic failure; and splenomegaly may be associated with splenic hemangiosarcoma. The presence of peripheral edema or dull lung sounds on auscultation (pleural effusion) may indicate that the clinician should focus on hypoproteinemia or vasculitis rather than on intraabdominal vascular pressure changes as a cause of ascites.

The ease with which ascites is diagnosed depends on the extent of fluid accumulation. If a large volume is present, the diagnosis is readily made on physical examination. A fluid wave may be palpable if the abdomen is ballotted. With one hand on each side of the abdomen, the abdominal wall is gently tapped with the fingers of one hand. If a large amount of fluid is present, the clinician will feel a sensation of fluid movement with the other hand.

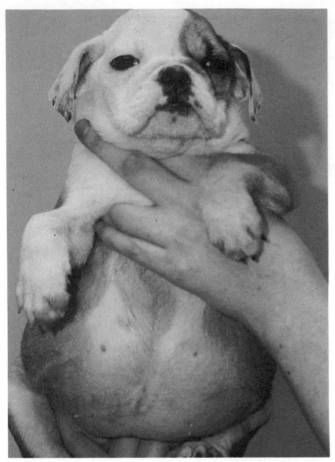

Figure 1—Bulldog puppy with ascites secondary to congenital pulmonic stenosis and right-sided heart failure.

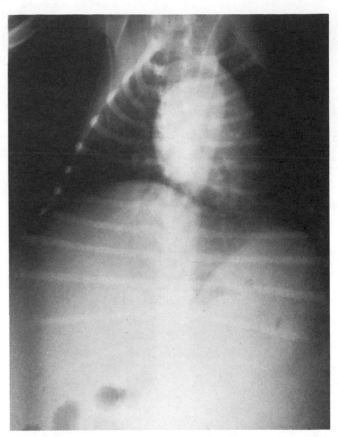

Figure 2—Plain radiograph demonstrating the loss of abdominal detail and increased intraabdominal pressure characteristic of peritoneal effusion.

In some cases (especially if the patient is recumbent), fluid movement may enable the clinician to visualize rippling of the abdominal wall after ballottement. The presence of a small amount of abdominal fluid is much more difficult to recognize; but, because analysis of the fluid can be diagnostically useful, fluid recognition and sampling may be vital in managing difficult cases.

Four major systemic effects of ascites are recognized. The effects are influenced by the type and volume of fluid as well as by the speed with which it accumulates. The first effect of ascitic fluid is physical: a large volume may increase intraabdominal pressure and thus decrease cardiac venous return and cardiac output.[4] Decreased cardiac output may lead to decreased perfusion of visceral organs and the periphery. The presence of fluid also may put pressure on the diaphragm (Figure 2) and lead to hypoventilation or excessive panting.[4]

As fluid accumulates in the peritoneal cavity, there may be significant loss of blood, fluid volume, or protein from the circulation. If fluid accumulates rapidly without allowing time for equilibration with the effective circulating blood volume, significant losses can lead to cardiovascular collapse and shock. Hemoperitoneum after trauma is an extreme example that is easily appreciated clinically.[5] Less obvious but equally significant are losses of fluid and albumin that can occur during such exudative processes as peritonitis; these losses often contribute to circulatory collapse, hypoproteinemia, and edema formation.[6,7]

If ascitic fluid contains vasoactive substances, cytokines, or eicosanoids, these substances may contribute to ongoing cardiovascular collapse. This process may occur in some animals with septic peritonitis or necrotizing pancreatitis, or even in the presence of necrotic abdominal neoplasms.[6,8] Activation of the coagulation cascade by inflammatory conditions may contribute to morbidity by inducing coagulopathy or disseminated intravascular coagulation.

Inflammatory conditions and increases in intraabdominal pressure may be associated with abdominal pain, which may affect morbidity by increasing heart rate and blood pressure.[9,10] This type of pain may be difficult to recognize clinically and is thus often untreated.

DIFFERENTIAL DIAGNOSIS

Initial analysis of the peritoneal fluid can be very helpful in formulating a differential diagnosis. Fluid should be analyzed as soon as possible after collection. Routine analysis

TABLE I
Peritoneal Fluid Analysis

Type of Effusion	Gross Appearance	Total Protein (g/dl)	Nucleated Cell Count (µl)	Cytology
Exudate	Opaque, serosanguinous	> 2.5	> 5,000	Neutrophils, macrophages, and mesothelial or neoplastic cells
Pure transudate	Clear, watery	< 2.5	< 1,000	Occasional neutrophils, macrophages, or mesothelial cells
Modified transudate	Serosanguinous	2.5 to 6.0	250 to 20,000	Macrophages, mesothelial cells, neoplastic cells, and neutrophils
Chyle	Milky	2.5 to 6.0	250 to 20,000	Lymphocytes, neutrophils, and macrophages
Hemorrhage	Red (blood)	3.5 to 7.5	1,000 to 20,000 (depends on peripheral cell count)	Erythrocytes, neutrophils, macrophages, mesothelial cells, or neoplastic cells

includes gross appearance, total protein and specific gravity determination, packed cell volume (PCV), red blood cell and nucleated cell counts, and differential cell counts and cytology.[1] Selected samples can be cultured for aerobic and anaerobic bacteria and/or fungi.[1,11]

BIOCHEMICAL ANALYSIS can be performed to detect the presence of triglycerides (chylous effusions),[1,12] amylase and lipase (pancreatitis),[3] bilirubin (ruptured gallbladder), or creatinine and potassium (ruptured bladder).[3] Other analyses that are occasionally performed include protein electrophoresis (feline infectious peritonitis).[13] Fluid is then categorized based on its characteristics (Table I); this information is used to direct diagnosis and therapy. Several types of fluid may be present.

Hemorrhage

The diagnosis of blood in the peritoneal cavity is based on finding sanguinous fluid with a packed cell volume and total protein similar to that of peripheral blood. If significant blood loss has occurred and fluid resuscitation has been performed, the fluid in the peritoneal cavity may have a higher packed cell volume than that of the periphery.[5] In most cases (unless acute, massive hemorrhage has occurred within the previous 45 minutes), the blood does not clot because defibrination and platelet destruction occur quickly when blood remains within a body cavity for a significant period.[14]

Trauma is a common cause of hemoperitoneum; rupture of such abdominal organs as the liver or spleen may be accompanied by tears in major abdominal blood vessels and subsequent hemorrhage.[5] Other elements in the differential

diagnosis include ruptured neoplasms (e.g., splenic hemangiosarcoma)[15] and erosion of blood vessels by neoplasm growth (e.g., vena caval rupture caused by pheochromocytoma).[16] Miscellaneous causes include splenic torsion, coagulopathy (e.g., coumarin toxicity), and thrombosis or occlusion of the blood supply to a major organ.

Many patients with traumatically induced hemoperitoneum stabilize with fluid resuscitation and/or blood transfusion and do not require further diagnostic evaluation.[5] Animals with coumarin toxicity may require vitamin K_1 administration and transfusions to supply coagulation factors. Other causes of hemoperitoneum (e.g., neoplasia, splenic torsion, or thrombosis) may necessitate surgical exploration and correction.

Exudates

Exudate is an effusion with a total protein greater than 2.5 g/dl (Table I). The fluid is usually opaque, and cell counts are usually high (greater than 5000/µl) but variable.[1] Exudative fluid may form fibrin clots after aspiration. Cytologic examination generally demonstrates the presence of neutrophils, macrophages, occasional mesothelial cells, or neoplastic cells[1] (Figure 3A). The presence of exudative fluids usually indicates a generalized inflammatory response of the peritoneum. The inflammation causes increased serosal permeability and vasculitis, which is accompanied by loss of fluid, protein, and cells into the peritoneal cavity.[7,8,17]

If bacteria or fungal elements are evident in the fluid, a diagnosis of septic peritonitis can be made (Figure 3A). If the neutrophils are apparently toxic or degenerative, septic peritonitis may be present, even in the absence of obvious bacteria. Septic peritonitis can occur secondary to rupture of bowel, abscesses (pyometra or prostatic), or extension of

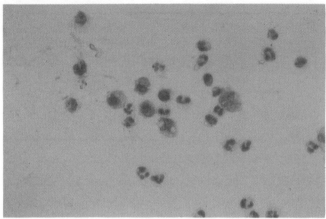

Figure 3A

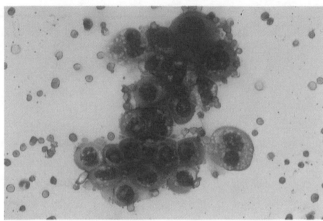

Figure 3B

Figure 3—Cytologic evaluation of peritoneal fluid may demonstrate its origin: (**A**) shows toxic and degenerative neutrophils and macrophages as might occur in septic peritonitis, and (**B**) shows metastatic adenocarcinoma cells in peritoneal fluid.

infection from an adjacent site. The presence of bacteria in peritoneal fluid usually warrants immediate surgical exploration to locate the source.

Exudates may be sterile, such as those associated with feline infectious peritonitis,[17] urine or bile peritonitis, or necrotizing pancreatitis.[7] Medical diagnostic methods (e.g., biochemical evaluation of serum and fluid, serum titers, ultrasonography, and radiographic contrast studies) may be required to evaluate these causes of peritoneal exudative responses. Other causes of sterile exudates include neoplasms (carcinoma, lymphosarcoma, or sarcoma), which may be detected as masses via abdominal palpation or ultrasonography or as exfoliated cells on cytologic evaluation of fluid samples.[1] In some cases, surgical abdominal exploration is required to diagnose the cause of exudative peritoneal fluid.

Modified Transudates

The most common type of ascitic fluid is a modified transudate. Modified transudates are often serosanguinous in appearance and have total solids between 2.5 and 6.0 g/dl (Table I). Cell counts vary from 250 to 20,000/μl.[1] Modified transudates are sterile. Cytologic analysis demonstrates macrophages and mesothelial cells as the predominant cell type and relatively few neutrophils.[1]

Modified transudates can result from any condition that obstructs the caudal vena cava or hepatic vein. Impaired blood flow through the hepatic sinusoids results. Increased production of hepatic lymph occurs because of filtration of blood under pressure into Disse's spaces.[11] Intrahepatic venous hypertension then causes hepatic lymph to leak from the surface of the liver via hepatic lymphatics, producing an ascitic fluid that is relatively high in protein. The formation of ascitic fluid is exacerbated by the presence of hypoproteinemia or conditions that lead to increased vascular permeability (vasculitis).

The following conditions are the most common causes of the formation of modified transudates: congestive right-sided heart failure,[11] pericardial tamponade,[11] and constriction or kinking of the caudal vena cava or hepatic vein.[18–20] Obstruction to venous flow also may accompany such neoplastic conditions as bile duct carcinoma, hepatoma, or other abdominal neoplasms that compress the great veins[11] (Figure 3B), or may be associated with various hepatopathies.[21] Diagnostic efforts should be directed toward evaluating venous return to the heart and cardiac function. This may require contrast angiography and/or cardiac ultrasonography. Biochemical evaluation of hepatic function is vital in determining whether hepatic disease is present. Abdominal ultrasonography may help in visualizing masses or neoplasms and in assessing the structure of the hepatic parenchyma.

THE UNDERLYING CAUSE of the modified transudate must be addressed when therapy is considered. If ascitic fluid is not impairing function, it is more appropriate to direct therapeutic measures to the underlying cause rather than to the fluid itself. Because it is often difficult to correct the cause of the problem, symptomatic management may be considered. Such diuretics as furosemide are the cornerstone of symptomatic therapy but should be initiated with care because they may produce hypovolemia and cardiovascular collapse before they eliminate ascitic fluid. Ancillary therapeutic measures may include steps to increase plasma protein concentration or such cardiac inotropes as digoxin to improve cardiac output in the presence of failure of the right side of the heart.

Pure Transudates

Pure transudates are clear, watery fluids (Table I). They

commonly have low total protein (less than 2.5 g/dl) and very few cells (less than 1000/µl).[1] The most important factor that contributes to a transudative process is hypoproteinemia, which may accompany chronic hepatic disorders, protein-losing nephropathy or enteropathy, malnutrition, or protein loss from wounds or effusions. If hypoproteinemia is the cause of transudative ascites, serum albumin concentrations usually drop below 1.0 to 1.5 mg/dl before ascites is evident; peritoneal fluid is then often accompanied by peripheral dependent edema.[22] If generalized edema is associated with peritoneal effusion, diagnostic efforts should be directed toward evaluation of the underlying cause of hypoproteinemia.

WHEN A PURE transudate accumulates only in the peritoneal cavity, without evidence of peripheral edema or pleural effusion, vascular hydrostatic pressure changes in the peritoneal cavity must be contributing to fluid accumulation.[23,24] Increases in pressure in the caudal vena cava usually cause accumulation of modified transudate by leakage of hepatic lymph. Increases in pressure in the portal vein, however, cause accumulation of low-protein fluid by leakage through the vessel wall.[23,24] Increased portal pressure is common in dogs with chronic hepatic disease, hepatic arteriovenous fistulas,[25] or portal venous thrombosis.[26]

Effusion occurs in dogs with chronic hepatic disease because hypoalbuminemia decreases the oncotic pressure holding fluid in the portal vein; the combination of decreased oncotic pressure and increased portal hydrostatic pressure leads to effusion. This is exacerbated by expanded plasma volume, which results from sodium retention caused by increased sympathetic nervous stimulation, increased renin–angiotensin activity and subsequent increased aldosterone release, and decreased production of natriuretic hormone.[27,28]

Clearly, multiple factors operate in the formation of ascitic fluid in patients with hepatic disease and/or portal hypertension. The type of ascitic fluid produced depends greatly on the type of pressure changes in the portal versus hepatic venous system, the serum albumin concentration, and the extent of activation of the renin–angiotensin and antidiuretic hormone systems. Animals with hepatic disease thus may present with peritoneal effusions that are modified or pure transudates.

Therapy depends on the type of hepatic disease and, especially, whether it can be corrected. If treatment of the underlying process is impossible, symptomatic therapy may include such diuretics as furosemide and spironolactone (which inhibits aldosterone and thus decreases sodium retention), therapeutic paracentesis, or dietary sodium restriction.[29] It should be remembered that some therapeutic agents (e.g., corticosteroids) used to manage chronic hepatic disease may exacerbate fluid retention.[29,30]

Chylous Effusions

Chylous effusions are characterized as milky effusions that are otherwise similar to modified transudates.[1] Chylous effusions often contain lymphocytes and may be confirmed by analysis of fluid triglyceride concentrations, which should be higher than 100 mg/dl.[1,12] Ether or chloroform solvent extraction should result in clearing of the fluid.[12] Chylous abdominal effusions are uncommon compared with chylous thoracic effusions.[12]

Chylous effusions form because of obstruction of lymphatic drainage, rupture of a major lymph vessel, or lymphangiectasia.[2,12] They may accompany neoplasms or other mass lesions that obstruct lymph flow.[12] Chylous effusions also occur with feline infectious peritonitis, feline cardiomyopathy, and constrictive pericarditis.[12] Trauma may lead to thoracic duct rupture and subsequent chylous ascites. Congenital anomalies reportedly cause chylous effusions in children but rarely in dogs.[12] Therapy depends on the underlying cause; surgical exploration or lymphangiography may be warranted if diagnosis cannot be made by noninvasive means. Biopsy of the intestine to check for the presence of lymphangiectasia may be helpful in some cases.

DIAGNOSTIC WORKUP

Confirmation of the presence of fluid may be sought via radiographic techniques. Plain abdominal radiographs may demonstrate a diffuse loss of peritoneal serosal detail in the presence of fluid[31] (Figure 2). Plain radiographs often are not otherwise useful diagnostically because details cannot be discerned: masses and organ shapes are often obscured. In abdominal radiographs from some animals (e.g., young puppies), decreased amounts of intraperitoneal fat can mimic the presence of fluid. The sensitivity of plain radiographs in detecting the presence of fluid may be improved by positioning the patient in sternal recumbency at a 45° angle with the head elevated, allowing the fluid to pool between the urinary bladder and abdominal wall.[31]

ABDOMINAL ULTRASONOGRAPHY is more sensitive than plain radiography in the diagnosis of ascites.[31] Using ultrasonography, the presence of a large amount of fluid can be easily and noninvasively confirmed, and otherwise unrecognizable small volumes of fluid may be detected[31] (Figure 4). Abdominal ultrasonography also allows the clinician to evaluate thoroughly the abdominal organs (e.g., the spleen and liver). In some cases, the technique may be used to guide needle aspiration of small, localized pockets of fluid.

Abdominal paracentesis should be performed in patients in which ascites is suspected. Because small amounts of air may escape into the peritoneal cavity when the procedure is performed, it is advisable to obtain abdominal radiographs

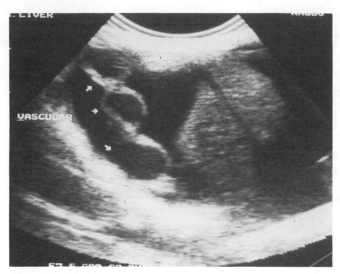

Figure 4—Abdominal ultrasonography can be used to demonstrate the presence of peritoneal fluid. Evident are large vascular structures located between the right side of the liver and the diaphragm in the case example (a four-month-old miniature schnauzer with a hepatic arteriovenous fistula).

before paracentesis.[1] This may avoid a diagnostic dilemma caused by the presence of free air in the peritoneal cavity. Several techniques are available for paracentesis. The procedure should be as aseptic as possible, with all sites clipped and surgically scrubbed.

If a large volume of fluid is present, a sample may be easily obtained using a 20- to 22-gauge needle and a 10-cc syringe slowly inserted on the abdominal midline at the level of or slightly caudal to the umbilicus.[32,33] This procedure may be performed with the patient restrained in lateral recumbency or standing. If a smaller amount of fluid is present or if the fluid is loculated, a single tap may not yield a sample. In such cases, the needle may be inserted in several locations until a sample is obtained; a four-quadrant approach is commonly attempted. Abdominal ultrasonography may help in guiding the needle to aspirate a very small volume of fluid.[31]

MOST PATIENTS with peritoneal effusions do not require complete drainage of the effusion. If the underlying cause of ascites can be corrected, the fluid, cells, and protein may be partially reabsorbed into the vascular space. In the case of hemorrhage, for example, as many as 50% of the red blood cells can reenter the circulation.[34] Significant protein loss can occur in association with removal of a large volume of fluid.[35]

In some patients, an increase in intraabdominal pressure may be a factor that prevents further accumulation of fluid or blood; if removed, fluid may rapidly reform.[36] Another consideration is the speed with which fluid is removed—in some situations, a sudden decrease in intraabdominal pressure can lead to acute fluid shifts, cardiovascular collapse, and shock.[35,37] If, however, the volume of fluid is large enough to cause respiratory compromise, the clinician may elect to drain the fluid partially until respiration is no longer compromised.

To remove a large volume of fluid, an over-the-needle venous catheter may be placed in the peritoneal cavity to allow drainage or aspiration of fluid.[32,33] The polyethylene catheter is less traumatic than a needle and less likely to lacerate abdominal organs once in position. The catheters can kink (cutting off fluid flow) or be collapsed by the abdominal musculature. They also can be easily occluded by fibrin tags or omentum in the peritoneal cavity. To minimize catheter plugging, extra side holes can be cut near the tip of the catheter before placement.

A second technique that facilitates effective drainage of a large volume of fluid is the placement of a peritoneal dialysis catheter,[32,33] which can be maintained for a longer period than an intravenous catheter. Peritoneal dialysis catheters are unlikely to collapse or kink and are less likely to become occluded than regular intravenous catheters.

BOTH TYPES of catheter can be used to infuse fluid in order to perform diagnostic or therapeutic peritoneal lavage. Diagnostic peritoneal lavage may be helpful in obtaining samples in patients with small amounts of fluid that cannot otherwise be easily collected. Warmed saline (20 ml/kg) is infused through the catheter into the peritoneal cavity, the patient may be gently rolled, and a sample is aspirated and analyzed.[33,38] Often, only a small amount of fluid can be reaspirated. Therapeutic peritoneal lavage may be performed in an attempt to relieve the pain and inflammation associated with peritonitis.[39]

Once the presence of a peritoneal effusion has been confirmed and a sample of the fluid has been obtained and analyzed, further diagnostic evaluation can proceed (Figure 5). A patient with a hemorrhagic effusion may require coagulation testing, abdominal ultrasonography to detect abdominal masses, and/or chest radiographs to check for metastatic disease. The exudative effusion may require culture; further workup for the patient might include serum titers, contrast radiographic studies, or exploratory laparotomy.

Patients with modified transudates might benefit from echocardiography, chest radiography, electrocardiography, contrast angiography, abdominal ultrasonography, or hepatic function studies. Pure transudates may warrant assessment of serum oncotic pressure, contrast angiography, or abdominal ultrasonography. Patients with chylous effusions may require exploratory surgery, intestinal biopsy, or lymphangiography.

CASE EXAMPLE

Signalment. The patient was a four-month-old, 3.2-kilo-

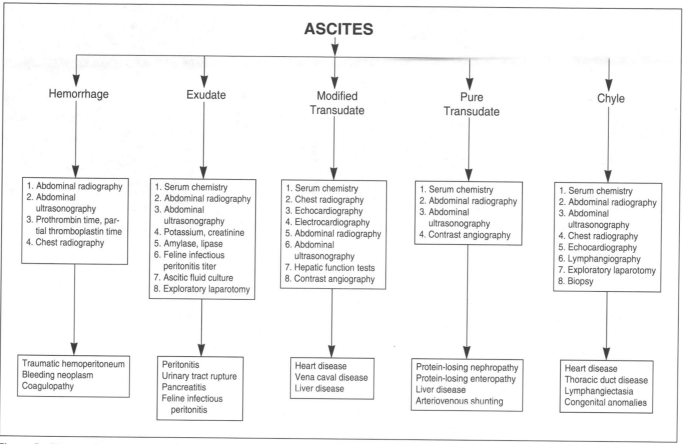

ASCITES

Hemorrhage	Exudate	Modified Transudate	Pure Transudate	Chyle
1. Abdominal radiography 2. Abdominal ultrasonography 3. Prothrombin time, partial thromboplastin time 4. Chest radiography	1. Serum chemistry 2. Abdominal radiography 3. Abdominal ultrasonography 4. Potassium, creatinine 5. Amylase, lipase 6. Feline infectious peritonitis titer 7. Ascitic fluid culture 8. Exploratory laparotomy	1. Serum chemistry 2. Chest radiography 3. Echocardiography 4. Electrocardiography 5. Abdominal radiography 6. Abdominal ultrasonography 7. Hepatic function tests 8. Contrast angiography	1. Serum chemistry 2. Abdominal radiography 3. Abdominal ultrasonography 4. Contrast angiography	1. Serum chemistry 2. Abdominal radiography 3. Abdominal ultrasonography 4. Chest radiography 5. Echocardiography 6. Lymphangiography 7. Exploratory laparotomy 8. Biopsy
Traumatic hemoperitoneum Bleeding neoplasm Coagulopathy	Peritonitis Urinary tract rupture Pancreatitis Feline infectious peritonitis	Heart disease Vena caval disease Liver disease	Protein-losing nephropathy Protein-losing enteropathy Liver disease Arteriovenous shunting	Heart disease Thoracic duct disease Lymphangiectasia Congenital anomalies

Figure 5—Diagnostic workup of patients with ascites.

gram, intact female miniature schnauzer (Figure 6).

History. There was gradual abdominal distention, decreased appetite, and occasional vomiting of one-month duration.

Physical Examination. The patient was a thin, potbellied pup with a poor haircoat. The abnormal findings were tachycardia (166 beats/min), slightly thready pulses, muscle wasting, and a distended abdomen (abdominal organs unpalpable) with a palpable fluid thrill.

Initial Workup. The workup consisted of complete blood count, chemistry screen, urinalysis, fecal examination, abdominal and chest radiographs, and abdominal paracentesis for fluid analysis. The complete blood count demonstrated a packed cell volume of 28% (normochromic, normocytic, nonregenerative; normal is 37% to 55%) but was otherwise nonremarkable. Abnormal values on the chemistry screen were alanine transaminase 190 IU/L (normal is 13 to 57 IU/L), serum alkaline phosphatase 464 IU/L (normal is 35 to 169 IU/L), cholesterol 147 mg/dl (normal is 150 to 250 mg/dl), and albumin 2.1 g/dl (normal is 2.7 to 3.6 g/dl). The fecal examination and urinalysis were unremarkable; urine specific gravity was 1.038. Chest radiographs were normal, but abdominal radiographs demonstrated a distended abdomen with marked peritoneal effusion obscuring the abdominal viscera (Figure 2).

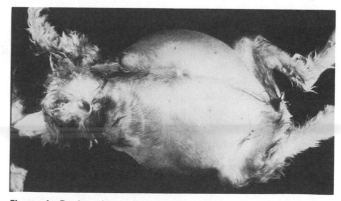

Figure 6—Postmortem picture of the case example.

On abdominal paracentesis, several milliliters of fluid were easily obtained. Analysis of the fluid was consistent with a pure transudate (specific gravity was 1.005, and total protein was less than 2.5 g/dl). The elevations of alanine transferase and serum alkaline phosphatase, combined with the decreases in serum albumin and cholesterol, suggested hepatic dysfunction. The low-protein transudate indicated that the cause of the effusion might be portal hypertension, probably combined with hypoalbuminemia-induced decreases in plasma oncotic pressure.

Further Diagnostic Efforts. To further evaluate liver

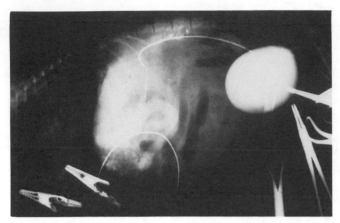

Figure 7—Celiac arteriogram in the case example, demonstrating blood flow from the hepatic artery to the portal vein via a distended, tortuous arteriovenous fistula.

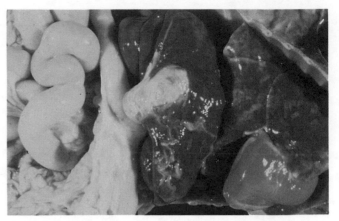

Figure 8—Necropsy findings of the hepatic arteriovenous fistula in the case example.

function, serum bile acids were submitted. Preprandial bile acids were 90 μmol/L (normal is 5 μmol/L), and postprandial bile acids at two hours were 41.8 μmol/L (normal is 10 μmol/L). These results demonstrate an impairment in the enterohepatic cycle of bile acids. On abdominal ultrasonography (Figure 4), a large amount of anechoic fluid was found and multiple large vascular structures were evident near the right liver lobe. A tortuous, large vascular structure was located between the right liver and diaphragm.

BASED ON the abnormal chemistry and ultrasonography findings, a congenital vascular anomaly was suspected. Portosystemic shunting usually does not cause portal hypertension and ascites, however, because the portal vein is emptying into the low-pressure venous system. A more complex vascular anomaly thus was likely. A caudal vena cavagram was performed but was nondiagnostic. The patient was anesthetized, and a celiac arteriogram was performed (Figure 7). Immediately after injection of the dye into the celiac artery, numerous abnormal tortuous vascular structures were evident emptying into the caudal vena cava between the diaphragm and third lumbar vertebra.

Clinical Diagnosis. Hepatic arteriovenous shunt was the diagnosis. Blood was flowing from the hepatic artery, through the portal vein, and into the caudal vena cava. In light of the extent of the vascular abnormalities and the poor prognosis, the owner elected euthanasia.

Necropsy Findings. Extensive portacaval shunting and an arteriovenous fistula from the hepatic artery to the dilated portal vein were found (Figure 8). Histopathologic examination of the liver demonstrated severe diffuse portal fibrosis and mild multifocal chronic active cholangiohepatitis.

Conclusion. In this case, an arteriovenous fistula caused increased hydrostatic pressure in the portal vein; this pressure, combined with hypoalbuminemia, resulted in the formation of a pure transudate. Fluid analysis was helpful in predicting the location of the vascular anomaly.

SUMMARY

Ascites is a common presenting sign associated with several disease processes. Because ascites always indicates an underlying disease process and is not a diagnosis in itself, clinicians should remember to evaluate each patient carefully to determine the underlying cause of fluid accumulation. When recognized, ascites can serve as a useful aid because the type of fluid present may provide valuable clues to assist clinicians in reaching a diagnosis.

ACKNOWLEDGMENTS

The authors thank the Pathology Department and the Section of Radiology, Department of Clinical Studies, School of Veterinary Medicine, University of Pennsylvania, for their assistance in preparing the figures that illustrate the case example.

About the Authors

Drs. King and Gelens are affiliated with the Department of Clinical Studies, School of Veterinary Medicine, University of Pennsylvania, Philadelphia, Pennsylvania. Dr. King is a Diplomate of the American College of Veterinary Internal Medicine.

REFERENCES

1. Meyer DJ, Franks PT: Effusions: Classification and cytologic examination. *Compend Contin Educ Pract Vet* 9(2):123–128, 1987.
2. Ettinger SJ: Ascites, peritonitis, and other causes of abdominal enlargement, in Ettinger SJ (ed): *Textbook of Veterinary Internal Medicine*, ed 3. Philadelphia, WB Saunders Co, 1989, pp 131–138.
3. MacIntire DK: The acute abdomen—Differential diagnosis and management. *Semin Vet Med Surg (Small Anim)* 3(4):302–310, 1988.
4. Cullen DJ, Coyle JP, Teplick R, Long MC: Cardiovascular, pulmonary, and renal effects of massively increased intra-abdominal

pressure in critically ill patients. *Crit Care Med* 17(2):118–121, 1989.

5. Mongil CM, Drobatz KJ, Hendricks JC: Traumatic hemoperitoneum in 28 cases: A retrospective review. *J Vet Emerg Crit Care*, submitted for publication.

6. Amundsen E, Ofstad E, Hagen PO: Experimental acute pancreatitis in dogs: Hypotensive effect induced by pancreatic exudate. *Scand J Gastroenterol* 3:659–664, 1968.

7. Schaer M: Acute pancreatitis in dogs. *Compend Contin Educ Pract Vet* 13(12):1769–1780, 1991.

8. Takada Y, Appert HE, Howard JM: Vascular permeability induced by pancreatic exudate formed during acute pancreatitis in dogs. *Surg Gynecol Obstet* 143:779–783, 1976.

9. Johnson JM: The veterinarian's responsibility: Assessing and managing acute pain in dogs and cats. Part I. *Compend Contin Educ Pract Vet* 13(5):804–807, 1991.

10. Sackman JE: Pain: Its perception and alleviation in dogs and cats. Part I. The physiology of pain. *Compend Contin Educ Pract Vet* 13(1):71–75, 1991.

11. Greene CE: Ascites: Diagnostic and therapeutic considerations. *Compend Contin Educ Pract Vet* 1(9):712–718, 1979.

12. Fossum TW, Hay WH, Boothe HW, et al: Chylous ascites in three dogs. *JAVMA* 200(1):70–76, 1992.

13. Shelly SM, Scarlett-Kranz J, Blue JT: Protein electrophoresis on effusions from cats as a diagnostic test for feline infectious peritonitis. *JAAHA* 24:495–500, 1988.

14. Crowe DT: Autotransfusion in the trauma patient. *Vet Clin North Am [Small Anim Pract]* 10(3):581–597, 1980.

15. Hosgood G: Canine hemangiosarcoma. *Compend Contin Educ Pract Vet* 13(7):1065–1075, 1991.

16. Bouayad H, Feeney DA, Caywood DD, Hayden DW: Pheochromocytoma in dogs: 13 cases. *JAVMA* 191(12):1610–1615, 1987.

17. Grahn BH: The feline coronavirus infections: Feline infectious peritonitis and feline coronavirus enteritis. *Vet Med* 86:376–393, 1991.

18. Cornelius L, Mahaffey M: Kinking of the intrathoracic vena cava in five dogs. *J Small Anim Pract* 26:67–80, 1985.

19. Miller MW, Bonagura JD, DiBartola SP, Fossum TW: Budd-Chiari-like syndrome in two dogs. *JAAHA* 25:277–283, 1989.

20. Crowe DT, Lorenz MD, Hardie EM, et al: Chronic peritoneal effusion due to partial caudal vena caval obstruction following blunt trauma: Diagnosis and successful surgical management. *JAAHA* 20:231–238, 1984.

21. Cohn LA, Spaulding HA, Cullen JM, et al: Intrahepatic post-sinusoidal venous obstruction in a dog. *J Vet Intern Med* 5:317–321, 1991.

22. Weech AA, Snelling CE, Goettsch E: The relation between plasma protein content, plasma specific gravity and edema in dogs maintained on a protein inadequate diet and in dogs rendered edematous by plasmapheresis. *J Clin Invest* 12:193–216, 1933.

23. Johnson SE: Portal hypertension. Part I. Pathophysiology and clinical consequences. *Compend Contin Educ Pract Vet* 9(7):741–748, 1987.

24. Johnson SE: Portal hypertension. Part II. Clinical assessment and treatment. *Compend Contin Educ Pract Vet* 9(9):917–928, 1987.

25. Bailey MQ: Ultrasonographic findings associated with congenital hepatic arteriovenous fistula in three dogs. *JAVMA* 192(8):1099–1101, 1988.

26. Willard MD, Bailey MQ, Hauptman J, Mullany T: Obstructed portal venous flow and portal vein thrombus in a dog. *JAVMA* 194(10):1449–1451, 1989.

27. Lieberman FL, Denison EK, Reynolds TB: The relationship of plasma volume, portal hypertension, ascites, and renal sodium retention in cirrhosis: The overflow theory of ascites formation. *Ann NY Acad Sci* 170:202–212, 1970.

28. Grauer GF, Nichols CER: Ascites, renal abnormalities, and electrolyte and acid/base disorders associated with liver disease. *Vet Clin North Am [Small Anim Pract]* 15(1):197–214, 1985.

29. Magne ML, Chiapella AM: Medical management of canine chronic hepatitis. *Compend Contin Educ Pract Vet* 8(12):915–921, 1986.

30. Strombeck DR, Miller LM, Harrold D: Effects of corticosteroid treatment on survival time in dogs with chronic hepatitis: 151 cases. *JAVMA* 193(9):1109–1113, 1988.

31. Henley RK, Hager DA, Ackerman N: A comparison of two-dimensional ultrasonography and radiography for the detection of small amounts of free peritoneal fluid in the dog. *Vet Radiol* 30(3):121–124, 1989.

32. Crowe DT: Diagnostic abdominal paracentesis techniques: Clinical evaluation in 129 dogs and cats. *JAAHA* 20:223–230, 1984.

33. Hunt CA: Diagnostic peritoneal paracentesis and lavage. *Compend Contin Educ Pract Vet* 2(6):449–453, 1980.

34. Clark CH, Woodley CH: The absorption of red blood cells after parenteral injection at various sites. *Am J Vet Res* 20:1062–1066, 1959.

35. Cruikshank DP, Buchsbaum HJ: Effects of rapid paracentesis—Cardiovascular dynamics and body fluid composition. *JAMA* 225(11):1361–1362, 1973.

36. Zink J, Greenway CV: Intraperitoneal pressure in formation and reabsorption of ascites in cats. *Am J Physiol* 233:H185–H190, 1977.

37. Kowalski HJ, Abelman WH, McNeely WF: The cardiac output in patients with cirrhosis of the liver and tense ascites with observations of the effect of paracentesis. *J Clin Invest* 33:768–773, 1954.

38. Henneman PL, Marx JA, Moore EE, et al: Diagnostic peritoneal lavage: Accuracy in predicting necessary laparotomy following blunt and penetrating trauma. *J Trauma* 30(11):1345–1355, 1990.

39. Willauer CC, Gregory CR, Parker HR: Treatment of peritonitis with the Parker peritoneal dialysis catheter. *JAAHA* 24:546–550, 1988.

Vomiting: A Clinical Approach

Gary W. Thayer, DVM, MS
Diplomate, ACVIM
Assistant Professor
Department of Small Animal Medicine
College of Veterinary Medicine
University of Georgia
Athens, Georgia

Vomiting dogs are commonly presented to the small animal practitioner for diagnosis and therapy. The vomiting patient is challenging in that it may be difficult to assess the need for in-depth diagnostic procedures, as opposed to symptomatic therapy, to assure the well-being of the patient. Vomiting is less common in the cat. The objectives of this review are to define vomiting and differentiate it from regurgitation, describe the vomiting reflex and the mechanical events of vomiting, discuss the secondary effects of profuse or persistent vomiting, and present a diagnostic and therapeutic plan for the vomiting patient.

Vomiting vs. Regurgitation[1]

It is important for the clinician to differentiate between vomiting and regurgitation because each is indicative of diseases of different organs of the gastrointestinal tract. Vomiting is associated with abnormalities of the stomach and small intestine. Regurgitation suggests a pathological condition of the oral cavity, pharynx, or esophagus.

Vomiting is defined as the ejection of stomach contents from stimulation of a neural reflex that has synaptic centers in the brain. The vomiting act is accomplished through contraction of the diaphragm and abdominal muscles. Vomiting is preceded by hypersalivation, repeated swallowing, and retching. The vomitus will usually have an acid pH and contain partially digested food. It may be bile stained, indicating reflux from the duodenum.

Regurgitation is the retrograde movement of food and fluid from the oral cavity, pharynx, and esophagus. The food and fluid move by gravity, as is determined by body position. Regurgitated food will be undigested and may have a neutral pH depending on the composition of the diet. The food material may have a cylindrical shape given it by the esophagus. Dyspnea or cough is more likely to be associated with regurgitation.

The Vomiting Reflex and the Mechanical Events of Vomiting[2]

Most of the receptors of the vomiting reflex are found in the abdominal viscera. The largest number are found in the duodenum. Acute distention or mucosal irritation of the duodenum can result in vomiting. In addition, receptors are present in the stomach, jejunum, ileum, pancreas, liver, and genitourinary tract. Most of the afferent pathways from the stomach and duodenum are in the vagus nerves. The afferent nerves from the other viscera are in the sympathetic trunks.

Afferent nerves from abdominal viscera synapse in the vomiting center of the medulla. Afferent input also comes to the vomiting center from higher centers in the brain, as is evidenced by stress-induced vomiting of wild animals which acts as a protective escape mechanism. A third source of afferent activity to the vomiting center is the chemoreceptor trigger zone (CRTZ), located on the floor of the fourth ventricle. The CRTZ is stimulated by blood-borne substances such as apomorphine, uremic toxins, cardiac glycosides, and toxins from other infectious or metabolic diseases. The afferent input of motion sickness reaches the vomiting center through the CRTZ. The CRTZ can be thought of as a receptor because the vomiting center must be functional for the animal to vomit when the CRTZ is stimulated.

The motor efferent nerves of the vomiting reflex are the spinal and phrenic nerves which innervate muscles of the diaphragm and abdominal wall. The autonomic activity of the vagal parasympathetic nerves and splanchnic sympathetic nerves mediates motility changes in the esophagus, esophageal sphincters, stomach, and duodenum. The autonomic activity is not essential for the vomiting act. Cranial nerves IX and X mediate activity of the larynx.

The mechanical events of vomiting begin with hypersalivation, followed by repeated swallowing and relaxation of the gastroesophageal sphincter. Then, retching begins, characterized by forceful contractions of the muscles of the diaphragm and abdominal wall with the glottis closed. The proximal small intestine and gastric antrum contract, forcing their contents into the body of the stomach where movement is inhibited. The gastroesophageal sphincter moves into the thoracic cavity, causing it to be incompetent and allowing gastroesophageal reflux. Motility is inhibited in the esophagus and pharyngoesophageal sphincter. As vomitus passes through the pharynx, the orifice of the nasopharynx closes, preventing nasal regurgitation. There is no reverse peristalsis in the stomach or small intestine. The driving force for expulsion of the stomach contents is contraction of the muscles of the diaphragm and abdominal wall.

Diagnostic Plan

After establishing that the patient is vomiting, as defined above, the diagnostic plan begins with a more detailed history, including duration and frequency of vomiting. Persistent or frequent vomiting is more likely to be associated with systemic disease or a severe gastrointestinal lesion. The characteristics of the vomitus (bile stained, bloody, containing foreign material) are helpful in localizing the lesion and determining its severity. The relationship to eating or drinking may be

important in that a shorter interval between vomiting and these events generally indicates that the lesion is situated higher in the gastrointestinal tract. History suggesting primary disease of other body systems (e.g., polydipsia and polyuria, neurological signs) cannot be ignored. The vaccination history of the patient is important in ruling out an infectious disease as the cause of vomiting. The patient's environment and management determine the possibility of ingestion of a foreign body or toxin or potential exposure to an infectious disease. Changes in a patient's diet can suggest a dietary allergy.

A complete physical exam should follow the history taking. Information gathered in the history can point to potentially abnormal organ systems. Signs of systemic disease such as dehydration, hypotension, or fever must be noted, and abdominal palpation should be carefully performed. Abdominal pain may be associated with pancreatitis, gastrointestinal obstruction, mesenteric abscess, peritonitis, or neoplasia. Abdominal masses may be the result of a foreign body, neoplasia, or intussusception.

The minimum data base for acute vomiting should include a complete history taking and physical examination. If no significant abnormalities are present and no signs of systemic disease are seen, the patient should be treated symptomatically. If signs of systemic disease are present, the data base must be expanded to include a complete blood count; serum biochemical profile including blood urea nitrogen, blood glucose, serum glutamic-pyruvic transaminase (SGPT), serum alkaline phosphatase, sodium, potassium, chloride, total protein, albumin, serum amylase and lipase (if pancreatitis is thought likely); urinalysis; and survey abdominal radiographs.

Persistent vomiting requires a more complete minimum data base. It should include the history, physical examination, serum biochemical profile (as previously described), complete blood count, urinalysis, determination of arterial blood gases (if possible), and survey abdominal radiographs. Following assessment of the information acquired for the minimum data base, endoscopy, contrast radiography, exploratory celiotomy, and biopsy of abnormal structures may be necessary to provide a definitive diagnosis. Many of the conditions that cause acute vomiting can become chronic and result in persistent vomiting. Some potential causes for acute and persistent vomiting are listed in Table I.

Secondary Effects of Persistent Vomiting

Vomiting results in dehydration because of the loss of dietary intake and water loss in secretions of the gastrointestinal tract. In a 20 kg dog, gastrointestinal secretions can total 3 liters daily. Prerenal azotemia may develop if dehydration is prolonged. Hypochloremia and, less commonly, hyponatremia are a result of loss of gastric secretions and dilution due to drinking water.

TABLE I

CAUSES OF VOMITING

I. Acute Vomiting
  A. Gastrointestinal causes
    1. Acute gastritis or enteritis
      a. Bacterial enterotoxins
      b. Ingested environmental toxin
      c. Drugs (aspirin)
      d. Ingested foreign bodies
      e. Parasites
      f. Viral enteritis
    2. Gastric outlet obstruction
    3. Small intestinal obstruction

  B. Nongastrointestinal causes
    1. Infectious diseases
      a. Canine distemper
      b. Canine hepatitis
      c. Leptospirosis
      d. Feline panleukopenia
      e. Canine parvovirus infection
    2. Noninfectious diseases
      a. Acute pancreatitis or pancreatic abscess
      b. Ketoacidotic diabetes mellitus
      c. Drug intoxication (narcotics, cardiac glycoside)
      d. Vestibular disturbances
      e. Central nervous system disorders
      f. Pyometra

II. Persistent Vomiting
  A. Gastrointestinal causes
    1. Chronic gastritis
      a. Hypertrophic
      b. Atrophic
    2. Neoplasia
      a. Stomach
      b. Small intestine
    3. Ulcers
      a. Stomach
      b. Duodenum

  B. Nongastrointestinal causes
    1. Noninfectious diseases
      a. Renal failure
      b. Hepatic disease
      c. Adrenocortical insufficiency

Hypokalemia results from loss of gastric secretions, renal losses, and an alkalosis-induced shift of potassium into the intracellular compartment. Renal losses occur because of a lack of hydrogen ions to exchange for sodium ions; therefore, potassium ions are exchanged in place of the hydrogen ions, resulting in increased excretion of potassium ions. Metabolic alkalosis results from loss of hydrogen ions in gastric secretions and retention of bicarbonate by the kidney in an attempt to maintain electrical neutrality in the presence of hypochloremia. Paradoxical aciduria results due to an increase of plasma anions, other than chloride and bicarbonate, being excreted in the urine. These anions are poorly reabsorbed, thus requiring an obligatory excretion of a cation. The cation in this situation is hydrogen due to the influence of aldosterone which promotes maximal sodium reabsorption.[3] Therefore, in the vomiting animal, the urine pH is not a reliable indicator of the animal's acid-base status.

In patients in which duodenal contents reflux into the stomach and loss of bicarbonate ion exceeds that of hydrogen ion, metabolic acidosis is observed.[4] This is most often seen when lesions are distal to the stomach and when no obstruction of the pylorus is present. Metabolic acidosis must be considered in two special situations: (1) in chronic vomiting patients with persistent bile-stained vomitus, suggesting duodenal gastric reflux, and (2) when severe diarrhea accompanies the vomiting, allowing loss of bicarbonate ion in the feces.

Therapy

Vomiting is a clinical sign, not a definitive diagnosis. Therefore, every effort should be made to identify the underlying cause so that specific therapy can be employed. Symptomatic therapy should be (1) reserved for the patient in which the specific cause cannot be identified or (2) used in combination with specific therapy to correct or prevent the secondary effects of persistent vomiting.

Symptomatic therapy for acute vomiting includes fasting and withholding water for 24 hours in an attempt to (1) rest the gastrointestinal tract from physical trauma and (2) eliminate the stimulation of secretions of the gastrointestinal tract, which could further damage an already abnormal mucosa. If necessary, fluids are administered parenterally. After 24 hours, if the vomiting has stopped, the animal should be allowed to drink small amounts of water. If no vomiting occurs, feeding can be started with small amounts of a bland diet composed of carbohydrate (rice) with a small amount of animal protein low in fat given four to six times daily for one to two days; then, the patient's standard diet can be resumed.

It may be desirable to stop the vomiting pharmacologically to prevent the continued loss of fluids and electrolytes. This can be accomplished most effectively with phenothiazine antiemetics. These compounds inhibit neural transmission through the vomiting center and the CRTZ. Phenothiazine antiemetics depress centrally mediated pressor reflexes and are peripheral alpha-adrenergic blockers, which results in hypotension. Therefore, they should not be used in dehydrated or hypovolemic patients. Examples of these compounds are chlorpromazine[a] and thiethylperazine,[b] administered at 0.5 mg/kg every 12 hours and at 0.2 to 0.4 mg/kg every 8 to 12 hours, respectively, as needed.

Antihistamine antiemetics block neural transmission through the CRTZ and from the vestibular apparatus. They are effective in preventing vomiting due to motion sickness or in those cases in which drugs or toxins are selectively stimulating the CRTZ. Anticholinergic agents (atropine) act by decreasing spasm of

---

[a]Thorazine®, Smith, Kline & French Laboratories, Philadelphia, PA 19101.
[b]Torecan®, Boehringer Ingelheim Ltd., Ridgefield, CT 06877.

the stomach and small intestine, thereby reducing the stimulus to vomit. They are usually not effective. Protectives or antacids act by soothing irritated mucosal surfaces, which reduces stimulation of vomiting receptors. This is accomplished by reducing the back flow of hydrochloric acid into the mucosa. They are probably not effective except in some cases of acute gastritis or duodenitis.

When vomiting persists, fluid and electrolyte disturbances result, as previously explained. The goal of fluid and electrolyte therapy is to correct the existing dehydration and electrolyte disturbances, to replace continued losses, and to supply maintenance requirements. In the vomiting animal, when blood gases and electrolytes cannot be evaluated, Ringer's solution is the fluid of choice because it is an isotonic, balanced electrolyte solution with no alkalizing agent (lactate) which can aggravate an existing metabolic alkalosis. As the fluid therapy replaces the chloride deficit, the retention of bicarbonate by the kidney stops and the metabolic alkalosis resolves. As the pH returns to normal, the availability of hydrogen ions prevents the excretion of potassium by the kidney, and renal losses of potassium no longer occur. Hydrogen ion diffuses into cells, promoting the release of potassium. Ringer's solution contains only physiologic amounts of potassium. If hypokalemia is present, potassium ions must be supplemented.[5c]

Cimetidine, an H_2 blocker (15 to 20 mg/kg, tid, IM) which reduces hydrochloric acid secretion in the stomach, can be beneficial in decreasing the loss of hydrogen and chloride in gastric fluids.[6] If the cause or clinical signs (bile-stained vomitus, severe diarrhea, increased respiratory rate) of vomiting suggest metabolic acidosis, a fluid such as lactated Ringer's solution, which contains an alkalizing agent (lactate), is the fluid of choice. Other solutions are available which contain the alkalizing agents acetate and gluconate.[d] Bicarbonate ion may be supplemented according to the formula $0.3 \times$ body weight (kg) $\times$ the deficit of HCO_3^-.[e]

Prophylactic antibiotic therapy should be used when a severe mucosal lesion that would potentially subject the patient to bacteremia is suspected. In these patients, both aerobes and anaerobes are potential invaders. Therefore, antibiotics against both gram-negative aerobes (kanamycin) and anaerobes (penicillin) should be used. They should be administered parenterally to avoid further irritation of the gastrointestinal tract and to assure adequate absorption for effective blood levels.[7]

[c]Tagamet®, Smith, Kline & French Laboratories, Philadelphia, PA 19101.

[d]Multisol®-M and Multisol®-R, Abbott Laboratories, N. Chicago, IL 60064; Plasmalyte®, Baxter/Travenol, Deerfield, IL 60015; Polysal®, Cutter Laboratories, Inc., Berkeley, CA 94710.

[e]$0.3 \times$ body weight (kg) is a measure of the volume of extracellular fluid. The bicarbonate deficit can be accurately obtained from a nomogram; however, for practical purposes, it is obtained by subtracting the patient's measured plasma bicarbonate concentration from the normal level (24).

REFERENCES

1. Strombeck, DR: *Small Animal Gastroenterology.* Davis, CA, Stonegate Publishing, 1979, pp 68-72.
2. Strombeck, DR: *Small Animal Gastroenterology.* Davis, CA, Stonegate Publishing, 1979, pp 73-77.
3. Gardham, JRC: Pyloric stenosis and paradoxical acid urine: An experimental study in dogs. *Br J Surg* 57:737,1970.
4. Moore, WE: Laboratory examinations, in Anderson NV (ed): *Veterinary Gastroenterology.* Philadelphia, Lea & Febiger, 1980, pp 45-46.
5. Finco, DR: Fluid therapy for profuse vomiting. *JAAHA* 8(2):200-205, 1972.
6. DeNovo RC: Personal communication, 1980.
7. Strombeck, DR: *Small Animal Gastroenterology.* Davis, CA, Stonegate Publishing, 1979, pp 98-109.

UPDATE

Abdominal ultrasound should be part of the diagnostic plan for persistent vomiting if acute pancreatitis or abdominal neoplasia is included in the differential diagnosis after the minimum data base is complete. Some obstructive lesions of the gastrointestinal (GI) tract can be visualized. If endoscopy is performed, it is imperative that the duodenum, esophagus, and stomach are examined.

Chronic inflammatory bowel disease can be added to the list of causes of persistent vomiting in Table I. Vomiting can also be a clinical sign of neoplasia of other abdominal organs (but not of the GI tract).

If an H_2 blocker is needed, ranitidine (a new alternative to cimetidine) can be administered at 1.1 to 4.4 mg/kg PO. Ranitidine is given every 12 hours.

Metabolic acidosis can usually be corrected by adequate fluid therapy and rectifying other electrolyte abnormalities. Bicarbonate ion should be supplemented only if blood gas data indicate that the metabolic acidosis is not being resolved by other fluid and electrolyte therapy.

Fecal Incontinence in Dogs and Cats

KEY FACTS

- Fecal incontinence is a life-threatening disease in dogs and cats.
- Extensive diagnostic effort to determine the cause of fecal incontinence in small animals may be necessary.
- Treatment of the primary cause of fecal incontinence may alleviate the condition; symptomatic medical and surgical therapy can be helpful.
- A better understanding of the physiology of fecal continence can improve therapy.

University of California, Davis
W. Grant Guilford, BPhil, BVSc

FECAL incontinence is the inability to retain feces. Whether defecation by a pet is considered appropriate primarily depends on the owner's conception of normal elimination behavior for that species. Unfortunately, fecal incontinence can have a disastrous ending for a household pet. Of the dogs and cats presented with fecal incontinence to the University of Missouri and University of California Veterinary Medical Teaching Hospitals, 50% were euthanatized within several days of presentation. This article considers statistics obtained from patient records at these two hospitals, describes the features of canine and feline fecal incontinence, and offers some suggestions for management of the condition.

INCIDENCE

The number of cats and dogs presented to the University of Missouri and University of California Veterinary Medical Teaching Hospitals because of fecal incontinence is small. Of 260,000 submissions during the past 10 years, fecal incontinence was the reason for presentation in only 43 animals. The number of cases was approximately the same for cats and dogs. There was no sex predilection, and the patients were between six months and 16 years of age; however, 50% of them were 11 years or older.

The number of cases recorded at the University of Missouri and University of California Veterinary Medical Teaching Hospitals may not be an accurate representation of the true incidence of fecal incontinence. The disorder is often accepted as an inevitable consequence of aging. Furthermore, owners often believe that the terms *incontinence* and *diarrhea* are synonymous, a misunderstanding that may only become apparent following careful questioning.[1] In addition, some veterinarians fail to diagnose fecal incontinence as a separate problem when presented with cases of severe spinal trauma or diarrhea because incontinence is considered an integral part of these conditions.

Two major types of fecal incontinence are recognized: reservoir incontinence and sphincter incontinence.[2] The anatomic structures believed to be involved in fecal continence are shown in Figure 1.

Reservoir Incontinence

A reservoir mechanism is essential for continence because the maximum period of voluntary contraction of the striated anal sphincter muscles is brief.[3,4] Reservoir incontinence results from a failure of the large bowel to adapt to and contain the colorectal content. Animals with reservoir incontinence usually sense the imminence of defecation.

Reservoir incontinence is most often characterized by frequent, conscious defecation and *not* by inadvertent anal dribbling. The ability of the large bowel to function as a reservoir adequately is affected by colorectal irritability, capacity, compliance, and motility as well as by the volume of feces.

Colorectal Irritability. Colorectal irritability causes an increased urge to defecate. Colonic irritability also may interfere with sphincter closure,[5] may decrease compliance, and may alter colonic motility.

Colorectal Capacity and Compliance. Excessive fecal volume overwhelms colorectal capacity, and poor compliance reduces colorectal capacity at a given intraluminal pressure. Removal of the proximal two thirds of the canine colon results in frequent passage of liquid or, at best, semiformed feces.[6] In contrast, subtotal colectomy in cats does not dramatically alter stool frequency or consistency.[7] Eventual development of what has been called *ileoanal continence* in colectomized humans following the gradual distention of the ileum has also been described.[8]

Colorectal Motility. Effective reservoir function is dependent on such colorectal motility mechanisms as segmental contractions and accommodation, both of which retard the transit of fecal material. Temporary retention of the stool facilitates the removal of fecal water, thereby reducing fecal volume. Accommodation is the receptive relaxation of the circular muscle of the colon during filling. This action inhibits propulsive colonic contractions[4,9,10] and prevents the development of increased intraluminal pressure that would challenge the sphincteric mechanisms.

Sphincter Incontinence

Sphincter incontinence is caused by failure of the sphincteric mechanisms to resist the propulsive forces of the rectum.[3,4] This condition is characterized by the involuntary passage of feces. Sphincter incontinence primarily depends on continence reaction, which is a reflexive or conscious contraction of the muscles of the external anal sphincter and the pelvic girdle in response to the presence of feces.[10]

Nervous Pathways of the Continence Reaction. Three afferent nervous pathways, each with different sensory triggers, apparently are involved in the continence reaction (Figure 2). The nervous pathway that is most important in the continence reaction is somewhat controversial. In humans, the majority of evidence suggests that the afferent nervous pathways are triggered either by stimulation of the anal epithelium or by stretching of the muscles of the pelvic girdle.[10-12] This issue has not been adequately addressed in dogs or cats.

THE HYPOGASTRIC NERVES, which transmit pain resulting from excessive dilation of the bowel,[13] probably do not have an important role in fecal continence. The information received from the three major afferent pathways is integrated in the sacral spinal cord. The reflex arc is completed by efferent nerve fibers to the muscles of the pelvic girdle (via the S3 and C1 nerves and, to a lesser extent, the S2 spinal nerves) and to the external anal sphincter (via the caudal rectal nerves, which are distal branches of the pudendal nerve).[14,15] There is very little information about the areas of the brain involved in the control of fecal continence and in the perception of the urge to defecate. Brain-stem centers similar to those that control micturition are believed to be important, however.[16]

Muscles of the Continence Reaction. In humans, the muscle group that is most important in the resistance of the anal canal to propulsive waves is apparently the puborectalis.[10] Contraction of the external anal sphincter can also raise pressure in the anal canal. The external anal sphincter and puborectalis muscle seem to be closely related and may actually be components of the same muscle group.[17] Apparently, these muscles are synergistic in action by serving as consecutive sphincteric muscle loops.[17] Partial fecal incontinence is probable if one muscle group malfunctions, and complete incontinence is likely if all muscle components fail.[17]

In dogs, the external anal sphincter probably plays an important role in fecal continence because experimental denervation of this muscle is usually followed by complete fecal incontinence.[18] This conclusion, however, is clouded by the fact that the sectioning of the pudendal nerves also deprives an animal of sensation of feces in the anal canal. Lack of sensation could in turn interrupt synergistic reflexive continence reactions by the muscles of the pelvic girdle following anal stimulation. Furthermore, neither complete removal of the external anal sphincter nor surgical splitting of the anus necessarily causes fecal incontinence.[19,20]

THE LEVATOR ANI MUSCLES may play a role in fecal continence in cats[21] and dogs. In dogs, the levator ani muscles apparently are the equivalent of the puborectalis muscles in humans.[9] Bilateral contractions of the levator ani muscles and, to a lesser extent, the coccygeus muscles laterally compress the rectum and depress the tail onto the dorsum of the rectum and anal canal.[15,21] Passage of feces into the caudal rectum and anal canal is thereby inhibited. Conversely, when the tail is elevated, as occurs with voluntary defecation, contraction of the levator ani muscles helps to evacuate feces from the caudal rectum.[15]

Other observations concerning the role of the levator ani muscles in canine fecal continence include (1) the absence of complete fecal incontinence in 33% of dogs with a denervated external anal sphincter[18]; (2) the observation of smaller-than-normal levator ani and coccygeus muscles in a tailless cairn terrier with fecal incontinence[22]; and (3) the small but significant incidence (both before and after surgery) of fecal incontinence in dogs suffering from perineal hernia, a condition in which deterioration of the levator ani muscles is common.[20,23,24] Although other explanations can be offered for these observations, the importance of the levator ani muscles to fecal continence in dogs and cats remains to be established.

Miscellaneous Factors. In addition to the continence reaction, other factors may contribute to sphincter continence.[25] In humans, the relative importance of these factors is controversial[25]; and in dogs it is poorly addressed.[9]

The internal anal sphincter, which is a thickening of the

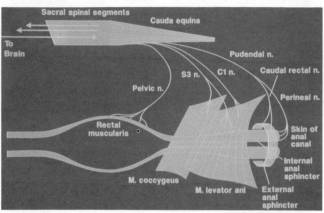

Figure 1—Schematic representation of the putative anatomic structures of fecal continence. (From Strombeck DR, Guilford WG: *Small Animal Gastroenterology*, ed 2. Stonegate Publishing, Davis, CA, 1990, p 405. Reproduced with permission.)

smooth muscle of the rectum,[9,26] apparently is important in maintaining the resting pressure of the anal canal. In humans or dogs, this muscle can relax in response to a propulsive wave or to slight distention of the rectum (rectosphincteric reflex).[10,26-28] Therefore, contraction of the internal sphincter is not likely to be important in maintaining continence when pressure in the rectum becomes high but may help guard against elimination of small amounts of liquid stool.[29] Relaxation of the internal sphincter following rectal distention shortens the functional length of the anal canal. The resultant contact of rectal contents with the highly sensitive anal skin[12] allows the animal to discriminate the material in the rectum (e.g., gas, fluid, or formed stool) and consciously reinforce the continence reaction.[12]

If low intrarectal pressures are maintained by effective reservoir function, passive factors are able to preserve some semblance of continence, even if the neuromuscular components of the sphincter mechanisms are damaged. Passive mechanisms include a flutter-valve–like action of the anorectum in response to increases in intraabdominal pressure,[25,30] the inherent resistance to expansion exhibited by any tissue in a collapsed state,[9,25] and the horizontal stance of the dog and cat.

CAUSES OF FECAL INCONTINENCE

Dysfunction of any of the anatomic structures that are listed on page 330 can predispose an animal to fecal incontinence. The causes of fecal incontinence are varied and are depicted in a separate listing on page 331.

Anal Diseases. Anorectal disease can interfere with sensory information from the anal epithelium as well as disrupt the integrity of the anal canal. A small percentage of dogs with perianal fistulas are presented with fecal incontinence.[31] Surgical repair of this condition is associated with a high rate of fecal incontinence.[31,32] As previously mentioned, complete surgical excision of the external anal sphincter as well as surgical splitting of the anus do not necessarily result in fecal incontinence.[19,20]

Colorectal Diseases. Colorectal diseases, such as colitis and neoplasia, can interfere with the reservoir function of the large bowel. Incontinence secondary to constipation is often called *overflow fecal incontinence*, which is the escape of loose feces that commonly surround an impacted fecal mass. This condition has been attributed to reflexive inhibition of the internal sphincter as a result of distention of the rectum with impacted feces (rectosphincteric reflex),[26,33,34] and to creation of a small gap in the anal canal caused by the pressure of the uneven distal extremity of the impacted fecal mass.[10]

Diseases or Diets That Increase Fecal Volume. Diarrhea can overwhelm colonic capacity. Large volumes of liquid feces place a strain on the reservoir and sphincter mechanisms and exacerbate fecal incontinence.[8,25,26]

Damage to the Muscles of Continence. Damage to the pelvic and the external anal sphincter muscles can interfere with the function of the effector organ of the continence reaction. Such damage can occur following trauma or denervation or as a result of myopathy.

Damage to the Somatic Peripheral Nerves. Damage to the pudendal nerve or to the S2, S3, or C1 spinal nerve can affect the afferent and efferent nervous tracts of the continence reaction (Figure 2). Trauma (especially surgical trauma), compressive lesions, polyneuropathies, and various other causes (see page 331) are responsible for the damage. Experimental bilateral sectioning of the pudendal nerves in dogs has produced complete fecal incontinence in two thirds of the dogs but compromises continence in all of them.[18] It is likely that partial functioning of the anorectal sensory and motor nerves would remain unless all peripheral nerves attendant to the area were simultaneously damaged. In humans, partial denervation of the external anal sphincter and the muscles of the pelvic girdle (such denervation can be caused by chronic straining at the stool or follow obstetric trauma) are believed to be important causes of fecal incontinence.[26,35]

Damage to Autonomic Peripheral Nerves. The pelvic plexus and nerves are closely related to the lateral aspects of the rectum and the dorsal aspect of the prostate.[36] These nervous tissues can be damaged by dysautonomia, abdominal trauma, and possibly obstipation or neoplasia. Damage to the pelvic plexus or pelvic nerves would interfere with the sensation of rectal fullness. In cats with dysautonomia, 20% have fecal incontinence.[37]

Cauda Equina Syndrome. Cauda equina syndrome is a well-recognized cause of fecal incontinence.[38] Damage to the cauda equina interferes with anorectal sensation and the motor control of the continence muscles. The syndrome has a variety of causes (see page 331) and a characteristic group of clinical signs, including priapism or paraphimosis, fecal and urinary incontinence, hindlimb weakness and self-mutilation, tail paralysis, and reduced or absent anal reflexes.[38,39]

Central Nervous System Injury. Even with complete decentralization, animals can usually defecate. The integrative capabilities of the well-developed intramural colonic nerve plexus make defecation possible.[40] Fecal incon-

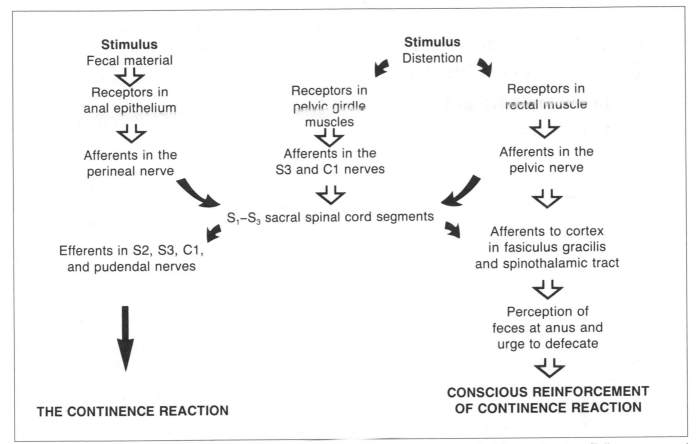

Figure 2—Hypothetical reflexes involved in the continence reaction. This figure was compiled from various conflicting papers and texts that deal with the problem of human and, to a lesser extent, canine incontinence. (From Strombeck DR, Guilford WG: *Small Animal Gastroenterology*, ed 2. Stonegate Publishing, Davis, CA, 1990, p 408.

tinence, however, is common in animals with central nervous system disease. Spinal, brain stem, or midbrain injury can interfere with the continence reaction or the animal's subconscious or conscious reinforcement of the reaction. Reinforcement is important when the rectal pressure markedly begins to exceed the pressure in the anal canal.[10,27]

ONLY severe transverse myelopathy or multifocal lesions would completely interrupt anorectal sensations because more than one area of the spinal cord is likely to be involved in the transmission of this sensation. If the cerebrum is damaged, the animal may not perceive anorectal sensation and therefore may lose house-training habits. Such states occur in animals affected by senility, certain metabolic disturbances, or organic brain disease. Examples of fecal incontinence in animals with central nervous system disease include congenital neural lesions of the Manx cat,[41] spina bifida and spinal dysraphism of the English bulldog,[42] distemper,[43] cervical meningioma,[44] degenerative myelopathy,[44] pituitary tumors,[45] and trauma.[44] In humans, lesions in the frontal cortex can cause fecal incontinence.[46]

Aging. Although aging is a common cause of fecal incontinence in humans[5] and dogs, the exact site of the defect

or defects is unknown. It is likely that multiple factors are involved. Suggested causes include senility, neuropathy, weakness and atrophy of the fecal continence muscles, diminished rectal compliance, and (in older patients) a higher incidence of diarrhea.[1,5,34] Diagnosis is by exclusion.

DIFFERENTIAL DIAGNOSIS AND DIAGNOSTIC TESTS

It is important that clinicians attempt to determine the site and the cause of fecal incontinence because the treatment regimen and prognosis vary considerably for the different conditions. To determine the cause, the clinician must first obtain a thorough history, perform a thorough physical examination, and (if necessary) complete a number of diagnostic tests. The diagnostic differentials for fecal incontinence are listed on page 332.

History. The patient history can help to differentiate between reservoir and sphincter incontinence and can assist in determining whether systemic diseases or poor diet, trauma, difficult whelping, drug or toxin exposure, or chronic constipation is involved. Reservoir incontinence caused by colorectal disease is often associated with clinical signs, such as tenesmus, frequent defecation, and blood-flecked or mucoid stools. Reservoir incontinence caused by an overwhelmed but normal colonic capacity is likely in animals with a history of dietary indiscretion or in

Anatomic Structures with a Confirmed or Possible Role in Fecal Continence

Reservoir incontinence
Rectum
Colon

Sensory triggers for continence reaction
Epithelium of the anal canal
Levator ani muscles
Coccygeus muscles
Rectal muscularis

Muscles of continence
External anal sphincter
Internal anal sphincter
Levator ani muscles
Coccygeus muscles

Passive factors
Interdigitating anal columns
Tissue of the anal canal

Peripheral nerves
Pudendal nerves
Perineal nerves
Pelvic nerves
Hypogastric nerves
Third sacral spinal nerves
First coccygeal spinal nerves

Central nervous system
Sacral spinal segments
Spinothalamic tracts
Fasciculus gracilis
Frontal cortex

those animals fed a low-quality high-fiber diet, the result of which can be a large volume of feces.

THE PRACTITIONER SHOULD ask the owner whether the animal consciously defecates (i.e., adopts a posture appropriate to defecation) and if so whether the time and place chosen are appropriate. Failure to attempt conscious defecation suggests a severe anorectal sensory derangement. Such animals usually have a history of unconscious anal dribbling that often occurs simultaneously with increased abdominal or rectal pressure, such as that

accompanying coughing or exertion. In a house-trained animal, conscious defecation at inappropriate times or places, without the associated distress and urgency of reservoir incontinence, is more suggestive of a behavioral problem. In a young animal, inappropriate defecation may be attributable to poor house-training techniques.

The practitioner should also inquire as to whether the animal has the ability to urinate normally. For an intact male, the practitioner also should ask whether the dog can attain an erection and subsequently achieve normal detumescence. Both micturition and erection rely on nervous pathways similar to those of fecal continence[47]; therefore, confirmation of concurrent abnormalities in these functions suggests that the fecal incontinence is of neurogenic origin.

Physical Examination. Close visual inspection of the anal area along with careful digital examination of the anorectum can facilitate detection of anorectal lesions. At this time, anal tone also can be assessed; however, anal tone is not a reliable measure of anal sphincter function,[1] possibly because a denervated external anal sphincter does not readily atrophy.[2]

Abdominal palpation can be helpful in assessing the colorectal content and bladder tone. Bladder tone can be altered by the presence of neurologic lesions. The skin of the hindlimbs also should be carefully examined for areas of self-inflicted trauma, which may indicate paresthesia; and the dorsal lumbosacral skin and musculature should be palpated for evidence of hyperesthesia. Hindlimb paresthesia and hyperesthesia are both suggestive of cauda equina syndrome.

Neurologic Examination. A thorough neurologic examination that includes evaluation of gait, cranial nerve function, myotatic reflexes, and postural reactions is an integral part of the workup. Depressed myotatic reflexes of the hindlimbs can occur in animals with lumbosacral spinal lesions, cauda equina syndrome, polyneuropathy, neuromuscular junction disease, or myopathy. Special attention should be given to the presence or absence of the anal reflex, the rectal-inflation reflex, the pudendal-anal (bulbocavernosus) reflex, and the animal's conscious perception of perineal and anorectal sensations.

The anal reflex is evaluated by pricking or pinching the perianal skin and observing contraction of the anal sphincter. The rectal-inflation reflex is induced by placing a Foley catheter in the caudal extremity of the rectum and inflating the catheter with 15 to 30 ml of air. This procedure induces anal contraction in dogs[48] and humans.[3] The pudendal-anal reflex is evaluated by applying digital pressure to the penis while observing for anal contraction. All three reflexes assess sacral spinal segments, motor neurons in the pudendal nerves, and the external anal sphincter. The anal and pudendal-anal reflexes test perineal nerve afferents, whereas the rectal-inflation reflex may test pelvic or S3 and C1 nerve afferents (Figure 2). These reflexes are usually preserved in patients with suprasacral spinal transverse myelopathy, whereas the conscious perception of perineal and anorectal sensations (induced by the inflated Foley catheter) is not.

Possible Causes of Fecal Incontinence[a]

Anorectal disease
Lacerations
Neoplasia
Anal sac removal
Perianal fistulas and fistula repair
Perineal hernia repair
Rectovaginal fistula

Colorectal disease
Proctitis
Colitis
Neoplasia
Constipation

Myopathy or neuromuscular junction disorders
Trauma
Myopathy[b]
Myasthenia[b]

Peripheral neuropathy
Trauma
Drug induced
  (e.g., vincristine sulfate)
Polyneuropathies
Dysautonomia
Chronic tenesmus[b]
Obstetric trauma[b]
Diabetes mellitus[b]
Pelvic radiation[b]

Cauda equina syndrome
Congenital vertebral malformations
Compressive vertebral malformations
Traumatic vertebral damage
  (e.g., sacrococcygeal subluxation)
Lumbosacral instability
Anomalous lumbosacral vertebral
  nerve roots
Infection
Neoplasia
Vascular compromise

Central nervous system disease
Congenital (e.g., spina bifida)
Traumatic
Infectious (e.g., distemper)
Degenerative myelopathy
Vascular compromise
Neoplasia
Confusional states

Miscellaneous
Aging
Constipation
Loose fecal consistency
Increased fecal volume
Anuria

[a]From Strombeck DR, Guilford WG: *Small Animal Gastroenterology*, ed 2. Stonegate Publishing, Davis, CA, 1990, p 408. Reprinted with permission.
[b]Causes of fecal incontinence documented only in human literature.

MANY MALE DOGS CAN BE manually stimulated to attain an erection. If erection and detumescence occur in a normal manner, the perineal nerves and the parasympathetic and sympathetic innervations of the genitalia as well as of the rest of the pelvic organs are probably intact. In contrast, failure of a male dog to attain an erection is not necessarily indicative of autonomic failure. Erection can be inhibited by many factors, such as fear.

Laboratory Data. A hemogram, serum chemistry profile, urinalysis, and fecal examination should be included in the workup of an animal with fecal incontinence. Such data may provide evidence of concurrent systemic or gastrointestinal disease.

Endoscopy. Colonoscopy or proctoscopy with biopsy is indicated if reservoir incontinence is suspected.

Radiography. Radiography is a very helpful aid in diagnosing the cause of fecal incontinence. Lateral and ventrodorsal survey films of the lumbosacral vertebral column should be taken. Lesions of significance include vertebral deformations, spina bifida, lumbosacral dislocations, diskospondylitis, severe spondylosis, and disk protrusions. Radiographs of the stressed lumbosacral spine also can help in diagnosing lumbosacral instability.

Myelography is valuable for the diagnosis of lesions that affect the spinal cord and the cauda equina.[49] Epidurography, diskography, or intraosseous caudal vertebral venography can also be used to detect compressive lesions of the cauda equina. These specialized techniques, however, require skill and experience to perform and interpret.[50-56] Intraosseous venography is the least desirable of

Differential Diagnosis of Fecal Incontinence[a]

History
Physical examination
Neurologic examination
Perception of perineal and anorectal
    sensation
Perineal reflex
Pudendal-anal reflex
Rectal-inflation reflex
Manual stimulation of erection

Data base
Complete blood count
Serum chemistry profile
Urinalysis
Fecal

Radiography
Lumbosacral survey radiographs
Radiographs of the stressed
    lumbosacral area
Myelogram
Epidurogram
Diskogram
Intraosseous vertebral venogram
Computerized axial tomography

Electrodiagnostics
Conventional electromyography
Single-fiber electromyography
Anal mapping
Pudendal-anal reflex
Pudendal and perineal nerve motor
    latencies
Spinal motor latencies
Hindlimb nerve conduction velocities
    and evoked potentials

Cerebrospinal fluid tap
Fluid analysis
Distemper titer

Colonoscopy

Anorectal/colorectal pressure profiles

Surgical exploration

[a]From Strombeck DR, Guilford WG: *Small Animal Gastro-enterology*, ed 2. Stonegate Publishing, Davis, CA, 1990, p 409. Reprinted with permission.

these techniques. Computer-assisted tomography is the technique of choice for the location of soft tissue masses in the spinal canal.

Neurodiagnostics. Electrodiagnostic evaluation of an animal with fecal incontinence can greatly facilitate diagnosis. Electromyographic examination of the continence muscles can reveal evidence of denervation or myopathy.[57] Electromyography can also be used to determine which areas of a damaged sphincter contain normal muscle. Such anal mapping can help the surgeon during subsequent surgical repair.[26] In humans, single-fiber electromyography is believed to be a useful technique to detect chronic denervation and reinnervation of the muscles of continence.[26]

Assessment of the pudendal-anal reflex can be made more objective by electrophysiologic evaluation (Figure 3).[58] As stated, this reflex assesses the integrity of the perineal and pudendal nerves and the sacral segments involved.

Two techniques have been developed to assess motor nerve conduction to the muscles of continence in humans.[59] These techniques involve either transrectal stimulation of the pudendal nerve or transcutaneous stimulation of spinal nerve motor roots. Electromyography and the measurement of nerve conduction velocities and evoked potentials in the hindlimbs are warranted if polyneuropathy, polymyopathy, or cauda equina lesions are suspected. Lumbosacral spinal taps may be a helpful diagnostic procedure. A cerebrospinal fluid examination can include a cerebrospinal fluid distemper titer. If the dog's cerebrospinal fluid distemper titer is higher than the serum distemper titer, a diagnosis of distemper encephalomyelitis is probable.[43]

Manometry and Miscellaneous Diagnostic Evaluations. Anal and colorectal pressure profiles are useful tools in the diagnosis of fecal incontinence in humans. These tests, however, have not been used in veterinary medicine. Manometry can be used to evaluate the degree of impairment of anorectal tone and to check the function of the internal and external anal sphincters. This technique also can be used as a baseline for objective comparison of the results of therapy.[1,11,26,34]

OTHER TESTS HAVE been used to assess fecal incontinence in humans. These procedures include measuring what volume of saline rectal infusion is required before the patient senses rectal distention, measuring the volume of saline a patient can retain in the rectum, and assessing the weight required to draw a spherical object out of the rectum.[1] The application of these tests to veterinary patients is limited by lack of patient cooperation.

Surgery as a Diagnostic Tool. In some cases, surgery may be required to obtain a diagnosis. Biopsy of muscle and the exploration and biopsy of inaccessible masses in the spinal or pelvic canals are examples.

TREATMENT
Before fecal incontinence can be treated, the veterinarian

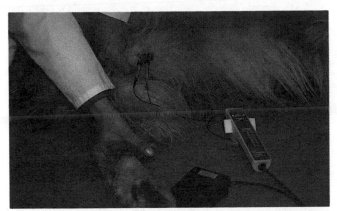

Figure 3—Electrodiagnostic evaluation of the pudendal-anal reflex. The stimulating electrodes are applied to the penis. Recording electrodes are inserted into the external anal sphincter. (Courtesy of Dennis O'Brien, DVM, PhD, University of Missouri)

should discuss with the owner the public health risks of canine and feline feces. If appropriate precautions regarding handling and disposal of the feces are taken, the risks are minimal.

Treatment of the Primary Cause. Therapy for fecal incontinence is more likely to be successful if the primary cause has been identified. For example, resolution of incontinence may follow successful treatment of diarrhea if the cause of the diarrhea.[8,25] Surgical reconstruction of the anal canal, decompressive and/or stabilization spinal surgery, antineoplastic drugs, antiinflammatory agents, anthelmintics, antibiotics, laxatives, and changes in diet all can be appropriate therapy in different situations.

Symptomatic Surgical Management. In humans, surgical treatment of intractable sphincter incontinence is used to reestablish the anal canal within the pelvic girdle, restore anorectal angulation, repair the anal sphincter, reduce the anal sphincter diameter by sphincteroplasty, or replace the muscles of continence with polymeric silicone material or autogenous muscle grafts.[5,11,34,59] In dogs, fascial slings have been used for the treatment of fecal incontinence, but they tend to loosen over time.[60,61] Surgical implantation of a perianal silicone elastomer sling, however, has proven valuable in resolving fecal incontinence in dogs.[18] In humans, the ileal J-pouch anal anastomosis has had a 92% continence rate when severe colorectal disease has necessitated extensive resection of the colon and rectum.[8]

Symptomatic Medical Management. The goals of electing symptomatic medical management are to reduce fecal water content, decrease fecal bulk, slow colonic transit time, and increase external anal sphincter tone.

Nutritional Therapy. The amount of dietary residue should be adjusted to maximize stool retention time, thus reducing stool frequency and increasing the time for desiccation of the stool. Low-residue diets, such as cottage cheese and rice, can reduce fecal volume by up to 85% as well as reducing the frequency of defecation.[62]

Pharmacologic Therapy. Bowel transit time can be slowed by the use of such opioids as diphenoxylate hydrochloride (Lomotil®—G.D. Searle & Company) and loperamide hydrochloride (Imodium®—Janssen Pharmaceutica). These drugs promote segmental contractions of the bowel and thereby decrease the transit time and allow greater resorption of fecal water. When used in humans, these opioids also increase the tone of the anal sphincter.[63] They can be given for prolonged periods with little development of tolerance to their effects.[63] In humans, loperamide hydrochloride has been shown to have an antisecretory action.[64] Because both drugs are available in liquid form, administration to small animals is facilitated; however, neither drug is licensed for use in dogs and cats. Furthermore, both drugs can cause constipation. If either drug is used, I recommend a dose of 1 mg/10 kg for diphenoxylate hydrochloride or 1 mg/30 kg for loperamide hydrochloride; both doses are based on label recommendations for use in humans. Both drugs can be given initially every eight hours and as needed thereafter for as long as signs persist.

Induced Defecation. The use of daily warm-water enemas administered in a place where defecation is appropriate can be used in animals with a dedicated and competent owner. Many animals can be induced to defecate by the insertion and inflation of a Foley catheter in the rectum. This technique does not produce conscious defecation in animals with anorectal anesthesia but can often produce involuntary rectal evacuation, a phenomenon also described in humans suffering from traumatic spinal lesions.[27] In animals with chronic posterior paralysis caused by damage to the spinal cord, a minor stimulus (such as a light toe pinch or warm washcloth) to the hindlimbs or perineum may stimulate appropriate elimination (i.e., the mass reflex).

Training. Training procedures can also be used as treatment of fecal incontinence. Humans have been retrained to sense the stool by developing a conditioned reflex. Varying degrees of inflation with a catheter coupled with a verbal warning that the catheter is being inflated are used to develop the reflex.[65,66] Eventually, the patient can discriminate much smaller degrees of catheter inflation. Although it is difficult to imagine this type of biofeedback being used in veterinary medicine, many animals can be trained to defecate on command. If this procedure can be achieved in an incontinent animal, then regular and appropriate evacuations of the bowels could be maintained.

Placement. It may be possible to avoid euthanasia for animals that have a satisfactory quality of life despite unmanageable fecal incontinence. The owner should consider confining the animal to the yard or finding a new home for it.

CONCLUSION

Fecal continence is maintained by a synergistic combination of colorectal, sphincteric, and passive mechanisms. Fecal incontinence has a variety of anal, gastrointestinal, or neuromuscular causes, some of which are curable. In most cases, appropriate therapy can considerably improve the incontinence.

ACKNOWLEDGMENTS

The author would like to acknowledge the technical assistance and advice of Dennis P. O'Brien, DVM, PhD, and Paul W. Dean, DVM, of the University of Missouri, College of Veterinary Medicine, Columbia, Missouri, and Steven Petersen, DVM, Donald R. Strombeck, DVM, PhD, and Joe P. Morgan, DVM, VetMedDr, of the University of California, Davis, California, in the preparation of this manuscript.

About the Author

Dr. Guilford, who is a Diplomate of the American College of Veterinary Internal Medicine, is affiliated with the Veterinary Medicine Teaching Hospital and Department of Physiology, University of California, Davis, in Davis, California.

REFERENCES

1. Read NW, Harford WV, et al: A clinical study of patients with fecal incontinence and diarrhea. *Gastroenterology* 76:747-756, 1979.
2. Gaston EA: The physiology of fecal continence. *Surg Gynecol Obstet* 87:280-290, 1948.
3. Gaston EA: Physiological basis for the preservation of fecal continence after resection of rectum. *JAMA* 146:1486-1489, 1951.
4. Karlan M, McPherson RC, Watman RN: An experimental evaluation of fecal continence—sphincter and reservoir—in the dog. *Surg Gynecol Obstet* 108:469-475, 1959.
5. Goldberg SM: Anal incontinence, in Goldbery SM, Gordon PH, Nivatongs S (eds): *Essentials of Anorectal Surgery*. Philadelphia, JB Lippincott Co, 1980, pp 282-290.
6. Peck DA, Hallenbeck GA: Fecal continence in the dog after replacement of rectal mucosa with ileal mucosa. *Surg Gynecol Obstet* 119:1312-1320, 1964.
7. Bright RM, Burrows CF, Goring R, et al: Subtotal colectomy for the treatment of acquired megacolon in the dog and cat. *JAVMA* 188:1412-1416, 1986.
8. Pemberton JH, Kelly KA: Achieving enteric continence: Principles and applications. *Mayo Clin Proc* 61:586-599, 1986.
9. Ashdown RR: Symposium on canine recto-anal disorders. 1. Clinical anatomy. *J Small Anim Pract* 9:315-322, 1968.
10. Scharli AF, Kiesewetter WB: Defecation and continence: Some new concepts. *Dis Colon Rectum* 13:81-107, 1970.
11. Parks A: Anorectal incontinence. *Proc R Soc Med* 68:681-690, 1975.
12. Duthie HL, Bennett RC: The relationship of sensation in the anal canal to the functional anal sphincter: A possible factor in anal continence. *Gut* 4:179-182, 1963.
13. deLahunta A: *Veterinary Neuroanatomy and Clinical Neurology*. Philadelphia, WB Saunders Co, 1977, pp 288-295.
14. Martin WD, Fletcher TF, Bradley WE: Innervation of feline perineal musculature. *Anat Rec* 180:15-30, 1974.
15. Evans HE, Christensen GC: *Miller's Anatomy of the Dog*, ed 2. Philadelphia, WB Saunders Co, 1979, pp 331-337.
16. deLahunta A: *Veterinary Neuroanatomy and Clinical Neurology*. Philadelphia, WB Saunders Co, 1977, pp 110-124.
17. Shafik A: A new concept of the anatomy of the anal sphincter mechanism and the physiology of defecation. *Invest Urol* 12:412-419, 1975.
18. Dean PW, O'Brien DP, Turk AM, et al: Silicone elastomer sling for fecal incontinence in dogs. *Vet Surg* 17:304-310, 1988.
19. Crighton GW: Surgical removal of the anal ring in the dog. *Vet Rec* 73:416-417, 1961.
20. Harvey CE: Treatment of perineal hernia in the dog—A reassessment. *J Small Anim Pract* 18:505-511, 1977.
21. Martin WD, Fletcher TF, Bradley WE: Perineal musculature in the cat. *Anat Rec* 180:3-14, 1974.
22. Hall DS, Amann JF, Constantinescu GM, et al: Anury in two cairn terriers. *JAVMA* 191:1113-1114, 1987.
23. Burrows CF, Harvey CE: Perineal hernia in the dog. *J Small Anim Pract* 14:315-322, 1973.
24. Cranfield RB, Bellenger CR: Perineal hernia, in Slater DH (ed):
    Small Animal Surgery. Philadelphia, WB Saunders Co, 1985, pp 886-899.
25. Duthie HL: Anal continence. *Gut* 12:844-852, 1971.
26. Wunderlich M, Parks AG: Physiology and pathophysiology of the anal sphincters. *Int Surg* 67:291-298, 1982.
27. Frenckner B: Function of the anal sphincters in man. *Gut* 16:638-644, 1975.
28. Strombeck DR, Harrold D: Anal sphincter pressure and the rectosphincteric reflex in the dog. *Am J Vet Res* 49:191-192, 1988.
29. Schuster MM: Tests related to the colon, rectum, and anus, in Berk JE (ed): *Gastroenterology*, ed 4. Philadelphia, WB Saunders Co, 1985, pp 388-401.
30. Phillips SF, Edwards DAW: Some aspects of anal continence and defaecation. *Gut* 6:396-406, 1965.
31. Harvey CE: Perianal fistula in the dog. *Vet Rec* 91:25-32, 1972.
32. Vasseur PB: Perianal fistulae in dogs: A retrospective analysis of surgical techniques. *JAAHA* 17:177-180, 1981.
33. Nicholls J, Glass R: *Coloproctology*. Berlin, Springer-Verlag, 1985, pp 42-46.
34. Schoetz DJ: Operative therapy for anal incontinence. *Surg Clin North Am* 65:35-46, 1985.
35. Bartola DCC, et al: The role of partial denervation of the puborectalis in idiopathic faecal incontinence. *Br J Surg* 70:664-667, 1983.
36. Evans HE, Christensen GC: *Miller's Anatomy of the Dog*, ed 2. Philadelphia, WB Saunders Co, 1979, p 576.
37. Sharp NJH, Nash AS: Feline dysautonomia, in Kirk RW (ed): *Current Veterinary Therapy. IX*. Philadelphia, WB Saunders Co, 1986, pp 802-804.
38. Lenehan TM: Canine cauda equina syndrome. *Compend Contin Educ Pract Vet* 5(11):941-951, 1983.
39. Tarvin G, Prata RG: Lumbosacral stenosis in dogs. *JAVMA* 177:154-159, 1980.
40. De Groat WC, Booth AM, et al: Neural control for the urinary bladder and large intestine, in Brooks C, Koizumi K, Sato A (eds): *Integrative Functions of the Autonomic Nervous System*. Tokyo, University of Tokyo Press, 1979, pp 50-67.
41. Kitchen H, Murray RE, Cockrell B: Animal model for human disease. Spina bifida, sacral dysgenesis, myelocele. Manx cats. *Am J Pathol* 68:203-206, 1972.
42. Wilson JW, Kurtz HJ, Leipold HW, et al: Spina bifida in the dog. *Vet Pathol* 16:165-179, 1979.
43. Guilford WG, Shaw DP, O'Brien D, et al: Fecal incontinence, urinary incontinence and priapism associated with multifocal distemper encephalomyelitis in a dog. *JAVMA*, in press.
44. Guilford WG: Unpublished data. University of California, Davis, CA, 1988-1989.
45. Feldman EC, Nelson RW: Hyperadrenocorticism, in *Canine and Feline Endocrinology and Reproduction*. Philadelphia, WB Saunders Co, 1987, pp 137-194.
46. Andrew J, Nathan PW: Lesions of the anterior frontal lobes and disturbances in micturition and defecation. *Brain* 87:233-262, 1964.
47. De Groat WC, Booth AM: Autonomic systems to the urinary bladder and sexual organs, in Dyck PJ (ed): *Peripheral Neuropathy*, ed 2. Philadelphia, WB Saunders Co, 1984, pp 285-299.
48. Guilford WG: Unpublished observations in a series of 10 dogs, University of California, Davis, CA, 1988.
49. Lang J: Flexion-extension myelography of the canine cauda equina. *Vet Radiol* 29:242-257, 1988.
50. Klide AM, Steinberg SA, Pond MJ: Epiduralograms in the dog: The uses and advantages of the diagnostic procedure. *J Am Vet Radiol Soc* 8:39-44, 1967.
51. Bartels JE, Hoerlein BF, Boring JG: Neuroradiography, in Hoerlein BF (ed): *Canine Neurology*, ed 3. Philadelphia, WB Saunders Co, 1978, pp 114-117.
52. Morgan JP: Vertebral column, in *Radiology in Veterinary Orthopedics*. Philadelphia, Lea & Febiger, 1972.
53. Oliver JE, Lorenz MD: Confirming a diagnosis, in *Veterinary Neurologic Diagnosis*. Philadelphia, WB Saunders Co, 1983, pp 110-114.
54. McNeel SV, Morgan JP: Intraosseous vertebral venography: A technic for examination of the canine lumbosacral junction. *J Am Vet Radiol Soc* 19:168-175, 1978.
55. Hathcock JT, Pechman RD, Dillon AR, et al: Comparison of three radiographic contrast procedures in the evaluation of the canine lumbosacral spinal canal. *Vet Radiol* 29:4-15, 1988.
56. Sisson AF, LeCouteur RA, Ingram JT, Park RD: Diagnosis of cauda equina abnormalities in dogs using electromyography, discography,

and epidurography. *Proc ACVIM*:1031, 1989.

57. Swash M: Anorectal incontinence: Electrophysiological tests. *Br J Surg* 72:s14–s15, 1985.

58. O'Brien DP, Dean PW: Pudendo-anal (bulbocavernosus) reflex electrophysiology in the dog (abstract). *Proc ACVIM*:1988.

59. Hakelius L, Gierup J, Grotte G: Urinary (and fecal) incontinence in children: Treatment with free autogenous muscle transplantation. *Prog Pediatr Surg* 17:155–167, 1984.

60. Lumb WV: Surgical treatment of fecal incontinence. *JAAHA* 12:666, 1976

61. Leeds EB, Renegar WR: A modified fascial sling for the treatment of fecal incontinence—Surgical technique. *JAAHA* 17:663–667, 1981.

62. Guilford WG: Unpublished data from a crossover study of six dogs, University of California, Davis, CA, 1988.

63. Jaffe JH, Martin WR: Opioid analgesics and antagonists, in Goodman-Gilman A, Goodman LS, et al (eds): *The Pharmacological Basis of Therapeutics*. ed 7. New York, MacMillan Co, 1985, p 503.

64. Kastrup EK, et al: *Drug Facts and Comparisons*. Philadelphia, JB Lippincott Co, 1985, pp 1243–1247.

65. Marzuk PM: Biofeedback for gastrointestinal disorders: A review of the literature. *Ann Intern Med* 103:240–244, 1985.

66. Buser WD, Miner PB: Delayed rectal sensation with fecal incontinence. *Gastroenterology* 91:1186–1191, 1986.